Surgical problems in children

Recognition and referral

Surgical problems in children
Recognition and referral

HOWARD C. FILSTON
M.D., F.A.C.S., F.A.A.P.

Associate Professor of Pediatric Surgery and Pediatrics,
Chief of Pediatric Surgical Service, Department of Surgery,
Duke University Medical Center, Durham, North Carolina

with Foreword by
SAMUEL L. KATZ, M.D.

with **578** *illustrations*

The C. V. Mosby Company

ST. LOUIS • TORONTO • LONDON   1982

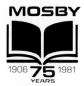

MOSBY
1906 **75** 1981
YEARS

A TRADITION OF PUBLISHING EXCELLENCE

Editor: Karen Berger
Manuscript editor: Judith Bange
Design: Susan Trail
Production: Ginny Douglas

Copyright © 1982 by The C.V. Mosby Company

Printed in the United States of America

The C.V. Mosby Company
11830 Westline Industrial Drive, St. Louis, Missouri 63141

Library of Congress Cataloging in Publication Data

Filston, Howard C.
    Surgical problems in children.

    Bibliography: p.
    Includes index.
    1. Children—Surgery.   2.   Diagnosis, Surgical.
I.   Title.   [DNLM: 1.   Physicians, Family.   2.   Surgery
—In infancy and childhood.   WO 925 F489sa]
RD137.F47   617′.98   81-11121
ISBN 0-8016-1574-7   AACR2

GW/CB/B   9   8   7   6   5   4   3   2   1   03/D/317

Contributors

JOHN W. DUCKETT, M.D.

Associate Professor of Urology,
The University of Pennsylvania School of Medicine, and
Director of Pediatric Urology, Children's Hospital of Philadelphia,
Philadelphia, Pennsylvania

HOWARD C. FILSTON, M.D.

Associate Professor of Pediatric Surgery and Pediatrics,
Chief of Pediatric Surgical Service, Department of Surgery,
Duke University Medical Center,
Durham, North Carolina

W. JERRY OAKES, M.D.

Assistant Professor of Neurosurgery and Pediatrics,
Department of Surgery, Duke University Medical Center,
Durham, North Carolina

ROBERT J. RUDERMAN, M.D.

Assistant Professor of Orthopedic Surgery and Pediatrics,
Department of Surgery, Duke University Medical Center,
Durham, North Carolina

PETER W. WHITFIELD, M.D.

Formerly Fellow in Pediatric Orthopedics,
Department of Surgery,
Duke University Medical Center,
Durham, North Carolina

ROBERT H. WILKINS, M.D.

Professor of Neurosurgery and Chairman,
Division of Neurosurgery, Department of Surgery,
Duke University Medical Center,
Durham, North Carolina

To

Scott, Timothy, and **Megan Lee—**

whose father loves them

Foreword

As Dr. Filston points out in the Preface, this book has been written for primary care physicians who will first see the infants, children, and adolescents whose problems may need surgical evaluation. In the normal flow of child health care, it is the primary care physician who is responsible initially for recognizing as early as possible the onset of a condition that may require surgical consultation and, perhaps, surgical intervention. Unless the primary care physician is alert to the early clinical presentation of these conditions, the patient's likelihood of an optimal result may be compromised if undue delay is allowed.

With the information that Dr. Filston has assembled here, much of it based on his own personal experience, the primary care physician should be able to recognize early those conditions which merit surgical attention. He should also be able to serve as a member of the patient care team during further evaluation and preoperative management, to participate in the immediate postoperative care with supportive therapy of various types, and to recognize any late postoperative complications.

It has been my pleasure and privilege to work with Dr. Filston for five years in connection with his role as a member of the Departments of Surgery and Pediatrics at Duke University Medical Center. In addition to his obvious technical skills as a pediatric surgeon, the most outstanding features that he demonstrates as a teacher and clinician are clarity, dedication, and sensitivity. He teaches the same principles of pediatric surgery presented in this book to medical students, residents, and graduate physicians representing the disciplines of pediatrics, family practice, and general and thoracic surgery. Nurses and physicians' associates benefit similarly from his extraordinary skills as a graphic and convincing teacher. Always his focus is on the patient for the attainment of ideal results—possible when diagnosis is early, treatment is appropriate, and supportive care is optimal. He is uncompromising in his quest for this level of care for every infant, child, or adolescent who comes to his attention. The introduction of a subclavian line is performed with the same painstaking, precise, and sensitive approach that he uses in the operative suite for a complicated intestinal resection.

The collaboration in authorship of key sections of the book by Drs. Ruderman and Whitfield, Oakes and Wilkins, and Duckett attests further to the quality Dr. Filston demands in all his attentions to the needs of pediatric patients. These clinical colleagues have added their keen perspectives to the breadth and excellence of this volume. If in his written words Dr. Filston can convey a fraction of the impact of his actions and spoken words, this will be a book of enduring value to all those physicians who include in their practice the primary care of children.

Samuel L. Katz, M.D.
Professor of Pediatrics and Chairman,
Department of Pediatrics,
Duke University Medical Center,
Durham, North Carolina

Preface

Today almost every major teaching center and children's hospital can provide safe, sophisticated surgical care for children. Innumerable lesions in infants, once highly lethal, can be treated with the expectation of a successful outcome. The evolution of pediatric surgery as a specialty, the rapid advances of neonatology, the development of safer anesthetic programs for children by highly trained individuals familiar with the special needs of infants and children, and the rapid improvement in critical care knowledge and methodologies for infants and children have all contributed to this progress. Within the surgical subspecialties, other individuals have taken special interest in children's lesions and have added further surgical accomplishments.

Sadly, however, many infants and children fail to benefit from these advances, either because of diagnostic failure by the primary care physician (whether pediatrician or family practitioner) or because of insufficient knowledge regarding the proper surgical approach on the part of both the primary care physician and the surgical consultant.

A wealth of texts and an entire journal (the *Journal of Pediatric Surgery*) are devoted to the surgical aspects of care for infants and children. This book has been written to help primary care physicians recognize and evaluate surgically treatable lesions and to give them some knowledge of the overall dimensions of care required, the proper procedures to be performed, and the prognosis and success rates to be anticipated and attained. The book is age group and symptom oriented to help primary care physicians know what to think of and when.

Each section contains separate discussions of the urologic, orthopedic, and neurosurgical lesions common to that age group, written by appropriate subspecialists in these fields. Where appropriate, the discussions of individual lesions are subdivided to discuss etiology, clinical presentation, evaluation, referral, medical versus surgical treatment, surgical options, the postoperative course, the prognosis to be expected, complications, and important aspects of follow-up.

The contributors and I hope that this work will provide primary care physicians with much of the information they need to recognize the lesions in children that have surgical implications. Guidelines for expeditious evaluation are presented, and an outline of the overall surgical management is included. Some suggestions regarding the level of surgical expertise required are provided to help primary care physicians make the wisest possible choice of surgical consultant.

Finally, enough information about the complexities and prognosis of the surgical procedures is included to enable primary care physicians to advise parents intelligently. Obviously, this work bears the strong influence of our experience and preferences. Other equally knowledgeable and experienced surgeons may differ in details of surgical management and preferred procedures. We have written to give primary care physicians information and guidelines, not to dictate the specifics of surgical care.

Dr. Samuel L. Katz, Professor and Chairman of the Department of Pediatrics at Duke University Medical Center was the catalyst for this book, for he was the first to point out the need for a text directed to the primary care physician. In the presentation of one's own understanding of a field, the continuing debt owed to one's teachers and peers remains ever obvious. My appreciation is, therefore, expressed to Dr. C. Everett Koop, Dr.

Harry C. Bishop, and Dr. Dale G. Johnson, who provided me with an initial, firm foundation at the Children's Hospital of Philadelphia, and to Dr. Robert J. Izant, Jr., whose valued association as teacher, research director, associate, and friend for so many years provided a standard of excellence and an atmosphere of excitement.

Dr. David C. Sabiston, Jr., Professor and Chairman of the Department of Surgery at Duke, has created an atmosphere of excellence in which pediatric surgery can flourish and the individual can pursue his own academic and clinical goals.

The temptation to mention the names of many is great, but one fears that by mentioning some, one will exclude others—and there is seemingly no end to the advancements being made in pediatric surgery, pediatric anesthesiology, pediatric radiology, neonatology, and general pediatrics and in the surgical subspecialties, as evidenced by the urologic, neurosurgical, and orthopedic sections of this work. Many of the names are to be found among the references and suggested texts. My thanks to all for their many contributions to the care of children with surgical problems.

I appreciate the help of my contributors, who were willing to spend their valued time on yet another writing project. Dr. John W. Duckett has made remarkable contributions to pediatric urology in the past several years, and his help in getting the urology sections together is greatly valued. Dr. W. Jerry Oakes, with the collaboration of Dr. Robert H. Wilkins, has compiled what may be the most complete and comprehensive discussion of neurosurgical lesions in children available for the primary care physician.

As one surveys children's surgical lesions from the neonatal period to adolescence, orthopedic problems, often serious in the neonate, become increasingly more numerous in late childhood and adolescence. Dr. Robert J. Ruderman, assisted by

Dr. Peter W. Whitfield, has encompassed these entities with emphasis on the primary care physician's role and needs.

Dr. Donald Kirks of the Pediatric Radiology Division at Duke was a great help in selecting radiographs, but he and his colleagues Dr. David Merten, Dr. Herman Grossman, and Dr. Eric Effmann contributed as well by their high clinical and academic standards and their ever present and knowledgeable consultations.

Dr. Edmond Bloch, Chief of Pediatric Anesthesia at Duke, is a constant source of support and knowledge. He graciously reviewed the anesthesia comments in the introductory section of the book.

Mr. Charles Lewis of the Audiovisual Department at Duke has again been a great help to me with the illustrations.

Ms. Karen Berger, Ms. Judith Bange, and Ms. Carol Trumbold have been most patient, supportive, and enthusiastic editors and are outstanding representatives of their publisher.

My wife, Nancy, always deserves the lion's share of credit for my endeavors—for her constant support and for the atmosphere of love and understanding that pervades our home.

Ms. Barbara Shaw, my very competent and enthusiastic secretary, has worked extremely hard and long to produce a manuscript from the "goulash" of tapes and scratchings with which I bombarded her.

Finally, this book was written to help primary care physicians in their struggle to sort out serious surgical illness from the overwhelming array of nonspecific complaints with which they are presented. They have my admiration and respect for their continuing vigilance in the face of such a burden of less serious ills and upsets with similar symptoms.

Howard C. Filston

Contents

Surgical problems in children

Recognition and referral

SECTION ONE

General considerations

This section provides a general discussion of some of the management concepts and concerns with which the primary care physician may become involved in the process of providing ongoing medical coordination for the patient undergoing a surgical procedure. An experienced pediatric surgeon will usually handle the overall management of the patient, but most other surgeons will depend on the primary care physician for ongoing consultative advice and medical support for the patient. Although many of the procedures and considerations are common to other pediatric medical problems, the primary care physician must have some appreciation of the modifications necessary for the surgical problem. In addition, this section contains suggested techniques that have been found helpful in optimizing care and minimizing complications. It begins with a discussion of the surgical environment, emotional support for children, and interaction with parents.

CHAPTER 1

The surgical environment and emotional support for the patient and parents

HOWARD C. FILSTON

It is amazing how long it has taken the medical community to recognize the dependence of children on their parents for emotional support in times of stress. We have maintained our sterile hospital environments, limiting parental visiting in the name of efficiency, at the expense of the emotional needs of the infant, young child, and even teenager. Obvious as is the dependence of the healthy child on parental support as he faces new and threatening experiences, it should be ever so much clearer that in sickness the child must have the constant reassurance that can be provided only by the continual presence of a trusted parent. For the child facing surgery, with all the mysteries and fears that it involves, such continual parental presence and support is of primary importance. Second in importance is the presence of other children enduring and surviving similar experiences. The child can relate to them and gain confidence from their successful results.

The child who must undergo major surgery and the complexities of postoperative care will probably experience more threatening procedures and encounter greater numbers and varieties of hospital staff personnel than will the child with a single medical illness.

Although many aspects of modern medical therapy arouse anxiety and involve threatening procedures, the surgical environment provides an anxiety-provoking atmosphere and an assurance of some pain for almost every patient. It is of paramount importance, therefore, that every person with whom the child interacts be understanding of and attuned to the emotional and physical needs of children at various ages. Each individual must realize the fearsomeness of even minor, painless procedures and take the time to soothe the child's fears and explain what must be done. Truthfulness and concern are the watch words. The best emotional support for the child is a friendly and concerned attitude on the part of all the individuals involved. The overriding concern should be to provide the child with explanations commensurate with his ability to understand, to provide him with the ongoing support of his parents whenever this is feasible, and to deal with him in a truthful and straightforward manner. Hurtful procedures should not be made light of, nor should they be presented as overly threatening. For the child who has reached the age of basic communication and understanding, straightforward explanations, including the facts that pain is to be expected and that control is necessary, will usually produce a cooperative patient. For the infant or toddler, the constant presence of his parents and the caring attitude on the part of family members and nurses will minimize the fear and pain the child experiences.

For the child who is able to understand simple but honest explanations of the procedures, a considerate but firm attitude on the part of the personnel and a sympathetic reassurance and support for the child's attempts at control will usually see the child through these anxiety-producing procedures. A little planning on the part of the personnel involved can result in a great deal of satisfaction for them as they take the child through a threatening surgical environment and procedure in a manner that the child finds acceptable and tolerable. If the entire anesthesia-surgical-nursing team makes the effort, in most cases anesthesia can be successfully induced in a well-controlled, cooperative patient who goes to sleep without undue anxiety or hysterics. This achievement on the part of the staff is a source of pride for them, and the control and accomplishment exhibited by the child is a source of pride for him that should be acknowledged and rewarded.

It should be appreciated that the child may see hurtful procedures as punishment for real or imagined transgressions. The child must be reassured that the pain is part of a necessary procedure and not something inflicted on him as punishment. The realization of attendant guilt may go far toward helping the parents and staff to understand transient personality changes in the child undergoing traumatic procedures.

For the child undergoing prolonged hospitalization, constant reaffirmation of the continuation of his existence is mandatory. A play therapy program is essential and should include schooling as well as play commensurate with the child's interests and physical ability to tolerate it. Play should range from simple games at the bedside to participation in activities in a play area with other children when tolerated.

When this kind of emotional support is provided, most children will see the surgical experience as a reasonably tolerable one; they will look on the staff as friends and enjoy return visits. When a child looks forward to return visits to the hospital, the staff can take pride in having achieved the emotional support that was the goal.

The physical environment must be tailored to children's needs and interests. Bright, cheery colors; play areas; toys; and comfortable clothing make the child feel relaxed and more at home. The simple act of wearing a surgical cap with familiar Sesame Street, Disney, or Peanuts characters portrayed on it will serve to remove some of the harshness from an otherwise cold and threatening environment. A transportation attendant who talks to the child, holds him, and tells him stories en route from the ward to the operating room will do more toward delivering a patient suitable for anesthetic induction than all the premedication available.

A superbly skilled surgical technician with an international reputation can certainly see any child through surgery safely and expect a successful outcome. A well-trained and competent surgeon who also understands the human needs of the child and who works with a concerned and caring team can achieve similar technical results while making the overall experience for the child and family an emotionally acceptable one. However, the primary care physician must not be deluded into believing that these factors will take care of themselves. Only enlightened surgical leadership can influence the otherwise efficiency-oriented operating room staff to take the extra time and effort needed to support the emotional needs of children.

A child should be able to come through a surgical experience having had the reassurance of his parents' constant attendance, the friendship and concern of a sympathetic and knowledgeable hospital staff, the comfort of attractive physical surroundings, and freedom from exposure to the agonies of adult illnesses and discomfitures. Achievement of this goal requires prior thought and preparation, continual staff education and encouragement, a vigilance for truthfulness, and a commitment toward the goal on the part of all concerned. The primary care physician should demand and accept no less for his young patients.

INTERACTING WITH PARENTS

It is the primary care physician who refers the child and therefore the parents to the surgical consultant, and it is through this physician's faith in the consultant that the parents' confidence in the surgeon is established. A surgeon who is experienced in the care of children will also be experienced in the care of their parents and will recognize that the patient is only one of a group of people whom he must communicate with and satisfy. Surgeons used to dealing with adults generally have only peripheral conversation with family members in most instances, the major thrust of explanation and decision making being with the patient himself.

However, in dealing with the child up until the midteenage years, the surgeon must not only gain the child's trust but must also gain the parents' trust and satisfy their questions and explanations, for it is their moral and legal responsibility to make decisions for the child. This is a burdensome responsibility for many parents, because they recognize that they are thrusting pain, discomfort, and risk on another individual and realize that it may be their own desires rather than the child's that are foremost in the decision-making process. Obviously, the more critical the illness and the more directly indicated the procedure, the easier these decisions are to make. Nevertheless, the parents will require support and explanation; and they may continue to rely on the primary care physician to provide it, particularly if the surgeon is uncommunicative.

The primary care physician must avoid committing the surgeon beyond retraction to a course before the consultation takes place. At times the surgical consultant may not think that surgery is indicated or may believe that further evaluation is indicated or that a different diagnosis is involved. If this relationship is to be a consultative and cooperative one, the surgeon must be given leeway to act as a consultant rather than a technician. Generally, it is better for the surgeon to discuss the details of the procedure and the attendant indications, risks, and alternatives. On the other hand, if the primary care physician knows that the surgeon is unlikely to communicate adequately with the parents, the former may be forced into an explanatory role. The parents will rely on whomever they can to provide them with the explanations and information they seek.

I have found that once a primary care physician opts for a surgical course of therapy, the physician tends to downplay the attendant risks. However, most parents appreciate a frank discussion of the problem, the indications for surgery, the alternatives, and the risks involved—conveyed in terms that they can understand. To tell parents that their child may die during anesthesia is a threatening statement, although a true one. The parents have no way of putting this statement into perspective. It is highly unlikely that the child will die during anesthesia, but one cannot tell the parents that it cannot happen. This type of information should be couched in terms the parents can relate to. To tell parents what they already know—that the child can die during anesthesia—reinforces their anxieties concerning a preknown truth and heightens the risks in their minds. On the other hand, to tell parents that anesthesia is generally safe but that nothing in life is 100% safe, that the child may die during the trip home—just as the child may die during anesthesia—and that both are unlikely, with the former being more likely than the latter puts perspective on the situation for most parents. It recalls to them that life has its uncertainties, but

it does not make the risk of death during anesthesia seem a probability rather than a minor possibility.

Of course, when the surgical procedure is a major, life-threatening one or the underlying disease has made the child a high risk for both anesthesia and surgery, the risks are obviously increased; and these increased risks must be conveyed to the parents.

Most parents prefer a reasonably complete discussion of the surgical procedure and a reasonable analysis of its chance of success. It is not fair for the surgeon or primary care physician to overstate the chances of failure in a procedure that should be highly successful; on the other hand, the surgeon should make the parents aware of the limitations of a surgical procedure in a given situation and give an honest evaluation of the chances of success and failure, the hoped-for gains, and possible complications. Doing so will provide the best basis for the ongoing relationship required to see the child through the surgical procedure and the postoperative period. The primary care physician who is thrust into the role of providing this communication for the parents, should try to the best of his or her ability to give them the necessary information and evaluation. On the other hand, the primary care physician should avoid this type of detailed discussion and evaluation if it will be subsequently provided by the surgeon, since even similar explanations coming from two different persons can be highly confusing and may sound contradictory. Many otherwise cooperative and devoted parents may become highly hostile and antagonistic in a setting where too many individuals are trying to explain the same procedure to them. The array of helpful persons who may feel called on to perform these tasks in the modern hospital setting may range from the surgeon, to the surgical resident, to the primary care physician, to the primary care resident, to the social worker, to the nurse, to the nursing student, to the medical student, to the play therapist, and on down the line.

The overriding consideration must be to ensure that the parents have the opportunity to have their questions answered and that open lines of communication are maintained. The time allotted in providing this opportunity for the family will pay great dividends in ensuring their cooperation and understanding of the complexities of modern surgical care for children. Complications do occur with the best of treatment and with the most care-ful and thoughtful decision making. The parents who have been dealt with straightforwardly and honestly—who have had the opportunity to make their decision with a balanced discussion of the hoped-for gains and attendant complications—will be best able to accept the complications that may arise, knowing that the decision was made in the child's best interest and with the careful advice and concern of the attending physicians. On the other hand, if the parents believe that they were forced into a decision that they hesitated to make, with an inadequate understanding of the complex-ities and with little knowledge of the possible com-plications, they will be hostile and antagonistic to-ward any ensuing complications or catastrophies. Although an occasional parent is so immature that he or she cannot handle a decision when risks are presented, such individuals are in the minority, and their existence does not warrant keeping in-formation from the overwhelming majority of par-ents who can handle the decision-making process in a mature way.

CHAPTER 2

Anesthetic considerations

HOWARD C. FILSTON

Pediatric anesthesia is an evolving subspecialty. It requires considerable time and experience to reach a degree of proficiency in the anesthetic management of children. The younger the infant, the more specialized the techniques, and the more necessary that the anesthesiologist be experienced in the care of children.

PREOPERATIVE VISIT FROM THE ANESTHESIOLOGIST

Successful anesthesia for the child begins with a preoperative visit by the anesthesiologist, at which time the anesthesiologist should make the child's acquaintance and hopefully win his trust and friendship. All the premedication in the world will not accomplish as much in quieting the child's fears and anxieties and in achieving his cooperation with the anesthetic manipulations as will the presence of a friendly, previously encountered, and trusted physician. A truthful but simple explanation of the procedures involved along with assurances that the child will not ''wake up'' during anesthesia and surgery, that he will feel no pain during the procedure, that he will awaken again, and that the anesthesiologist will be there, constantly caring for him, are important emotional supports for the child. Although the parents' questions should be answered frankly and simply, medicolegally necessary explanations about the risks of death and dire complications should probably be discussed outside of the child's hearing— but not in such a way as to be secretive and arouse the child's suspicions. Although truthfulness about what will happen in the operating room is extremely important, the child is in no position to interpret the necessary explanations of minor risks and may see them as more significant than they really are. The child should be spared these anxieties.

ANESTHETIC PROCEDURES

The amount of premedication necessary to quiet a really anxious and out-of-control child may carry with it the risk of untoward respiratory depression. Therefore, only mild sedation is advisable. Many times, a well-controlled and properly prepared child can reach the operating room with no premedication whatsoever and cooperate with the procedures, which were previously explained to him, to the point of helping to put himself to sleep by holding the mask, breathing regularly, and cooperating with the manipulations of the anesthesiologist. When atropine is needed for blockage of vagal effects or control of secretions, it can be given after the intravenous line is established; for the young child who cannot tolerate the establishment of an intravenous line prior to induction of the anesthetic, atropine can be given imtramuscularly as a premedication so that the vagal effects will be blocked during induction.

Establishment of an intravenous line

An intravenous line is an excellent safeguard for all general anesthesia; it provides a ready route for the administration of anesthetic agents—especially muscle relaxants, which may be essential in the event that emergency intubation becomes necessary. Certainly, the muscle relaxant facilitates an easy, atraumatic intubation, although it is essential that prior to administration, the anesthesiologist is assured that easy access to the airway is possible or that ventilation can be accomplished by bag and mask. We have favored the establishment of intravenous access for even simple procedures such as herniorrhaphies.

Maintenance of an airway

Maintenance of an airway is the primary consideration in anesthesia of children. Children have few myocardial complications unless they become hypoxic. Arrhythmias are rare and myocardial infarcts essentially unknown in the anesthesia of children, but obstruction of the airway with resultant hypoxia and myocardial depression and arrest is a continuing threat. We prefer to intubate almost all children receiving general anesthesia unless the surgical procedure is an exceedingly short one, such as a needle biopsy of an abdominal viscus, in which little draping takes place and the overall time that the patient is under anesthesia is short. Even though such procedures as herniorrhaphies may take as little as 20 to 30 minutes of operating time, the total time of anesthesia from induction to awakening usually approaches an hour; and maintenance of a good airway throughout this period is best accomplished by intubation.

It has been our experience that the least accomplished and least experienced anesthesiologists are the ones most likely to favor nonintubation techniques, whereas those with the greatest skill and experience with children favor the most meticulous procedures with the greatest number of fail-safe mechanisms built in. Anesthesia of the young child is no place for a cavalier or know-it-all attitude. The fact that the child is physiologically healthy and presents the anesthesiologist with the lowest possible risk of untoward events makes safe and successful anesthesia even more mandatory for this age group. The standard against which pediatric anesthesia must be judged is essentially zero mortality and morbidity.

The choice of agents and techniques varies considerably and should be the domain of the anesthesiologist based on his experience and preferences. Nevertheless, modern pediatric surgical anesthesia is more than just keeping the patient anesthetized. The refined surgical techniques that have evolved over the last 15 to 20 years are highly dependent on good relaxation of muscles, allowing small incisions and careful dissection in a well-controlled operative field.

Management of fluid and electrolyte replacement

Management of intraoperative fluid and electrolyte replacement as well as blood replacement should be a combined venture of the anesthesiologist and surgeon; but in a well-coordinated team effort, much of this responsibility intraoperatively falls to the anesthesiologist. A surgeon who must be overly concerned with these areas of patient care will be distracted from the meticulous and demanding technical procedure. Careful monitoring of blood loss and an estimation of fluid loss from exposure of the intestines will guide the program of replacement. Lost blood should be carefully collected and measured in small-volume traps in the suction line so that the seemingly small volumes of shed blood that may represent major portions of the infant's blood volume can be appreciated. Washing the soiled sponges in known volumes of water followed by colorimetric analysis can give the clinician very accurate estimations of small-volume blood losses.

During intrathoracic procedures, coordination between the anesthesiologist and the surgeon will allow frequent interludes in the surgical procedure during which the anesthesiologist can inflate the deflated lung, improving gas exchange and avoiding postoperative atelectasis.

Awakening of the patient

Probably the most dangerous period of the anesthetic procedure is that of the discontinuance of anesthesia and awakening of the patient. It is at this point that careful judgment on the part of the attending anesthesiologist will identify the ideal time for removal of the endotracheal tube. This should be done when the child is in good control of his reflexes, is performing his own ventilation adequately, has had his secretions aspirated from both his airway and his hypopharynx, and is beyond the point where light stimulation may send him into laryngobronchial spasm. An alternative method is to extubate the child while he is still deeply anesthetized and bring him up into a lighter plane by mask ventilation. This is dependent on the prior confirmation during induction that mask ventilation can be successfully accomplished and on the assurance that postoperative supervision of the airway will be meticulous.

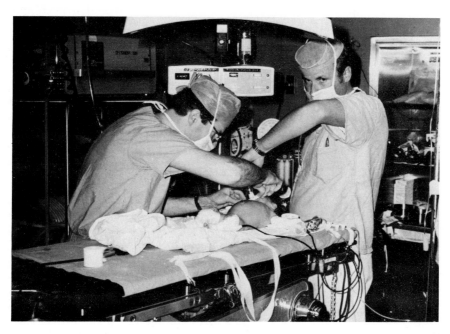

Fig. 2-1. Overhead warmer in place above the operating table as the infant is prepared for anesthesia and surgery. (From Filston, H. C., and Izant, R.: The surgical neonate: evaluation and care, New York, 1978, Appleton-Century Crofts.)

Transport of the patient

Another danger point in the anesthetic experience is the period of transport from the operating room to the recovery room or the ward. Particularly for the neonate, it is often safer to transport him back to the intensive care nursery still intubated, even though he is ventilating well. Because of the marked effects of hypothermia on the infant's respiratory drive, and because of the frequent persistent effects of relaxing agents, it is not unusual for the neonate to become apneic after a period of seemingly adequate spontaneous ventilation. Hospital corridors and elevators are poor places for managing an hypoxic cardiorespiratory arrest. We have considered it far better to transport most of these infants back to the intensive care nursery intubated; at that point, they can be either extubated in a surrounding equipped to deal with any untoward occurrences, or mechanical support can be continued until they have recovered further and can maintain their own ventilatory function adequately.

For the older infant and child, careful evaluation of respiratory function before leaving the operating room and careful observation during the short trip to the recovery room and thereafter are essential. Particularly if the child has had a procedure requiring manipulation of the airway, or if a traumatic intubation was experienced, careful observation of continued airway patency is essential under the direction of experienced recovery room personnel and an attending anesthesiologist.

Management of the newborn

Finally, for the management of the newborn in the operating room, the anesthesiologist must attend to careful maintenance of body temperature and fluid and electrolyte balance. Heat loss can be partially prevented by keeping the infant in the warm transport device until time for induction of anesthesia and by utilizing a warming mattress beneath the patient and an overhead radiant warmer during preinduction and induction (Fig. 2-1). For some tiny infants, the overhead warmer must be maintained during the surgical procedure itself, despite its encumbrance, or the rapidity of heat loss in the air-conditioned room will be excessive. A facility to warm the operating room individually will help to offset this tendency, but excessive warming is intolerable to the surgical staff in their heavy gowns. Nonetheless, the overriding consideration must be to maintain the child's temperature at normal levels, for the effects of hypothermia on perfusion and respiratory function cannot be tolerated. In addition, the anesthetic gases must be warmed and humidified to avoid cooling the child with cold, dry inspired gases.

Even with all of these considerations, the tiny premature infant will often lose 1° or 2° C of body heat during a long surgical procedure. Recognition of this problem will lead the anesthesiologist to maintain control of the airway and return the infant to the intensive care nursery while the infant is still being ventilated through the endotracheal tube. There, the infant can be mechanically ventilated until he is rewarmed and the integrity of his own ventilatory drive is ensured.

LOCAL ANESTHESIA FOR CHILDREN

A word should be said about local anesthesia for minor procedures in children. The primary requirement for successful local anesthesia is a cooperative patient. Most children will not be able to maintain the degree of control required to allow sterile preparation of an area, maintenance of a sterile field, injection of a local anesthetic agent with its attendant initial pain, and the threatening manipulations of the surgical procedure with its attendant implements and noises. It is difficult for a mature adult to maintain self-control under such circumstances, and to ask it of a young child is unrealistic. Thus, these procedures usually are attended by attempts to quiet the child with tranquilizers and analgesics, many of which will only increase the child's anxiety and make him less able to control his responses. Tranquilization or analgesia to the point of absolute control usually requires dosages that threaten a child's respiratory integrity and risk a respiratory arrest. Under these circumstances, local anesthesia becomes more dangerous than well-controlled general anesthesia.

This is not to say that many minor procedures, such as suturing of lacerations, cannot be accomplished by a surgeon who is willing to take the time to gain the child's trust, explain the manipula-

tions, and sustain the child's control with constant reassurance. Suturing of most lacerations, however is a far simpler procedure than even the most minor elective surgical procedures, such as resection of minor skin tags and tumors. Since these latter procedures involve fresh incisions, they are attended by considerable fresh bleeding, which requires hemostasis, time for ligatures, and the placement of several layers of sutures. Most lacerations are already under hemostatic control by the time of medical attention, and the number and complexity of manipulations required is considerably less.

It is far better to ensure that a safe general anesthetic can be given to the child and then perform the surgical procedure under ideal conditions. If safe general anesthesia cannot be guaranteed, it is better to delay the procedure or send the child to a facility where such competent anesthesia can be achieved.

SPECIAL CONSIDERATIONS

Finally, a word should be said about procedures such as needle biopsies of intrathoracic or intraperitoneal organs in the awake child. The safety of needle biopsy is dependent on controlled respiratory arrest so that the viscus being penetrated will not move while the sharp needle point is within it. The mature older child or adult can be counted on to hold his breath while the needle is being manipulated if the procedure is carefully explained and if adequate local anesthesia has been utilized. This is asking too much of the younger child and is impossible for the infant; thus, such procedures performed in this manner in these age groups carry with them a higher risk of laceration and its attendant severe hemorrhage. We have, therefore, discouraged the use of local anesthesia for such procedures in age groups in which we cannot be assured that the child's cooperation can be maintained and relied on; we have preferred to perform the same procedure under a short period of carefully applied, well-controlled general anesthesia with assured respiratory control.

CHAPTER 3

Vascular access

HOWARD C. FILSTON

PERCUTANEOUS VENIPUNCTURE

Facility at venipuncture in a child is a skill that comes primarily with repetition and experience. Nevertheless, the ability to achieve venous access must be part of the armamentarium of any physician faced with caring for a child, for the acute situation that would require rehydration or blood loss replacement may occur at any time.

Once one accepts the fact that venipuncture in a child can be achieved in essentially the same manner as venipuncture in an adult, a great array of vessels is available. Generally, the veins on the dorsum of the hand or those in the antecubital fossa are utilized. A proper-size soft tourniquet is essential, and it should be placed fairly close to the point of venipuncture. One of the most important factors is to have the vein stretched, and to achieve adequate stretch of the veins in a young infant so that the vein does not simply fold away from the advancing needle point may require considerable flexion of the wrist beyond that usually necessary in the adult. The following material, excerpted from a 1971 article in *Pediatrics,* describes a technique for venipuncture utilizing a plastic cannula sheath. The principles apply to any type of plastic catheter insertion with a needle stylet; but the principle of utilizing the bevel down is equally applicable to the butterfly or scalp vein needle and is perhaps more essential when a metal needle is being utilized, because the perforation of the back wall of the vessel by the needle tip makes advancement of the needle into the lumen of the vessel impossible. When a plastic cannula is utilized, it can often be manipulated into the vessel after the needle stylet is withdrawn, even though the needle stylet penetrated the back wall of the vessel.

Equipment

1. A 20- or 22-gauge percutaneous venous cannula constructed as a tapered plastic sheath surrounding a removable metal stylet with syringe attached. This is referred to subsequently as the percutaneous venous cannula.
2. An 18-gauge needle.
3. A padded arm-board splint.
4. Antiseptic solution for preparation of the skin.
5. Standard intravenous fluid administration set with pediatric control chamber.
6. A short segment of extension tubing or "T-connector" for the intravenous tubing.
7. Usual tourniquet, tape, and fluids for intravenous therapy.

Venipuncture technique

Because success with this technique requires meticulous attention to seemingly obvious points, discussion of details and equipment used is essential.

The antecubital veins of the forearm are preferred but the veins on the dorsum of the hands or ventral surface of the wrist are used frequently, especially in smaller infants. Antiseptic solution is used on both the patient and the physician's palpating finger. The site must then be dried with sterile gauze to allow traction during insertion. A soft padded arm-board approximately 10 by 20 cm is used. Rolled gauze padding is used behind the elbow to hyperextend the antecubital fossa. Waterproof tape is essential. The arm-board is then taped to the table or mattress for complete immobilization of the extremity. The baby is placed on the table so that with the arm extended, there is still room for the physician to stabilize his hand on the table surface. A medium-sized rubber band is an ideal tourniquet (Fig. 3-1).

Many products for percutaneous venous cannulation are available on the market, but the one chosen must have the following features:
  a. An inner metal needle as stylet with a clear cham-

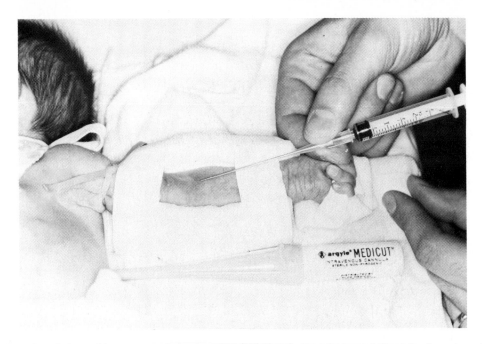

Fig. 3-1. Infant with arm extended on an arm board and properly immobilized for insertion of the needle stylet plastic cannula system into the antecubital vein. Note the rubber band serving as a tourniquet. (From Filston, H. C., and Izant, R.: The surgical neonate: evaluation and care, New York, 1978, Appleton-Century-Crofts.)

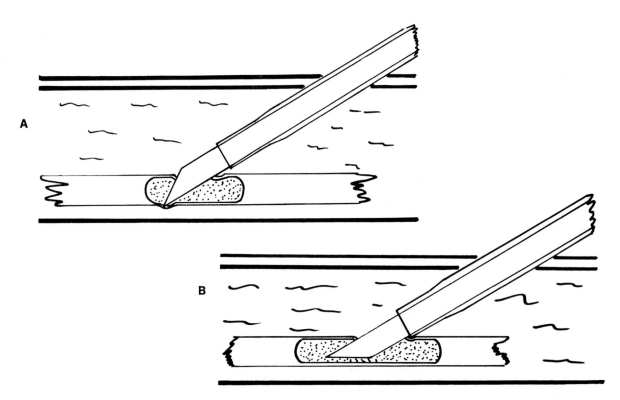

Fig. 3-2. A, When the needle is inserted with the bevel up, the point of the needle may pass through the back wall of the vessel before the plastic cannula enters the lumen of the vein. **B,** With the bevel down, the lumen of the needle remains within the lumen of the vessel without the point of the needle traversing the back wall of the vessel, so that aspiration of blood will indicate a successful venipuncture. (From Filston, H. C., and Johnson, D. G.: Pediatrics **48:**896, 1971. Copyright American Academy of Pediatrics 1971.)

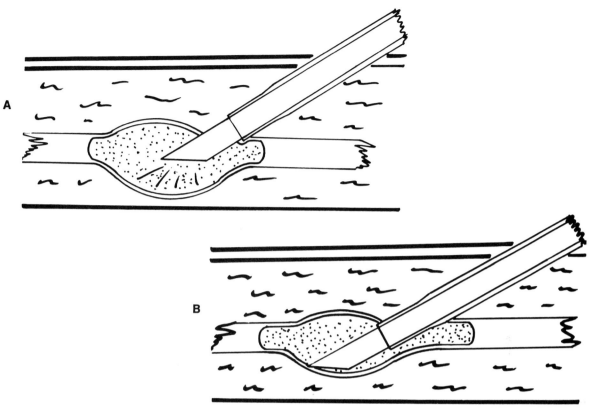

Fig. 3-3. A, Reinjection of the blood will dilate the vessel, providing additional room for further insertion of the needle point, allowing the following plastic catheter to enter the vessel before the point of the needle traverses the back wall of the vein, as illustrated in **B.** (From Filston, H. C., and Johnson, D. G.: Pediatrics **48:**896, 1971. Copyright American Academy of Pediatrics 1971.)

ber in the hub for early detection of aspirated blood.

b. An outer plastic cannula that is gently tapered at the distal end to permit easy insertion into tiny veins.

c. A tapered hub end that is an integral part of the cannula. This eliminates the connection of catheter to metal hub with its risk of disconnection and embolism.

d. An attached syringe with an airtight connection to the stylet hub.

A standard 18-gauge needle is used to puncture the skin approximately 1 cm from the proposed site of venipuncture and in line with the direction of the vein. The percutaneous venous cannula is then inserted, *bevel down,* through the skin puncture site and advanced slowly toward the vein. Negative pressure is applied to the barrel of the syringe and the clear chamber observed for the first sign of blood aspiration as the cannula is advanced. The importance of inserting the needle with the bevel down is shown in Fig. 3-2. In a small vein the point of a needle inserted with the bevel up

passes through the back wall of the vessel before the lumen of the needle reaches the lumen of the vein. Thus, by the time the blood is aspirated into the syringe and success of the venipuncture is recognized, the needle has passed through both walls of the vein. When the needle is inserted bevel down, the point advances into the lumen of the vein in line with the lumen of needle. Therefore, blood aspiration is apparent in the hub chamber before the back wall is pierced, and the cannula can then be advanced into the lumen of the vein.

The cannula must be advanced slowly in fractions of a millimeter. The index finger of the opposite hand is used to palpate the relationship between the needle point and the vein. The venipuncture is performed directly into the upper surface of the vein.

Once successful entry is confirmed by the return of blood into the viewing chamber of the needle hub, approximately 1 ml of blood is withdrawn into the syringe. The hand holding the syringe is carefully braced against the table top and the thumb of that hand used to reinject the blood into the vessel, thus distending it.

Simultaneously, the hand advances the whole syringe, needle, and plastic catheter as a unit forward a few millimeters into the lumen of the vein. This allows the plastic catheter with its slight "lip" to puncture the vein wall and enter the lumen while the needle tip is advancing easily into the blood-distended lumen ahead of it (Fig. 3-3). Usually a distinct "pop" can be felt as the catheter traverses the vein wall. If this step is omitted, the catheter is merely pushed forward after the needle enters the vein, the edge of the catheter will push the vein wall off the end of the needle, and the procedure will fail. Once the plastic catheter has entered the vessel lumen, the inner needle stylet can be withdrawn and the catheter advanced inward until the flare of the hub binds at the skin puncture site. When the procedure is successful, a free flow of blood from the catheter hub is noted after removal of the stylet. If no such flow is present, either the catheter never entered the lumen or the entire cannula has traversed both walls and the vessel has been transfixed by the catheter. If the latter is the case, a successful cannulation can usually be salvaged by slowly withdrawing the plastic catheter (without reinserting the stylet) until a free flow of blood is noted. Rotation and advancement of the catheter will then place it into the lumen properly. Free flow of blood will persist. If the catheter has not entered the lumen at all, free blood flow may be noted when its tip is opposite the needle puncture site, but after rotation and readvancement the blood flow will again cease.

Antibiotic ointment is used to cover the puncture site on the skin and is covered with a small "Band-aid" dressing. If the catheter is allowed any room to slide back and forth, it will soon leak. The arm is therefore coated with tincture of benzoin solution and a long strip of waterproof tape is used to secure the catheter. Additional strips of tape are then used to further anchor the catheter. Immobilization is accomplished by readjusting the padded arm-board splint. The child must not be allowed to flex at the elbow, as this will crimp or break the plastic catheter. Rolls of 4 × 4 gauze sponges are placed along each side of the arm, bridging the elbow. The arm-board splint is then taped in place. To facilitate daily solution and tubing changes, a "T-Connector"* is inserted into the cannula and the IV line then connected into this. In this manner, the IV bottle, tubing, and administration set can be changed daily without disturbing the catheter. If the IV tubing is connected directly into the catheter, the motion of changing the tubing connection will enlarge the venipuncture and cause leakage. It is mandatory to inspect the cannula daily to be certain that it is still functioning properly and phlebitis is not developing. It is usually unnecessary to untape the cannula completely to make this inspection.

*TM Abbott Laboratories, North Chicago, Illinois 60064.

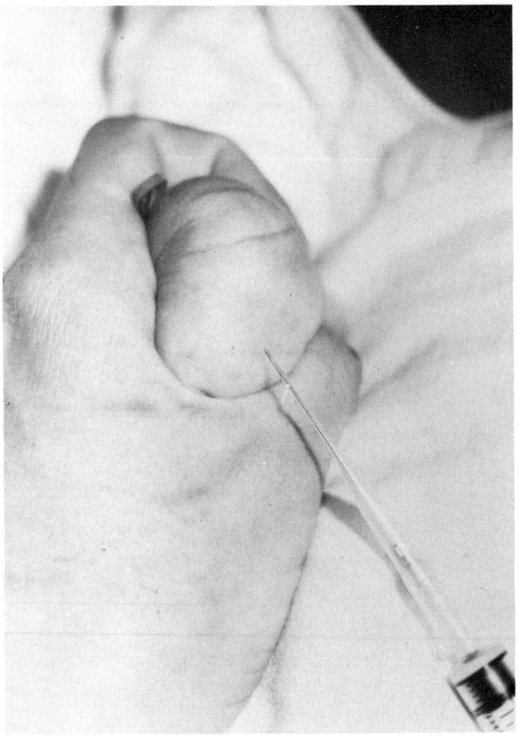

Fig. 3-4. The infant's hand and wrist are grasped in the physician's hand so that the hand is folded firmly against the ventral surface of the wrist, providing a firm stretch for the tiny veins on the dorsum of the hand prior to insertion of the plastic cannula with its needle stylet. (From Filston, H. C., and Johnson, D. G.: Pediatrics **48:**896, 1971. Copyright American Academy of Pediatrics 1971.)

Frequently, in tiny infants, the vessels on the dorsum of the hand or ventral surface of the wrist are more easily cannulated. In these cases, the arm is not attached to a board until successful cannulation is accomplished. The infant's hand is held by the physician in such a way as to put maximum stretch on the vein. For the dorsum of the hand, this requires complete flexion of the infant's wrist such that the ventral surfaces of the hand and fingers appose the ventral forearm (Fig. 3-4). The physician must not place his hand between the infant's forearm and ventral hand surface as this will leave the veins too lax.*

*From Filston, H. C., and Johnson, D. G.: Percutaneous venous cannulation in neonates and infants; a method of catheter insertion without "cutdown," Pediatrics **48:**896, 1971. Copyright American Academy of Pediatrics 1971.

INCISIONAL CUTDOWN

Unless the physician has become adept at utilizing a plastic cannula needle stylet system, he should probably not attempt it under duress. In an emergency the ability to do an expeditious cutdown for vascular access must remain the cornerstone of such therapy. Any vein can be cutdown on, and a general knowledge of areas where veins are prominent is helpful. However, the classic access point is at the greater saphenous vein at the ankle. This vein can be localized by making a point that is 1 cm anterior and 1 cm superior to the medial malleolus. A transverse incision covering 0.5 to 0.75 cm should then be made in the skin just through the dermis with a scalpel, and a pair of scissors or a mosquito hemostat should be used to spread the wound open. A deep cut with a knife blade should be avoided, because it may transect the vein and injure tendons or nerves or other vessels in the area. Once the skin is open, the fine-pointed mosquito hemostat should be pushed firmly down into the deep tissues of the wound and then turned toward the opposite corner of the incision and pulled up. The vessels, with their high content of elastic tissue, will not be injured by such a maneuver; and the other tissue will tear and fall away. If the incision is placed in the proper location and this maneuver is performed with adequate dissection deep into the soft tissues, the saphenous vein should be contained in the curve of the hemostat as it is elevated out of the wound. It is not necessary to ligate the vein proximal to the venipuncture or to make an incision in the vein. Once the vein is located, a ligature can be passed around it loosely for traction and the needle or plastic cannula passed directly into the vessel while it remains filled with blood. This maneuver facilitates the venipuncture, and a larger-bore cannula can be placed within the vein. Once an incision is made into the vessel and the blood is emptied from it, the vessel shrinks down in size and a considerably smaller cannula must be utilized. If the incision in the skin has been made small enough, the tissues will still support the cannula adequately without suturing the vein around it. The cannula can then be taped in place as though a percutaneous puncture had been performed, thus preserving the vein for subsequent use.

ARTERIAL CANNULATION

If emergency access to the arterial system is necessary in an infant beyond the age in which umbilical artery cannulation is feasible, the radial artery is easily accessible and the complications associated with cannulation of this vessel are minimal. If the pulse can be felt, a small incision can be fashioned in the same way as described for the saphenous vein access. A similar procedure— dissecting deep into the soft tissues with a fine-pointed mosquito hemostat, turning the hemostat, passing across the extent of the incision, and bringing up all the tissue—will usually bring up the elastic artery, which can then be cannulated in a similar fashion without being ligated.

Finally, adequate taping, the most important part of which is a strip of waterproof tape that runs from the needle or cannula directly across the puncture site or incision and up along the extremity, followed by subsequent cross-taping, will hold the cannula well seated into the vessel. Adequate immobilization of adjacent joints will prevent kinking or crimping of the catheter and will help to maintain the vascular access for the period of time necessary. Utilization of 1 unit of heparin per milliliter of fluid will not interfere with clotting mechanisms but will help maintain the integrity of the vascular access.

CHAPTER 4

Management of fluids and electrolytes

HOWARD C. FILSTON

Ideally the decisions relating to the volume and makeup of fluid and electrolyte solutions for replacement preoperatively and postoperatively should be made by the surgical team, since the team can evaluate these requirements in the light of the extent of the disease process found and the extent of trauma sustained by the surgical manipulations themselves. Too often, however, the surgical team is incapable of making these judgments accurately because of a lack of knowledge or experience in dealing with the child, and the primary care physician's own knowledge of the requirements is needed to augment that of the surgical team. The primary care physician in this position must be willing to learn a great deal about the requirements for vascular volume maintenance and the potentially extensive fluid requirements that may accompany certain disease states and certain surgical procedures. In order to comprehend fully these requirements, the primary care physician must have some knowledge of the underlying physiologic theory by which the decisions regarding fluid and electrolyte requirements are made.

The primary goal of all fluid and electrolyte therapy in the management of the surgical patient is to maintain the vascular volume. If the vascular volume is maintained, it can be assumed that the general state of hydration of the body is adequate and that vital organs will be perfused. It is this perfusion that must be ensured. If perfusion fails, anaerobic metabolism is substituted for the normal aerobic processes, and ultimately damage to vital enzyme systems takes place. In addition, direct injury to capillary epithelium results in additional shifts of fluid into the extravascular space, further interfering with normal tissue-organ perfusion.

PHYSIOLOGIC CONCEPTS OF VASCULAR VOLUME REPLACEMENT

For many years, including the recent past, the blood pressure measurement was the primary modality for monitoring the state of volume replacement. Reliance on the blood pressure measurement led to the use of pharmacologic agents such as pressors to maintain the pressure at normal levels. The presence of a normal blood pressure is still often invoked as an indication that volume replacement is adequate. However, the following example should illustrate the fallacy of relying on the blood pressure measurement as an indication of vascular volume.

If all of the small-vessel volume were removed from the system, and the blood from the heart entered the major aortic vessels, shunted back to the vena cava, and returned to the heart, a volume of blood representing only a small percentage of the total body volume could maintain adequate filling of the vessels, so that a normal blood pressure would be recorded. Yet, this situation would represent a total lack of perfusion of the vital organs and tissues of the body as well as a markedly reduced vascular volume.

Although this case is extreme, it does illustrate that the compensatory mechanisms that come into play when vascular volume is reduced will shunt blood past vital organs and tissues and enable a markedly reduced volume to still maintain normal blood pressure. Thus, a normal blood pressure measurement does not ensure that adequate perfusion of all vital tissue is maintained.

Perfusion of the kidneys, on the other hand, as represented by a continued adequate urine output, is a good monitor of vascular perfusion; for although urine output may be maintained in the

16

face of some reduction in vascular volume, it will quickly diminish and stop altogether when significant reductions in vascular volume have taken place. Thus, the continued output of an adequate urine volume is the best indicator of adequate tissue organ perfusion in the body. However, the validity of certain assumptions must be ensured for kidney function to be used as a reliable indicator of the adequacy of vascular volume. These are that the heart is functioning normally, that there is no intrinsic pathologic state involving the kidney that is altering the urine output, that there are no abnormal secretory substances such as antidiuretic hormone or an excess of aldosterone upsetting the normal responses of the body to changes in vascular volume, and that basic liver function is maintained, so that these substances are normally sustained or degraded as necessary. When these assumptions cannot be totally relied on, some other monitor in addition to urine output is required, such as indwelling catheters monitoring the function of the right and left sides of the heart. Generally for children, right-sided heart monitoring in the form of a central venous pressure line is all that is required unless some marked pathophysiology of cardiac functioning can be identified or is suspected.

Once it is understood that vascular volume and perfusion (rather than the simple maintenance of "normal" blood pressure) are the goals, then some idea of the potential sources of loss must be appreciated. The most obvious source of vascular volume deficiency is external blood loss. Volume replacement is obviously necessary and is usually provided.

PHYSIOLOGIC CONCEPTS OF MAINTENANCE OF OTHER FLUIDS

Other fluids can be lost from the body and represent a sizable portion of vascular volume. Severe diarrhea with tremendous losses of fluid and electrolytes in the stool is a well-known source of volume deficiency to the pediatrician, and replacement of such external losses is clearly necessary. Severe vomiting, losses from fistulas such as biliary and pancreatic fistulas, and excessive fluid and electrolyte loss due to perspiration are other sources of loss to the external environment.

Every patient has a basic need for free water replacement to make up for losses sustained by exhalation of water vapor from the lungs and evaporative losses of fluid from the body's surface.

These insensible losses have been studied and measured, and formulas can be utilized to replace the needs adequately. The most difficult concept to grasp with regard to the needs of the surgical or trauma patient is the requirement for replacing fluids that are still in the body. This so-called third-space concept evolved over a period of years, with much experimental work contributing to its evolution. In the 1940s Wiggers,[6] in a series of experiments, showed a high mortality in dogs associated with hemorrhage leading to marked falls in blood pressure, even though the lost blood was replaced with the animal's own blood in equivalent volume—a concept designated as irreversible shock. Subsequent research looking for some "x factor" in the shock state that caused the irreversible nature of the shock was extensive but unsuccessful. In the 1950s in Boston in Moore's laboratory,[2a] extensive metabolic research regarding traumatized patients revealed the presence of high levels of aldosterone and antidiuretic hormone; and from these experiments it was concluded that traumatized patients, including those having undergone major surgical procedures, have an inappropriate secretion of salt- and water-retaining hormones and therefore cannot tolerate salt and water loads following surgery. This conclusion led to the designation of inappropriate antidiuretic hormone (ADH) secretion and to a program of management that involved primarily salt and water restriction in the postoperative period. However, many patients went into renal failure and succumbed to generalized hypoperfusion in a prolonged shocklike state.

Many experiments related to shock research in the late 1950s and the early 1960s culminated in the work of Shires,[3,4] who demonstrated that repeating Wiggers' experiments with hemorrhaging dogs and replacing the same volume of blood augmented with various volumes of balanced salt solution led to a high survival rate in the dogs. This demonstration emphasized the concept of third-space losses within the body and the need to replace a greater volume of fluid than that actually measured as loss during the acute hypovolemic phase. The reason for this need becomes clear when the preceding discussion of the effects of hypoperfusion is taken into account. As blood is lost from the vascular space, vasoconstrictive compensatory mechanisms come into play; these mechanisms shunt blood from vital tissues and lead to anaerobic metabolism in those cells. As a result, capillary membrane damage ensues and acid waste products build up. When the volume of lost blood is replaced, restoration of flow to these tissues leads to leakage of fluid out of the damaged capillary membranes and to diffusion of these acid waste products back into the general systemic circuit. The seemingly restored vascular volume is depleted once again of its fluid phase, and the shock state is maintained. Marked hypovolemia persists, with restoration of vasoconstriction and resumption of anaerobic metabolism and its resultant injury to vital tissues and organs. In addition, the acidosis in the systemic circuit may depress pulmonary and cardiovascular functioning and lead to further hypoperfusion of vital structures. Thus, what starts out as a simple, direct, measurable blood loss may end up in sizably greater volume deficits in the total body.

Timely replacement of blood loss tends to offset this secondary fluid requirement, but such requirements must be kept in mind whenever replacement of blood loss is delayed long enough to allow hypoxic tissue injury. Thus, one aspect of third-space fluid loss is loss through damaged capillary membranes as a result of hypoxic tissue damage from hypoperfusion. There are other, more common sources of such loss, however. The third space essentially represents any compartmentalization or sequestration of fluid within the body that is not immediately recoverable to the vascular volume by simple hydrostatic and osmotic forces.

The most frequent example of such a loss is that into the lumen of the bowel during the neurogenic ileus that develops during and after intra-abdominal surgical procedures or as a result of abdominal trauma. The lumen of the bowel can be likened to the hole in a doughnut, which is both inside and outside the doughnut. Running from the stoma of the mouth to the stoma of the anus, the lumen of the intestine can be likened to a cylinder. Ordinarily, fluids lost into the proximal aspect of this long cylinder are recovered continuously in the distal aspect by absorption. Thus, the liters upon liters of extracellular fluid that enter the lumen of the bowel daily, representing many times the normal vascular volume, are continuously recovered; and the net loss from the gastrointestinal tract amounts to a mere fraction of a liter daily.[1] However, whenever fluids are lost into the lumen of the bowel as a result of mechanical obstruction distally or as a result of

the adynamic ileus that results from intraperitoneal manipulations, these fluids become sequestered and not immediately recoverable. The fact that they will be easily recovered in a few days, when the motility of the bowel is restored, is inconsequential to the dynamic requirements of the vascular volume in the immediate intraoperative and postoperative periods. Thus, hypovolemia and hypoperfusion can result from the shifting of fluid into the lumen of the bowel and from the inability of the normal hydrostatic and osmotic forces to recover it back into the vascular volume despite a deficit resulting therein. This third space loss must be replaced if normal volume is to be maintained and restored and normal perfusion is to be ensured.

Understanding of this particular example will make obvious the unreliability of body weight as a measure of vascular volume replacement. In fact, in the postoperative period the patient who sustains a third-space shift will *gain* weight if vascular volume is adequately restored, since the *lost* volume is still contained within the body. If this concept is not grasped, and reliance is placed on a fluid management program that views weight gain as an indication of fluid overload, hypoperfusion and the injurious effects of hypoxia to the vital tissues will result.

MAINTENANCE REQUIREMENTS FOR FLUIDS AND ELECTROLYTES

Once these basic physiologic concepts are understood, a plan of management for the surgical patient can be easily developed. The 24-hour fluid requirements for a surgical patient consist of maintenance fluids, replacement of measured losses, and replacement of those third-space shifts that can be identified. Since maintenance requirements are dictated by insensible losses and the need for an adequate urine output, formulas have been developed that describe these requirements accurately. For the adult they amount to roughly 1,500 to 2,000 ml of water and a certain amount of salt replacement in the form of sodium chloride and potassium chloride. Various formulas based on weight or surface area have been derived for the child. The formula we have utilized is one presented in 1952 by Wallace[5]; this formula represents the caloric requirements of a hospitalized child whose kidneys are functioning in the mid-range of concentrating ability—a comfortable level without excessive demands for concentration or dilution. It states that the daily fluid and caloric requirements are equal to 100 ml minus three times the age in years times the weight in kilograms (100 ml − [3 × age in years] × wt in kg). Since we generally adhere to a minimum volume of 1,500 ml of maintenance fluid for an adult, when this formula calculates to 1,500 ml, we adhere to that volume. The child, in addition, has a requirement of 3 mEq of sodium and chloride per kilogram and 2 to 3 mEq of potassium per kilogram daily. It should be recognized that the maintenance requirement is generally one for free water, but this free water can be utilized as a vehicle for carrying in the needed milliequivalents of electrolytes. Since normal saline solution provides 154 mEq of electrolytes per liter, or 15.4 mEq of electrolytes per 100 ml, and since the young child will receive approximately 100 ml/kg, the electrolyte requirement of 3 mEq of sodium and chloride per kilogram can be provided by placing it into the 100 ml/kg that the child will receive; thus, there should be 3 mEq of sodium and chloride and 2 mEq of potassium in each 100 ml that the child will receive for each kilogram of body weight. A solution of one-fifth normal saline contains 3 mEq of sodium and chloride per 100 ml and therefore is the most ideal solution for administering this requirement. A solution of one-fourth normal saline, which is more widely available, is also acceptable, since it provides 3.8 mEq of sodium and chloride per 100 ml and therefore per kilogram.

It must be appreciated that once the volume of free water or hypotonic electrolyte solution calculated for the patient has been administered, no additional volumes of hypotonic solution are required, nor should they be given. Certainly, they should not be substituted for those volumes of replacement solutions that can be identified as measured losses or as third-space shifts. All of these requirements represent losses of extracellular fluid in one form or another and are therefore replaceable only by balanced electrolyte solution or by solutions of greater osmotic concentration, such as those containing colloid. Substitution of hypotonic solutions for these requirements will result in dilution of intravascular osmotic forces and a shift of fluid out of the vascular space into the extravascular tissues, representing an inefficiency of replacement. Thus, greater volumes will be required to achieve replacement of vascular volume, resulting in greater

edema of the surrounding tissues. Although this may be of little consequence in some tissues and organs, it can be of vital concern if excess volume shifts into the interstitial spaces of the lung, resulting in interference with gaseous diffusion, particularly of oxygen from the alveolus to the capillary. For some patients with borderline pulmonary function, such an additional insult may tip the balance in the direction of ventilatory failure. In fact, for the patient who can be identified as having a preexisting deficit of intravascular oncotic pressure, such as patients with liver disease with marked hypoalbuminemia or patients who have already sustained marked blood loss, the provision of replacement solutions in the form of colloid-containing solutions may be essential for adequate volume replacement without undue fluid shifts.

Most measured losses can be approximated with the aid of some knowledge of the makeup of the gastrointestinal fluids. Losses from the stomach are primarily hydrochloric acid with sodium, potassium, and chloride. Provision of adequate chloride is essential to the maintenance of acid-base equilibrium; and if no potassium can be administered, normal saline will be needed to give adequate chloride replacement. If the patient can tolerate potassium administration, a solution made up of half normal saline with 30 mEq of potassium chloride per liter will provide 75 mEq of sodium, 30 mEq of potassium, and 105 mEq of chloride—an adequate gastric replacement solution.

For all losses from the gastrointestinal tract beyond the pylorus, some solution approximating extracellular fluid is essential. Thus, Ringer's lactate, which is a balanced salt solution containing 130 mEq of sodium, 105 mEq of chloride, 4.5 mEq of potassium, and 27.5 mEq of lactate, will provide excellent replacement for extracellular fluid losses both externally and into third-space compartments. Fallacies related to the use of Ringer's lactate solution include the following: potassium administration is dangerous (this is not valid, since the potassium content is equal to that of the extracellular fluid shifted); Ringer's lactate is more expensive than sodium chloride solution (this is not true); and finally, the body cannot handle the lactate, and the lactate represents an acid load (this is not true, because the lactate will be metabolized to bicarbonate and provide a balanced basic replacement solution). Losses represented by diarrhea or by fluids lost from fistulas or ostomies approximate extracellular fluid in their electrolyte content and are best replaced with a balanced salt solution.

All internal shifts or so-called third-space losses are made up of extracellular fluid, and their replacement must be in a balanced salt solution. Again, the replacement of these losses with a hypotonic solution will result in an inefficient filling of the vascular space and a shift of fluid into the extravascular tissues to the detriment of vital organ functioning. It is ironic that it is often the physician who is overly concerned about excess volume administration who errs on the side of providing a hypotonic solution in excess, thereby creating the very fluid shifts he is concerned about avoiding.

To develop an intelligent program of fluid and electrolyte management for the surgical patient, we still need to know the volume of urine required. It has been shown that 1 to 2 ml/kg/hr, or approximately 40 ml/kg/day, is a urine output that will allow the kidney to function in the midrange, avoiding demands for extreme concentration and extreme dilution.[5] It must be appreciated that not only must we work to achieve this urine volume, but once it has been achieved, we must be ready to cut back on fluid administration to hold the volume down to this level if excess fluid with the risk of fluid overload is to be avoided.

The following is a method for roughly approximating the amount of fluid required for replacing the third-space shifts in various intraperitoneal procedures. This method relates the extent of disease and surgical manipulation within the peritoneal cavity to the child's size by means of the maintenance requirement formula. Thus, the child is given an extra one fourth of his maintenance volume for each quadrant of the peritoneal cavity involved with either the disease process or the surgical manipulation.[2] By this system, for example, an appendectomy for acute unruptured appendicitis would require an additional one fourth of the volume for the surgical manipulation in the right lower quadrant and an additional one fourth of the maintenance volume for the disease in the right lower quadrant. By the same token, a generalized peritonitis due to perforated appendicitis in which an appendectomy is performed would require four additional one-fourth volumes for the generalized peritonitis and one additional one-fourth volume for the appendectomy, or five-fourths additional volume above the maintenance

requirement for the disease process and the surgical manipulation. This replacement fluid, which replaces the internal or third-space losses, *must be in the form of balanced electrolyte solution and not in a maintenance type of hypotonic solution,* as discussed above.

It must be understood that all attempts to replace third-space shifts are guesses or *estimates,* since all attempts to measure these shifts by various tracer elements have met with failure. The third-space shifts are an ongoing dynamic process, and the areas of sequestration are unpredictable. On the other hand, we are not interested in measuring the third-space volume so much as we are interested in maintaining an adequate vascular volume; therefore, we rely on the urine output to tell us when the vascular volume is adequate. Depending on the rate of vascular volume replacement, the vascular volume may be maintained at an adequate level even though all of the third-space shifts have not been replaced. Thus, if we direct our attention to maintaining vascular volume and continue this attention until the diuretic phase is entered at 48 hours or so following surgery or trauma, we will maintain adequate replacement and do not need to be concerned about measuring third-space volumes directly.

Perhaps if we now take an example and follow it through, it will help to emphasize the above-discussed principles. Let us say that a 4-kg, 3-day-old infant develops signs and symptoms of necrotizing enterocolitis with gastric retention of bile-stained fluid, abdominal distension, and the passage of seedy, blood-streaked stools. Despite nasogastric decompression, the institution of antibiotic therapy, and adequate fluid and electrolyte administration, the child's abdominal distention suddenly increases and abdominal radiographs demonstrate the presence of free intraperitoneal air. With the diagnosis of perforation secondary to necrotizing enterocolitis, abdominal exploration is planned. In the management of fluid and electrolytes, attention must be directed toward preoperative replacement therapy, so that the child enters the anesthetic phase with an adequate vascular volume. This can be initially accomplished by a push of 20 ml/kg, which represents one fourth of the child's vascular volume of 80 ml/kg. If adequate time is available, additional balanced electrolyte solution should be administered to achieve and maintain an adequate urine output.

Following surgery, if we were to write the child's 24-hour fluid requirements, the following considerations would apply.

First, the child's maintenance is defined by the formula: 100 ml minus 3 times his age in years times the weight in kilograms, which is 100 minus 3 times 3/365, or essentially 100 ml times 4 kg or 400 ml of fluid for maintenance, which is to be given as 5% dextrose/one-fifth normal saline solution. In addition, assuming that the child's nasogastric losses will be approximately 3 to 4 ml/hr, he will be given 100 ml of 5% dextrose/one-half normal saline solution containing 3 mEq of potassium chloride. Finally, the child's disease process involves his entire peritoneal cavity, and at the time of surgery his entire colon is involved with extensive necrotizing enterocolitis with multiple perforations; it is elected to perform a total colectomy. Thus, both the child's disease process and his surgical procedure involve all four quadrants of his peritoneal cavity, he will therefore require eight fourths of his maintenance volume, or an additional 800 ml of fluid in the form of 5% dextrose in Ringer's lactate for his third-space requirements. Therefore, the child's total fluid requirements are 800 ml of 5% dextrose in Ringer's lactate, 400 ml of 5% dextrose/one-fifth normal saline solution, and 100 ml of 5% dextrose/one-half normal saline solution with 3 mEq of potassium chloride—or a total

of 1,300 ml to be administered in 24 hours. This is roughly 55 ml/hr; and because we want the child's vascular volume replaced as early as possible, we will begin by giving him a volume of the 5% dextrose in Ringer's lactate until his urine output is established, after which we will mix in the various fluid formulas over the 24-hour period. Administration of the fluid volume will begin at the rate of 55 ml/hr, and the child's urine output will be watched. With his weight of 4 kg, the child's urine output should be between 4 to 8 ml/hr (40 ml/kg/day), and we will increase or decrease the rate of fluid administration to keep his urine output within those limits. If his urine output exceeds the range desired, we will slow down the rate of fluid administration and in essence effectively eliminate some of the fluid by the end of the 24 hours. If, on the other hand, this rate of fluid administration does not achieve a urine output of between 4 to 8 ml/hr, we will give the child an additional push of 20 ml/kg of balanced salt solution; and if this does not raise his urine output to the desired level, we must then question whether some of our assumptions are incorrect. If this point is reached, additional monitoring will be needed to evaluate the state of replacement of the child's vascular volume, which will require the placement of a central venous pressure monitoring catheter, preferably percutaneously by the subclavian route (Fig. 4-1).

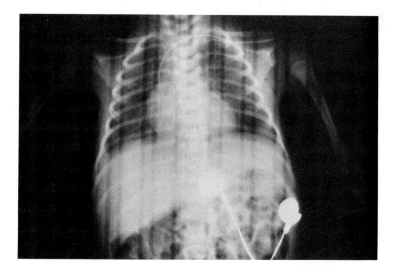

Fig. 4-1. Chest x-ray film showing a central venous catheter properly positioned in the superior vena cava by the percutaneous route into the subclavian vein. (From Filston, H. C., and Izant, R.: The surgical neonate: evaluation and care, New York, 1978, Appleton-Century-Crofts.)

If we cannot provide ourselves with a central venous monitoring catheter, then we do not know whether the child's inability to achieve an adequate urine output represents a persistent deficit of vascular volume or whether there is, in fact, adequate or even excess replacement of vascular volume and either inappropriate ADH or cardiovascular insufficiency is affecting the child's urine output. In addition, in conditions of sepsis, renal function may be abnormal, and if the child sustains severe preoperative hypovolemia, his renal functioning may be in question. Evaluation of the extent ot the child's tissue edema will not tell us accurately the state of his vascular volume, for it is possible to have marked edema secondary to capillary leakage from hypoperfusion injury and still have an inadequate vascular volume. As noted previously, comparing the child's operative weight with his preoperative weight will also fail to tell us the state of his vascular volume. Thus, if the child does not respond directly to the fluid administration defined by the preceding calculations and principles, we cannot intelligently manage him without a central monitor.

Once more, it must be emphasized that if the urine output exceeds the level desired, the volume of fluid administered should be slowed appropriately to eliminate some of the fluid; it should be recognized that the estimation utilized to arrive at the volume of replacement necessary is subject to considerable error in either direction.

SPECIAL CONSIDERATIONS

Additional considerations in managing the child's fluids include the following:
1. All fluids should contain at least 5% dextrose to supply the child with adequate calories for normal metabolic functioning.
2. Blood and colloid replacement should be elected where the red blood cell count or albumin concentration is insufficient for normal physiologic functioning. In this regard, consideration must be given to maintaining an adequate intravascular oncotic pressure to lessen the shift even of balanced salt solutions out of the vascular space into the extravascular tissues.
3. Most of the principles and examples given in the preceding discussion assume that the child begins with a normal level of serum electrolytes. If the child begins in a hyponatremic or hypochloremic state, some of

the maintenance requirements can be given as balanced salt solution or as normal saline to carry in additional electrolytes to correct the deficiency. By the same token, if the child begins in a hypertonic state with sodium concentration in the range of 150 to 160 mEq/liter and chloride concentration from 110 to 120 mEq/liter, more dilute solutions can be administered in place of the balanced electrolyte solutions to reduce the hypertonicity. These are the exceptions to the principles for administration of specific fluid types previously outlined.

Although the concepts discussed previously and the fluid volumes and types illustrated may be unfamiliar to the average primary care physician in dealing with more medically oriented diseases, the principles are sound and tested over many years and the fluid administration program has proved successful in hundreds of patients undergoing surgery, ranging in age from the tiniest premature infant to the adolescent.

One word about electrolyte balance is essential. It must be recognized that there is a balance of sodium and potassium across electrically active membranes maintained by an active energy-requiring process. Sodium is maintained as the primary extracellular cation and potassium as the primary intracellular cation. When the level of either changes, the other must respond to maintain the balance. Thus, typically when the serum sodium level falls, potassium shifts out of the cell to equalize the total cation balance across the membrane. If no potassium is lost from the body, the serum potassium level will rise; and a serum sodium level of 130 mEq/liter would be associated with a serum potassium level of over 5 mEq/liter. When, under circumstances of hyponatremia, the serum potassium level is normal or slightly low, total body potassium must be deficient, and replacement of potassium along with replacement of sodium is essential; otherwise, the resultant correction of sodium deficit will result in a shift back of potassium into the cell, and the serum potassium level will fall. Since hypokalemia may interfere with normal cardiac mechanisms, particularly when they are affected by drugs such as some of those used during anesthesia, such hypokalemia may be detrimental to the patient.

An example of this is the child who has pyloric stenosis with a history of profuse vomiting over a period of time. Often he has a serum sodium level in the 120s, a chloride level in the high 70s, and a potassium level in the range of 3 to 3.5. If the true total potassium deficit represented by this slight hypokalemia is not appreciated, correction of sodium and chloride deficits along with the fluid deficit in this patient will result in a rehydrated patient with a normal serum sodium level, a normal serum chloride level and a serum potassium level in the range of 1.9 to 2.5. The alert anesthetist would refuse to put this patient under anesthesia until this potassium deficit was corrected, resulting in an excessive preoperative hospital time. The unalert anesthetist may create considerable problems for the child by going ahead with anesthetic administration under these circumstances.

The primary care physician who understands the principles and theory underlying this practical fluid management program for the immediate intraoperative and postoperative period will also learn to recognize those nonsurgical disease states such as severe diarrhea and generalized peritonitis that may be associated with internal fluid shifts and realize the importance of adequately balanced electrolyte replacement therapy rather than the hypotonic solutions commonly used for restoration of fluid balance in these patients.

Although the most frequent situation in which the primary care physician is called on to administer fluids to the surgical patient is in relation to intra-abdominal procedures in which these needs are fairly obvious, the primary care physician must also be alert to the situations in some of the subspecialty surgical procedures performed in children that may, in essence, re-create Wigger's shock experiments. Any procedure that results in extensive blood loss that is not replaced in a timely fashion will, in essence, re-create such a hypovolemic state. Although subsequent blood replacement may restore the actual volume of blood lost, the ensuing fluid losses from the damaged capillary membranes and the acidosis that occurs as a result of restoration of flow to hypoxic tissues may lead to subsequent recurrent hypovolemic hypoperfusion and hypoxia. Recognition of these states is essential if tragic complications of such procedures as spinal fusion for scoliosis and extensive reconstructive plastic surgery procedures are not to result. The primary care physician attuned to this problem can contribute much in recognizing the needs of the patient for adequate fluid volume replacement in addition to blood, as indicated by careful urine output monitoring. Discussions of these problems with the subspecialty surgeon and the attending anesthesiologist can do much to prevent their occurrence by making these individuals aware of the need for timely blood replacement during and after the surgical procedure. When such large-volume blood losses are kept up with, the hypoperfusion damage to the capillaries does not take place and the requirements for extra fluid administration never occur.

REFERENCES

1. Drucker, W. R., and Wright, H. K.: Physiology and pathophysiology of gastrointestinal fluids. In Current problems in surgery, Chicago, 1964, Year Book Medical Publishers, Inc.
2. Filston, H. C., and Izant, R. J., Jr.: The surgical neonate, New York, 1978, Appleton-Century-Crofts, p. 8.
2a. Moore, F. D.: Metabolic care of the surgical patient, Philadelphia, 1959, W. B. Saunders Co.
3. Shires, T.: The role of sodium-containing solutions in the treatment of oligemic shock, Surg. Clin. North Am. **45:**365, 1965.
4. Shires, T., and others: Fluid therapy in hemorrhagic shock, Arch. Surg. **88:**688, 1964.
5. Wallace, W. M.: Quantitative requirements of the infant and child for water and electrolyte under varying conditions, Am. J. Clin. Pathol. **23:**1133, 1953.
6. Wiggers, C. J.: Physiology of shock, New York, 1950, The Commonwealth Fund, p. 138.

CHAPTER 5

Management of feedings

HOWARD C. FILSTON

POSTOPERATIVE MANAGEMENT OF THE INTESTINE AND REINTRODUCTION OF FEEDINGS

When abdominal surgery has been performed, and often when surgery has been performed that only abuts against the peritoneum, such as herniorrhaphies or extensive retroperitoneal dissections, including those involved in thoracolumbar spine surgery, postoperative ileus may develop. This is somewhat of a misnomer, since a true adynamic ileus of the small intestine rarely results. Such a complication, which is classically represented by dilated loops of small intestine in a ladderlike pattern filling the entire peritoneal cavity and showing extensive air fluid levels, is more likely to result from a secondary insult such as the development of sepsis or an intra-abdominal abscess. It has been shown that peristalsis continues in the small intestine even after extensive intra-abdominal surgery and that feedings can be provided by continuous infusion into small-caliber jejunal feeding tubes shortly after surgery.[1,4,6,10]

Nevertheless, it is well known that feedings by mouth or gastrostomy tube are not tolerated following such surgery because of gastric retention and the likelihood of subsequent emesis. Thus, the true source of feeding disabilities in the postoperative period seems to be a gastric atony leading to gastric dilatation and then perhaps secondarily to reflux small bowel dysfunction.

Nasogastric decompression of the stomach is, therefore, essential in the postoperative period whenever either a significant intra-abdominal exploration has been performed, a significant degree of intraperitoneal inflammation exists from the disease process, or extensive hemorrhage or dissection adjacent to the peritoneal surface makes such gastric atony likely. Because small infants are notorious air swallowers, especially during crying episodes, we tend to err on the side of using nasogastric decompression liberally in younger patients. Failure to provide this decompression may lead not only to gastric dilatation with vasovagal complications, including a prolonged adynamic ileus, but may lead to regurgitation and aspiration soilage of the tracheobronchial tree.

In tiny infants, especially, a single nasogastric tube may be inadequate to decompress swallowed air. When the infant swallows air and is lying supine, the air tends to rise to the anterior surface of the stomach beneath the abdominal wall. The nasogastric tube lies posteriorly, where it is effective in draining liquids, but may fail to remove the air, which may then be pushed on into the small intestine and lead to secondary small bowel dilatation. Particularly in such entities as necrotizing enterocolitis or after treatment of ischemic injury from malrotation and volvulus, it is essential to ensure that the blood supply to the already-compromised intestine is well maintained. Dilatation leads to an inadequate blood supply to the antimesenteric aspect of the intestine because the vasa recti (end arteries) of the blood supply coming from the mesenteric side of the bowel have a poor anastomotic overlap at the antimesenteric border. Severe distention may stretch and compress these small vessels, leading to severe secondary ischemia. We have found that a double-tube technique using a nasogastric tube to drain liquid and a sump-type tube in the midesophagus to decompress swallowed air provides better over-all decompression and, in fact, frequently leads to an airless abdomen. A gastrostomy tube positioned through the anterior abdominal wall and into the anterior surface of the stomach can also be used effectively to decompress all of the air from the patient's gastrointestinal tract if the tube is hung loosely from an overhead support and left open to the air. This allows all of the air in the stomach to rise up through the tube and out into the atmosphere. An airless abdomen on the abdominal radiograph is a common finding in patients with gastrostomy tubes in place.

The amount of secretions coming from the gastric tubes is helpful in making the determination of when to begin utilizing the gastrointestinal tract postoperatively. Usually, about 48 hours after surgery gastric atony improves and the secretions begin to empty from the stomach. This can be tested by removing the suction from the tube and letting it drain by gravity into a container. If doing so causes a marked decrease in the volume of secretions, the secretions are passing through. If the amount of secretions still remains high, even with gravity drainage, intermittent clamping of the tube will ensure that the tube is not simply draining off all of the secretions from the posterior aspect of the stomach. Periods of 2 to 4 hours of clamping followed by irrigation to ensure that the tube is still patent and then 15 minutes of suctioning may show a dramatic decrease in the volume of secretions and indicate that the gastrointestinal tract is ready for use. If under these circumstances the secretions remain high, gastric emptying is still impaired.

With tiny infants, particularly premature ones whose gastrointestinal tracts have never been utilized, we prefer to hang the tube from an overhead support with an open syringe barrel attached. This allows a chamber into which gastric secretions can reflux, helping to prevent regurgitation and aspiration (Fig. 5-1). Once the secretions are decreased, small increments of feedings can be placed into the chamber and the tube can be aspirated prior to each additional feeding to ensure that large volumes of retained feedings are not building up in the stomach. Again, this procedure serves as a protection against the complications of aspiration. Once this source of feeding is tolerated, the tube can be removed and the child begun on nipple feedings.

Such a system is unnecessary and cumbersome

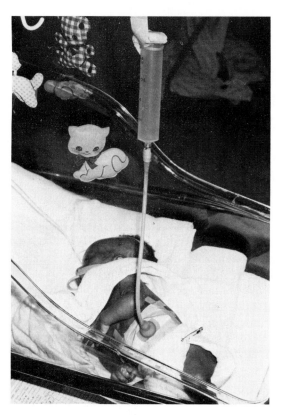

Fig. 5-1. Method of management of a gastrostomy tube. The open syringe barrel attached to the tube allows for a chamber into which gastric secretions can regurgitate if the infant increases his intra-abdominal pressure or tries to vomit.

in the older infant and child, and once the patient has demonstrated that he is handling his own gastric secretions, the tube can be removed and oral feedings begun. Because of the continued propensity of infants and toddlers to swallow air when they cry, it is important to begin liquid feedings in this age group at the time the nasogastric decompression is discontinued. Leaving the patient NPO for a period after removal of the decompressing tube may lead to air swallowing during crying, and the lack of burping may lead to gastric dilatation and subsequent complication of adynamic ileus.

Once clear liquids have been tolerated, the patient can progress quickly to a full liquid diet and then to a bland diet. Most hospitals consider a soft diet, which is the typical diet ordered next, to be simply an edentulous diet. The term *soft* really has nothing to with the quality of the food provided. Thus, the patient may be presented at his first postoperative meal with a plate of highly seasoned spaghetti, whereas what he would really tolerate best would be some poached eggs with toast and jelly or a hamburger patty with mashed potatoes. Thus, specific diet orders must be written for the patient; we usually consider that a diet progression similar to what one would follow after a severe bout of gastroenteritis is a reasonable one for the postoperative patient.

INTRODUCTION OF FEEDINGS FOR THE INFANT WITH SHORT BOWEL SYNDROME OR SEVERE ISCHEMIC INJURY

The management of the patient with significant deficiencies of intestinal length due to loss from malrotation and volvulus, to multiple or extensive areas of atresia, or to resection of extensive areas involved with necrotizing enterocolitis is a challenging undertaking that sometimes seems to be a mixture of science and witchcraft. Any patient who has lost extensive intestinal length from any of the above causes or who has had an ischemic injury to the bowel that may have damaged or destroyed the mucosal integrity must be managed along the lines outlined herein. These patients may lack adequate mucosal area for handling the osmotic loads presented by normal feedings and may lack any or all of the necessary digestive enzymes for handling the complex molecules of normal nutrition. It has been shown that even losses of intestine amounting to well over 80% of the jejunum and ileum can be tolerated and associated with successful reestablishment of gastrointestinal nutrition.[2,7,9] The adaptive capacity of the intestine is remarkable, but it must be supported and nurtured patiently. Obviously, the child's needs for nutrition during this period of adaptation must be met by parenteral nutrition, and we have generally preferred total central parenteral nutrition for this support. We found that any injury of this type requires at least 3 weeks for adequate healing. The basic principles of wound healing would dictate that true healing does not take place in less time than this, although partial reepithelialization may occur. Such epithelium is extremely sensitive to reinjury, however.

Once it is demonstrated that the child can handle his gastric secretions, glucose can be used to attain a moderate volume of feeding, with the utilization of an open-tube, open syringe barrel technique with hourly feedings and aspiration before each feeding, as discussed previously. A partially digested formula such as Nutramigen (a mixture of casein hydrolysates, disaccharides, and partially digested fats) can then be given in a reduced strength, such as one eighth of the standard 20 calories/ounce concentration. Such dilution is particularly important in predigested formulas, because their osmolalities may be twice the normal osmolality of extracellular fluid (Table 5-1). Although the exact mechanisms are not fully understood, the introduction of highly osmolar solutions into the gastrointestinal tract may lead to reinjury of the epithelium, perhaps by ischemia resulting from a rapid outpouring of fluid from the adjacent vessels with subsequent hypovolemia and arterial venous bypass secondary to vasoconstriction. Regardless of the exact mechanism, such hyperosmolar feedings can cause damage that may produce a serious if not irremediable setback for the child.

Progression with increasing the concentration should be slow, depending on the extent and seriousness of the bowel injury. For severe losses of length or obvious severe ischemic injuries, progression may be in increments of one-eighth strength every 2 to 3 days; before raising the concentration, one should ensure that the child's stooling pattern does not indicate an intolerance. Progress is usually easily made until a five-eighths or three-fourths strength formula is reached. At this point, the osmolality is increasing considerably; great care should be utilized and longer intervals provided, especially if the child's stools begin to show an increased volume or fluidity. The utiliza-

Table 5-1. Osmolalities of common infant formulas (20 Kcal/ounce)

Formula	Osmolality
Breast milk	300
Cow's milk	288
SMA-20	300
Enfamil	290
Similac	290
Nursoy	244
ProSobee	258
Isomil	224
Nutramigen	443
Pregestimil	590
Portagen	236

tion of a few extra days at this point may prevent a severe setback requiring additional weeks or months to overcome a secondary insult.

If the introduction of the formula is unsuccessful, in that the patient immediately has high-volume stool losses, a careful analysis of the content of the stool for carbohydrates, fats, and proteins along with electrolytes will give some idea of the type of dysfunction that is ensuing. If significant nutrients are being lost, a more highly digested formula such as Pregestimil (a mixture of amino acids, medium-chain triglycerides, and glucose) may be necessary. On the other hand, the loss of significant electrolytes in a high-volume liquid stool suggests that the bile salts are not being well handled. This is often true if the distal ileum and ileocecal valve have been resected. In this case, either cornstarch or cholestyramine may bind the bile salts and overcome the cathartic effect of the bile salts entering the colon.[5] Cholestyramine should be introduced in small amounts and gradually titrated until the volume of stool is reduced. Great care must be utilized to ensure that the cholestyramine does not completely bind up the liquid in the intestine and leave a totally obstipated infant. We have had one tiny premature infant who required laparotomy and surgical removal of a cholestyramine cast of the small intestine. This complication is rare, however, in patients with severe postresectional or postischemic diarrhea.

Specific enzyme deficiencies, including lactase and disaccharidase deficiencies, are common after such injuries.[3] Usually provision of a predigested formula will overcome such problems quickly.

Even children with the most extensive intestinal losses can be maintained until adaptation occurs. We have successfully rehabilitated an infant with only 6 cm of jejunum and 13 cm of ileum with an intact ileocecal valve back to normal gastrointestinal functioning. Wilmore[9] has reported rehabilitation of a child with 15 cm of small bowel and an intact ileocecal valve, and there are probably many patients who have adapted with even less. Nevertheless, we still consider total loss of the jejunum and ileum to be a situation that does not warrant institution of prolonged support mechanisms.

Once the infant has tolerated a full-volume, full-caloric load of the predigested formula, he can be maintained on the formula until he has established a good weight gain. Over-hasty attempts to progress the infant to a standard infant formula may produce a severe setback, and in the infant with a more seriously injured intestinal tract, such an attempt should not be made until several months of demonstrated normal functioning on the special formula have passed. Careful mixture of small parts of standard formula with the predigested formula can then be instituted, and if any change in bowel habits is obvious, the attempt should be abandoned for a time. Once the child is tolerating the predigested formula well, he will usually tolerate introduction of rice cereal and bananas. There is no hurry to introduce additional solid foods until several months of normal bowel functioning have been achieved.

The ultimate measurement of the adequacy of bowel function after extensive resections is, of course, the rate of growth and development. We have found that generally once full-caloric feedings are tolerated, nutritional maintenance has not been a major problem. However, children who lack a distal ileum may have long-term problems with vitamin B_{12} absorption.[8] Such problems take considerable time to develop, and studies of vitamin B_{12} levels or monitoring of blood counts in the first few months after surgery may not be properly indicative. Some have felt that the easiest approach is to give these children routine vitamin B_{12} injections three or four times a year. Although once-yearly injections may be adequate, such a long interval may lead to loss of follow-up and failure to get the yearly injection. Iron and calcium metabolism may also be interfered with, and almost assuredly these children will have more than moderate difficulty in handling gastrointestinal viral or bacterial illnesses. The primary care physician must be prepared to hospitalize these patients early in the course of such illnesses and support them with intravenous fluid and electrolyte mixtures so that severe dehydration and hypovolemia do not lead to additional ischemic insults to the intestine during the healing phase.

We have generally found that infants who have totally failed to recover intestinal function after prolonged attempts at reintroduction of feedings have some other underlying lesion, such as a congenital infection with cytomegalic virus or an ongoing septic source that is providing an ongoing injury and interfering with normal healing and adaptation. Such additional disease entities should be carefully sought in any patient who is not showing reasonable progress with healing and adaptation under the conservative management program described above.

The management of a child with a severe intestinal loss is a complex problem and requires the experience and judgment of experienced neonatologists and pediatric surgeons for successful management. The time involved is extensive, but the rewards in seeing a child who had a seemingly irreparable intestinal injury survive are inestimable.

REFERENCES

1. Andrassy, R. J., and others: The role and safety of early postoperative feeding in the pediatric surgical patient, J. Pediatr. Surg. **14:**381, 1979.
2. Bell, M. J., and others: Massive small-bowel resection in an infant; long-term management and intestinal adaptation, J. Pediatr. Surg. **8:**197, 1973.
3. Howat, J. M., and Aaronson, I.: Sugar intolerance in neonatal surgery, J. Pediatr. Surg. **6:**719, 1971.
4. Nachlas, M. M., and others: Gastrointestinal motility studies as a guide to postoperative management, Ann. Surg. **175:**510, 1972.
5. Nagaraj, H. S., and others: Oral cholestyramine and paregoric therapy for intractable diarrhea following surgical correction of catastrophic disease of the GI tract in neonates, J. Pediatr. Surg. **11:**795, 1976.
6. Shoemaker, C. P., and Wright, H. K.: Rate of water and sodium absorption from the jejunum after abdominal surgery in man, Am. J. Surg. **119:**62, 1970.
7. Tepas, J. J., III, and others: Total management of short gut secondary to midgut volvulus without prolonged total parenteral alimentation, J. Pediatr. Surg. **13:**622, 1978.
8. Valman, H. B., and Roberts, P. D.: Vitamin B-12 absorption after resection of ileum in childhood, Arch. Dis. Child. **49:**932, 1974.
9. Wilmore, D. W.: Factors correlating with a successful outcome following extensive intestinal resection in newborn infants, J. Pediatr. **80:**88, 1972.
10. Wright, H. K.: Nutrition in stress: role of absorption. Postgraduate course: Pre- and postoperative care, American College of Surgeons Clinical Congress, Miami, 1974.

CHAPTER 6

Management of tubes and drains, including gastrostomies

HOWARD C. FILSTON

MANAGEMENT OF TUBES AND DRAINS

The management of tubes and drains can be based on very simple principles but often presents considerable mystery and confusion to the physician. Even many surgeons have no idea other than that "they have always done it that way" as to why they remove drains at certain times. The principles are simple. If one is draining for a particular entity, the drain remains as long as the entity may be present. Thus, a drain left because of the possibility of postoperative hemorrhage can usually be removed within 24 to 48 hours if no hemorrhage is evident. By that time the vasoconstrictive and clotting mechanism should have ensured that no further bleeding will ensue. If one is draining for a potential leak from a structure such as a closed-off cystic duct stump, the closed end of a duodenal stump after a gastric resection, or a portoenterostomy such as that performed for biliary atresia, the drain must remain as long as the potential for breakdown is present. If the possibility of leakage is very remote, perhaps the drain should not have been placed at all. To ensure that any subsequent leak will drain to the outside, a sinus tract must be allowed to form from the source of the potential drainage to the skin.

Remembering from basic science the principles of wound healing,[1] one may recall that during the first few days after a wound an inflammatory reaction is occurring, consisting first of polymorphonuclear leukocytes and then of macrophages debriding and cleaning the wound. From 3 to 5 days or so, a phase of capillary ingrowth occurs, which

forms granulation tissue. At about 7 days, fibroblasts proliferate in the wound; and from then until 21 days or more, fibroblasts invade the granulation tissue and lay down collagen. Somewhere from 7 to 10 days, enough collagen is laid down in the tract and enough epithelialization achieved that the tract will remain open if the drain or tube is removed. However, to be absolutely certain that the tract remains open, a minimum of 3 weeks must pass; even then, unless complete epithelialization of the tract has occurred, the tract will likely close if no drainage occurs. Removal of drains and tubes, thus, can be based on these principles of wound healing superimposed on a consideration of the likelihood of drainage to occur at any given time following the surgical procedure.

If one has placed a gastrostomy tube or a cecostomy tube, one must wait for 3 weeks to remove the tube, even though no further use for the tube remains. This is so because premature removal of the tube may cause separation of the involved viscus from the abdominal wall, and the resulting leakage from the stoma in the viscus may cause peritonitis or abscess formation. By 3 weeks, sufficient scarring of the viscus to the abdominal wall should have occurred that removal of the tube will not be accompanied by a falling away of the viscus from the abdominal wall; any leakage can then occur to the cutaneous surface. The stoma will usually heal with the passage of additional time.

MANAGEMENT OF GASTROSTOMIES

Various tubes are used when the gastrostomy is initially performed. A frequent choice is that of a mushroom catheter, which has a flared end that holds the tube in place, preventing its dislodgement. A modification of this tube is the Malecot catheter, which has a less rigid flare than the mushroom and is more easily dislodged. These tubes usually remain in place fairly well unless they are inadvertently dislodged, and they are less likely than a Foley catheter to be pulled down the gastrointestinal tract. However, they may be very difficult to replace if they are inadvertently dislodged from the stomach, and the replacement of this type of tube before strong healing of the gastric wall to the abdominal wall has occurred may result in tearing of the gastric wall away from the abdominal wall. Therefore, this type of tube should not be reinserted unless at least 4 weeks of healing have taken place after the performance of the gastrostomy. Even then, tearing of the stoma with subsequent leakage into the peritoneal cavity is a definite risk. We prefer to insert a Foley catheter if the original tube is dislodged. A complication, as noted, of a Foley catheter, however, is that the stomach misinterprets the balloon on the Foley catheter as a bolus of food and catches it in the peristaltic wave. The balloon is passed across the stomach and through the pylorus and into the duodenum, and the tube may be pulled well down into the intestinal tract. The Foley balloon may then obstruct the duodenum, leading to the unusual situation in which feedings pass through the Foley catheter and progress down the jejunoilium, but the child vomits all of his gastric secretions. Any vomiting that occurs while a gastrostomy tube is in place, particularly if the tube is a Foley balloon catheter, should lead to investigation of the position of the catheter.

A simple method of maintaining the catheter in its proper place in the stomach and avoiding the passage of the balloon down the duodenum is to pass the catheter through a regular feeding nipple with the nipple pointing toward the proximal end of the catheter so that after the catheter is passed into the gastrostomy stoma and the Foley balloon inflated, it can be pulled back until it abuts against the gastric wall. The nipple, with its flange, is then pushed down until it fits snugly against the abdominal wall. This maneuver holds the gastric and abdominal walls trapped between the Foley balloon and the flange of the nipple, and the tight hold of the nipple itself on the catheter prevents it from sliding further into the stomach.

A clean gauze bandage should be then placed beneath the flange of the nipple to prevent irritation of the abdominal wall, and this bandage should be changed at least daily. The skin around the stoma should be cleaned with peroxide and a mild ointment applied beneath the bandage. The parents may be taught how to reinsert the Foley catheter and inflate the balloon so that they can reinsert the tube if it becomes inadvertently dislodged. The tube must be reinserted fairly soon after dislodgement, or the stoma will close down considerably and a much smaller tube may have to be utilized. Occasionally such an occurrence results in an inadequate tube for feeding purposes.

REFERENCE

1. Madden, J. W.: Wound healing: biologic and clinical features. In Sabiston, D. C., Jr., editor: Davis Christopher textbook of surgery, Philadelphia, 1977, W. B. Saunders Co., pp. 271-294.

CHAPTER 7

Management of an enterostomy

HOWARD C. FILSTON

The idea of an ostomy often strikes dread into the minds of parents and often leads to considerable resistance on the part of the referring physician. Perhaps the connotation of the ostomy as a device for bypassing cancer of the bowel and its relative permanency in the adult experience is the cause of this consternation. An ostomy in the typical infant, of course, has none of these connotations and is usually used to bypass an obstructed bowel or, as in the case of necrotizing enterocolitis, a destroyed segment of bowel; there is the very strong supposition that the ostomy will be temporary and that reconstruction of the entire intestine and resumption of normal functioning can be expected in the near future. Therefore, ostomies in infants can usually be presented as temporary devices that will be eliminated at the time of definitive surgery for such lesions as Hirschsprung's disease and imperforate anus. Usually, the correction will have been achieved before the age of toilet training. Care of an ostomy in infancy is not difficult. It may, in fact, be easier to keep the child with an ostomy clean than to clean the buttocks and genitalia of a soiling un-toilet-trained infant.

Ostomies are usually performed as bypassing loop ostomies or as end ostomies with or without an accompanying mucous fistula of the proximal end of the distal or bypassed bowel. Regardless, we prefer to mature the ostomy so that the mucosa is turned back and sutured to the skin. This leaves a small "bud" protruding from the abdominal wall, which functions well and is particularly adaptable to the use of collecting devices.

Complications of ostomies include bleeding from the mucosal surface or from granulation tissue at the skin mucosal interface, prolapse or intussusception of the ostomy, retraction of the ostomy into the peritoneal cavity, stricture of the bowel just proximal to the ostomy or stenosis of the ostomy itself, and, the most universal complication, that of breakdown of the skin surrounding the ostomy.

Bleeding is common and can usually be controlled by simply applying pressure with a gauze sponge until it ceases. Prolapse is usually the result of the bowel having been markedly dilated and hypertrophied at the time the ostomy was performed and then, after the decompression achieved by the ostomy, shrinking back down to normal size; the stoma is too large for the bowel, allowing it to herniate or intussuscept through the overly large abdominal wall stoma. Reduction usually can be accomplished easily, but reprolapse is common. When this occurs and is a moderate nuisance, the definitive procedure can often be advanced in time. Stricture usually results from ischemic injury to the bowel and is common in such lesions as necrotizing enterocolitis. It is unusual in the loop colostomies performed for temporary diversion for Hirschsprung's disease or anorectal agenesis (imperforate anus). Stomal stenosis can usually be prevented by taking an adequate resection of the fascial layers for the stoma. This complication is unusual in the usual loop colostomy. Retraction of the ostomy into the peritoneal cavity can be prevented by careful suturing of each layer of the abdominal wall to the bowel and by the use of a skin bridge passed beneath the loop through the mesentery.

The recent use of a protective adhesive layer that surrounds the ostomy and is tightly adherent to the surrounding skin combined with the application of a collecting bag held to the adhesive layer with a karaya seal have almost eliminated problems with skin breakdown. These materials are well worth their added expense to protect the abdominal wall surrounding the ostomy. Unless one has experienced the frustrating and continual problems of skin breakdown that occurred prior to the use of these materials, they are not readily appreciated. Nevertheless, they have made ostomy maintenance in infants a remarkably easy procedure.

Functional problems with ostomies may occur, particularly when there is some degree of stenosis or bowel obstruction near or proximal to the ostomy. This is particularly true with ileostomies. Short-term gastrointestinal illnesses caused by bacterial or viral infection may result in severe diarrhea out of proportion to what would be experienced by a child without an ostomy. The physician must be prepared to admit the child and maintain his hydration and electrolyte balance with intravenous fluid therapy. Persistence of diarrheal stools beyond the time that seems reasonable for

an acute illness should lead to investigation for a partial bowel obstruction. This entity may cause marked flora changes in the intestinal bacteria, leading to consequent changes in the bile salt and bile acid makeup of the intestinal contents. Such changes may produce a cathartic effect with severe loss of fluids and electrolytes through the ostomy. Realization that the ostomy patient is at greater risk for having dehydrating diarrheal illnesses should lead the physician to early evaluation and admission to the hospital.

The best support for parents dealing with a child with an ostomy is the ready availability of an ostomy therapist, either a nurse clinician or technologist, who has extensive experience and knowledge about ostomy care and malfunction. These individuals will often make themselves available to parents on a 24-hour call basis. They relieve the physician of much of the burden, while they provide the parents with additional support through the time during which the child must maintain the ostomy.

CHAPTER 8

Management and late complications of wounds

HOWARD C. FILSTON

MANAGEMENT OF WOUNDS

A brief idea of the principles of management of various wounds may be helpful to the primary care physician. The body will heal any wound through its normal mechanisms. Even losses of significant portions of the abdominal wall will eventually heal by contracture, granulation tissue, scar formation, and subsequent epithelialization. Such healing may take weeks to months to occur. The surgical management of wounds is an attempt to optimize the rate of healing and to minimize scar formation for functional and cosmetic reasons. The usual management of a clean wound is by primary suture closure. The principles involve achieving hemostasis and careful apposition of all layers of the depth of the wound to obliterate dead space into which fluid may leak, leaving a nonvascularized site for bacterial contamination. When contamination of the wound has occurred or tissue has been devitalized, cleansing of the wound must be accomplished to remove any foreign particles and any devitalized tissue must be debrided. The goal here is to provide careful apposition of viable tissue, obliterating any dead space with its potential for hematoma or seroma and subsequent abscess formation.

The choice of sutures is often an idiosyncrasy of the surgeon, but there is certainly some justification for using absorbable suture material such as catgut in wounds that may be contaminated and in which one does not wish to leave a permanent foreign body. Careful apposition of the deeper tissues with well-placed buried sutures will allow the use of fine suture material and tiny sutures loosely tied on the skin, which will minimize scar-

ring and leave a fine, cosmetically acceptable scar.

Wounds that are frankly contaminated can be treated by a technique known as delayed primary closure. This technique is utilized in a wound in which the surgeon would like to achieve primary closure for its cosmetic effects and rapid healing but is concerned about the possibility of infection developing in the wound. The deeper layers of muscle and fascia are closed in the usual fashion, but the subcutaneous tissue and skin are left open and packed with a gauze pack usually soaked in an antiseptic solution such as povidone-iodine. In 3 or 4 days, this packing is removed and the wound is inspected. If it appears clean, healthy, and vascularized, a secondary closure of the superficial tissues and skin is accomplished. If there is evidence of exudate suggesting infection, the wound is treated as described below for infected wounds and allowed to close by secondary intention.

Clearly infected wounds are left open and packed and repacked, and various debriding agents such as hydrogen peroxide may be useful in cleaning up the debris. The eventual goal is to produce a wound that is filled with healthy, deep pink to red granulation tissue that will then be replaced by scar tissue and finally epithelialize. It is important that the wound heal from the inside to the outside. If the skin is allowed to fall together and an epithelial bridge is formed, a dead space, which will fill with serous fluid and become infected, may result. The packing serves to keep the wound open; and by gradually reducing the amount of packing, either by utilizing less with each repacking or by packing it once and gradually removing small amounts of the packing, one will cause the deeper levels of the wound to fill in first.

Wounds on the extremities, especially those near joints, are subject to considerable disrupting forces. Immobilization is an important part of treatment of such wounds, and splints and casts and bulky dressings should be used liberally in children to protect these wounds during healing. If immobilization is not assured, the sutures must be left in for intolerable periods, during which the risks of infection along the suture tract increase and the scar laid down around the sutures leaves an unsightly sinus tract as a permanent record of the location of the sutures. If the sutures are removed at the standard time, the wound is likely to dehisce because of the stresses applied to it.

Additional considerations in the care of wounds will be found in Chapter 20 in the section on the child from 2 to 12.

LATE COMPLICATIONS OF SURGICAL WOUNDS

The primary care physician should have some understanding of the late complications of surgical wounds, for it is to this individual that the parents may turn when such complications arise. Serious postoperative infection in a wound will usually have occurred by 7 to 10 days following surgery. Dehiscence is most unlikely after this period of time, because the degree of fibroblast infiltration and collagen formation during the second week following surgery is extensive; certainly, by the third week sufficient collagen formation and organization has taken place that the wound can be considered solid. Common complications somewhat later, after successful initial wound management, include areas of fat necrosis with subsequent infection and breakdown, and so-called suture abscesses. Both of these problems result from the presence of material that is essentially an unvascularized foreign body that harbors infection. Primary epithelialization over an area of fat necrosis may be followed by a softening and liquefaction of the fat with subsequent abscess formation, and the child may have a localized area of thinning out of the epithelium over an obvious pocket of fluid. Usually, simple drainage (achieved by opening the epithelial bridge), the placement of a small amount of sterile packing or a wick, and treatment of the wound with peroxide and antiseptic solution will lead to successful healing.

Suture abscesses may result from bacterial con-

tamination of the interstices of braided sutures. Such abscesses are rarely a primary contamination of the sutures; rather, they may represent a secondary wound contamination resulting in harboring of the organisms in the suture interstices. More likely, there is a moderate inflammatory or foreign body reaction to the suture material with secondary bacterial invasion and abscess formation. Usually the suture becomes free floating due to the inflammatory process disconnecting the suture material from the tissue. The abscesses appear as localized areas of pustule formation along the wound and can usually be cleared up quickly by breaking the epithelium and removing the suture with a hemostat. When the suture is deeply buried, a sterile crochet hook will often hook the loop of the suture and allow its easy extraction.

Most often, only an isolated suture abscess forms; occasionally, however, the initial abscess is the harbinger of a long series of suture abscesses in which all of the sutures are eventually extruded. Occasionally it is necessary to reanesthetize the child, reopen the wound, and remove all of the suture material.

Another complication is the presentation of a ventral hernia in an abdominal wound, representing dehiscence of the deeper layers of a closure with an intact and healed superficial wound. These hernias do not carry the threat of evisceration, but they usually represent an area of weakness and will require repair at some later time. They are unusual occurrences in transverse incisions and in pediatric surgery in general.

A common complaint after surgery is the development of paresthesia in the wound several weeks following its successful closure. Such a development represents regrowth into the area of small nerve endings that were divided at the time of the incision. Examination of the wound to ensure that no point tenderness or inflammatory signs are present (suggesting a wound infection) is all that is necessary, followed by reassurance to the patient that these feelings are normal and will eventually disappear. Severe, persistent pain in an incision unattended by inflammatory signs may represent the entrapment of a sizable sensory nerve in a suture. This occurrence is most common in the inguinal area, where the ilioinguinal nerve may be entrapped in the suture deep in the repair. The symptoms usually lessen with time, but occasionally it is necessary to explore such a wound and free the entrapped nerve.

SECTION TWO

The newborn

CHAPTER 9

General considerations

HOWARD C. FILSTON

MATERNAL-FETAL HISTORY

The maternal-fetal history may contain clues leading to early diagnostic evaluation that, in turn, may identify the infant who is at risk for having significant surgical anomalies. Hydramnios in the mother is a classic clue to difficulties in the infant. Although certain maternal entities may lead to hydramnios, and other infant entities, such as erythroblastosis fetalis, may be associated with hydramnios, approximately 15% of infants born to mothers with an excess of amniotic fluid will have anomalies of the upper gastrointestinal tract, producing obstruction.[7] Among these are esophageal atresia with or without tracheoesophageal fistula, duodenal atresia including annular pancreas, and upper jejunal atresias.

The infant swallows amniotic fluid throughout the latter part of gestation. The fluid passes through the infant's gastrointestinal tract and is reabsorbed in the jejunum and ileum and excreted from the infant's kidneys back into the amniotic fluid, completing the circle. An obstruction high enough in the gastrointestinal tract to make significant reabsorption of the amniotic fluid impossible may lead to hydramnios in the mother.

When hydramnios has been present in the mother, the evaluation of the infant is simple; a radiopaque tube is passed through the nose or mouth of the infant into the stomach and its position confirmed by x-ray examination. This procedure will rule out or confirm an esophageal atresia; and either on this radiograph or one taken a short time subsequently, the gas pattern should determine whether there is passage of air through most of the small intestine (Fig. 9-1). If a normal gas pattern develops, high intestinal obstruction can be ruled out as the cause of the hydramnios. Obviously,

this evaluation does not rule out distal bowel obstructions, but these are not usually associated with maternal hydramnios.

The small-for-gestational-age infant is more likely than any other to be associated with congenital anomalies.[10] Abnormal presentations of the infant and difficult passage through the birth canal may also be associated with abnormalities in the infant, usually in relation to masses such as sacrococcygeal teratomas or in relation to abnormal head positions.

Infants of diabetic mothers, in addition to being large, have a significant incidence of small left colon syndrome, a variant of the meconium plug syndrome in which the infant fails to pass meconium in the first 24 hours of life and has a small spastic colon distal to the splenic flexure.[5,9] Often it is very difficult to stimulate defecation in these infants, and they may require a water-soluble contrast enema to loosen up the inspissated meconium and initiate bowel movements. Occasionally, colostomy is required because of persistent obstruction.

A history of alcohol or drug ingestion by the mother during pregnancy may also be associated with anomalies in the infant.[4]

Finally, some anomalies tend to be repetitive, familial, or hereditary, so that the history of a prior sibling with chromosomal abnormalities or congenital defects should alert the obstetrician and pediatrician to the possibility of anomalies in the infant in question. The evolution of perinatal medicine as a combined discipline offers the potential for significant advances in the prenatal identification of infants with anomalies. Ultrasonography has been reported to be capable of recognizing in utero such anomalies as duodenal atresia, gastro-

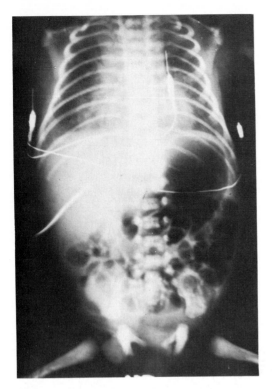

Fig. 9-1. Abdominal film of a newborn infant 20 minutes after delivery by cesarean section showing a well-established small bowel gas pattern and demonstrating the rapidity with which the normal bowel gas pattern develops.

schisis, and diaphragmatic hernia when factors such as maternal hydramnios indicate the possibility of a lesion in the infant.[12,13]

SURGICAL CONSIDERATIONS IN THE NEWBORN EXAMINATION

A complete physical examination of the newborn is obviously essential, and certain aspects of the physical examination will elicit surgically correctable anomalies. Sacrococcygeal teratoma usually presents as a mass arising from the coccyx and extending out from the area between the coccyx and the anus. It may be more to one side or the other and involve the buttock. Few other lesions present in the newborn period in this area; occasionally, however, differentiation from a low sacral myelomeningocele or a lipoma of the cauda equina may be difficult. The entire spine, from the base of the skull to the tip of the coccyx, should be inspected and palpated, with the examiner searching for masses or defects such as encephaloceles and myelomeningoceles. The skin surface should be carefully inspected and any evi-

dence of hemangiomas or other lesions noted. Facial anomalies, especially clefts, are usually apparent; and clefts of the palate can be palpated or visualized on examination of the oral pharynx.

Low-set ears have frequently been associated with severe renal anomalies, so that their presence should lead to an evaluation of urinary tract function (Fig. 9-2, *A*).

The neck should be inspected and palpated for masses and tracheal deviation. The shape and development of the jaw should be noted, since a small, regressive jaw is consistent with Pierre Robin syndrome and may be associated with severe obstructive respiratory difficulties (Fig. 9-2, *B*). Cleft palate frequently accompanies this syndrome. The presence of cyanosis, especially when it is accompanied by respiratory distress, should lead to immediate evaluation of the child's airway and chest, including an immediate chest radiograph. Cyanosis unassociated with respiratory distress is usually the result of congenital heart disease, and early consultation with a pediatric cardiologist is indicated.

Defects of the abdominal wall are apparent at birth. They may involve complete evisceration of the bowel, as in gastroschisis or ruptured omphalocele; or they may, as in an intact omphalocele, represent a defect of the abdominal wall formation, but with containment of the viscera in the peritoneal sac. Early differentiation of these two entities is important for proper resuscitation and treatment. Wrinkling and laxity of the abdominal wall suggest the prune-belly syndrome and its associated severe abnormalities of the urinary tract. A thorough, gentle examination of the child's abdomen will demonstrate any organ enlargement or abnormal masses that may be present. Both kidneys of the newborn infant can usually be palpated and should be differentiated from any abnormal masses present in the upper quadrants.

In the examination of the genitalia in the male infant, it should be noted if hydroceles are present, since the notation of their presence at birth will be important in decisions regarding subsequent treatment. The presence and position of the testicles should be noted. The perineum should be inspected and the presence of a normally patent anus confirmed. The anus may be gently probed with a thermometer or clamp to confirm patency, but no attempt to open a fistula should be made, since doing so may significantly alter the proper therapy

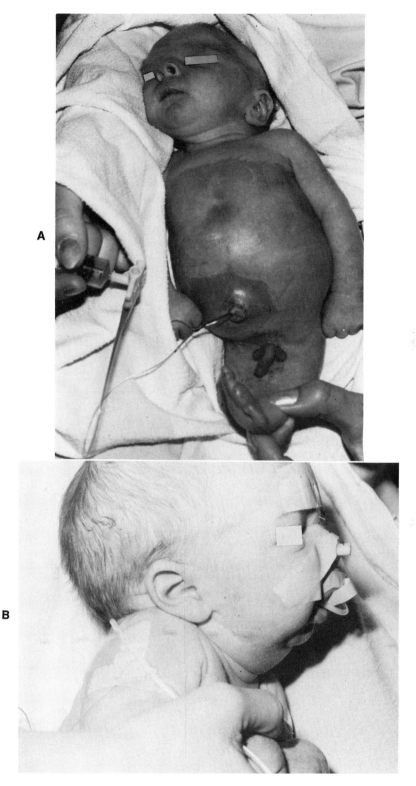

Fig. 9-2. A, Infant with multiple anomalies including renal agenesis. Note the low-set ear. **B,** Infant with Pierre Robin syndrome. Note the underdeveloped mandible. A nasohypopharyngeal tube is in place to release the suction and prevent the tongue from being "swallowed," obstructing the airway.

for any anomaly that may be present. In the female infant, the perineum should be inspected to make sure that it is normal in appearance and that both a urethral orifice and a vaginal introitus are present. Again, the anal area should be evaluated.

Finally, the limbs should be evaluated for the presence of normal bony structures, a full complement of digits, and normal range of motion of all the joints. Of particular importance is proper evaluation of the hip joint to make sure that congenital dysplasia of the hips is not present. Such evaluation requires "frog legging" of the child; that is, testing the ability of the legs to be placed in full flexion and external rotation at the hips.

DIAGNOSTIC CLUES IN THE NEONATAL NURSERY
Respiratory distress; coughing with feedings

Most children who have respiratory distress in the immediate newborn period will have hyaline membrane disease or some other medically treatable respiratory problem, such as meconium aspiration. However, certain surgically treatable diseases and lesions also present with respiratory distress in the newborn period, and only early chest x-ray evaluation will identify them for proper resuscitation and therapy. Among these are diaphragmatic hernias, lobar emphysema, pneumothorax, and, more rarely, sequestration of the lung and bronchogenic cysts. The child with really severe respiratory distress including dyspnea and cyanosis in the newborn period should be suspected of having a congenital diaphragmatic hernia, an expanding lobar emphysema, or a tension pneumothorax, all of which require urgent and well-planned therapy.

The child with mild respiratory symptoms exacerbated by feedings (particularly if the child coughs with feedings) should be suspected of having an esophageal atresia or a pure tracheoesophageal fistula without esophageal atresia. Finally, mechanical obstructions of the airway, including lesions of the nasopharynx (choanal atresia), occasional masses in the hypopharynx obstructing the glottis, and cysts and maldevelopments of the tracheobronchial tree may produce severe respiratory distress.

Failure to pass urine or stool

The child's failure to pass urine or stool is an obvious indication of maldevelopment of the urinary or gastrointestinal tract, but these signs are frequently overlooked. It should be the policy of every newborn nursery to have the nurses record at 24 hours whether or not the child has passed urine and stool. The child should urinate within the first 24 hours of life and usually will do so within the first 12.[3] Ninety-eight percent of normal full-term children pass meconium within the first 24 hours of life, and well over 90% of normal premature infants pass meconium within 36 hours (Table 9-1). Sick premature infants in an intensive

Table 9-1. Times of first void and first stool in 500 infants*

		395 Full-term infants		80 Preterm infants		25 Postterm infants	
	Hours	No. of infants	Cumulative %	No. of infants	Cumulative %	No. of infants	Cumulative %
Time of first void	In delivery room	51	12.9	17	21.2	3	12.0
	1 to 8	151	51.1	50	83.7	4	38.0
	9 to 16	158	91.1	12	98.7	14	84.0
	17 to 24	35	100.0	1	100.0	4	100.0
	>24	0	—	0	—	0	—
Time of first stool	In delivery room	66	16.7	4	5.0	8	32.0
	1 to 8	169	59.5	22	32.5	9	68.0
	9 to 16	125	91.1	25	63.8	5	88.0
	17 to 24	29	98.5	10	76.3	3	100.0
	24 to 48	6	100.0	18	98.8	0	—
	>48	0	—	1	100.0	0	—

*Adapted from Clark, D. A.: Pediatrics **60:**457, 1977. Copyright American Academy of Pediatrics 1977.

care nursery may fail to pass stool during this period of time and require further observation but will not prove to have such a high incidence of significant anomalies.

When a child fails to urinate during the first 24 hours of life, his state of hydration should be assessed and the amount of his fluid intake evaluated; if these are adequate, further evaluation for the presence of kidneys and their drainage tracts should be undertaken.

The child who fails to pass meconium during the first hours of life has a good chance of having Hirschsprung's disease. In their evaluation of Hirschsprung's disease, Swenson, Sherman, and Fisher showed that 94+% of the children they studied with Hirschsprung's disease failed to pass meconium during the first 24 hours of life.[11] As noted above, 95% of normal newborns will pass meconium during that period. Other obstructive anomalies of the gastrointestinal tract will also be found in children who fail to pass meconium during the first 24 hours of life.

Salivation

The child who blows bubbles in the newborn period and has obvious difficulty handling his saliva probably has an obstruction of the esophagus. The most likely reason is esophageal atresia. A radiopaque catheter should be passed through

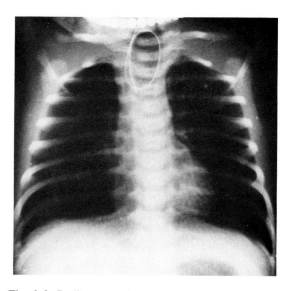

Fig. 9-3. Radiopaque tube coiled in the blind pouch of an infant with esophageal atresia. The presence of gas in the stomach confirms the presence of a distal tracheoesophageal fistula.

the nose or mouth a distance premeasured to reach the child's stomach. If the catheter reaches an obstruction considerably short of this distance, or if it passes the required distance, an x-ray film of the chest and abdomen should be obtained to evaluate the position of the tube. Tubes have been known to coil in the blind proximal pouch of esophageal atresia, leading to the erroneous assumption that the esophagus is patent (Fig. 9-3). It is also possible for a tube to pass down the trachea, out the tracheoesophageal fistula, into the distal esophagus, and on into the stomach (Fig. 9-4), giving the false impression, both by external appearance and by abdominal radiograph, of successful passage through the esophagus. Since about 90% of infants with esophageal atresia have the classic variety with a blind proximal pouch and the distal esophagus connecting to the membranous trachea just above the carina and thence onward to the stomach (Fig. 9-5), this configuration should be assumed until a less common variety is clearly defined.[6]

Vomiting and distention

Vomiting and distention are obviously the common signs of bowel obstruction. The normal newborn may spit up feedings, but real vomiting suggests obstruction. Distention of the abdomen in the newborn period suggests a low intestinal obstruction. Even the passage of meconium does not rule against congenital obstruction of the gastrointestinal tract, because meconium is generated throughout gestation and the child probably passes it through to the anus and on into the amniotic fluid during gestational life.[8] If the gastrointestinal tract becomes obstructed in the mid- or late gestational period, meconium may have reached the colon and be beyond the site of obstruction.

Bilious vomiting should always suggest obstruction. Although occasionally a child with sepsis, severe congenital heart disease resulting in failure, or simply extensive vomiting may regurgitate bile, the overwhelming number of infants who vomit bile or back significant quantities of bile up into the stomach to be aspirated through a gastric tube will have mechanical obstruction. It is far safer to assume that the child with bilious vomiting has mechanical obstruction than to assume otherwise. Early onset of vomiting, particularly bile-stained vomiting, suggests an upper gastrointestinal obstruction. Failure to pass stool and distention without vomiting or significant amounts of bilious

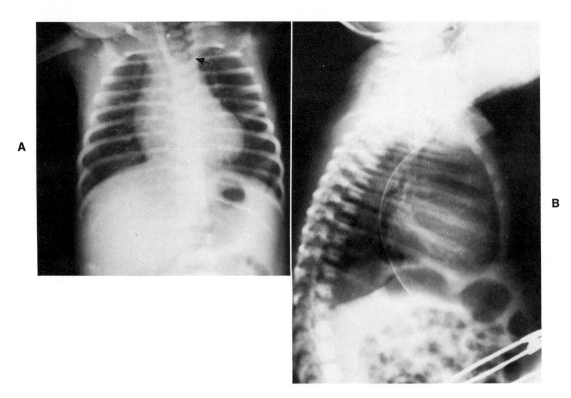

Fig. 9-4. A, A fine radiopaque catheter has passed down the trachea, out through the fistula, down the esophagus, and into the stomach. Without careful perusal of the radiograph, the blind esophageal pouch (arrow) and the wayward course of the catheter might be missed. **B,** Lateral view. A second catheter is now coiled in the blind proximal esophageal pouch. (From Gwinn, J. L., and others: Radiologic case of the month: atresia of the esophagus with tracheoesophageal fistula, Am. J. Dis. Child **126:**621, 1973. Copyright 1973, American Medical Association.)

aspirate suggest a lower gastrointestinal obstruction. After the distention has been present for hours or days, subsequent vomiting, including bile-stained vomiting, may occur even in children with lower gastrointestinal obstruction.

Late-onset obstruction

Late-onset obstruction is an extremely significant surgical lesion, because the child who once demonstrates patency of his gastrointestinal tract and then becomes obstructed cannot have a simple congenital atresia as the cause of the obstruction. Although congenital stenoses of the gastrointestinal tract do occur, they are infrequent entities. The most likely cause of an obstruction presenting after patency of the gastrointestinal tract has been demonstrated is a mechanical obstruction occurring after birth, the most likely cause of which is malrotation with volvulus and strangulation of the mesentery. The initial patency of the gastrointestinal tract is indicated by the passage of transitional stools, a mixture of meconium with feedings, the passage of air through the gastrointestinal tract, or the passage of a marker such as charcoal or radiographic contrast medium instilled from above. As noted previously, the mere passage of meconium does not guarantee patency of the entire gastrointestinal tract.

Hematochezia

The presence of blood in the stools may be an entirely benign finding and may be due to swallowed maternal blood. On the other hand, it may be the first indication of a serious abnormality. Today, the most common entity associated with blood in the stools is neonatal necrotizing enterocolitis. Initially, a seedy yellow, often watery stool with streaks of blood is passed. Subsequently, the

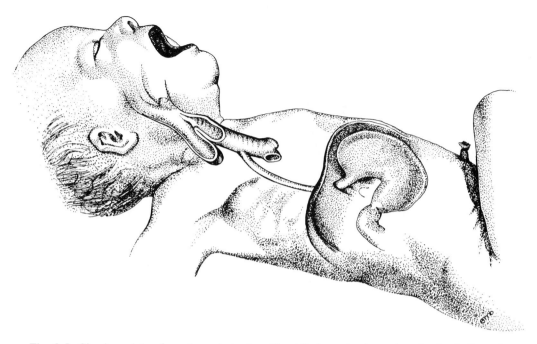

Fig. 9-5. Classic variety of esophageal atresia with a blind proximal pouch and a fistula from the distal esophagus entering the membranous trachea just above the carina and connecting the stomach to the tracheobronchial tree.

blood becomes more mixed with the stools and the stools become more mucoid. Associated findings are those of distention of the abdomen, bile-stained vomitus, or bile-stained gastric aspirate. Systemic manifestations include bradycardia, apnea, and inability to maintain body temperature. Marked abnormalities of the coagulogram and platelets may accompany the lesion as severe sepsis leads to disseminated intravascular coagulopathy. Hematochezia may also accompany malrotation with volvulus and strangulation of the mesentery. Vomiting of bile-stained material is usually an earlier and more prominent feature of malrotation. Finally, hematochezia may be associated with such simple lesions as fissures and irritation of the rectal mucosa. Maternal blood as the source of hematochezia can be easily ruled out by performing an Apt test.[1]

Palpable masses

The palpable masses that are likely to be found in the newborn period are those in the neck and abdomen. Cystic hygromas frequently present in the newborn period. These are large cystic masses that usually deviate the head and face to the opposite side and generally occur in the area of the posterior triangle of the neck, although they may extend anteriorly. There may be a bluish discoloration in the cyst, especially if hemorrhage occurs into the cyst fluid. Although hemangiomas may be noted in the newborn period, they usually are more obvious later in infancy.

Neuroblastomas and Wilms' tumor are probably present at birth, but they are infrequently found on the newborn physical examination. However, a retroperitoneal or flank mass should be carefully differentiated from a normal kidney, which is usually palpable in a newborn. It there is a question that a mass is not a normal organ, it should be evaluated at once; for early detection is important in most of these lesions, especially the malignant ones. Cystic masses in the peritoneal cavity may represent urinary tract anomalies such as hydronephrosis and hydroureter, or they may be mesenteric cysts or duplications. The latter are usually freely movable within the peritoneal cavity, and this sign helps to differentiate them from the fixed retroperitoneal masses that characterize tumors.

Finally, although most sacrococcygeal teratomas will be visible in the newborn period, some of them are imbedded in the buttock and must be palpated to be appreciated. Occasionally, they

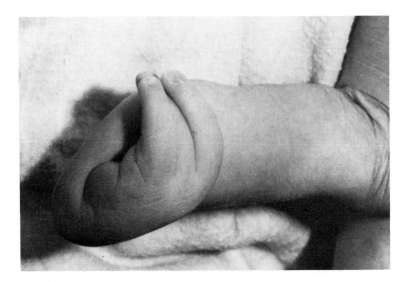

Fig. 9-6. Limb deformity accompanying imperforate anus, an example of the VATER or VACTEL complex.

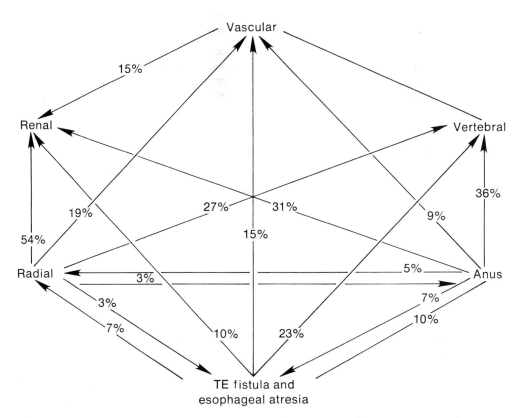

Fig. 9-7. Six categories of VATER association anomalies. Approximate percentages of concurrence are given. (Modified from Barnes, J. C., and Smith, W. L.: The VATER ASSOCIATION, Radiology **126:**445, 1978.)

present entirely as intrapelvic masses and will not be seen at all externally. These masses usually should be discovered on the first well-baby examination, when a careful rectal evaluation should be accomplished.

Visible lesions

The most apparent visible lesions are the facial anomalies, the spinal dysrhaphic anomalies, and the defects of the abdominal wall. The latter include prune-belly syndrome, gastroschisis, omphalocele, and exstrophy of the bladder. Limb anomalies may accompany other internal anomalies and may be part of the VATER or VACTEL complex[2] (Figs. 9-6 and 9-7), which includes anomalies of vertebral, anal, tracheoesophageal, and renal origin or those of vertebral, anal, cardiac, tracheoesophageal, and limb origin, respectively. Imperforate anus with or without a fistula is a visible anomaly, and one should appreciate the fact that imperforate anus is associated with esophageal atresia and duodenal atresia in a more than random association. When imperforate anus in a female infant is associated with only one perineal orifice, hydrometrocolpos should be suspected, especially if an abdominal mass arising from the pelvis is palpable.

REFERENCES

1. Apt, L., and Downey, W., Jr.: Melena neonatorum; the swallowed blood syndrome, J. Pediatr. **47:**6, 1955.
2. Barnes, J. C., and Smith, W. L.: The VATER association, Radiology **126:**445, 1978.
3. Clark, D. A.: Times of first void and first stool in 500 newborns, Pediatrics **60:**457, 1977.
4. Clarren, S. K., and Smith, D. W.: The fetal alcohol syndrome, N. Engl. J. Med. **298:**1063, 1978.
5. Davis, W. S., and Campbell, J. B.: Neonatal small left colon syndrome, Am. J. Dis. Child. **129:**1024, 1975.
6. Holder, T. M., and others: Esophageal atresia and tracheoesophageal fistula: a survey of its members by the Surgical Section of the American Academy of Pediatrics, Pediatrics **34:**542, 1964.
7. Lloyd, J. R., and Clatworthy, H. W., Jr.: Hydramnios as an aid to the early diagnosis of congenital obstruction of the alimentary tract: a study of the maternal and fetal factors, Pediatrics **21:**903, 1958.
8. Matthews, T. G., and Warshaw, J. B.: Relevance of the gestational age distribution of meconium passage *in utero,* Pediatrics **64:**30, 1979.
9. Philippart, A. I., Reed, J. Q., and Georgeson, K. E.: Neonatal small left colon syndrome, J. Pediatr. Surg. **10:**733, 1975.
10. Sweet, A. Y.: Classification of the low-birth-weight infant. In Klaus, M. H., and Fanaroff, A. A., editors: Care of the high-risk neonate, Philadelphia, 1979, W. B. Saunders Co., p. 82.
11. Swenson, O., Sherman, J. O., and Fisher, J. H.: Diagnosis of congenital megacolon: an analysis of 501 patients, J. Pediatr. Surg. **8:**587, 1973.
12. Touloukian, R. J., and Hobbins, J. C.: Maternal ultrasonography in the antenatal diagnosis of surgically correctable fetal abnormalities, J. Pediatr. Surg. **15:**373, 1980.
13. Wrobleski, D., and Wesselhoeft, C.: Ultrasonic diagnosis of prenatal intestinal obstruction, J. Pediatr. Surg. **14:**598, 1979.

CHAPTER 10

Specific problems

HOWARD C. FILSTON

DIAPHRAGMATIC HERNIA OF BOCHDALEK

Clinical presentation. When a newborn with a diaphragmatic hernia of Bochdalek has symptoms in the early neonatal period, he faces a prohibitive mortality. If most of the bowel is in the chest through a posterolateral defect in the diaphragm and the lungs are hypoplastic, symptoms usually develop immediately. Apgar scores are usually very low, and the 5-minute score is often worse than the 1-minute score.

Possible findings on physical examination include dyspnea, cyanosis, and rapid progression to total cardiovascular collapse. Since the defect occurs on the left side ten times as frequently as it does on the right, dextrocardia is a common finding on auscultation of the chest. Breath sounds are usually diminished or absent on the side of the hernia. The abdomen is scaphoid, indicating the absence of the bowel from the peritoneal cavity. Since this deformity is usually an isolated one, associated abnormalities are infrequent.

Variations in presentation. All infants with a diaphragmatic hernia are not symptomatic in the immediate newborn period. In fact, in some infants, months or even years may pass without the defect being discovered. These variations in the degree of cardiopulmonary insufficiency are probably related to the extent of pulmonary hypoplasia and the amount of bowel in the chest. Whether pulmonary hypoplasia is a primary phenomenon accompanying the diaphragmatic defect or a secondary one related to the interference with lung development caused by compression by the bowel in the pleural space is not known. It can be produced in the fetal lamb by creating a dia-

phragmatic defect at an appropriate stage of gestation.[42,81] If the latter is the cause, the timing and degree of intestinal herniation could well affect the extent of the hypoplasia. Certainly, the degree of pulmonary hypoplasia is the most significant determinant of the onset of symptoms and the likelihood of successful treatment.

Evaluation. Evaluation required for these children is a simple chest radiograph to confirm typical findings of bowellike contents in the chest with a sparsity to absence of bowel gas pattern in the abdomen and the typical dextrocardia of the left-sided defect. For the symptomatic newborn with these findings, further diagnostic evaluation is contraindicated. Be aware, however, that when the chest radiograph is obtained very early after birth, the amount of gas in the intestine may be limited and the bowel may look like a more solid mass in the chest (Fig. 10-1).

Differential diagnosis. A major problem in differential diagnosis is that of lobar emphysema. This is less likely to lead to acute respiratory failure in the newborn period and, in fact, usually presents later in infancy. When it does present symptoms in the immediate newborn period, they are usually milder than those of diaphragmatic hernia. Initially. lobar emphysema presents as a hazy opacity of the chest on the involved side, usually the left. Gradually, over a period of days, the haziness clears and the emphysematous nature of the problem becomes apparent (Fig. 10-2). On the other hand, an early chest film in diaphragmatic hernia will usually show some gas in the otherwise opacified hemithorax, since it would be most unusual for no gas to work its way through the bowel. A repeat chest film a short time later

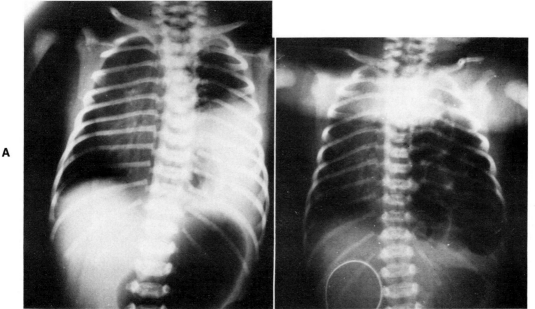

Fig. 10-1. A, Left diaphragmatic hernia of Bochdalek before significant entry of air into the herniated bowel. There is a mass effect in the left side of the chest with a shift of the mediastinum, an apparent dextrocardia, and an absence of bowel gas in the abdomen other than the stomach bubble. **B,** Subsequently, air has entered the herniated bowel and the more typical appearance of bowel loops in the chest is seen.

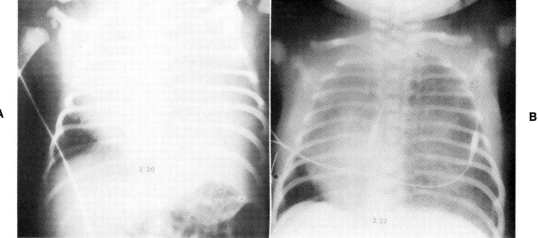

Fig. 10-2. A, Radiograph of an infant with respiratory distress showing an opacified left lung and an apparent shift of the mediastinum to the right with a normal bowel gas pattern in the abdomen. As fluid is gradually cleared from the lung parenchyma, the overexpanded nature of the left lung becomes evident and congenital lobar emphysema can be suspected **(B).**

may help to clarify the problem, but it is best to assume that the infant in severe respiratory distress with such a picture has a diaphragmatic hernia.

Resuscitation. Resuscitation for the infant with a diaphragmatic hernia requires considerable judgment as to the best means of respiratory management. Of utmost importance is good decompression of the gastrointestinal tract by an oral or nasogastric tube that is well functioning and kept on reliable suction. If the infant can be stabilized by simply adding oxygen to the ambient air, endotracheal intubation can sometimes be avoided; but one should err on the side of providing endotracheal intubation for good ventilatory control. Mask and bag ventilation is absolutely contraindicated, for it will fill the child's gastrointestinal tract with air, further compromising his ventilation and circulation. On the other hand, once he is intubated, the infant should be ventilated with great care inasmuch as his hypoplastic lungs are highly susceptible to rupture with attendant tension pneumothorax. Immediate bilateral tube thorocostomies may be required under such circumstances, and some authorities have suggested that these be provided prophylactically.[104] Arterial blood gases should be obtained and acidosis corrected appropriately.

Referral. Referral should be urgent and directed to the most totally capable facility available. If these children are to survive, they will require sophisticated postoperative management with numerous indwelling central monitoring lines and a critical balance of cardiotonic and pulmonary vasodilating agents. Cardiac catheterization facilities may be required for the placement of pulmonary artery catheters; and, of course, experienced surgical and anesthetic management are mandatory.

Medical versus surgical treatment. There is no medical treatment for the newborn who is acutely ill with a diaphragmatic hernia; surgical repair is mandatory as soon as resuscitation is achieved. The older infant who is discovered incidentally on chest radiograph to have a diaphragmatic hernia should be referred urgently, but not necessarily as an emergency, for competent surgical care. Even when the child survives weeks or months without symptoms, the threat of cardiopulmonary collapse from the expansion of the bowel in the chest is ever present.

Surgical options. Surgical options relate primarily to the timing of the surgical procedure in

the course of resuscitation and stabilization of the infant. Repair of the diaphragmatic hernia can be accomplished either by thoracotomy or laparotomy, and studies of comparable series of patients using each approach have failed to show significant differences.[49,108] Occasionally, inadequate development of the peritoneal cavity may require evisceration of the bowel into a prosthetic pouch with gradual reduction of this evisceration back into the peritoneal cavity after repair of the diaphragm. Although total nonfixation of the mesentery is the rule in this lesion, too much has been made of the value of laparotomy in providing treatment for this associated entity. Adhesions probably adequately fix the bowel loops in either approach, preventing volvulus of the mesentery in most cases.

Postoperative course. The postoperative course for infants symptomatic from a diaphragmatic hernia in the first few hours of life is often a stormy one, with the mortality approaching 50% to 75%.[28,88] When the infant has sustained severe preoperative hypoxia, postoperative difficulties may result, primarily from fluid leakage from capillaries damaged by the hypoxic insult and the consequent inability of the infant to maintain sufficient vascular volume. When the hypoxic insult involves the pulmonary tissue itself, there may be severe interstitial pulmonary edema or a "shock lung."

Unfortunately, even infants who have been well managed preoperatively, so that severe hypoxic damage has been avoided, frequently follow a progressive downhill course postoperatively. It has been postulated that pulmonary arteriolar hypertension develops in the hypoplastic ipsilateral lung.[27] The resulting increased resistance in the pulmonary circuit leads to shunting of the right-sided heart outflow through the ductus arteriosus, which remains potentially patent for many days after birth.[23]

The problem has so far eluded solution, and a prospective national study is now being conducted by the Surgical Section of the American Academy of Pediatrics. Therapeutic manipulations aimed at solving the problem of pulmonary hypertension have included the use of vasodilator substances (chosen for their relative selectivity of the pulmonary circuit) and ligation of the ductus. These techniques require extensive monitoring and a team approach utilizing the talents of the pediatric cardiologist, the pediatric surgeon, and the neonatologist. Some progress is being made, and some children who would previously have fallen into the irretrievable category are now being saved.

Prognosis. The prognosis for the child symptomatic from a diaphragmatic hernia within the first few hours of life remains extremely guarded at this point. For the child who survives beyond the first day of life before becoming symptomatic, the mortality falls to almost zero when the child is properly managed.

Important aspects of follow-up. For the child who survives the pathophysiologic insults of a diaphragmatic hernia and its postoperative complications, long-term follow-up is essential. Persistent pulmonary hypertension may lead eventually to right-sided heart failure. A chest radiograph should be obtained at any sign of recurrent pulmonary symptoms to rule out recurrence of the diaphragmatic defect. Also, any symptoms of abdominal pain, distention, or vomiting should be investigated for signs of strangulating mechanical bowel obstruction, either from volvulus of the poorly attached mesentery or from postoperative adhesions.

OTHER DIAPHRAGMATIC DEFECTS

Other lesions of the diaphragm that may be symptomatic in the newborn period are eventration of the diaphragm, either congenital or acquired, paraesophageal or hiatal hernias, and hernias through the anterior substernal foramen of Morgagni. Hiatal hernias are discussed later in the chapter along with gastroesophageal reflux.

Eventration

Congenital eventration of the diaphragm appears to be a failure of formation of the muscular central portion of the diaphragm or an atrophy of the diaphragmatic muscles. Acquired eventration of the diaphragm may be due to trauma to the phrenic nerve roots during delivery or to injury to the phrenic nerve during intrathoracic surgical procedures. Regardless of its etiology, the diaphragm fails to function as a muscular organ and instead moves passively with respirations, causing paroxysmal and counterproductive motions interfering with normal respiration. Rarely is this lesion acutely symptomatic in the immediate newborn period. It can be differentiated from diaphrag-

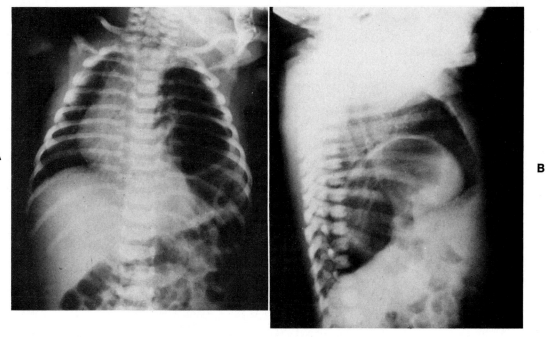

Fig. 10-3. A, Eventration of the left hemidiaphragm is recognized by the elevation of the gastric air bubble in an otherwise normal abdominal gas pattern. The true position of the diaphragm is better revealed in **B,** the lateral film, which clearly shows the elevation of the hemidiaphragm. (From Filston, H. C., and Izant, R.: The surgical neonate: evaluation and care, New York, 1978, Appleton-Century-Crofts.)

matic hernia of Bochdalek by the presence of two diaphragms on the lateral film and a relatively normal bowel gas pattern in the abdomen (Fig. 10-3). A more superior position of the gastric bubble and splenic flexure of the colon indicate the abnormally high position of the diaphragm. When the right side is involved, of course, the liver will be high in the abdomen, occupying the lower part of the right thoracic space.

Eventration may interfere with good ventilation and lead to atelectasis or recurrent pneumonia. In an infant with borderline pulmonary function, the presence of eventration may be enough to tip the balance against the infant's ability to sustain

his own ventilation. There are some differences of opinion as to whether all of these defects need surgical therapy,[120] but many feel strongly that most of these children have ventilatory difficulty and that all of them should have their diaphragms plicated.[14]

The surgical therapy is straightforward and involves plication of the diaphragm, either by excising the central portion and tightly closing the diaphragm or by folding over and suturing the diaphragm in a pleat. This procedure eliminates the paradoxical motion and allows better filling of the lung on the side of the eventration.

Generally, the prognosis for these children is

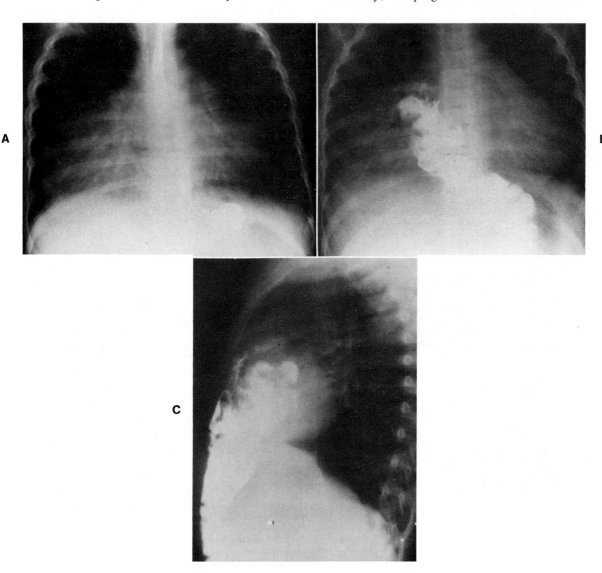

Fig. 10-4. A, Normal barium swallow and gastric position in an infant with opacification of the right hemithorax. A subsequent barium enema study **(B)** shows herniation of the colon into the right mediastinum, confirmed as a hernia through the foramen of Morgagni on the lateral view **(C).**

good and they maintain long-term satisfactory respiratory function. Occasionally, the diaphragm again stretches up and additional plications may be needed. When the cause is a transient injury to the phrenic nerve, eventual recovery of function may be anticipated.

Hernias through the foramen of Morgagni

Hernias through the foramen of Morgagni are unusual lesions[4,54] and often are found because the infant has had chest radiographs for some other reason (Fig. 10-4). They may cause mild respiratory symptoms, but because the herniation is primarily beneath the pericardium into the mediastinum, there is far less interference with ventilatory function than with either the diaphragmatic hernia of Bochdalek or with eventration of the diaphragm. These lesions warrant eventual repair, but rarely is such a repair urgent; any other problem the infant may exhibit can usually be given priority over these lesions.

LOBAR EMPHYSEMA

Clinical presentation. Another entity that presents with varying degrees of respiratory distress and may be acutely symptomatic in the newborn period is lobar emphysema.[45,53] It is unusual for this entity to present with severe respiratory symptoms in the immediate newborn period, and rarely does it present with the overwhelming respiratory distress characteristic of so many infants with diaphragmatic hernia. The usual findings are those of a child with some mild respiratory dysfunction who, on radiography of the chest, may show either a large air-filled hyperlucent area on one side of the chest or, earlier, a cloudy opacity of that side of the chest (Fig. 10-2). There is usually some shift of the mediastinum. Decreased breath sounds on the side of the emphysematous lobe with dextrocardia if the involved side is on the left may be appreciable. Symptoms progress in severity over the first days or weeks of life.

Evaluation and differential diagnosis. If the hyperlucent lobar distribution is already apparent, no further workup is necessary. The left upper lobe is most commonly involved; the left lower lobe the least.[52] In cases with opacity due to fluid-filled alveoli that have not yet been resolved, differentiation from congenital adenomatoid degenerative disease is necessary. Observation with respiratory support and serial chest films will usually show clearing of the fluid and delineate the distribution of the process.

Referral. Whether or not to refer the infant to a major center depends to some extent on the degree of difficulty the child is having. However, these children may progress rapidly to severe respiratory embarrassment and require full-scale respiratory support and subsequent urgent surgery. Therefore, unless these support modalities are immediately available, the child should be referred to a major center. He should be accompanied by a knowledgeable medical or paramedical individual who can maintain respiratory support and augment it during transport, if necessary.

Medical versus surgical treatment. These cases require judgment as to whether continued medical management or surgical intervention will provide the best therapy. Ravitch believes that surgery is always imperative.[89] Where respiratory distress is minimal and improving, the child can be supported and watched carefully.[30] At times the process will improve and go on to clear without surgical intervention. On the other hand, when marked overexpansion of the lung is present at birth and there is severe shifting of the mediastinum to the contralateral side, improvement is

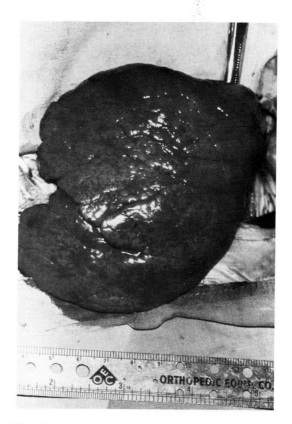

Fig. 10-5. At surgery the overexpanded left upper lobe of the infant in Fig. 10-2 is seen just before resection.

less likely and urgent excision of the overexpanded lobe may be needed.

Surgical options. There are few surgical options, for if surgical intervention is necessary, lobectomy is the procedure of choice (Fig. 10-5).

Postoperative course. Once lobectomy is accomplished, the postoperative course is usually benign and the child can be expected to be discharged from the hospital within a week if all other systems are normal.

Prognosis. The prognosis for the child with an isolated lobar emphysema is excellent.

Important aspects of follow-up. Important aspects of follow-up include inquiry into and examination for any signs of respiratory distress. Repeat chest films at intervals over the next year will demonstrate any involvement of other lung segments.

Complications. Complications in the immediate postoperative period may include pneumothorax and even bronchopleural fistula formation, but these severe complications of adult thoracic surgery are extremely unusual in the child.

Differential diagnostic entity. The primary differential diagnostic entity of lobar emphysema is congenital adenomatoid degenerative disease, which involves the lung diffusely and may involve all lobes on both sides (Fig. 10-6). This lesion, though milder in onset than acute lobar emphysema, may be more debilitating in the long run because of the extensive degenerative changes in the smaller bronchioles and alveoli of the lung. When the disease is limited to specific lung segments, excision may leave the child with more normal pulmonary function.

PNEUMOTHORAX (AIR BLOCK SYNDROME)

Pneumothorax (air block syndrome) is the most common surgically significant entity in the newborn period that involves the respiratory system.

Etiology and clinical presentation. Possible findings may range from incidental discovery on chest x-ray examination in a totally asymptomatic patient with a minimal degree of pneumothorax or pneumomediastinum, to a variety of presentations with varying degrees of respiratory distress, to severe acute pulmonary collapse in complete bilateral pneumothorax (Fig. 10-7). This lesion may result from hypoplastic development of the lung, may arise spontaneously, or (commonly in the modern neonatal era) may result from extensive support programs for premature infants with severe respiratory distress syndrome. Air block syndrome results from rupture of alveolar membranes due to high pressures.[38] Differential com-

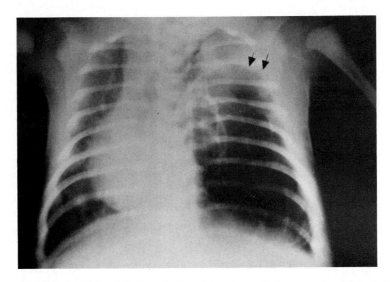

Fig. 10-6. This entity, which might be mistaken for a congenital eventration of the left hemidiaphragm, is actually a congenital adenomatoid degeneration of the lung. Most of the lung fields are involved with the disease process, and the line that could be mistaken for elevation of the left hemidiaphragm (arrows) is actually the interlobar fissure. (From Filston, H. C., and Izant, R.: The surgical neonate: evaluation and care, New York, 1978, Appleton-Century-Crofts.)

pliance in the neonatal lung can lead to overexpansion of some segments when the need for large air volumes and end-expiratory pressure arises due to hyaline membrane disease, meconium aspiration, or other causes. Air block syndrome can present as pneumomediastinum, pneumothorax (unilateral or bilateral), pneumopericardium, and, occasionally, secondary pneumoperitoneum.[70] Pneumopericardium may produce acute tamponade and cardiovascular collapse.

Evaluation. When the child is asymptomatic or only mildly dyspneic, chest x-ray examination will confirm the entity. Occasionally, the question of pneumothorax is equivocal on the plain anteroposterior (AP) chest film, and in these cases lateral and decubitus films may be definitive. These views are also essential in differentiating pneumopericardium from pneumomediastinum.

Referral. The minor degrees of pneumothorax that do not seem to be increasing and show no evidence of tension can be watched expectantly without tube thoracostomy, but the availability of this procedure must be ensured and the child followed with serial chest x-ray films. Persistent pneumothorax that is not responding may require referral to a major center.

Medical versus surgical treatment. If the pneumothorax involves only minimal collapse and the child is relatively asymptomatic, it can be watched and reevaluated by serial chest x-ray films. The major decision to be made is whether or not tension pneumothorax is present. Mere entry of air into the pleural space and collapse of the lung is usually associated with only minimal distress unless the child already has respiratory impairment from other causes. On the other hand, the forceful entry of air into the pleural space accompanied by a continued air leak and no source of escape leads to tension with shifting of the mediastinum as well as compromise of the contralateral lung and even of venous return to the heart (Fig. 10-8). Once tension pneumothorax is evidenced by shifting of the mediastinum or overexpansion of the pleural outline on the involved site, immediate tube thoracostomy is indicated. Short-term temporary emergency decompression can sometimes be achieved by placing a large-bore plastic cannula of the type used for vascular cannulation into the pleural space and aspirating the air. This procedure will not succeed in overcoming a major lung leak, however. Pneumopericardium requires immediate relief. Needle aspiration through the left parasternal area near the xyphoid may be lifesaving. Continuous tube decompression may then be required. Prophylactic tube thoracostomies, bilaterally, are probably in-

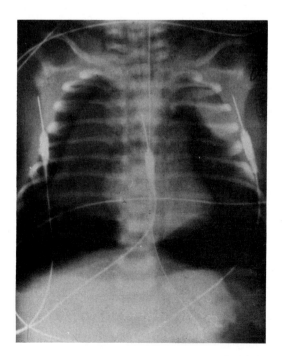

Fig. 10-7. Bilateral tension pneumothorax secondary to air block syndrome resulting from hypoplastic lungs.

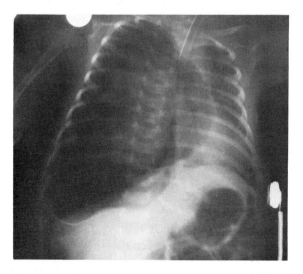

Fig. 10-8. Right tension pneumothorax compressing the left lung and shifting the mediastinum of this infant. There is essentially complete collapse of the right lung.

dicated as well, since pneumothorax usually follows soon after pneumopericardium. Pneumomediastinum alone needs no treatment, but pneumothorax may follow and should be watched for.

Once definite pneumothorax with complete collapse of one lung is evidenced, tube thoracostomy through the fourth intercostal space in the anterior axillary line should be achieved with a No. 12 French plastic chest tube. The common practice in adults of placing chest tubes for air decompression in the second intercostal space in the midclavicular line is dangerous in infants, because so much critical vascular and neural anatomy lies within a few millimeters of this point. Satisfactory decompression can always be achieved through the safer lateral and lower approaches.

Postoperative care. Following achievement of tube thoracostomy, the tube should be placed to underwater seal, and if this does not succeed in reexpanding the lobe, suction should be applied and maintained until the tube stops bubbling air. At this point a short period of underwater seal should be reinstituted and a chest x-ray film observed for reaccumulation of the pneumothorax. Once the lung is up and stable, the tube may be removed. A postextubation film should be obtained to ensure that the pneumothorax has not recurred.

Prognosis. The prognosis for the child with a pneumothorax that responds to treatment is excellent, and there should be no long-term problems. In the child whose pneumothorax is due to severe hypoplastic lung, treatment may be unsuccessful; and if both lungs are involved, death must be expected. Severe cases of air block syndrome may lead to such severe pneumothorax that even multiple tube thoracostomies bilaterally will fail to control the tension.

A recent report documents ten cases in which thoracotomy and suture of the lung leaks resulted in the survival of nine infants.[39]

AIRWAY OBSTRUCTION

Etiology and clinical presentation. Any child who has dyspnea must be evaluated for airway obstruction. One must never assume that dyspnea is due to respiratory distress syndrome or hyaline membrane disease. The ability of the infant to ventilate must always be ascertained as the initial evaluative step. A common cause of airway ob-

struction is the *Pierre Robin syndrome,* in which the child's lower jaw structure is underdeveloped and the tongue falls back and obstructs the hypopharynx. With swallowing, the tongue is sucked down into the hypopharynx so hard that the child cannot ventilate. These symptoms represent the extreme cases of this syndrome, however. Many children with Pierre Robin anomalies have only mild symptoms. The symptoms may be progressive, however.

Choanal atresia is another rare lesion caused by lack of perforation of the nasopharyngeal septum. Because the neonate is an obligate nose breather, ventilation is severely interfered with. Resuscitation can usually be accomplished by placing an oral airway or, if necessary, by intubating the child. The inability to pass a small tube through the nares into the hypopharynx helps to confirm the suspected diagnosis; and, if necessary, a small amount of contrast material can be injected to further demonstrate the obstruction.

Benign tumors may arise in the hypopharynx or in the trachea itself and obstruct the airway. *Cysts* in the trachea may enlarge rapidly and occlude the airway, and these may be present at birth (Fig. 10-9). Anomalous development of the tracheal cartilages accompanied by softening and deformity may lead to collapse of the trachea with deep inspiration. This, too, may be progressively symptomatic.

Evaluation. For all of these entities, evalua-

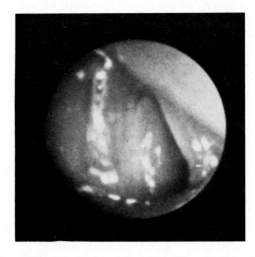

Fig. 10-9. Obstructing left subglottic cyst distorting the left vocal cord, as seen through the telescopic bronchoscope.

tion must include careful consideration of all the parts of the ventilatory system, including the jaw structure, the tongue, the nasopharynx, the hypopharynx, the larynx, the trachea, and the bronchi. Laryngoscopy and bronchoscopy are often required for definitive diagnosis. Lateral films of the neck may be helpful in showing obstructive lesions of the upper airway.

Referral. Early referral of infants with this type of distress is essential so that they can be sent to a center where competent specialists are available to evaluate the hypopharynx, the larynx, and the tracheobronchial tree. Special instruments with optical telescopes are usually needed for satisfactory evaluation of the infant airway. Surgical subspecialists familiar with adult airway problems may not have adequate experience to make correct judgments regarding the management of such lesions in the infant. Referral to a major center capable of taking care of surgical problems of all types in the infant age group is essential.

Medical versus surgical treatment. In the Pierre Robin deformity, those infants with mild symptoms may be managed by careful positioning of the infant, usually in the prone position, and occasionally by the placement of a decompressing tube into the hypopharynx or upper esophagus to protect the child against sucking the tongue down the esophagus with resultant obstruction of the airway.[110] Other children with this entity may require suturing of the tongue to the lip, and occasionally tracheostomy may be required when the airway cannot be maintained by other means.[66,122]

Provision of an oral airway or endotracheal intubation is preferable to blind puncturing of the nasal septum for initial management of choanal atresia, since the septum may be quite thick and require more sophisticated surgical management for successful reconstruction.

For those infants with obstructions of the airway by neoplastic masses, tracheostomy is usually required in the newborn period. Rarely can successful surgical excision be accomplished in one step, and the integrity of the airway is compromised while the entity remains. Most benign tumors and cysts can be excised endoscopically through the instrument channel of the Storz telescopic bronchoscope. Such excision may, however, require multiple-stage procedures. Before any attempt at excision is made, careful preop-erative evaluation is necessary to be certain that there is no major vascular component to the lesion.

Lesions of the hypopharynx can often be removed by direct surgical access through a lateral pharyngotomy.

Postoperative care. The tracheostomy can usually be removed once the lesion is controlled. The fear of decannulation problems has been shown to be unfounded when the tracheostomy is performed and managed and the decannulation program attended to by physicians knowledgeable in the overall management of infant tracheostomies.[33,93]

Prognosis. The long-term prognosis in most of these lesions is excellent once an airway is restored. The lesions are usually benign and do not recur. Even the severe Pierre Robin deformities usually improve with growth and age.

Important aspects of follow-up. Important aspects of follow-up include careful bronchoscopic evaluation of the tracheobronchial tree before any attempt is made at decannulation of the tracheostomy. Subsequent reevaluation at intervals to ensure that the lesion is not re-forming and that granulation tissue is not threatening to obstruct the trachea at the level of the tracheostomy stoma is essential.

Complications. Long-term complications of stricture formation are ever a potential hazard when any manipulation of the infant airway has taken place. Fortunately, with experienced management these are unusual.

STRIDOR

Etiology, clinical presentation, and evaluation. Although stridor is a common complaint in infancy and is usually due to tracheomalacia, laryngomalacia, or tracheal compression by an aberrant arch vessel, stridor is an infrequent finding in the immediate newborn period. When it is present, it will often be caused by a hypopharyngeal or subglottic benign tumor such as a hemangioma or a laryngeal cyst.[56] This symptom should lead to early evaluation by laryngoscopy and bronchoscopy, but this procedure must be accomplished by an anesthesia team competent to deal with the infant airway and by a surgeon with the instruments and experience needed to deal with such lesions and to perform a proper infant tracheostomy, which may be urgently required if the lesion is completely obstructing. Furthermore, manipulation may cause edema of the partially obstructing lesion, leading to complete occlusion, so that inappropriate manipulation by unskilled and inexperienced personnel is contraindicated.

Tracheomalacia may be of varying degrees. It may produce only occasional stridor on exertion, or it may cause intermittent airway obstruction during normal breathing.

Most typically, laryngomalacia is a narrowing of the base of the epiglottis so that it becomes "omega shaped" and can be pulled down over the glottis with deep inspiration. This condition rarely gives significant obstruction but does cause noticeable stridor. It is the most common finding when laryngoscopy and bronchoscopy are performed in older infants who have stridor, but it is usually not symptomatic in the immediate newborn period.

Medical versus surgical treatment. Some hemangiomas will respond to alternate-day steroid therapy, and if the lesion is not immediately life threatening, such treatment may be given a brief trial.[34] Other lesions such as cysts and specific malformations of the airway must be treated in such a way as to ensure the child's survival. For example, tracheomalacia causing intermittent airway obstruction during normal breathing would require a tracheostomy. A properly performed infant tracheostomy has an insignificant complication rate and a low incidence of inability to decannulate the infant when the entire care of the tracheostomy and its decannulation are in the hands of knowledgeable individuals. In the past, infant tracheostomy led to considerable morbidity and continues to have considerable morbidity in the hands of the inexperienced surgeon. Nevertheless, tracheostomy is protective; and it allows time for a planned and, if necessary, staged excision of any hypopharyngeal or subglottic lesions. This careful and considerate approach gives the best chance for the infant to have a successful recovery and useful airway.

Complications. Long-term complications in the airway are stenosis of the subglottic area and decannulation problems. The most common cause of stenosis is prolonged endotracheal intubation with a too large and too tightly fitting endotracheal tube.[65] This problem can be almost completely eliminated if attention is given to a properly fitting tube. Remember, the subglottic or cricoid

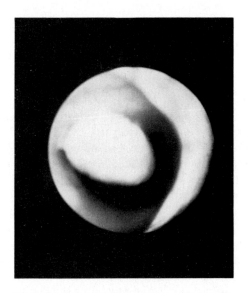

Fig. 10-10. Granuloma obstructing most of the tracheal lumen arising from the superior edge of the tracheostomy stoma site, as seen through the telescopic bronchoscope. (From Filston, H. C., and Izant, R.: The surgical neonate: evaluation and care, New York, 1978, Appleton-Century-Crofts; courtesy Dale G. Johnson, M.D., Salt Lake City, Utah.)

area of the infant airway is the narrowest portion, unlike in the adult, in whom the cords are the narrowest part of the airway. Decannulation problems mean that the child's airway is not capable of sustaining ventilation without the tracheostomy. If all upper airway lesions have been resolved, the most likely reason for a decannulation problem is the presence of a granuloma at the superior margin of the tracheostomy stoma (Fig. 10-10). We believe that all children with tracheostomies should be bronchoscoped to evaluate the airway thoroughly before any attempts at decannulation are made. If a granuloma is present, it can be excised either transtracheally or by excising the entire stoma and the granuloma incontinuity with it.

MISCELLANEOUS CONDITIONS OF THE CHEST AND AIRWAY
Chest wall deformities

Common deformities of the chest such as pectus excavatum and pectus carinatum are rarely associated with symptoms. Their presence in the newborn period, therefore, should cause little concern. Only major rib deficiencies causing flail chest deformity are likely to cause any real dyspnea. Obviously, extreme lesions such as complete

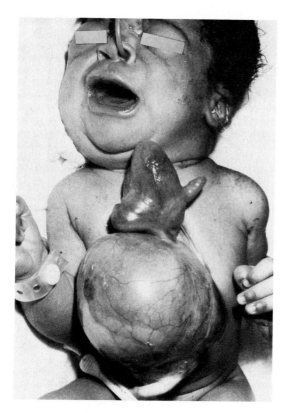

Fig. 10-11. Ectopia cordis, sternal cleft, and ompha-locele.

sternal clefts and ectopia cordis present major difficulties for the child's cardiorespiratory function (Fig. 10-11).

Cleft palate and cleft lip

Cleft palate and cleft lip are obvious at birth and are readily found on the newborn physical examination. Because of their monstrous appearance, children with cleft lip are usually referred early to a neonatal center. Failure to identify a cleft palate on initial physical examination may lead to aspiration problems in the infant.

Most surgeons who deal extensively with these lesions prefer to repair the cleft lip in the early neonatal period, whereas they postpone cleft palate repair until the second year of life. Often a prosthesis is fashioned to tide the child through this waiting period. These lesions are best managed by a team approach that includes a plastic surgeon, orthodontist, dentist, speech and hearing therapist, and social workers so that the child is cared for in a comprehensive clinic atmosphere. Cosmetic repair of cleft lip has progressed to the point where

most individuals have a perfectly normal appearance following surgical correction, and the gratitude of the parents for the early repair is inestimable.

After repair of the cleft palate, some swallowing discoordination may persist, with spillage of swallowed oropharyngeal contents into the nasopharynx and occasional expulsion through the anterior nares. Speech difficulties are probably the most common long-term problems with these lesions, and it is for this reason that the comprehensive approach is so useful.

Tongue-tie

Another lesion that is common is that of persistent subglossal frenulum, or tongue-tie. When the frenulum extends to the tip of the tongue, the child may have trouble protruding the tongue beyond the teeth. Many children have been subjected to surgery because of concern over speech difficulties related to this lesion. Despite the frequency of tongue-tie, the incidence of speech defects due to this lesion is low. We generally prefer to have the child's speech development evaluated by a competent speech and hearing therapist before proceeding with surgery. When, according to the speech and hearing therapist, the frenulum is interfering with the child's speech development, simple clipping is usually inadequate; a definitive surgical procedure that incises the frenulum transversely and sutures it longitudinally to lengthen the frenulum and allow further protrusion of the tongue is required. This procedure usually requires general anesthesia.

ANOMALIES OF THE ESOPHAGUS
Esophageal atresia

Clinical presentation. The first clue to esophageal atresia in the infant may be the recognition of hydramnios in the mother. As noted previously, an excess of amniotic fluid suggests an obstruction in the upper gastrointestinal tract of the infant. This prevents the passage of the amniotic fluid through the infant's gastrointestinal tract, reabsorption back into the infant's circulatory system, and excretion through his kidneys into the urine and back to the amniotic fluid. Obstruction to the gastrointestinal tract above the upper to middle jejunum may be associated with hydraminos. This finding is not a universal one, however; only about 15% of infants with esoph-

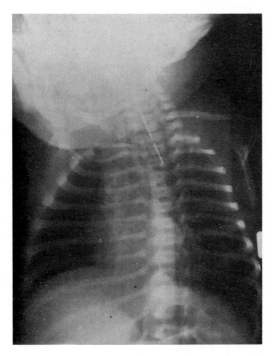

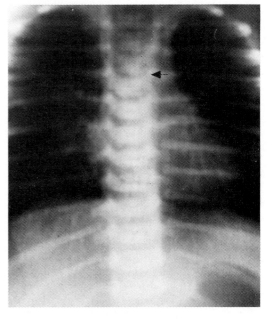

Fig. 10-12. A radiopaque catheter stops in the upper mediastinum, indicating the extent of the blind upper pouch of an esophageal atresia. The presence of a fistula between the distal esophagus and the tracheobronchial tree is confirmed by the air in the gastrointestinal tract.

Fig. 10-13. Esophageal atresia. The arrow points to the lower end of the blind proximal esophageal pouch. The presence of a tracheoesophageal fistula between the distal esophagus and the tracheobronchial tree is confirmed by the air in the gastrointestinal tract.

ageal atresia are said to be associated with maternal hydramnios. The low incidence may be due to the ability of the amniotic fluid to pass down the trachea and out through the distal esophagus, through the fistula, and into the stomach.

Physical findings are those of increased salivation and bubbles combined with an inability of the child to swallow water.

Evaluation. At the recognition of any of these findings, a radiopaque tube of fairly substantial size, such as a No. 10 or 12 French, should be passed gently into the hypopharynx and into the esophagus. It should be advanced until an obstruction is encountered, at which point a chest x-ray film should be obtained (Fig. 10-12). It should then be ascertained whether the tube reaches the stomach and whether it appears to pass through the normal channels. A blind eosphageal segment filled with air may be recognized in the neck and upper mediastinum (Fig. 10-13). Occasionally a small tube may pass through the larynx, down the trachea, and out through the fistula into the stomach (see Fig. 9-4). Enough of the upper abdomen should be included on the film so that the

presence of bowel gas can be noted. If esophageal atresia is demonstrated and bowel gas is present, the classic variety of atresia associated with a distal tracheoesophageal fistula is confirmed. Were this not true, no gas would be present in the abdomen. This configuration is the most common variety, being found in 85% to 95% of cases. The above-recommended evaluation confirms the diagnosis, and no further diagnostic studies are necessary. Particularly, radiographic contrast material should not be used, because it may be aspirated from the proximal pouch into the trachea, causing aspiration pneumonia. This is particularly likely to be true if water-soluble contrast is used, since its high osmolarity injures the ciliated respiratory epithelium. If there is doubt about the diagnosis, further evaluation should consist of endoscopy with the Storz telescopic bronchoscope, which will easily confirm the presence of the tracheoesophageal fistula. The blind proximal eosphagus can also be demonstrated by this means. The rare proximal fistula between the upper esophagus and the tracheobronchial tree can also be found on endoscopy.

Further evaluation should be undertaken to ascertain the state of the child's pulmonary system. Assurance that the child does not have severe aspiration pneumonia is necessary. This can be accomplished by finding the lungs to be clear to auscultation and on chest x-ray examination and, most important, by demonstrating the child's ability to achieve a Po_2 of 60 mm Hg or higher in room air on an arterial blood gas evaluation.

Referral. This evaluation is best left to a major pediatric surgical center, and the child should be referred as soon as the diagnosis is confirmed with a radiopaque catheter. Endoscopy without the Storz telescopic bronchoscope is hazardous and is likely to be undependable. The child should be transported in the prone, head-up position to prevent regurgitation of gastric secretions from the stomach up the distal esophagus into the trachea through the tracheoesophageal fistula (Fig. 10-14). The proximal pouch should be decompressed by good suction on the nasoesophageal tube.

Surgical options. Surgical options are defined primarily by the size of the infant and the state of health of his lungs. Our preference is for primary repair of any infant who satisfies the above criteria for good pulmonary function, particularly that of achieving a Po_2 of 60 mm Hg in room air. This is true regardless of the infant's size, but some pediatric surgeons still opt occasionally for a staged approach to the infant weighing under 1,600 to 1,800 g.[59,119] This consists of initial gastrostomy with the infant under local anesthesia followed by thoracotomy and division and ligation of the fistula. Subsequently a second thoracotomy is done for anastomosis of the esophageal segment after the child has reached an adequate weight. However, it has been shown that the child often does poorly with this staged management, and we concur with those who believe that all children who are candidates for primary repair on the basis of pulmonary function should have the complete repair at the initial operation.

Criteria for primary repair of esophageal atresia with a tracheoesophageal fistula

1. The chest is clear to auscultation and on x-ray examination.
2. The arterial Po_2 is 60 mm Hg or higher in room air.
3. Adequate operative, anesthetic, nursing, and postoperative pulmonary support are readily available.

If the child does not meet the criteria for initial primary repair, a gastrostomy for decompression of the stomach should be achieved with the child under local anesthesia. The child should then be placed prone with the head up and a total parenteral nutrition catheter placed for nutritional maintenance. Vigorous pulmonary therapy should then be afforded while nutritional maintenance is achieved, and this therapy should be continued until such time as the child does satisfy the criteria for primary repair. This may take as long as 3 weeks when severe aspiration pneumonia is present.

Surgical options also relate to the type of anastomosis that is performed. We prefer a division and suture of the tracheal end of the fistula followed by simple end-to-end anastomosis of the esophageal segments. Successful end-to-end anastomosis should be achievable in the majority of cases.

Postoperative course. Although much has been written about problems in the postoperative period, these should be unusual. Stenoses should be rare in a carefully performed end-to-end anastomosis in which the mucosa is carefully approximated. Stenosis usually results from failure to include the mucosa on both sides of the anastomosis in the sutures or from leakage from the suture line with resultant infection and hypertrophic granulations.

The postoperative course in these children should usually be benign. They are usually not fed enterally until the fifth postoperative day. If the extrapleural chest tube is not showing any signs of leaking saliva, a barium swallow is then obtained; and if an intact anastomosis is demonstrated, the tube can then be pulled and the child begun on oral feedings.

Prognosis. The prognosis for these children is excellent. Although discordant peristaltic waves can be demonstrated on cinefluorography, most of the time these children swallow quite well. They are somewhat more prone to obstruction and may have more frequent choking episodes than normal children. They are particularly unable to handle foreign bodies that may be ingested during the infant and toddler years.

Important aspects of follow-up. Important aspects of follow-up include recognition and treatment of the common problem of gastroesophageal reflux. Although this entity is becoming recognized as a fairly common problem in general, it is frequently associated with esophageal atre-

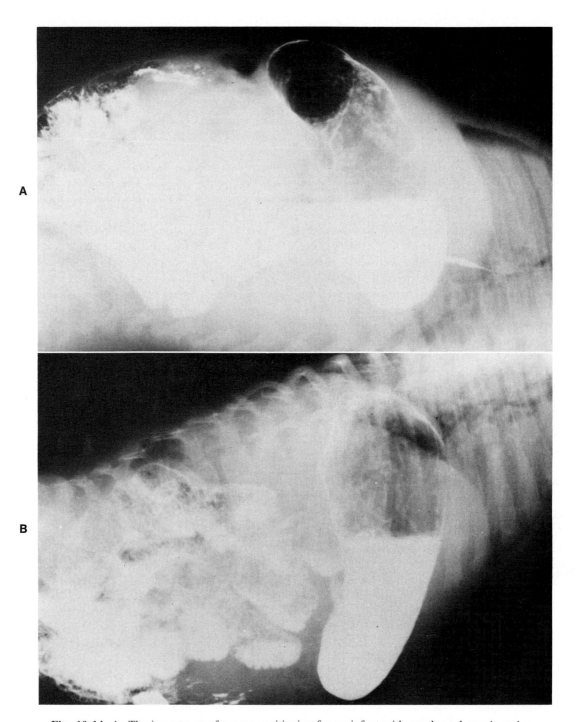

Fig. 10-14. A, The importance of proper positioning for an infant with esophageal atresia and a distal tracheoesophageal fistula is shown by this film of the infant lying supine with contrast material in the stomach. Note the ease with which the contrast material refluxes into the distal esophagus. With the infant prone and head up **(B),** the contrast material pools anteriorly, away from the esophagus, and reflux is less likely. (From Filston, H. C., and Izant, R.: The surgical neonate: evaluation and care, New York, 1978, Appleton-Century-Crofts; courtesy Dale G. Johnson, M.D., Salt Lake City, Utah.)

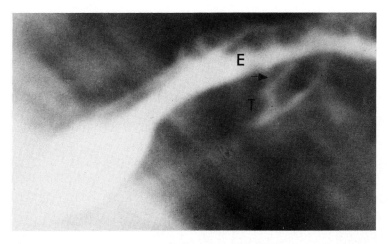

Fig. 10-15. Cine–barium esophagogram of an infant with a questionable recurrent tracheoesophageal fistula after repair of esophageal atresia and tracheoesophageal fistula. The esophagus *(E)* and trachea *(T)* are indicated on the film along with the questionable fistulous connection (arrow). The fact that contrast material has refluxed into the proximal esophagus (left) with possible aspiration and filling of the "pit" of the old fistula makes accurate identification difficult. (From Kirks, D. R., and others: A.J.R. **133:**763, 1979. Copyright © 1979, American Roentgen Ray Society.)

sia.[3,103] These infants are generally placed in infant seats so that they are maintained in the upright position continuously over the several weeks to months after surgery. If aspiration pneumonia or obvious vomiting and regurgitation are occurring, evaluation for gastroesophageal reflux by cine-esophagography should be performed. The differential diagnosis of this type of postoperative problem includes recurrent tracheoesophageal fistula by refistulization between the two suture lines: that from the fistulous closure in the trachea and that at the anastomosis of the esophageal segments. Esophagography can be equivocal or misleading in this entity, inasmuch as the child may regurgitate and aspirate while being evaluated (Fig. 10-15). Balloon catheters have been used to prevent reflux into the larynx during the cine-esophagograms, and recently the use of angiographic catheters has been found to be helpful in cannulating the recurrent fistula (Fig. 10-16, *A* and *B*).

Although endoscopy with the optical telescopic bronchoscope is highly successful for identification of the initial fistula, it too, may be equivocal in evaluating the child for a recurrence. The pit-like diverticulum of the trachea where the fistula occurred is always present, and it may be difficult to ascertain whether it still communicates with the esophagus (Fig. 10-16, *C*).

On a long-term basis, the possibility of stenosis must be kept in mind, although its incidence should be low. Any signs that the child is having difficulty is ingesting food should be evaluated by esophagoscopy and barium swallow. The mere presence of a constricted area on the barium swallow does not confirm that there is an anatomic stricture; whether one is present or not should be evaluated by cinefluoroscopy and, if necessary, esophagoscopy. These strictures, if not resulting from severe anastomotic breakdown, usually respond satisfactorily to one or more dilatations.

Other, less common lesions. Less common related lesions include the pure esophageal atresia without a tracheoesophageal fistula that is found in 5% to 10% of patients in most series of esophageal atresias. These infants present symptoms similar to those of the classic variety, but on chest and abdominal radiography the blind upper esophageal pouch is associated with an airless abdomen (Fig. 10-17), demonstrating the absence of a fistula between the tracheobronchial tree and the distal eosphagus. Referral is somewhat less urgent for these children, inasmuch as the gastric secretions cannot reach the tracheobronchial tree. Their primary risk is that of aspirating saliva from the blind proximal pouch. This risk, of course, is increased if the child is fed.

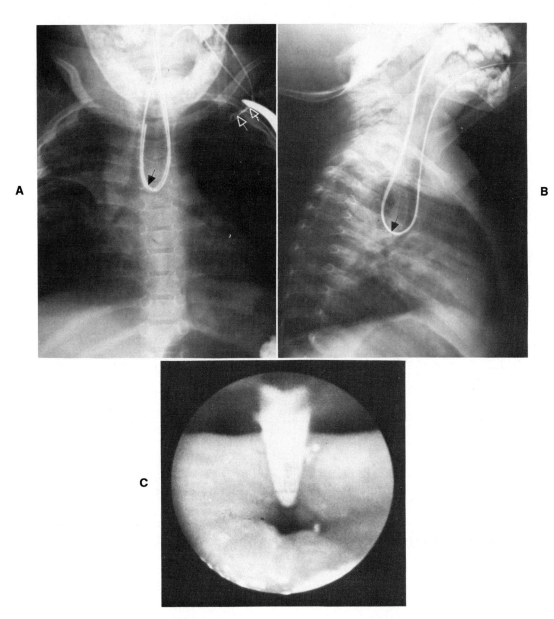

Fig. 10-16. A, Anteroposterior (AP) chest radiograph with a selective catheter and guide wire passing through the tracheoesophageal fistula (arrow). Nasoesophageal and orotracheal ends of guide wires are secured externally (open arrows). **B,** The lateral chest radiograph demonstrates the course of the selective catheter and guide wire from the nasopharynx to the esophagus, across the fistula (arrow), into the trachea through the larynx, and out the mouth. **C,** Telescopic endoscopic view of the "pit" at the site of the previous tracheoesophageal fistula. A ureteral catheter is being used to probe the pit, but no definite fistula can be identified. (**A** and **B** from Kirks, D. R., and others: A.J.R. **133:**763, 1979. Copyright © 1979, American Roentgen Ray Society.)

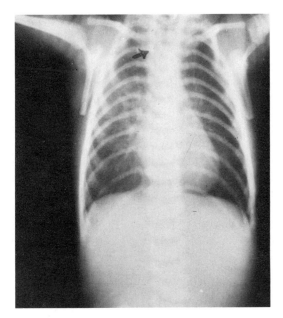

Fig. 10-17. Esophageal atresia without a tracheoesophageal fistula is diagnosed by the blind proximal esophageal pouch and the absence of air in the gastrointestinal tract. The arrow identifies the inferior aspect of the pouch. A radiopaque tube, which has pulled back from the inferior aspect of the pouch, can just be seen at the top of the film. (From Filston, H. C., and Izant, R.: The surgical neonate: evaluation and care, New York, 1978, Appleton-Century-Crofts; courtesy Dale G. Johnson, M.D., Salt Lake City, Utah.)

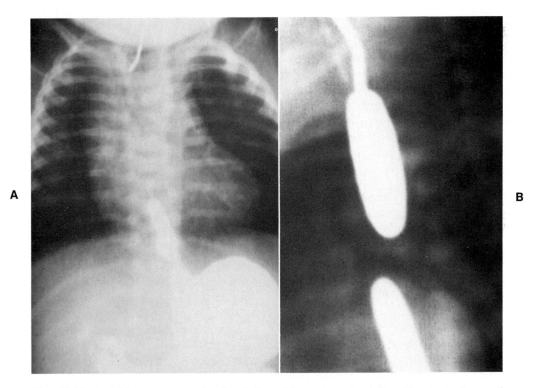

Fig. 10-18. A, Initial contrast study of an infant with esophageal atresia without a tracheoesophageal fistula, revealing a wide gap between segments. **B,** With metal dilators, segments can be stretched close to one another, eventually allowing primary repair.

When this lesion is demonstrated by the presence of the radiopaque catheter stopping in the blind proximal pouch, careful physical examination of the child becomes essential, since this variety of the lesion is more likely to be associated with other congenital anomalies and with major syndrome complexes such as chromosomal abnormalities.

Once the entity is demonstrated, referral to a major center for further therapy is indicated. The usual surgical program consists of initial gastrostomy, which may then be followed by radiographic studies to demonstrate the extent of the distal esophagus. Almost always, the gap between the two segments of esophagus is considerable on initial contrast evaluation, but no conclusion about primary repair should be made until the gastrostomy has healed enough to allow a dilator to be passed through it into the distal esophageal remnant. A second dilator is then passed orally into the proximal pouch and the two remnants stretched toward one another[76] (Fig. 10-18). Gaps of 3 to 4 vertebral bodies have been bridged after prolonged stretching by adding circular myotomy of the proximal pouch at the time of anastomosis.

The decision as to whether to strive for a primary esophageal repair rather than an interposition of the colon or stomach requires experienced judgment. Cervical esophagostomy, which may interfere with the ability to stretch the proximal pouch, should be delayed until the infant has been evaluated by a knowledgeable pediatric surgeon. In the interim, the saliva can be managed by maintaining sump suction of the proximal pouch.

Tracheoesophageal fistula without esophageal atresia and laryngotracheoesophageal cleft

The common practice of calling infants with esophageal atresia "TEFs" leads to overemphasis on an entity that really is quite rare. As noted, most infants with esophageal atresia have a blind proximal pouch and a tracheoesophageal fistula connecting the distal esophagus with the tracheobronchial tree. The N-type tracheoesophageal fistula (or N-type TEF; often called H-type TEF) accounts for only about 1% of all patients categorized as having esophageal atresia. It is probably better categorized with the equally rare laryngotracheoesophageal cleft, rather than being included as a form of esophageal atresia, which it is not.

Clinical presentation. Infants with N-type TEF experience coughing and dyspnea with feedings, abdominal distention, and recurrent aspiration pneumonia. Their symptoms may progress to cyanosis with feedings and, depending on the degree of delay in making the diagnosis, a picture of chronic lung disease.

Patients with laryngotracheoesophageal clefts present a similar picture and, depending on the extent of the cleft, may undergo a rapid downhill course to collapse.[17,84] First- and second-degree clefts, which extend through only the larynx or the larynx and cricoid, respectively, present a picture similar to the N-type TEF. Clefts extending further down the trachea (third-degree clefts) and those extending the entire length of the trachea and involving either or both bronchi (fourth-degree clefts) lead to overwhelming aspiration pneumonia in the early newborn period.

Evaluation. Any child having a combination of symptoms that includes respiratory distress with or without cyanosis with feedings should be suspected of having either an N-type TEF or a laryngotracheoesophageal cleft, and evaluation should be accomplished expeditiously. In the past, confirmation of either of these entities was made difficult by the high rate of false-negative results with either the cine-esophagogram or routine bronchoscopy for the N-type TEF. In addition, laryngoscopy may fail to demonstrate a laryngotracheoesophageal cleft, because the posterior larynx may fall together, obscuring the cleft. Although the older literature has many articles debating the advantages of various diagnostic methods, the use of the modern telescopic bronchoscope, in sizes appropriate for newborns, has made the diagnosis of either of these lesions straightforward; and the success rate should be 100%[35] (Fig. 10-19). Bronchoscopy without these instruments has a 35% failure rate and is, therefore, of limited usefulness.[7]

Preoperative care. Whenever either of these lesions is suspected, the child should be protected by having a nasogastric tube placed in the stomach for continuous decompression and all oral feedings discontinued until investigation can be accomplished. The child should not be fed through the tube, because the frequent presence of gastroesophageal reflux in the infant may lead to aspiration, even of tube feedings.

Referral. Referral should be urgent and should be to a center where optical telescopic endoscopy with an appropriate-size infant scope can be accomplished. A contrast esophagogram should not

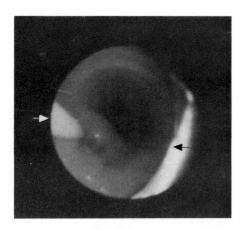

Fig. 10-19. Tracheoesophageal fistula without esophageal atresia (N-type TEF). The white arrow points to the ureteral catheter passed into the fistula from the tracheal side, and the black arrow points to the edge of the telescopic bronchoscope.

be obtained prior to telescopic esophagoscopy, because severe aspiration may occur if either of these lesions is present.

Medical versus surgical treatment. There is no medical treatment for these lesions, but if the child has already sustained severe injury to the lung from aspiration, it may be possible to protect the child from further aspiration while allowing clearing of the pneumonia. This is only possible in the N-type TEF and in first- and second-degree laryngotracheoesophageal clefts. In the more extensive clefts, continued aspiration of saliva will perpetuate the lung damage and urgent correction is indicated. If delay in surgical treatment is elected, the child should be maintained on total central parenteral nutrition and have a gastrostomy placed for constant emptying of the stomach. If clearing of secretions is a problem because of a deficient Valsalva capability of the child with the low-pressure shunt into the esophagus, a tracheostomy may be needed to allow adequate clearing of the pneumonic process.

Surgical options. Surgical therapy for the N-type TEF is generally possible through a supraclavicular cervical incision. The feasibility of this should be determined by judging the level of the fistula on esophagoscopy and bronchoscopy. Gans has pointed out that a catheter can be threaded through the fistula at the time of telescopic bronchoscopy to facilitate location of the fistula at surgery.[35] Rarely is a thoracotomy required to repair an N-type TEF.

First- and second-degree laryngotracheoesoph-

ageal clefts can usually be repaired through a lateral pharyngotomy. Until recently, only 33 cases of this lesion had been reported in the literature and only 8 successful surgical cures obtained.[17] Earlier diagnosis and a better understanding of this lesion combined with newer surgical approaches have led to improved survival in recent years.

The more extensive degrees of laryngotracheoeosphageal cleft, however, have not been repaired with such success and often the infant has such extensive damage to the lungs from the constant and immediate aspiration problems that survival is unlikely. Only earlier recognition and urgent surgical repair are likely to lead to greater survivors of this rare anomaly.

Postoperative course. The postoperative course after repair of an N-type TEF is usually short and uncomplicated. The small cervical incision usually heals readily, and the division and suture ligation of the two ends of the fistula is usually successful. The child can begin feeding a few days after surgery when a barium swallow confirms an intact repair. The incidence of recurrent tracheoesophageal fistula is far more frequent after repair of the classic esophageal atresia with distal tracheoesophageal fistula than it is after the N-type fistula repair.

For the child with minor degrees of laryngotracheoesophageal cleft, the postoperative course is also usually uncomplicated, although repair of this lesion is technically more difficult and the chances of failure greater. Postoperative bronchoscopy is, therefore, indicated to inspect the suture line before feedings are begun. If a prior tracheostomy has been necessary, it should be left in place until adequate healing of the repair has been assured.

Prognosis. The prognosis for children with these lesions depends primarily on the degree of lung damage occurring prior to repair. In the past, because of the difficulty in making the diagnosis of the N-type TEF combined with delays in thinking of it as a possibility, these children sustained frequent recurrent aspiration pneumonia and often succumbed to chronic lung disease. With the ease and safety of diagnosis afforded by the optical telescopic bronchoscope, this should no longer be a problem.

Important aspects of follow-up. Important aspects of follow-up include investigating any evidence of aspiration pneumonia for the possibility of persistence or recurrence of the fistula.

GASTROESOPHAGEAL REFLUX; HIATUS HERNIA

Gastroesophageal reflux is being recognized with increasing frequency as a cause of many symptom complexes in infancy.[19] The most obvious symptom of gastroesophageal reflux is vomiting. If the gastroesophageal reflux is severe enough, the vomiting may be so extensive that the child is unable to tolerate enough food to gain weight adequately and failure to thrive may present in the immediate newborn period as a major problem. Other presentations are those of aspiration pneumonia, asthmatic bronchitis, an allergy-type syndrome, and some unusual combinations of posturing and apparent mental aberrations.[15,50]

Since most infants with gastroesophageal reflux will not have symptoms until they are in the infant and toddler age group, an extensive discus-

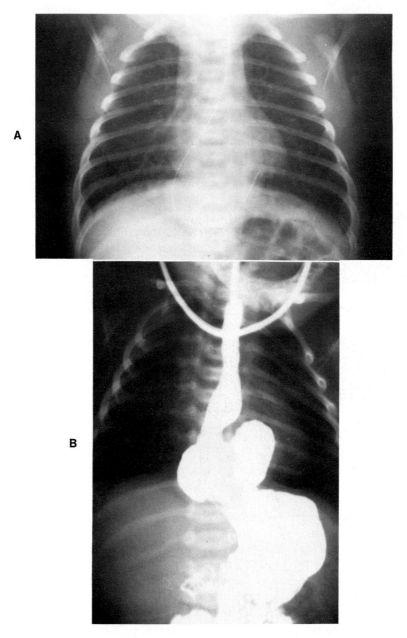

Fig. 10-20. A, Chest x-ray film showing the abnormal course of the nasogastric tube, suggesting herniation of the stomach. **B,** Contrast radiography confirming a hiatus hernia with the stomach partially herniated above the diaphragm. (Courtesy Donald Kirks, M.D., Durham, N.C.)

sion of gastroesophageal reflux is given in the infant and toddler section (Chapter 15). Nevertheless, it should be considered in the differential diagnosis of any newborn infant who has feeding difficulties represented by vomiting or regurgitation or the seeming inability to tolerate adequate amounts of feedings. It should also be considered in the differential diagnosis of any child with repeated aspiration problems or dying spells. Recently, some instances of sudden infant death syndrome have been related to gastroesophageal reflux causing laryngobronchospasm.[63]

Although hiatus hernia is thought to be a minimal part of the problem and many children with gastroesophageal reflux do not have a demonstrated hiatus hernia, in the newborn period hiatus hernia may be present and may allow the stomach to herniate into the chest (Fig. 10-20) and undergo volvulus. This possibility should be considered whenever gastric herniation through a hiatus hernia is identified. The mere presence of a hiatus hernia without gastroesophageal reflux is probably of little significance.

As indicated above, further discussion of gastroesophageal reflux can be found in Chapter 15 in the section on the infant and toddler. Additional comments regarding the complication of gastroesophageal reflux following surgery for esophageal atresia with tracheoesophageal fistula can be found throughout the book in discussions dealing with that entity.

Surgical treatment for hiatus hernia involving gastric herniation and volvulus (also known as the upside-down stomach), requires reduction of the stomach from the chest and closure of the hiatus. At the time, some procedure to ensure that adequate esophagus is held beneath the diaphragm should be added. Whether this should include a complete antireflux procedure such as fundoplication has not been determined by controlled series.

The prognosis for the child treated for a hiatus hernia should be excellent unless damage to the stomach from the volvulus and strangulation have already occurred. The long-term prognosis should be excellent if an adequate repair of the hiatus hernia is accomplished and particularly if an antireflux procedure is added. Otherwise, the child must be watched for a considerable period of time to ensure that gastroesophageal reflux does not persist or recur.

PYLORIC STENOSIS; PYLORIC ATRESIA; ANTRAL WEB

Pyloric stenosis, pyloric atresia, and antral web are lesions that are extremely rare in the newborn period. The child with *pyloric stenosis* generally begins to have symptoms at about the age of 3 weeks. Only occasionally does the child have the typical symptoms of pyloric stenosis earlier than that and very rarely before 10 days of life. Otherwise, the disease is no different in the newborn period than it is in the infant and toddler age group, and it is described at length in the infant and toddler section (Chapter 15).

Pyloric atresia is an extremely rare lesion; it has been reported in a few families but is generally an unusual lesion to encounter.[82]

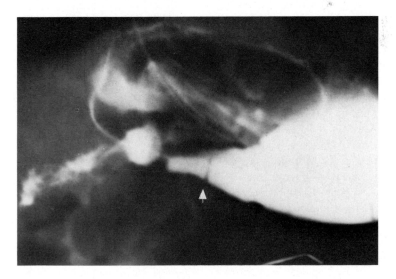

Fig. 10-21. The arrow indicates the antral web on this upper gastrointestinal study.

Antral web usually is diagnosed when an upper GI series is obtained in the infant and toddler age group by a physician looking for pyloric stenosis.[9,18,121] A line on the radiograph in the distal antrum in a child showing signs of gastric obstruction is usually interpreted as an antral web (Fig. 10-21). Further workup by endoscopy may or may not demonstrate the presence of the web. It may be hard to recognize through the gastroscope because it has a similar appearance to the entrance to the pylorus.

Many have thought that the antral web does not exist, but it has been found at surgery in children with persistent obstruction; and simple excision with pyloroplasty is usually curative. Surgery for this entity is indicated when a child with gastric outlet obstruction who has no evidence of a pyloric ''tumor'' is found to have a picture on the barium gastrogram of an antral web and fails to respond to attempts at smaller, frequent feedings over a short period of time.

DUODENAL ATRESIA; ANNULAR PANCREAS; MALROTATION

Etiology. Obstructions at the duodenal level introduce the whole subject of the common intestinal obstructions in the newborn period. Although many years have now passed since Louw and Barnard[68] and Nixon[78] demonstrated that atresias of the small intestine are generally due to vascular accidents occurring in utero, atresias of the duodenum have been left in a limbo of embryologic confusion. The etiology of duodenal atresia has been linked to the supposed solid-core phase of intestinal development, with the obstruction thought to be due to a failure of coalescence of the so-called chain of lakes.[74] This concept was previously invoked as the cause of all intestinal atresias. However, if this were true, one would expect to find duodenal atresias and stenoses occurring throughout the entire length of the duodenum; and such is not the case. When duodenal atresias or stenoses occur as isolated entities, they almost invariably occur at the area of the duodenum associated with the dorsal migration of the ventral anlage of the pancreas in association with an annular pancreas.[79] Thus, it would seem that duodenal atresia, duodenal stenosis, and annular pancreas are all part of the same phenomenon, the migration and fusion of the ventral anlage of the pancreas with the dorsal anlage to form the head of the pancreas.[105] By this theory, if the pancreas rotates and the band of tissue trailing around

the duodenum atrophies appropriately, no lesion will be produced. However, if pancreatic tissue is wrapped about the duodenum, either stenosis from an *annular pancreas* will be found and the pancreatic tissue wrapping the duodenum will be noted at surgery, or the pressure from the pancreatic tissue will cause necrosis, gangrene, atrophy, and atresia, either in the form of a mucosal web or a complete loss of the full-thickness bowel wall. In any case, the lesion will be found in the area of the second and third portion of the duodenum, the site of the migration of the pancreas.

The other common association with duodenal atresia and stenosis is that of *malrotation*. When the infant has complete obstruction of the duodenum in the immediate newborn period, annular pancreas and malrotation are approximately equal in incidence as the underlying cause. Malrotation is probably the most common etiologic entity for most intestinal atresias—a point that is little emphasized in the literature. When one looks for malrotation in association with atresias of the jejunum and ileum, one finds this association quite frequently (Fig. 10-22). If in utero vascular accidents are the causes of atresia, as they seem to be, then an entity such as malrotation, which oc-

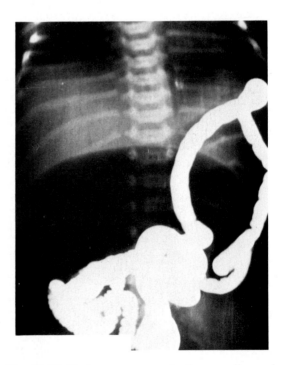

Fig. 10-22. Barium enema examination revealing malrotation as the probable cause of this upper gastrointestinal obstruction (jejunal atresia) in an infant with a complete bowel obstruction.

curs commonly and causes varying degrees of ischemic necrosis, would be expected to play a significant role in the etiology of atresia. Thus, to be safe, one must look at every obstruction in the infant as a potential malrotation with its implication of mesenteric volvulus and strangulation and not be lulled into complacency by such descriptive phrases as "partial malrotation" and "malrotation of the cecum or colon"—terms often used by the radiologist to describe the findings on barium enema examination. Malrotation should always be seen for what it is, a malfixation of the base of the mesentery with its attendant threat of volvulus of the entire small bowel mesentery and ischemic necrosis of the entire small intestine. Malrotation is a major cause of obstruction throughout infancy and the early childhood period, and a more extensive discussion of its anatomic defects will be found in the infant and toddler section (Chapter 15).

In the newborn period, malrotation must be seen as the underlying cause of many intestinal obstructions that present as duodenal, jejunal, and ileal atresias. In this light, one must consider the seemingly simple obstructions as potential dynamic ones in which further ischemic necrosis of the bowel may be occurring with loss of additional digestive and absorptive function. To explain this further, a simple atresia may be seen as one in which some pressure necrosis of the

segment of intestine occurred during development and left the child with either a weblike diaphragm across the bowel lumen, producing obstruction, or a complete segmental loss of the entire bowel. Nontheless, this is a stable situation and at birth the child is not at risk of losing additional length of intestine. However, if malrotation is the cause of such an atresia, the volvulus of the mesentery may still be strangling loops of intestine and further loss of vital intestinal length may occur if treatment is delayed. Delay in treatment of simple atresias may be warranted if the child has underlying respiratory or infectious problems that would make anesthesia and surgery especially hazardous. Before such delay is allowed, however, proof that malrotation is not involved as the underlying cause of the atresia must be obtained.

Clinical presentation. These duodenal obstructions present with a set of findings that are clearly recognizable. Often the mother will have hydramnios because of the inability of the swallowed amniotic fluid to reach the infant's reabsorptive segment of the intestine. This is true regardless of the cause of the duodenal obstruction. These children almost invariably vomit bile-stained fluid or have sizable amounts of material on gastric aspirate. The color of this fluid may vary from a golden yellow to a bright green. Abdominal distention may be minimal, since only the stomach and first and second portions of the duodenum

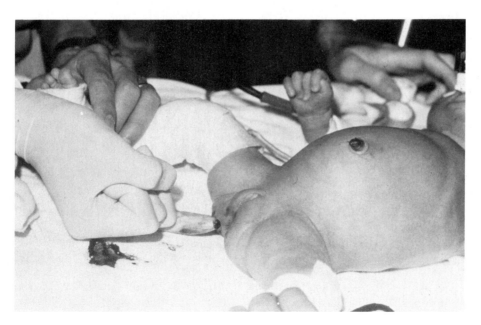

Fig. 10-23. Grossly bloody stool in this distended infant with bilious vomiting is an almost certain sign of volvulus secondary to malrotation.

are likely to distend. These organs often are intermittently decompressed by vomiting. Meconium passage may be delayed but the passage of meconium does not demonstrate intestinal patency, since the vascular accident leading to atresia may occur well after meconium begins moving through the intestinal tract. Thus, only the passage of transitional stools, air, or contrast media instilled from above clearly demonstrates continuity of the intestinal tract.

If malrotation is the cause of the duodenal obstruction, generalized abdominal distention may occur as the obstructed distal bowel loops, which are becoming ischemic, fill with fluid. Occasionally, these infants may pass bloody stools, which, in association with obstructive symptoms and bile-stained gastric content, should be an absolute indication of the cause of the problem (Fig. 10-23). This is no time to consider swallowed maternal blood as the cause of bloody stool in the infant.

Evaluation. Evaluation entails recognizing the significance of hydramnios in the mother and re-

sponding urgently to the presence of bile-stained vomiting or gastric aspirate in the child. Plain abdominal radiographs should be obtained, and these usually show the classic "double bubble" film representing dilatation of the stomach and first portions of the duodenum with complete obstruction beyond. This film is generally associated with duodenal atresia or annular pancreas, but from the preceding discussion it becomes obvious that any duodenal atresia may be malrotation until proved otherwise (Fig. 10-24). If a "double bubble" appearance is present on the plain film, no further workup is necessary if the infant can tolerate immediate surgery. However, if delay in surgery would be to the child's benefit, further radiographic evaluation should be undertaken. Although we generally have considered an upper GI series to be the best means of demonstrating the presence of malrotation by revealing the configuration of the C-loop of the duodenum and ensuring that the bowel crosses well back to the left behind the stomach to a normal position of the ligament of Treitz (Fig. 10-25), this procedure

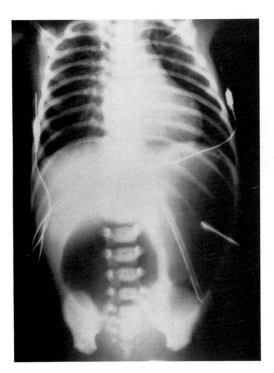

Fig. 10-24. Typical "double bubble" film of an infant with duodenal obstruction. Note the absence of other air in the abdomen and the marked dilatation of the duodenum.

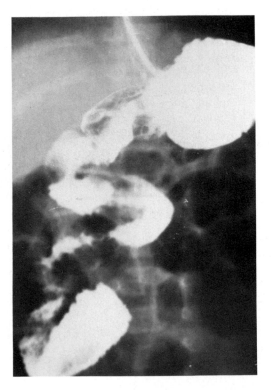

Fig. 10-25. Upper gastrointestinal examination revealing the failure of the duodenal C-loop to complete the crossover to the left upper quadrant and the jejunal pattern developing to the right of the spine. This demonstration of malrotation on the upper GI series is classic.

is impossible to achieve in complete duodenal obstruction. The barium enema, which may be fraught with hazardous misinterpretation, is in this instance the procedure of choice. When this procedure is chosen, great care must be taken to ensure that the pattern of the large bowel is entirely normal and that the cecum lies well down in the right lower quadrant and is of normal configuration (Fig. 10-26). Ideally, the appendix and ileocecal area should be identified to ensure that the loop of bowel interpreted as being cecum is, in fact, that entity. Even in the hands of the most experienced pediatric radiologist, misinterpretation of this configuration has led to missing malrotation.

Medical versus surgical treatment. These lesions all require surgical correction, but the simple atresias unassociated with malrotation can be managed medically for long periods of time if the infant's underlying condition would make surgery particularly hazardous. Under these circumstances, good decompression of the gastrointestinal tract should be achieved with a two-

tube system utilizing a sump tube in the esophagus and a drainage tube for the stomach. This ensures that swallowed air will not be trapped under the dome of the abdomen and continue to distend the child's intestine. Total parenteral nutrition can then sustain the child until his underlying condition improves and surgery is possible.

Surgical options. Surgical procedures utilized to correct duodenal atresia, duodenal stenosis, and annular pancreas depend on the degree of duodenal loss. For simple weblike atresias that do not involve the full thickness of the wall, a simple longitudinal incision with excision of the web and transverse closure of the incision may be all that is necessary. Usually, duodenal atresias and annular pancreas can be bypassed by a duodenoduodenostomy, anastomosing the proximal dilated portion of the duodenum to the next adjacent distal portion of the duodenum by a straightforward intestinal anastomosis. When the gap between the proximal and distal segments of duodenum is too great, a loop of proximal jejunum can be brought over to the duodenum and a duo-

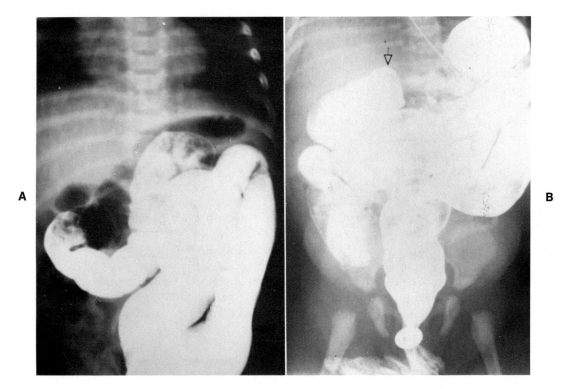

A

B

Fig. 10-26. A, Malrotation is clearly defined on this barium enema examination. **B** is more difficult to interpret. The arrow indicates the cecum in the right upper quadrant beneath the liver, but the filling of small bowel loops and overlapping of the sigmoid give the appearance that a normal colon pattern exists.

denojejunostomy achieved. Gastrojejunostomy is a less favored bypass procedure, because it fails to decompress the proximal duodenum, with its biliary and pancreatic secretions, adequately; in addition, it leaves the child with a potential for a marginal ulcer at the anastomosis.

The standard procedure for correction of malrotation is the Ladd procedure, named after Dr. William E. Ladd, one of the founding fathers of American pediatric surgery, who did so much to elucidate malrotation as a devastating malformation in infants.[62] This procedure consists of dividing numerous adhesions that hold the bowel in the malrotated position, in the process of which, adhesions holding the duodenum in an accordion and obstructive configuration are lysed. The duodenum is stretched out as much as possible so that it runs essentially down toward the right lower quadrant of the abdomen. The transverse colon and ascending colon are freed of adhesions and placed into the left side of the abdomen. This maneuver essentially opens the mesentery, broadening its base and putting it in a totally nonrotated configuration, eliminating the superimposition of the two points of normal fixation over the base of the superior mesenteric artery, the condition that leads to volvulus. Because the cecum ends up on the left side of the abdomen, appendectomy is almost always performed and may be accomplished either by standard amputation of the appendix and inversion of its base into a purse string in the cecum or by total intussusception of the entire appendix into itself and into the cecum with ligation of the base and purse string closure.[12,64] A gastrotomy is almost always performed and a Foley balloon catheter passed around the duodenum well into the jejunum. The balloon is then inflated and the catheter withdrawn so that if any webs were produced by the pressure of the malrotation on the duodenum, they will be demonstrated by the withdrawing of the balloon.[92,95] If such webs are found, duodenotomy is performed and the webs excised. The gastrotomy may be closed or a gastrostomy tube sutured in place and brought out through an abdominal stab wound.

Postoperative course. For simple atresias associated with an annular pancreas, the postoperative course may be benign and of short duration. Often these children can begin feedings by the end of the first postoperative week and will progress quite readily. However, others will show signs of delayed gastric emptying secondary to the persistent dilatation of the duodenum. It is probably best to keep the child well decompressed for a week or two to allow the duodenum to return to a more normal size and configuration and regain muscular tone. We prefer to test the child's ability to handle gastric secretion by elevating the orogastric or gastrostomy tube above the infant. The tube is attached to an open syringe barrel (see Fig. 5-1), which allows a safety chamber for regurgitation of retained gastric secretions and at the same time prevents continued drainage of all of the child's gastric secretions. If gastric secretions are obviously passing through into the intestine, small increments of feedings can then be added to the syringe barrel and rapid progress then achieved. Parenteral nutritional support through either a peripheral or central line should be provided if a delay in the resumption of gastrointestinal feeding is anticipated. We prefer to begin parenteral nutrition for all infants immediately following recovery from the acute surgical challenge, so that the infants do not sustain prolonged nitrogen depletion.

When malrotation has been involved with a duodenal obstruction, the postoperative course is highly variable, depending on the degree of bowel ischemia and intestinal loss. Obviously, when great segments of the intestine are lost, considerable time will be necessary for the short intestine to adapt to the osmotic demands of normal feedings. Nevertheless, with proper management, even infants who have lost all but a few centimeters of the intestine may adapt and be able to resume reasonably normal gastrointestinal function if given enough time and parenteral nutritional support. If the ileocecal valve has been spared, children may adapt with even as few as 6 to 7 cm of small intestinal length remaining. Wilmore has demonstrated that 30 cm of remaining intestine is generally adequate in most instances and that children with as little as 10 to 15 cm with an intact ileocecal valve can occasionally adapt with time. Such adaptation requires marked hypertrophy of the villous lining, and achieving this hypertrophy takes considerable time and gradual reintroduction of osmotic loads. Our plan of management for intestinal problems is discussed in general terms in Chapter 5 in the section of general considerations.

Prognosis. The prognosis for children with duodenal obstruction secondary to simple atresias is excellent, and they have little in the way of long-term problems. Problems that do occur are limited almost exclusively to those of intestinal adhesions with obstruction, which are common to all laparotomies. The prognosis for the child with intestinal loss due to malrotation and volvulus is dependent on the length of the intestine surviving, the functional viability of that intestine, and its ability to adapt over a period of time.

Important aspects of follow-up. Recognition of the constant risk of adhesive bowel obstruction in any child with a past history of a laparotomy should be of primary concern. In the immediate neonatal period hyperbilirubinemia is common in children with upper gastrointestinal tract obstructions and should be carefully monitored. The cause of this has been thought to be either a partial obstruction of flow through the common bile duct into the obstructed duodenum or some interference with the enterohepatic circulation of bile.

Although the Ladd procedure does not fix the bowel in any particular pattern, the likelihood of its finding its way back into the fixed configuration that leads to volvulus is low; volvulus following the Ladd procedure is an unusual occurrence.[11,29,111] The most important aspect of follow-

up for these children is proper reintroduction of gastrointestinal feeding.

JEJUNOILEAL ATRESIA

Etiology. As noted in the preceding discussion, atresias are generally thought to be due to vascular accidents occurring in utero. The causes of such vascular accidents are multiple, but malrotation and intussusception are two of the known causes of such ischemic necrosis. Anything causing kinking or pressure on the developing intestine may lead to pressure necrosis with either a mucosal necrosis and formation of a weblike scar or a loss of a complete segment of the bowel with or without the accompanying mesentery. Atresias due to acute angulation of the duodenojejunal junction at the ligament of Treitz, causing pressure necrosis and a web across the lumen, have been found. Malrotation may cause one or more areas of atresia to form, either because of pressure on the bowel loop itself from a mild volvulus or because of ischemia from vascular obstruction in the strangulated mesentery. Atresias may be single, isolated lesions or multiples ones, occurring

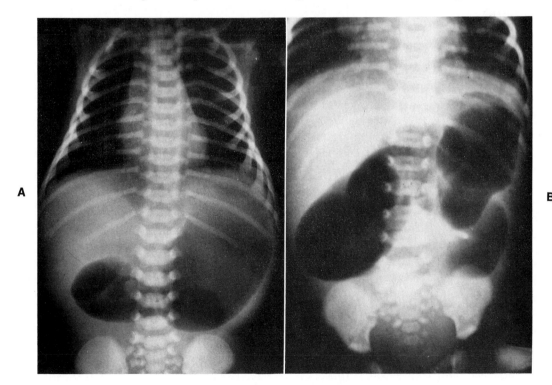

Fig. 10-27. A, A complete upper gastrointestinal obstruction is revealed on this plain abdominal x-ray film of an infant with jejunal atresia. As can be seen in Fig. 10-22, malrotation is one possible cause for such an occurrence. **B,** Radiograph of another infant with a high intestinal obstruction slightly further along the jejunum than in **A.** (From Filston, H. C., and Izant, R.: The surgical neonate: evaluation and care, New York, 1978, Appleton-Century-Crofts.)

throughout the entire small intestine. Multiple atresias are often associated with malrotation.

Clinical presentation. These entities generally present with a combination of bile-stained vomiting or gastric aspirate with abdominal distention, depending on the level of the atresia. Very high jejunal atresias may be associated with hydramnios in the mother. The passage of meconium does not rule out an atresia, but simply indicates that the vascular accident that underlies the atresia occurred later in gestation than the onset of passage of meconium through the intestine.

Evaluation and differential diagnosis. Evaluation consists of plain abdominal radiographs, which usually demonstrate intestinal obstruction with dilated bowel loops and air fluid levels on the upright film (Fig. 10-27). The level of obstruction can be estimated by the number of distended loops present on the film.

When only a few loops of dilated bowel are present and the obstruction is obviously high, further workup is unnecessary and the child can be taken directly to surgery for repair. If the child's underlying state of health makes surgery particularly hazardous so that delay would be beneficial for the child, further evaluation to rule out malrotation as the cause of the atresia must be undertaken (See the previous discussion on duodenal atresia.) When multiple loops of dilated bowel suggest a more distal obstruction, differentiation from large bowel obstructions may not be possible without further evaluation, which should generally consist of a contrast enema study. Since the differential diagnosis of distal atresias includes meconium ileus, Hirschsprung's disease, meconium plug, and small left colon syndrome, some estimate as to which of these entities is likely to be present must be made before the decision regarding the contrast enema is made. Particularly when meconium ileus is suspected, use of a water-soluble contrast material such as Gastrografin will be beneficial. (See the discussion on meconium ileus later in this chapter for elaboration on this point.)

Medical versus surgical treatment. If the plain x-ray films demonstrate a distal bowel obstruction and the contrast enema studies show a small, unused colon not participating in the dilatation, the diagnosis of ileal atresia can be made and surgery accomplished if the infant's underlying condition permits. Otherwise, the child can be sustained with decompression and nutritional support until any underlying condition making anesthesia

and surgery unduly hazardous has been corrected.

Surgical options. Surgical correction involves a simple end-to-end reanastomosis of bowel segments. However, there is usually marked disparity between the size of the proximal dilated distended loop of bowel and the distal, relatively unused segments (Fig. 10-28). Although an anastomosis can be readily accomplished between such disparate bowel segments, it usually is functionally inadequate. The overdistended distal end of the proximal segment may fail to contract well; when it does do so, it may dissipate a great deal of its peristaltic energy against the blind end of the distended loop. This situation is similar to the pragmatic problem of opening a clotted intravenous catheter using various sizes of syringes. It has generally been found that the small tuberculin syringe is most effective for such a procedure because all of the pressure exerted on the plunger of the syringe is directed at the hole in the needle. When a large syringe such as a 30- or 50-ml syringe is chosen, much of the pressure exerted on the plunger is dissipated against the large area of the distal barrel with only part of the pressure being directed at the needle hole. Similarly, the overdistended blind end of the proximal bowel absorbs much of the peristaltic force with only a fraction of the force being directed at the small anastomosis. Generally, therefore, it is best to resect a portion of the proximal bowel so that a less disparate anastomosis can be accomplished and the bowel utilized for the proximal segment of the anastomosis has better tone and presents less of an area for dissipation of peristaltic force.

Such resection may not be achievable when the atresia is high in the intestine, so that resection of the most proximal jejunum or duodenum would be required to achieve a proximal bowel of more normal caliber. Under these circumstances a prolonged period of postoperative nonfunction is to be anticipated, and good decompression of the proximal bowel must be achieved to allow toning up and shrinkage. We have found that this is best accomplished by placing a sump-type tube in the esophagus to minimize the amount of swallowed air reaching the stomach in combination with gastrostomy drainage of both the air and fluid from the stomach. A gastrostomy should almost invariably be performed when such a high atresia is encountered to allow efficient decompression of gas from the stomach. Three weeks of decompression may be needed before such children can begin enteral feedings. Prior to feed-

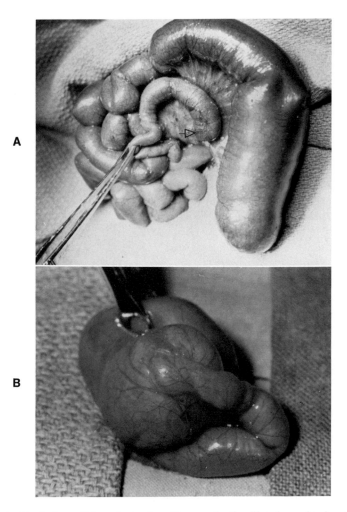

Fig. 10-28. A, Typical small bowel atresia with a markedly dilated proximal segment, a gap in the mesentery, and a much narrow "unused" distal segment. Note the marked disparity in the size of the two segments. The arrow marks the proximal end of the segment distal to the atresia. **B,** Intrinsic web atresia of the proximal jejunum. These lesions can often be handled by longitudinal enterotomy, excision of the web, and transverse closure.

ing, an upper gastrointestinal contrast study should be performed to ascertain that the anastomosis is open and that material passes readily through it from the proximal bowel.

For more distal atresias, such prolonged periods of nonfunction are less likely if resection of the overdistended segment has been possible. Gastrointestinal feedings can usually be started in these children by the end of the first week after surgery.

Complications. Complications generally are those of any bowel anastomosis and include leakage, stenosis, and prolonged failure to function. In the hands of experienced surgeons such problems are unusual.

One problem that may be troublesome and unique to the anastomosis of disparate-size bowel loops is that of the late blind loop syndrome. This was a common problem following anastomosis when the usual procedure was a side-to-side anastomosis, as originally advocated by Ladd and Gross.[40,62] Since the lumenal contents were being pushed distally in the proximal loop of intestine, they would encounter the blind end of the proximal loop. Only by spillover did they pass through the side-hole anastomosis. This situation led to continued pressure against the blind loop, further distending and elongating it until an area of sequestered bowel was developed that contained masses of nonprogressing lumenal content. Bacterial flora changes would then occur that interfered with the bile-acid, bile-salt balance, producing a catharsis-like effect on the distal intestine. The children often had frequent loose bowel movements and malabsorption syndrome. This kind of problem can still occur with the end-to-end anastomosis of disparate bowel loops because the overdistended proximal loop may be stretched to eventually produce a configuration similar to the side-to-side anastomosis.[79] Thus, the child who initially adapts to the surgical procedure and subsequently, months or years later, develops a picture of intestinal hurry and malabsorption should be investigated for such a complication.

Finally, the general problem of adhesive bowel obstruction must be again considered for any patient having had a previous laparotomy.

When multiple atresias are encountered, numerous bowel anastomoses may be required and some of the segments of intestine may not function well for prolonged periods. In addition, the overall length of remaining intestine may be inadequate and a short bowel syndrome postoperatively may require prolonged periods of adaptation with interim total parenteral nutritional support. Specific enzyme deficiencies such as those of lactase and disaccharidase are common following any intestinal problem in the newborn. The discussion of reintroduction of feedings in Chapter 5 in the section on general considerations should be consulted.

MECONIUM ILEUS

Clinical presentation. The term *meconium ileus* in most common usage implies the functional obstruction of the distal ileum due to inspissated intestinal contents in a child with mucoviscidosis or cystic fibrosis. The presentation of this disorder will differ from that of the simple intestinal atresias or functional colonic obstructions such as the meconium plug and small left colon syndrome or Hirschsprung's disease in that the abdomen is frequently distended at the time of birth (Fig. 10-29). In any case, distention is a major component of the illness, and bile-stained vomiting may ensue very early or somewhat later in the neonatal period. Meconium is never passed.

Evaluation. Plain abdominal radiographs have many similarities to those of distal small bowel and large bowel obstructions but show three distinct differences: a triad suggesting meconium ileus as the cause. These are disparity in the size of the distended loops, a muddy or bubbly appearance to the intestinal contents, and a sparsity or absence of air fluid levels on the upright film[71]

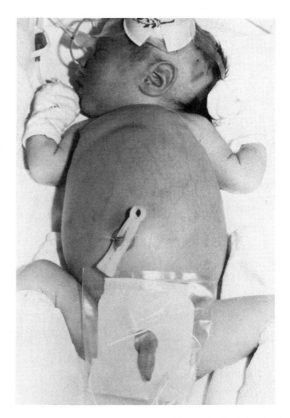

Fig. 10-29. This infant, born with marked abdominal distention, subsequently proved to have meconium ileus.

(Fig. 10-30). Thus, meconium ileus becomes the most likely diagnosis in the infant distended at birth who fails to pass meconium and who has evidence of a distal bowel obstruction with the triad of roentgenographic findings.

Medical versus surgical treatment. Such findings should then lead one directly to a full-strength Gastrografin contrast enema study in an attempt to reflux the material well up into the ileum. This procedure causes an inrush of extracellular fluid along the osmotic gradient to the hyperosmolar contrast material and eventual evacuation of the inspissated meconium.[80,118] Several attempts at filling and emptying may be required over a period of time to achieve successful correction. Because the hyperosmolar contrast medium leaches huge quantities of body fluid into the intestinal lumen, the child should be protected by a well-functioning, stable intravenous cannula and should be given sufficient replacement of balanced electrolyte solution to maintain an adequate urine output over the next 24 to 36 hours.[96] Absorption of the water-soluble contrast material with sub-

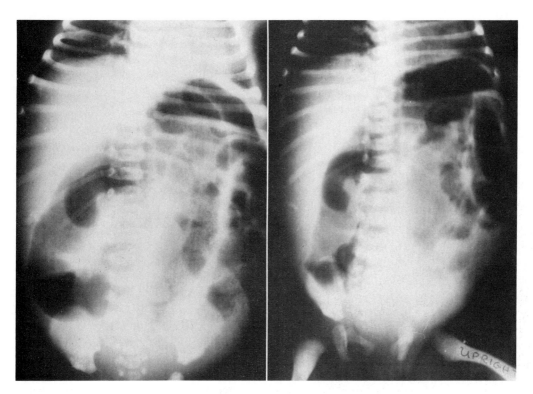

Fig. 10-30. Abdominal radiographs from an infant with meconium ileus. The triad of findings are disparity in the distention of the bowel loops, a bubbly or muddy appearance to the luminal contents, and sparsity of air fluid levels on the upright film. (From Filston, H. C., and Izant, R.: The surgical neonate: evaluation and care, New York, 1978, Appleton-Century-Crofts.)

sequent excretion through the kidneys will lead to a diuresis that will give a false impression of adequate hydration in the face of great losses into the intestinal lumen. The most critical periods are immediately following introduction of the Gastrografin into the ileal lumen and following the diuretic phase caused by excretion of the material. One should generally give the child a push of 20 ml/kg of balanced salt solution on introduction of the contrast material and then run it at two to three times the child's maintenance rate, monitoring the urine output carefully. Adjustments in the rate of intravenous fluid administration are made to keep the child's urine output at 2 ml/kg/hr.

Gastrografin has been the most consistently successful material for freeing up the inspissated meconium. Many substances were tried prior to the use of Gastrografin without consistent success. The small amount of detergent (polysorbate 80) breaks up the adhesions of the sticky meconium to the bowel wall and allows the hygroscopic effect of the hyperosmolar Gastrografin to liquify

the lumenal contents (Fig. 10-31). The introduction of barium or less concentrated water-soluble materials prior to the use of Gastrografin may prevent the Gastrografin from reaching the distal ileum and thus make the procedure unsuccessful.

Surgical procedures for this lesion were associated with a great deal of morbidity prior to the introduction by Bishop and Koop[13] of their ileo-ileostomy. If a Gastrografin enema is unsuccessful in overcoming the obstruction, if perforation or peritonitis make a Gastrografin enema contraindicated, or if a completely atretic segment of bowel makes decompression impossible, surgery should consist of a Bishop-Koop type of procedure, which involves resecting any nonviable or functionally questionable segments of intestine, bringing the distal ileum out as a "stovepipe" ileostomy and bringing the proximal ileum into the ileostomy segment end-to-side. This procedure allows the luminal stream to pass preferentially into the distal bowel, provides a vent to decompress the intestine, and facilitates irrigations

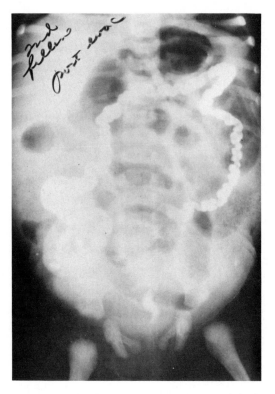

Fig. 10-31. Gastrografin enema on the infant shown in Fig. 10-30. Note the tiny colon with its beadlike inspissated mucus superimposed on the dilated small bowel. Successful evacuation of the inspissated meconium from the distal ileum was accomplished after several fillings and emptyings of the Gastrografin. (From Filston, H. C., and Izant, R.: The surgical neonate: evaluation and care, New York, 1978, Appleton-Century-Crofts.)

with material such as Gastrografin or acetylcysteine (Mucomyst).

Postoperative course. The postoperative period is usually uneventful if a successful procedure has been accomplished, but often several days of irrigations are required to free the inspissated meconium. Once the bowel is unobstructed, the ileostomy may close spontaneously or can be closed by a local procedure not requiring laparotomy.

Prognosis. The long-term outlook for the child depends on the degree of lung involvement with the basic underlying disease of cystic fibrosis. These children may have ongoing malabsorptive problems and may have recurrent intestinal obstructions from inspissated bowel content if pancreatic enzyme supplements are not provided. Meconium ileus equivalent is an obstruction of the distal bowel secondary to inspissated bowel

content occurring after the newborn period.[25] Although cystic fibrosis is still associated with a short life span and chronic illness, many children cared for in centers specializing in the care of cystic fibrosis are living longer and more satisfactory lives through modern therapy.

MECONIUM PLUG SYNDROME; SMALL LEFT COLON SYNDROME

The meconium plug and small left colon syndromes are being recognized with increasing frequency. They involve the inspissation of meconium in the distal colon.[22,26,31,112] Although some authors have considered these lesions to be distinct and separate entities, they appear to be part of a spectrum of disease involving functional obstruction of the distal colon with inspissation of mucus and meconium. The small left colon syndrome has a very distinctive pattern involving the distal colon from the splenic flexure to the rectum. The colon proximal to this level is dilated, whereas that segment distal to the splenic flexure is narrow and spastic in appearance.

Clinical presentation. These children usually fail to pass meconium. They gradually become distended. Vomiting, including bilious vomiting, may follow. Vomiting is usually a later symptom than in the higher intestinal obstructions. Attempts to stimulate passage of meconium with thermometers, tubes, and rectal examinations are usually unsuccessful or result in the passage of only a small amount of inspissated mucus and meconium. These maneuvers should generally be avoided, because they may lead to injury to the anorectum and they may mask the presence of Hirschsprung's disease. Infants of diabetic mothers have a high incidence of the meconium plug and small left colon syndromes.[85] Some have thought this incidence to be due to the differential effects of glucagon on various bowel segments; glucagon may be secreted in response to hypoglycemia in the infant of the diabetic mother.[58]

Evaluation and differential diagnosis. Plain abdominal radiographs may show a pattern difficult to differentiate from that of meconium ileus. There may be bubbly-appearing material in the bowel loops, but there is usually not a disparity in size; and if marked proximal distention occurs, air fluid levels should be present (Fig. 10-32).

This lesion is almost impossible to differentiate from Hirschsprung's disease on plain abdominal radiographs, and Hirschsprung's disease should

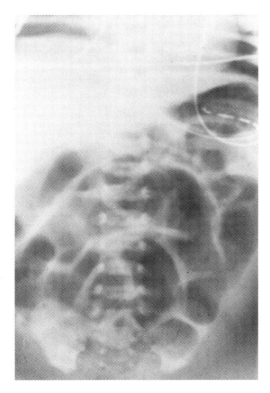

Fig. 10-32. Plain abdominal radiograph of an infant with small left colon syndrome showing multiple dilated loops of bowel. Remember that the large bowel cannot be distinguished from the small bowel on plain radiographs in an infant.

always be suspected in any child with symptoms of a large bowel obstruction that proves to be functional. The fact that the infant is one of a diabetic mother lessens the chance of Hirschsprung's disease and enhances the probability of meconium plug or small left colon syndrome. Nevertheless, Hirschsprung's disease may coexist in these infants.

The realization that these entities are functional does not lessen the risks of an obstructed bowel. Any cause of bowel obstruction can lead to the complications of proximal perforation, pseudo-membranous enterocolitis, or generalized stasis. These complications are contributed to by the buildup of bacteria in the obstructed intestinal lumen, destruction of the mucosal barrier, and possible ischemia of the antimesenteric wall of the bowel secondary to overdistention. These factors occurring in the immune deficient newborn may lead to overwhelming sepsis.

Care of these infants should include adequate decompression with oroesophageal and orogastric tubes (see Chapter 6 in the section on general considerations), maintenance of fluid and electrolyte balance by means of intravenous therapy, and usually coverage with broad-spectrum antibiotics to prevent sepsis from the intralumenal bacterial stasis.

Once the plain abdominal films have demonstrated a distal bowel obstruction, contrast enema studies should be obtained (Fig. 10-33). Because of concern that water-soluble contrast medium may mask the presence of Hirschsprung's disease, our pediatric radiologists prefer to begin these studies with barium. Once the meconium plug or small left colon syndrome is recognized, they then change to water-soluble contrast medium to aid the evacuation of the inspissated material. These enemas should be continued until the dilated proximal bowel is encountered. They need not be pushed further proximally. Attention must be paid to the fluid shifts that occur secondary to the presence of hyperosmolar water-soluble contrast medium in the intestinal lumen. Although these shifts are lessened by using less concentrated formulas, attention to fluid replacement is still required. The further proximally the enema progresses and the more contrast material utilized, the greater will be the fluid shift and consequent need for replacement. This replacement should be accomplished with balanced electrolyte solution rather than hypotonic electrolyte or sugar water solutions.

Referral. Because of the constant need to differentiate these entities from Hirschsprung's disease, because of the critical fluid management required to offset the effects of the water-soluble contrast material, and because even children with meconium plug and small left colon syndromes may require colostomy decompression, these children are best handled in a center that can provide experienced pediatric radiologic consultation as well as pediatric surgical support. Early referral will usually prevent the complications of perforation and generalized sepsis.

Medical versus surgical treatment. Although water-soluble contrast enemas will lead to evacuation in most of these infants, some will fail to evacuate or, having evacuated, will fail to maintain decompression despite repeated water-soluble enemas. Why some infants with small left colon syndrome have a persistent spastic obstructed colon is not yet understood. Nevertheless, some of these infants require temporary colostomy by-

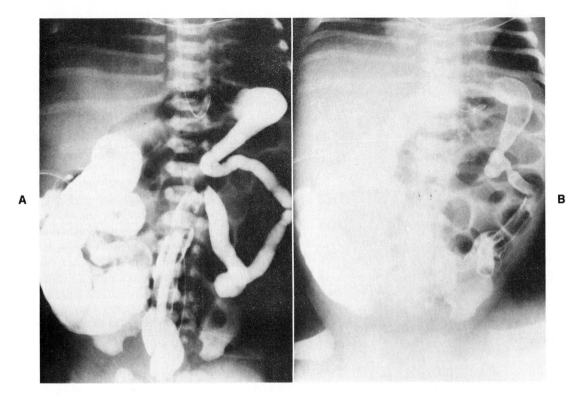

Fig. 10-33. A, Gastrografin enema study of an infant with small left colon syndrome. **B,** Emptying film on the same infant. (From Filston, H. C., and Izant, R.: The surgical neonate: evaluation and care, New York, 1978, Appleton-Century-Crofts.)

pass. Following subsequent rectal biopsy to rule out Hirschsprung's disease, they can usually be successfully relieved of their enterostomies at 3 to 4 months of age.

Surgical options. Surgical options are few; the standard surgical procedure is a decompressing loop colostomy performed at the transition between the dilated proximal bowel and the spastic distal segment. Colostomy in an infant is a significantly different procedure from that in an adult and requires considerably more suturing of the bowel loop to the abdominal wall.

Postoperative course and complications. Postoperatively, the hospital stay is usually short and the complications of colostomy when properly performed in a child are few. Occasional wound separations and infections occur that delay discharge. Rectal biopsy should generally be performed after a few months of colostomy bypass to ensure that Hirschsprung's disease does not underlie the functional obstruction. If the rectal biopsy proves to contain ganglion cells, the colostomy can usually be successfully closed.

Important aspects of follow-up. When the child responds to water-soluble enema therapy and evacuates the inspissated material, it is mandatory that the physician follow the child carefully to ensure that he maintains normal bowel function. Any persistence or recurrence of the constipation pattern should lead to reevaluation for Hirschsprung's disease. This should begin with a barium enema study and progress to rectal biopsy if indicated. These factors are stressed in the following discussion on Hirschsprung's disease. Particularly if the child is not an infant of a diabetic mother, some underlying cause for the inspissation should be sought. This cause will usually prove to be Hirschsprung's disease; but on rare occasions, cystic fibrosis presents with meconium obstruction in the colon. The more usual presentation of cystic fibrosis in a newborn, of course, is meconium ileus. It cannot be overstated that any child who has failed to pass meconium in the first 24 hours of life must be suspected of having Hirschsprung's disease until proved otherwise.

HIRSCHSPRUNG'S DISEASE
(AGANGLIONIC MEGACOLON)

Hirschsprung's disease is the most common cause of distal bowel obstruction in the newborn. Swenson has shown that 95% of infants with Hirschsprung's disease fail to pass meconium during the first 24 hours in the nursery, and his studies and studies by others of normal newborns have shown that 95% of normal newborns do, in fact, pass meconium spontaneously within the first 24 hours.[21] Premature infants who are otherwise well may show a delay of up to 36 hours; but by that time 90% of them have passed meconium. Sick tiny premature infants in the intensive care nursery may have considerable delay without implying any abnormality of the bowel. Thus, particularly the otherwise healthy full-term infant who fails to pass meconium within the first 24 hours has a high likelihood of having an abnormality of the bowel. Among these abnormalities, Hirschsprung's disease is prominent.

Misunderstandings about Hirschsprung's disease are still widely prevalent. Many still feel that this is a disease of the older child, whereas the above-noted statistics point to the fact that the vast majority of infants with Hirschsprung's disease will be symptomatic from birth. Others still make the mistake of thinking that the megacolon is the diseased bowel, whereas the distal narrowed bowel is the segment that is aganglionic. A brief discussion of the pathophysiology of Hirschsprung's disease may help to clarify and explain the clinical findings.

Pathophysiology. The bowel in Hirschsprung's disease is entirely normal except for an absence of the ganglion cells in the myenteric plexus and submucosal plexus of the intestine. These cells reach the intestine from their neural-crest origin in the embryo by migrating along the vagus nerve to that part of the bowel supplied by the vagus nerve and along pelvic parasympathetic nerves to the parts of the bowel supplied by these nerves.[51] Thus, the vagal distribution extends from the hypopharynx to the transverse colon just proximal to the splenic flexure, and the pelvic parasympathetic supply extends from this point to the anus. Although a theoretical "skip" area could exist between the distal-most vagal supply and the proximal pelvic parasympathetic supply, skip areas have only been reported on a few occasions in the literature.[72,114,115] The most typical pattern is that in which the ganglion cells are present all the way to the sigmoid colon; then, at some point in the sigmoid colon, they are absent and are absent on down to the anus. In fewer than 25% of patients the ganglion cells are absent proximal to the lowermost portion of the descending colon, and in less than 8% they are absent in the entire colon or more proximally in the intestine.[57]

The association of the ganglion cells with the parasympathetic nerve supply would lead one to believe that absence of the ganglion cells would lead to an absence of the parasympathetic supply and, thus, to an overactivity of the sympathetic supply, which would lead not to a spastic obstruction of the intestine but to relaxation of the loop of bowel. This, however, is not the case; and denervation of the intestine does not lead to Hirschsprung's disease. Recent evidence suggests that the ganglion cells are involved as intermediaries in coordinating an intramural relay system that governs the peristaltic waves.[94,116,117] This allows the bowel segment into which the bolus of stool is about to move to relax and accept the bolus followed by a contraction wave, which pushes it onward. The absence of ganglion cells and the concomitant absence of the nonadrenergic, noncholinergic mediator that has been identified in this role[91] leads to constant contraction of the segment of bowel and thereby to its inability to accept the bolus of stool. The segment of bowel that is normally innervated proximal to the aganglionic segment fills with stool and thus becomes distended; at the same time, it develops work hypertrophy of its muscular layers as it tries to force the lumenal contents into the obstructing distal segment. Thus, the megacolon is produced.

Clinical presentation. All newborn infants with Hirschsprung's disease do not fail to pass meconium in the first 24 hours, since approximately 6% of them do pass meconium. Occasionally, children with Hirschsprung's disease will have several normal bowel movements and may continue a normal stool pattern over several days. Others may show a picture similar to that of meconium plug or small left colon syndrome and then may establish a reasonably normal stooling pattern before becoming obstructed. Nonetheless, almost all infants with Hirschsprung's disease will have some symptoms of colorectal dysfunction in early infancy.

Clinically, the child with Hirschsprung's disease

will present a progressive pattern of distal bowel obstruction. Having failed to pass meconium, or having passed only small amounts, the child will become distended and usually will begin vomiting bile-stained material. The risks of perforation, sepsis, and pseudomembranous enterocolitis, mentioned in the discussion on the meconium plug and small left colon syndromes, are even more prevalent with Hirschsprung's disease.

Evaluation. A carefully performed barium enema on an *unprepared* bowel is the standard evaluation for the child with Hirschsprung's disease. Although careful attention to the filling phase is important, the emptying phase is of the most diagnostic value. With the tube out and the pressure relieved, the differential size between the proximal dilated bowel and the distal narrowed bowel may be appreciated, and a transition zone may be clearly seen (Fig. 10-34). However, this pattern may not be prominent in the newborn period. If a classic picture of Hirschsprung's disease is not present on evaluation of these films, no attempt to encourage or aid evacuation should be made and the child should be re-examined with plain abdominal radiographs in 24 hours to evaluate the degree of emptying of the bowel. Most normal children will empty most of the barium from the large intestine in 24 hours and certainly will have moved it around from its proximal extent well into the distal sigmoid and rectum. Failure to empty a barium enema in 24 hours is significant evidence of Hirschsprung's disease and warrants a rectal biopsy (Fig. 10-35). Rectal biopsy may be avoided and one may proceed directly to a decompressing colostomy if a classic pattern of differential size with transition zone is present on the initial radiographic study (Fig. 10-36).

Referral. The child with Hirschsprung's disease has a complex disorder that will require two or more surgical procedures during the first year of life. Thus, the child's surgical care from the beginning should be in the hands of a surgeon familiar with this disease, including its ramifications and treatment. Except in extreme emergencies, the initial colostomy should not be performed by a surgeon unfamiliar with the treatment of Hirschsprung's disease in a tiny infant. A serious mistake made in evaluation and early therapy in the disease may lead to subsequent failure to cure what is otherwise a highly curable lesion.

Medical versus surgical treatment. There is no medical therapy for Hirschsprung's disease, although many have tried constipation regimens with temporary success. However, such a regimen leaves the child at a constant risk for developing pseudomembranous enterocolitis, a devastatingly injurious illness that may persist and leave the child a colonic cripple even after definitive surgical therapy.

Although some surgeons may try to perform the definitive pullthrough procedure in the newborn period, there is little justification for doing so in the tiny newborn. A colostomy placed just proximal to the transition zone and confirmed to be in a segment of bowel containing ganglion cells will nicely decompress the child and allow normal nutrition and bowel function during the first year of life (Fig. 10-37). The child can then have a definitive procedure when he is a better risk for surgery and better able to withstand any minor degrees of contamination that may occur. Furthermore, his decompressed bowel is in better shape for the pull-through procedure. In addition, it can be more thoroughly cleansed and prepared for the surgical procedure so that any contamination that does occur will be minimal. Successful reconstruction when the child is 1 year of age still leaves him functioning normally well before the age of toilet training. Definitive surgical procedures for repair of Hirschsprung's disease and their postoperative course and prognosis are discussed in Chapter 15 in the section on the infant and toddler, since children usually undergo the procedure when they are in that age group.

Prognosis. The prognosis for children with this entity is excellent when a definitive pullthrough is accomplished by an experienced surgeon. Most children are restored to normal bowel function.

Complications. Complications of a colostomy performed in the infant are retraction of the colostomy into the peritoneal cavity, stricture of the ostomy stoma, bleeding from the exposed mucosa, and, not infrequently, prolapse of the proximal colostomy segment. Prolapse occurs when a colostomy is performed for Hirschsprung's disease because the dilated hypertrophied normal proximal segment shrinks back down to normal size, which may result in a redundant proximal loop that is too small for the original fascial stoma, allowing the bowel to herniate through the stoma and resulting in prolapse of the colostomy seg-

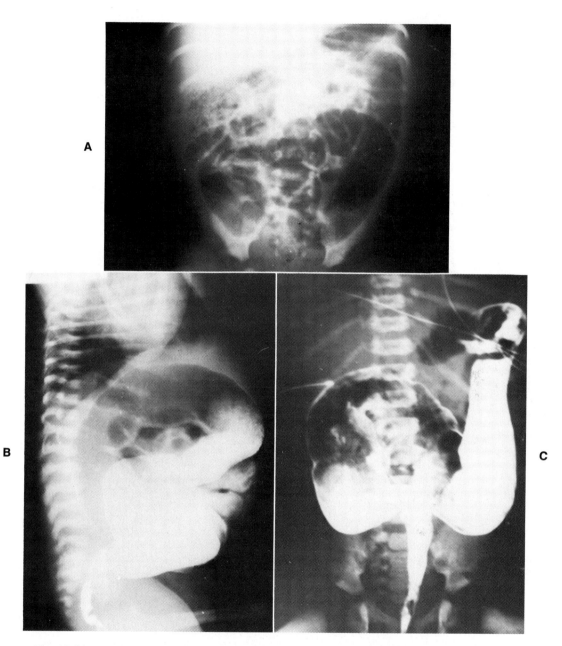

Fig. 10-34. A, Dilated loops of bowel on a plain abdominal radiograph of an infant with a probable distal bowel obstruction. This picture in an infant who fails to pass a stool in the first 24 hours of life should suggest Hirschsprung's disease. **B,** Clear-cut transition zone in the midrectum. **C,** A transition zone is seen at the junction between the distal sigmoid and the upper rectum, best appreciated on the AP film. It is important to recognize that the dilated hypertrophied sigmoid proximal to a transition zone in the upper rectum will stretch over to the right side and overlap the cecum. (**B** and **C** from Filston, H. C., and Izant, R.: The surgical neonate: evaluation and care, New York, 1978, Appleton-Century-Crofts.)

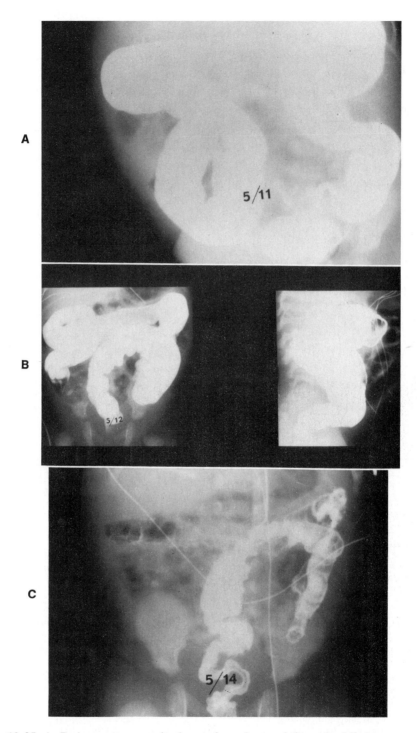

Fig. 10-35. A, Barium enema examination performed on an infant who failed to pass meconium spontaneously in the first 24 hours of life failed to reveal a definite transition zone, although one is suggested on the lateral view of the film dated 5/12. Note that by 24 hours after the initial study **(B),** little of the barium has moved around the colon, and at 72 hours **(C),** there is still significant retention of the barium. Subsequent rectal biopsy confirmed Hirschsprung's disease in this infant.

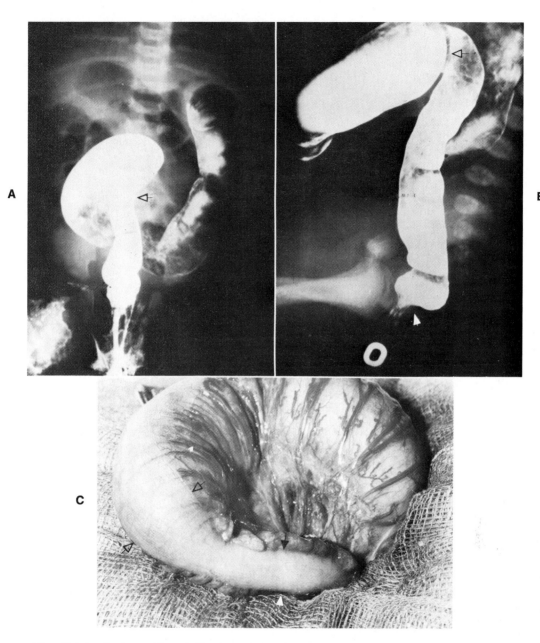

Fig. 10-36. AP **(A)** and lateral **(B)** films of the distal bowel in an infant who failed to pass meconium in the first 24 hours of life reveal a transition zone at the junction between the sigmoid and rectum (open arrow). This zone may be missed if attention is directed exclusively toward the rectal segment. In addition, the lateral film reveals the normal puborectalis sling ''cutoff'' indicated by the white arrow. This normal appearance is frequently misinterpreted as low-segment Hirschsprung's disease. **C,** The appearance of the transition zone at surgery. Note the marked hypertrophy and widening of the tinnea (open arrows) in comparison with that of the distal aganglionic segment (closed arrows).

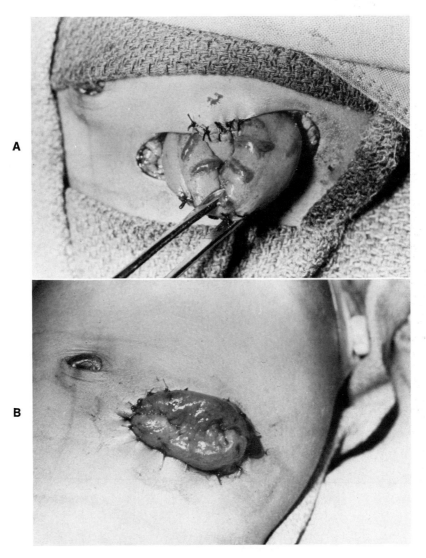

Fig. 10-37. A, Construction of the loop colostomy in the ganglion-containing bowel just proximal to the transition zone. All layers of the abdominal wall have been sutured to the loop of bowel, and a skin bridge has been passed through the mesentery beneath it. **B,** The colostomy has been opened and matured by suturing the edge of the bowel to the skin. It can then be fitted with Stomadhesive and a collecting bag.

ment. Most of these prolapses are minimal and can be controlled. If prolapse becomes a problem, the definitive procedure can be performed slightly earlier if the child is otherwise developing well and is in good health.

• • •

In summary, because Hirschsprung's disease is the most common cause of distal bowel dysfunction in the newborn, and because it has such a high degree of successful repair when it is properly handled from the beginning, it should be fore-

most on the list of diagnostic considerations when the physician encounters a child who fails to exhibit normal bowel function in the newborn period. Expeditious referral for diagnosis and therapy should be made.

COLONIC ATRESIA

Colonic atresia is an extremely rare lesion and is encountered only infrequently by the pediatric surgeon. The colon has an excellent anastomotic blood supply and is relatively fixed in an extended pattern in the peritoneal cavity. It is, therefore,

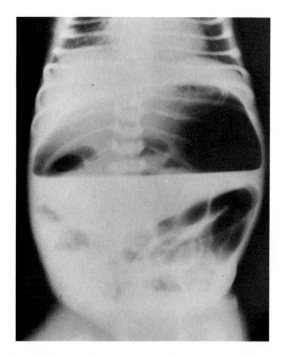

Fig. 10-38. Radiograph of an infant with distal bowel obstruction that proved to be colonic atresia. (From Filston, H. C., and Izant, R.: The surgical neonate: evaluation and care, New York, 1978, Appleton-Century-Crofts.)

less likely to sustain a vascular accident in utero than is the small bowel. Colonic atresia will present as a distal bowel obstruction with failure of the child to stool, abdominal distention, and subsequent vomiting, usually bilious. Plain abdominal radiographs will often show a very dilated loop of bowel that is obviously distal (Fig. 10-38). Otherwise, it appears similar to Hirschsprung's disease, small left colon syndrome, and meconium plug syndrome.

Barium enema studies will encounter a complete obstruction at the proximal extent of the collapsed distal segment, demonstrating the complete occlusion of the bowel, in contrast to such studies performed in Hirschsprung's disease and small left colon syndrome, where the barium can be refluxed into the proximal dilated segment.

Treatment can usually be achieved by primary resection and end-to-end anastomosis, but if the child is particularly ill or the bowel segments are particularly disparate, a temporary diverting colostomy may be indicated.

NEONATAL NECROTIZING ENTEROCOLITIS

The devastating bowel lesion of necrotizing enterocolitis in the newborn can be looked on as a disease of success; the successful treatment of premature infants who have been severely stressed by hypoxia or shock may subsequently be complicated by necrotizing enterocolitis. It is interesting that the lesion is not even referenced in the index of the 1969 edition of *Pediatric Surgery.*[75] Since that time it has been recognized with increasing frequency, so that in the past 5 or 6 years it has become one of the most frequent entities treated by the pediatric surgeon.

Etiology and pathogenesis. The exact etiology of the lesion is unknown, but laboratory research has demonstrated that a picture similar to it can be produced in a laboratory animal by stress consisting of severe hypoxia.[5] The pathogenesis is thought to be a stress injury resulting in a low-flow syndrome with shunting of blood from the intestine, leading to ischemic loss of the mucosal barrier and invasion of the bowel wall by bacteria from the lumen. These bacteria then colonize the bowel wall, leading to damage to the muscular structure of the wall and subsequent perforation. The concomitant absorption of the bacteria from the colonies in the bowel wall into the mesenteric portal venous system carries the bacteria to the liver and on into the general circulation, leading to overwhelming sepsis in the immune-deficient neonate. Other factors that have been suggested as contributing to the disease are a substrate provided by formula feeding, the lack of immune factors provided by breast milk, the osmotic effects of some of the formulas when given at full strength, and the additional ischemia to the antimesenteric side of the bowel resulting from gaseous distention secondary to ileus.[36,60,83]

Clinical presentation. The disease seems to present in three distinct patterns. The less common pattern is that of infants who are born having sustained severe stress and who show signs of intestinal disease on the very first day of life. These children usually show an extensive progressive ischemic necrosis of the bowel, leading to perforation, and are rarely salvageable. At the other extreme are infants who have weathered the early neonatal period and who are well beyond their initial stresses. Often these children are 3 or 4 weeks old and are in the less acute areas of the

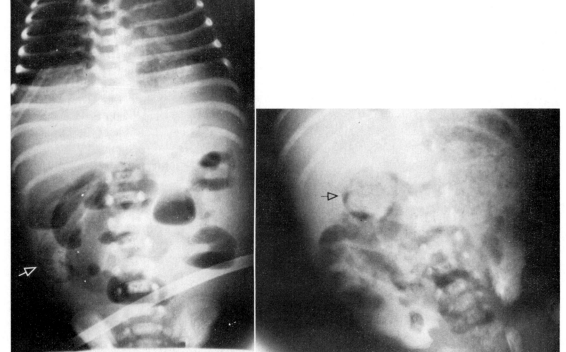

A

B

Fig. 10-39. Two excellent examples of pneumatosis intestinalis (arrows) diagnostic of neonatal necrotizing enterocolitis. Occasionally, only the "muddy" appearance noted in the left upper quadrant of **B** indicates the presence of necrotizing enterocolitis.

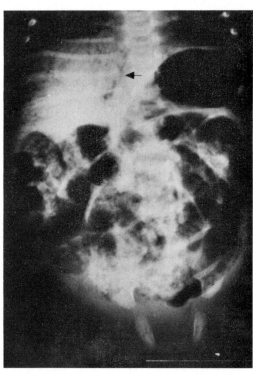

Fig. 10-40. Abdominal radiograph of an infant with severe necrotizing enterocolitis revealing portal vein gas (arrow). (From Filston, H. C., and Izant, R.: The surgical neonate: evaluation and care, New York, 1978, Appleton-Century-Crofts.)

nursery. For some unknown reason, they develop necrotizing enterocolitis and may, despite early medical therapy, go on to a severe pattern of disease with perforation. It is this group of infants that is often involved with epidemics, and some infectious agent has been sought for extensively in this population.

The typical infant with necrotizing enterocolitis, however, is the small premature infant who has had relatively minor but usually identifiable neonatal stress. Following initial stabilization of his vital signs and usually at a time when his respiratory support is becoming less intense, he develops a symptom complex that consists of loose, seedy stools streaked with blood; abdominal distention; and bilious vomiting or gastric aspirate. He may show a deterioration of his general stability accompanied by hypothermia, hypotension, bradycardia, and apnea.

Evaluation. Plain abdominal radiographs obtained early in the course of the disease may show only distended loops of bowel in a nonspecific "ileus" pattern, but frequently those experienced in evaluating this entity can identify the muddy or bubbly appearance of the intestinal contents, a disparity in the distention of the loops, and some thickening of the bowel wall suggestive of peritonitis.

The child may or may not progress to the classic finding of necrotizing enterocolitis: the presence of intraluminal air or pneumatosis intestinalis cystica. This finding represents the gas-forming bacteria in the wall of the bowel and is evidenced by a double contrast of air outlining the bowel wall (Fig. 10-39). Transport of these gas-forming bacteria to the liver through the mesenteric portal venous system may lead to outlining of the portal venous channels with air as well (Fig. 10-40). Although this pattern usually occurs in the more serious forms of the disease, it no longer has as serious a prognostic implication as was originally believed. Further deterioration may lead to perforation of the bowel, which may be recognized by a rapid increase in abdominal distention and loss of the normal liver dullness in the right upper quadrant. Radiographic evaluation at this point will usually show free peritoneal air, although it may be difficult to recognize on the supine plain film, since it is evidenced primarily by a bubble of gas overlying the usually opaque hepatic shadow. Air may also outline the

falciform ligament, and the cross striations of the overlying ribs may give the so-called football sign (Fig. 10-41). Free peritoneal air is more easily appreciated on a cross-table lateral or upright film, where the free air beneath the abdominal wall or beneath the diaphragm can be appreciated (Fig. 10-42).

Referral. Referral of the infant with necrotizing enterocolitis should be accomplished at the first signs of the disease, because the disease is a multisystem failure and the child may require the maximal support available in a major center. He should be protected during transport with the usual precautions of nasogastric decompression, warmth, and knowledgeable monitoring.

Medical versus surgical treatment. Most infants with necrotizing enterocolitis can be success-

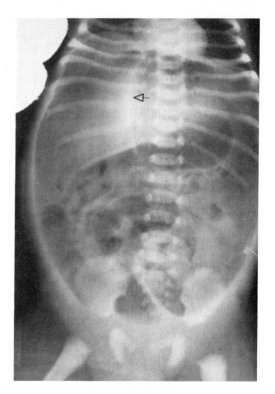

Fig. 10-41. Example of the "airdrome sign" of extensive pneumoperitoneum secondary to perforation of the gastrointestinal tract as seen on the supine abdominal radiograph. The "football sign," which is made up of air outlining the falciform ligament as it crosses the ribs on the right side is also obvious in this film (arrow). (From Filston, H.C., and Izant, R.: The surgical neonate: evaluation and care, New York, 1978, Appleton-Century-Crofts.)

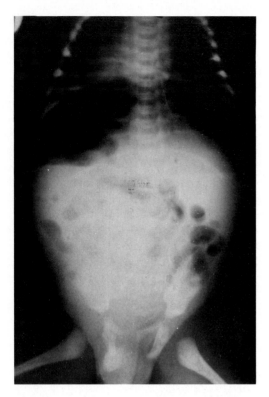

Fig. 10-42. Pneumoperitoneum is most easily demonstrated on an upright film. (From Filston, H. C., and Izant, R.: The surgical neonate: evaluation and care, New York, 1978, Appleton-Century-Crofts.)

fully managed if medical therapy is initiated early in the course of the disease. Successful management is less likely for the child with the rampant form of the disease that presents in the early hours of the newborn period. For the typical child, however, early recognition should lead to adequate intestinal decompression. Such decompression has usually required tubes in both the esophagus and the stomach to ensure that swallowed air does not progress along the bowel and maintain the distention, which may enhance ischemia. All gastrointestinal feedings should be discontinued; broad antibiotic coverage, usually consisting of ampicillin and gentamicin should be provided; and the child should be carefully monitored. General support is provided in the form of respiratory assistance, oxygen therapy, and intravenous fluid and electrolyte replacement and correction. Signs of overwhelming septic deterioration should be carefully sought and appropriate additional supportive therapy instituted. This therapy may involve blood or plasma transfusions, provision of platelets, additional antibiotic therapy, major fluid

administration, pharmacologic support of the cardiovascular system, diuretics, and exchange transfusions when disseminated intravascular coagulopathy complicates the picture.[41] Adequate monitoring must be provided in the form of arterial blood gas and blood pressure monitoring, dependable intravenous routes, and, occasionally, central venous pressure monitoring.

If the child can be maintained through the initial acute phase of the disease and free perforation or abscess formation avoided, the bowel will usually heal with adequate rest and maintenance of nutrition through total central or peripheral alimentation. We have favored the central route because of the ease of maintenance of the percutaneous subclavian catheters and the relatively low complication rates that we have encountered by our techniques.[32] Others have preferred to maintain nutrition through the use of total peripheral parenteral nutrition and intralipid supplements.[24] We have considered 3 weeks of bowel rest as a minimum for ensuring a low incidence of recrudescence of the disease, but others have been more aggressive in resuming feedings and have had apparently low complications.[8] Certainly, no feedings should be administered until all signs of sepsis have been abated, the child is stable, the abdominal distention is relieved, and the stools no longer contain blood. Regardless of when feedings are resumed, any sign of reappearance of the symptoms should lead to a further period of bowel rest and total parenteral nutrition.

Although we prefer that all children respond to medical therapy, surgical intervention is not infrequently required. We have found that early consultation between the pediatric medical and pediatric surgical services leads to an ongoing combined evaluation of the infant and optimizes the timing of surgical intervention. Obviously, for the child with free perforation, surgery is mandatory (Fig. 10-43). Identification of the child for whom surgery would be beneficial prior to frank perforation remains the difficult factor in providing care for these children. Exploration and resection of a segment of bowel with impending perforation leads to much less morbidity and is often lifesaving. It has generally been thought that those infants who have failed to respond to medical therapy during the first 24 hours are candidates for surgical exploration. Failure to respond may include failure of normalization of vital signs accompanied by persistent hypotension, hypo-

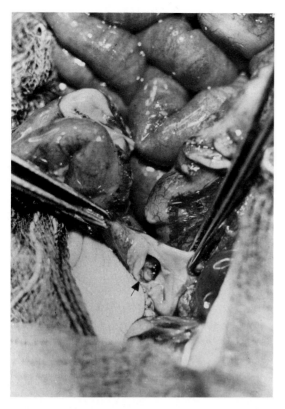

Fig. 10-43. Surgical view of an infant with a free perforation of the ascending colon from neonatal necrotizing enterocolitis. The severity of the process is shown by the almost complete destruction of the bowel and the large perforation (arrow). (From Filston, H. C., and Izant, R.: The surgical neonate: evaluation and care, New York, 1978, Appleton-Century-Crofts.)

thermia, bradycardia, and apnea; or it may involve the development of signs of peritonitis with persistent or increasing tenderness, edema, and erythema of the abdominal wall. The mere presence of pneumatosis or portal vein gas is not an indication for surgery, but the persistence of dilated loops in a fixed location with persistent pneumatosis has been an indication for surgical exploration and resection. Persistent acidosis indicates persistent bowel ischemia and has been a reasonably reliable indication for surgery.

Why not explore all of these children if perforation is such a common complication? A period of surgical aggressiveness in the early 1970s met with little success and led to confusion on the part of the surgeon encountering extensive diseased bowel with multiple areas of partial-thickness destruction. Resection and anastomosis of all of these lesions would be a formidable task, and

resection of long lengths of bowel containing multiple lesions would leave the child with a short bowel syndrome. Since we know that many of these lesions will heal without sequelae, it is best to reserve surgical intervention for the child who will sustain a severe complication without resection. That child has been difficult to identify. Our present program is to utilize a combined medical-surgical evaluation team and to explore all children with free perforations; all children developing a mass indicating abscess formation; all children who fail to improve after 24 hours of medical management, as indicated by continued deterioration or failure of improvement of vital signs and arterial blood gases and pH; and all children who develop signs of peritonitis while under medical management (see below). With this system, the child who remains a difficult decision is the child who was septic when necrotizing enterocolitis first ensued. This child may show deterioration from his systemic sepsis while his abdominal picture improves.

Neonatal necrotizing enterocolitis: indications for surgery

1. Free intraperitoneal air (perforation)
2. Physical signs of peritonitis
   a. Increasing abdominal tenderness
   b. Abdominal rigidity
   c. Edema and erythema of the abdominal wall
3. Progressive cardiorespiratory deterioration despite treatment for sepsis
4. Progressive or persistent metabolic acidosis
5. Physical examination or radiographic evidence of a mass

Prognosis. If the infant responds to medical therapy and becomes asymptomatic, he will usually go on to recover and his bowel function will be normal. Similarly, those children who are operated on and resected prior to frank perforation usually have a successful recovery. Mortality remains high for those children whose disease presents with the rampant progressive picture in the early newborn period and for those children who sustain free perforation. With better multisystem support, broad-spectrum antibiotics, and surgical resection and peritoneal lavage, improved survival rates have been achieved in recent years. The long-term prognosis and complications common to the child with surgical resection of the bowel depend on the extent of resection and the extent of severe damage to the mucosal lining of the intestine. Some of these children will have short bowel syndrome, and others will have an equivalent functional debility due to inadequate mucosal absorptive surface and function. With prolonged total parenteral nutrition, most of these children will ultimately adapt and gastrointestinal feeding can be resumed. Some may linger for many months and ultimately succumb, however.

Important aspects of follow-up. A small percentage of children who recover through medical therapy will have signs of intestinal obstruction several weeks or months later. Such obstruction may be due to adhesions, but it may also be due to stricture formation at the site of bowel damage from the necrotizing enterocolitis.[61,67] Early recognition of this complication will lead to surgical intervention with resection and anastomosis and usually a benign postoperative course.

Inadequate numbers of these children have been followed into late childhood and adulthood to determine whether they have bouts of colitis or other functional problems with their intestinal tract. In the short run, most of them have responded to medical therapy and have grown and developed normally in infancy and early childhood. Hopefully, in the near future, a better understanding of the pathogenesis of this disease may lead to prevention, at least of its most serious ravages. At this point early recognition affords the infant the best chance of successful response to medical management, avoiding the complications of the disease and the need for surgical intervention.

MISCELLANEOUS INTESTINAL AND ABDOMINAL ANOMALIES
Duplications and mesenteric cysts

Clinical presentation. Although duplications and mesenteric cysts are frequently listed as part of the differential diagnosis of abdominal conditions presenting in the newborn period, they are really quite rare. A freely movable palpable mass that seems to be intra-abdominal may be noted on physical examination. Characteristically, the cyst can be moved from one quadrant to another quite readily, unlike a retroperitoneal tumor (Fig. 10-44). Occasionally, a cyst may twist and strangulate its base, presenting with the symptoms of an acute abdominal condition. Duplications can obstruct the bowel, either by direct compression or by acting as the lead point of a localized vol-

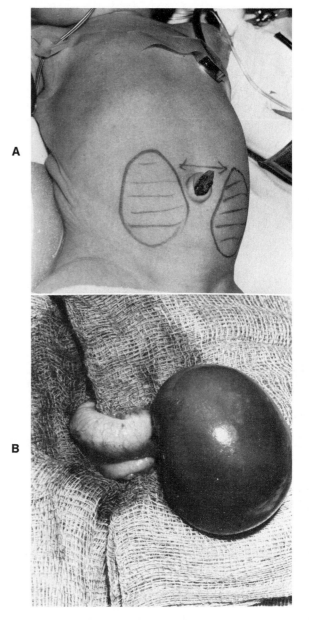

Fig. 10-44. A, The mobility of a mesenteric cyst or cystlike duplication within the abdominal cavity is illustrated by the abdominal markings. **B,** The lesion proved to be a cystlike duplication of the sigmoid.

vulus (Fig. 10-45). Duplications can also act as the lead point of an intussusception and may occasionally lead to gastrointestinal hemorrhage when they contain gastric mucosa.

Evaluation. Radiographic evaluation usually shows a mass effect on the plain x-ray film, and contrast studies usually show little more than a "draping" effect of the bowel over the mass (Fig.

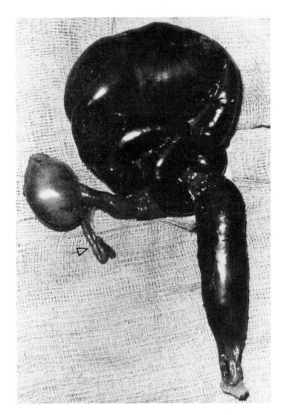

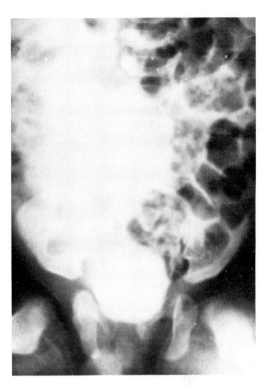

Fig. 10-45. Volvulus of this distal ileal duplication produced ischemic necrosis of a considerable segment of the distal ileum. The appendix is indicated by the arrow.

Fig. 10-46. Abdominal radiograph showing the "mass effect" of a mesenteric cyst.

10-46). When the duplication leads to an intussusception, this entity may be encountered on barium enema examination; and if bowel necrosis occurs from strangulation due to volvulus of a duplication, pneumatosis intestinalis may be evident on the plain film. Few duplications communicate openly with the main intestinal channel, so that contrast filling of the duplication is unusual (Fig. 10-47).

Surgical options. Treatment is universally surgical so long as the infant can tolerate anesthesia and surgery. Since resection and anastomosis of a sizable length of bowel may be required, the surgery should be performed by someone experienced in the anastomosis of neonatal intestine. Although usually duplications are short-segment, localized lesions, they have been known to extend for long distances; and duplications of the entire small intestine have been described.[123] Mesenteric cysts can often be excised; occasionally, however, this excision interferes with the blood supply to a segment of mesentery and requires excision of the adjacent loop of small intestine. Duplications can be excised similarly, with resection and primary anastomosis of the adjacent intestine. When resection of the normal bowel in continuity with the duplication would leave the child with a short bowel syndrome, an endo-intestinal stripping of the mucosa of the duplication can be performed as described by Wrenn.[123] This procedure eliminates the secretory epithelium and allows the residual muscular surfaces to scar together.

Postoperative course, prognosis, and follow-up. When the duplication is handled appropriately, the postoperative course should be benign and of short duration. The prognosis should be excellent so long as strangulation of sizable portions of the intestine has not occurred. In follow-up, the main consideration is that of intestinal adhesions, as it is after any other intra-abdominal procedure.

Duplications may fail to present with symptoms in the newborn period and may therefore be diagnosed in later childhood.

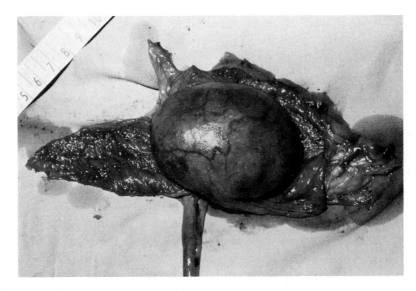

Fig. 10-47. Duplication of the cecum. The duplication bulges into the intestinal lumen but does not communicate directly with the main intestinal channel.

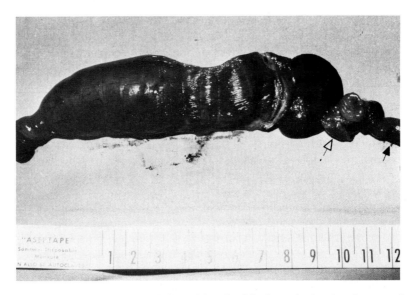

Fig. 10-48. Surgical specimen from an infant with a distal ileal atresia showing the opened proximal segment with meconium leaking from it. The proximal part of the distal segment (open arrow) is shown with intussuscepted Meckel's diverticulum (solid arrow).

Intussusception

Intussusception is a rare lesion in the newborn period but does occur occasionally. If it has occurred in utero, it may prove to be the cause of an intestinal atresia. Sometimes an intraluminal polyp or intussuscepted Meckel's diverticulum will prove to have been the leading point of an in utero intussusception. In these instances the patient has the signs and symptoms of an intestinal atresia. When the proximal portion of the distal bowel is opened, the intussuscepted leading point is found (Fig. 10-48).

A

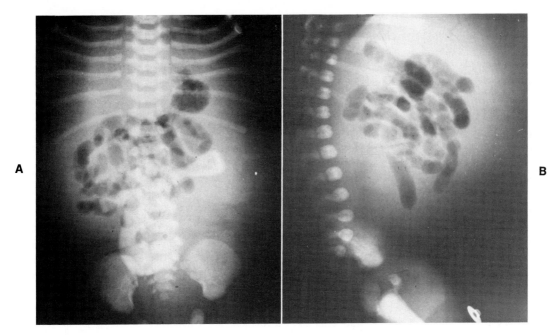

B

Fig. 10-49. AP film of an infant with ascites indicated by the central location of the bowel gas pattern surrounded by a hazy film of fluid **(A).** On the cross-table lateral projection **(B),** the bowel is seen floating up under the abdominal wall, completely surrounded by fluid. (Courtesy Donald Kirks, M.D., Durham, N.C.)

Since intussusception is such a rare lesion in the newborn period, the reader is referred to Chapter 15 in the section on the infant and toddler; it is in that age group that intussusception is common.

Neonatal ascites

The infant who is born distended is a rarity. Despite all the causes of intestinal obstruction, few lead to obvious distention at birth. Therefore, the list of entities to be thought of when an infant is born with abdominal distention is relatively short. Generally, distention present at birth is due to ascites rather than gaseous distention or obstruction of the intestinal tract per se. Entities that may produce ascites are complicated meconium ileus, meconium peritonitis representing free perforation in utero with subsequent ascites formation, ascites due to urinary tract obstructions and abnormalities, ascites associated with hydrometrocolpos and urogenital sinus abnormalities, and ascites as part of a generalized picture of edema associated with hydrops from either cardiac abnormalities or erythroblastosis fetalis.

Clinical presentation and evaluation. Ascites can be identified by a lack of the tympany that

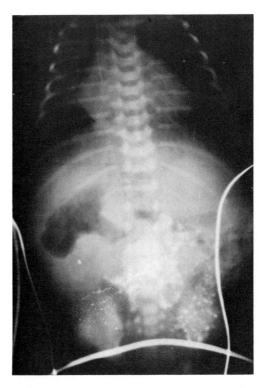

Fig. 10-50. Abdominal radiograph showing the calcifications of meconium peritonitis.

is usually present with gaseous distention of the bowel, by a shifting dullness on physical examination, and by the presence of a fluid haze on abdominal radiographs with the bowel gas pattern seemingly floating in the midst of hazy density. The latter may best be appreciated on cross-table lateral films where the air pattern of the intestine is pushed up under the anterior abdominal wall (Fig. 10-49).

Meconium peritonitis can usually be identified by the presence of calcifications on abdominal films (Fig. 10-50). The perforation that led to the meconium peritonitis may still be present or may have sealed. There may be intestinal obstruction, or the bowel may once again be in continuity. Investigation for the presence of a continued leak or obstruction should be undertaken. Hydrometrocolpos is recognized when the infant has a mass arising from the pelvis and the intestinal gas pattern is pushed into the upper abdomen beneath the diaphragm (Fig. 10-51). When hydrometrocolpos is associated with a urogenital sinus abnormality, the perineum contains only one outlet representing the urogenital sinus. Imperforate anus with rectovaginal fistula often accompanies

these lesions (Fig. 10-52). The urethra enters the proximal urogenital sinus. The ascites is due to urine and cervical secretions leaking out the fallopian tubes in a retrograde manner and into the peritoneal cavity, causing a chemical peritonitis with reactive ascites formation.[87]

When none of these distinct entities can be identified, it is probable that the urinary tract is responsible for the ascites. Evaluation of the urinary tract begins with a voiding cystourethrogram followed by an intravenous pyelogram. Common findings are bladder outlet obstructions such as are due to posterior urethral valves and major obstructions of the ureters. By no means, however, is urinary ascites a frequent accompaniment of obstructive uropathy.

Treatment. Treatment obviously depends on the specific entity responsible for the ascites. If none is identified, the infant should be given supportive care and observed for proper functioning of the urinary and intestinal tracts. If meconium peritonitis is identified and no lesion of the gastrointestinal tract is apparent, the infant should be treated with antibiotics to prevent secondary bacterial peritonitis in the inflamed peritoneal cavity.

Hydrometrocolpos with urogenital sinus abnormalities is a complex anomaly requiring prolonged skilled surgical treatment. Early referral is therefore mandatory. Often these children are mistakenly diagnosed as having ambiguous genitalia. Success in eventual reconstruction depends

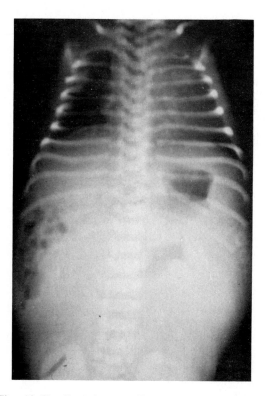

Fig. 10-51. Central mass effect of hydrometrocolpos seen on a plain abdominal radiograph with the bowel gas pushed up into the upper abdomen.

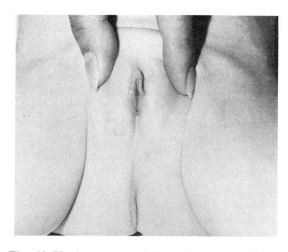

Fig. 10-52. Appearance of the perineum of an infant with hydrometrocolpos, a urogenital sinus deformity, and an imperforate anus with rectovaginal and urethrovaginal fistulas. (From Filston, H. C., and Izant, R.: The surgical neonate: evaluation and care, New York, 1978, Appleton-Century-Crofts.)

primarily on the integrity of the nerve supply to the perineum and the development of the pubo-rectalis and pubococcygeus muscular diaphragm. Colostomy diversion of the high rectovaginal fistula will enable most infants to thrive until subsequent planned reconstruction can be accomplished when the child is about 1 year of age. Occasionally the huge pelvic mass has led to severe obstructive uropathy with marked destruction of the kidneys, so that survival is impaired. In the usual case, however, the urinary tract recovers once the obstruction is relieved by decompressing the hydrocolpos.

When the ascites is due to urinary obstruction, initial diversion followed by reconstruction may be necessary. Posterior urethral valves can usually be resected, avoiding the need for complicated diversionary procedures.

Biliary atresia

Since biliary atresia is usually a lesion diagnosed after the immediate neonatal period, the major discussion of this entity belongs in the infant and toddler section among the findings at the first well baby visit (Chapter 14). It is introduced here only to emphasize that it is necessary to follow all infants with jaundice in the newborn period until their jaundice clears. The common habit of following the physiologic jaundice of the newborn only to the point where it "turns the corner" may lead to missing the early onset of biliary atresia. Most commonly, this entity presents with moderate jaundice when the child is 3 to 4 weeks of age. Until recent surgical improvements provided hope for at least a percentage of these infants, late diagnosis of this entity proved to be of little consequence. Today, however, when surgical intervention may lead to a marked prolongation of life for these infants, if not actual cure, late diagnosis may lead to a tragic early death. Thus, careful follow-up of neonatal jaundice to ensure that the bilirubin level becomes normal and thorough evaluation of any child whose jaundice recurs after the neonatal period or who develops jaundice after having none in the neonatal period should be mandatory.

IMPERFORATE ANUS

Imperforate anus is a relatively common newborn anomaly but is one of the most mishandled entities in all of pediatrics. The primary reason for this may well be the nomenclature, which leads the inexperienced physician to look for a true imperforate anus. A true imperforate anus, that is, the presence of an anus with a membrane obstructing it, is an uncommon lesion among entities in this group.

The subject of imperforate anus is best understood when the nomenclature is correctly presented. The lesions referred to as imperforate anus are actually either anal atresia or anorectal atresia. Therefore, absence of an anus is almost a sine qua non of the entity. The two lesions that the inexperienced primary care physician expects to find are, in fact, rare ones. The first of these is the anus with a cover or membrane obstructing it, known as a covered anus, which can be treated by simple rupture of the membrane connecting the well-formed perineal anus to the bowel. The second is actually a membranous atresia of the rectum with a well-formed anus, a most unusual entity. This latter anomaly probably does not belong in the imperforate anus classification, since it more accurately is a case of colorectal atresia similar to other atresias of the bowel and the anus is uninvolved. Because of the extensive anastomotic blood supply to the rectum and because intestinal atresias are due to vascular accidents in utero, it follows that rectal atresia would be an extremely rare entity.

Anal atresia and anorectal atresia, the common entities, imply a lack of formation of the anus. Thus, infants born with these lesions have no anus but may have a rudimentary dimple or cleft in the area of the normal anus. Anal atresias may be associated with perineal fistulas, whereas anorectal atresias are generally associated with fistulas into the urinary tract in the male or into the vagina in the female. Anal atresia can thus be differentiated from anorectal atresia at the 90% confidence level by demonstrating the presence of a perineal fistula. In the absence of a perineal fistula, it may be more difficult to demonstrate that the lesion is anal atresia rather than anorectal atresia.

Initial management. The absence of an anal opening means that the infant has a bowel obstruction. The presence of a fistula may be adequate to decompress the bowel, but this is not always the case, even when the fistula is at the perineal level. Thus, there is some urgency about treatment, but emergency surgery is rarely indicated. These infants can be maintained for many hours and even days by careful nasogastric decompression of the intestine, preventing overfilling with swallowed air; sustenance with either peripheral or central parenteral nutrition; and prevention of sepsis secondary to the obstruction with broad-spectrum antibiotics. This therapy will usually prevent the complications of obstruction such as sepsis, enterocolitis, and perforation and allow time for a careful, thoughtful evaluation of the lesion.

The importance of a correct decision as to the level of the bowel cannot be overemphasized. Little skill, judgment, or experience is required to achieve an anal opening to allow passage of stool to the environment. Many surgeons have taken great pride in rushing the hours-old newborn to the operating room and achieving a perineal opening with a satisfying burst of meconium. Such glory and satisfaction are short lived, however, since the child may soon demonstrate total and lifelong incontinence. Thus, the aim of therapy must be not only to achieve successful passage of stool to the environment, but a socially acceptable, functioning anus that is continent and responsive to the child's lifelong social needs. This goal may challenge the diagnostic acumen and experience of both the pediatric radiologist and pediatric surgeon and will demand the utmost in skill and judgment during the operative procedure itself.

Continence mechanisms. A brief review of the continence mechanism may help in understanding the anatomy and physiology of the anorectal mechanisms. When proper physiologic function is present, a gastrocolic or ileocolic stimulus results in a massive peristaltic movement of stool from the distal colon into the upper rectum.[46] In response to the entry of stool into the rectum, the internal sphincter, which represents a specialized portion of the circular muscle coat of the rectum, and the adjacent puborectalis sling relax. At the same time, there is a transient contraction of the external sphincter, preventing evacuation of stool. This produces a retrograde pressure gradient from the anus toward the rectum, which tends to push the stool back proximally for a brief period. Although the involuntary contraction of the external sphincter is transient, the individual can voluntarily increase the time during which this contraction occurs by consciously maintaining contraction of the external sphincter. If the individual desires to evacuate the stool, he relaxes the external sphincter and a second wave of contraction of the rectum will evacuate the stool with the help of Valsalva-type maneuvers of the abdominal musculature, which help to propel the

stool through the anus. If the individual desires not to pass stool at that time, maintenance of the voluntary contraction will lead to relaxation of the rectum and puborectalis sling and accommodation of the rectum so that the urgency sensation ebbs and the desire to defecate disappears.[98]

Between such times of maximum stimulus to defecate, continence is maintained by the combination of the resting tone of the external and internal sphincters and the closure and kinking of the distal rectum, produced by the slinglike puborectalis muscle, which is the central portion of the pubococcygeus diaphragm.[98] The efficiency of this system is impaired when sizable amounts of stool build up in the rectum itself, so that compression and kinking of the rectum by the puborectalis sling is no longer possible. This may lead to soiling as stool protrudes through the slightly patulous anus. Other factors in maintaining normal continence are the angles of the sigmoid-rectal junction and the colosigmoid junction, which tend to minimize the amount of stool moving through this area except at times of peristaltic action.

Anatomic deficiencies. Although external sphincter fibers may be present in the perineum of the child with an anal or anorectal atresia, they are usually in disarray and rarely can be fashioned into a circumferential sphincter. The child with an anal atresia usually has a functioning internal sphincter, so that the fashioning of the perineal stoma will leave him with both the internal sphincter and puborectalis sling functions for continence. Thus, for the child with a low-type anal atresia, construction of a pliable, adequately sized anal stoma becomes the major concern.

The child with an anorectal atresia presents a more complex problem. This child's bowel is atretic up to or above the puborectalis sling. Little internal sphincter is present, and the bowel must be pulled down through the lower pelvis to the perineum. Depending on the level of the atresia, more proximal bowel may have to be mobilized, and to avoid damage to the pelvic nerves running to the genitourinary mechanism, more proximal colon may have to be pulled through a tunnel of rectum in an endorectal pull-through fashion after the mucosa is stripped from the pelvic segment. This procedure leaves the individual with a segment of bowel that has little of the sensory and muscular function of a normal rectum. Thus, only the puborectalis sling remains to provide the child with continence. If the bowel is atretic

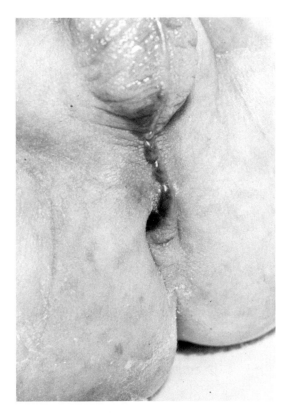 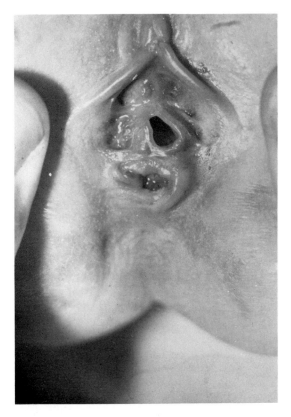

Fig. 10-53. Anal atresia with a deep perineal dimple and a fistula tract running along the perineal and scrotal raphe in a male infant. (From Filston, H. C., and Izant, R.: The surgical neonate: evaluation and care, New York, 1978, Appleton-Century-Crofts.)

Fig. 10-54. Anal atresia and an anal-vestibular or anal-fourchette fistula in a female infant. (From Filston, H. C., and Izant, R.: The surgical neonate: evaluation and care, New York, 1978, Appleton-Century-Crofts.)

to a level at or above the puborectalis sling, the puborectalis sling will probably have pulled forward against the next anatomic structure: the vagina in the female infant or the urethra in the male infant. The importance of pulling the bowel through the puborectalis sling in the proper relationship can, therefore, not be overemphasized. If the bowel is not pulled through anterior to the puborectalis sling, the child will have no continence function remaining.

Evaluation. Identification of the puborectalis sling from a perineal approach is difficult; the most successful procedure described has been the sacrococcygeal perineal approach described by Stephens and Smith.[109] When the atresia is proximal in the rectum and considerable mobilization must be achieved to reach the perineum, this approach is combined with abdominal mobilization of the proximal colon and an endorectal pull-through of the colon. Rectovaginal and recto-urethral or rectovesical fistulas are easily handled during the course of this procedure.

From the above discussion it is obvious that correct decisions in the newborn period are mandatory. The basic rule that must be held inviolate is that if the bowel cannot be clearly demonstrated to be a low-type anomaly, that is, anal atresia with the bowel having properly passed through the puborectalis sling, a colostomy must be performed in the newborn period for decompression; more thorough investigation can then be accomplished at leisure over the next several months without the pressure of an obstructed bowel forcing inappropriate and hasty actions. When a perineal fistula is present, either in the form of a direct opening on the perineum, as is common in a male (Fig. 10-53), or into the perineum, vestibule, or vulvar fourchette in a female (Fig. 10-54), it can generally be assumed that an anal atresia or low-type lesion is present. However, because a small percentage of infants with perineal fistulas may have higher lesions, contrast injection of the fistula should be performed to demonstrate that the fistula runs transversely; that the bowel is, in fact,

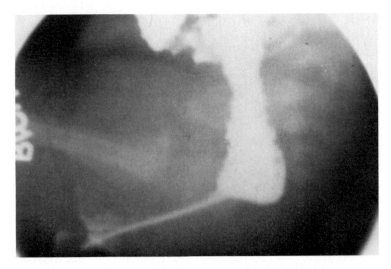

Fig. 10-55. Radiograph of an infant with a fourchette fistula who had an anorectal atresia with the bowel ending considerably more proximal than the perineal-type fistula would suggest.

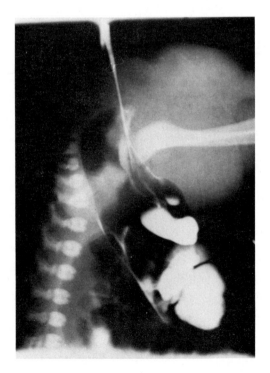

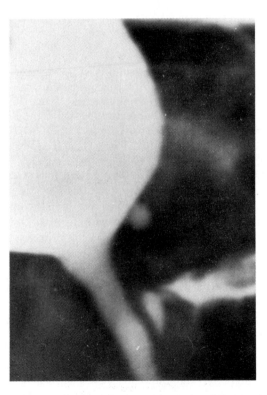

Fig. 10-56. Inverted radiograph with transperineal needle injection of the bowel clearly demonstrating the level of bowel when no fistula is available for injection.

Fig. 10-57. Voiding cystourethrogram showing the presence of a fistula from the distal rectum into the urethra in a male infant with anorectal atresia.

present immediately behind the perineum; and that no unusual pattern exists (Fig. 10-55).

If no fistula is present on the perineum, the safest course is probably to assume that the level is high and that initial treatment should be in the form of a diverting colostomy. However, if upside-down films of the pelvis suggest that the air column at the end of the rectum is close to the perineum and if appropriate measurements of the relationship of the bowel gas to various lines drawn through the ischium that have traditionally been used to judge the level of the puborectalis sling confirm the probability that this is an anal atresia or a low-type imperforate anus, needle puncture of the perineum to inject contrast medium into the rectum and allow thorough study of the configuration and level of the most distal bowel may be in order (Fig. 10-56). Reliance on the air-filled plain inverted radiograph may lead to erroneous conclusions if the child's Valsalva pressures push the bowel toward the perineum, stretching the puborectalis sling ahead of it.[106] The injection of contrast medium will allow a more prolonged evaluation of the distal bowel and its position relative to the perineum after the child has relaxed.

If no perineal fistula is present and the inverted films do not suggest a low lesion, a voiding cystourethrogram may be helpful in demonstrating the presence of a fistula into the urinary tract in the male infant (Fig. 10-57). Fistulas into the vagina and urinary tract generally represent cases of anorectal atresia, but occasionally the fistula will be found to run transversely from a very low situated bowel. Perhaps 10% of infants with such otherwise high-type fistulas simply have anal atresias with the bowel having passed properly through the puborectalis sling. When that situation is demonstrated, a perineal approach may accomplish successful repair.

From the preceding discussion it is obvious that these lesions are complex, requiring the experience of a surgeon who knows them well. In no way are they cases for the occasional surgeon of children. Even for a surgeon with years of experience, this entity remains a challenge, for new varieties are encountered frequently.

Surgical options. Surgical options relate to the timing of repair and to the handling of the more extensive rectal atresia. Anal atresias in male infants are usually repaired in the newborn period. The fistulas usually are small and inadequate to

convey stool over any period of time. Many surgeons advocate simple dilatation of the fistula, but we favor an operative anoplasty, tailoring the anus with a U-shaped posterior flap, which provides a more pliable anus that is less likely to form a stricture (Fig. 10-58). In the female infant with an anterior perineal or fourchette fistula, we have favored dilatation for a few months, followed at approximately 3 months of age by a perineal anoplasty. Many have advised a simple cutback procedure,[106] but we have favored transposing the anus from the fistula site back to the normal perineal site.[107]

For anorectal atresias, colostomy in the newborn period, followed by a sacroperineal approach to identification of the puborectalis sling is the favored approach. When the atresia is quite high, requiring abdominal mobilization of the colon, most physicians favor the procedure advocated by Kiesewetter[55] of stripping the mucosa from the pelvic segment and using this as a pull-through tunnel to bring the proximal colon through and thence through the previously identified pathway anterior to the puborectalis sling and on to the perineum. This maneuver protects the pelvic innervation of the genitourinary tract from inadvertent destruction. Miller and Izant[73] have shown that careful blunt dissection of the pelvic intestine will enable successful pull-through from the

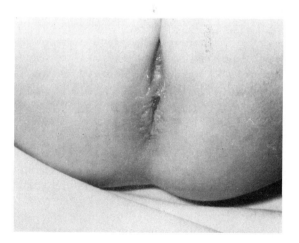

Fig. 10-58. Appearance of the perineum in a female infant who had a formal transposition of the anus with a U-shaped posterior flap anoplasty. Note that the anus tucks in well into the gluteal crease and that there is adequate anal tone.

sacroperineal approach without damage to the pelvic nerves. We generally use the sacroperineal approach for the so-called intermediate level lesions in which the bowel stops at the puborectalis sling and the degree of mobilization required to reach the perineum is minimal. When the lesion is high, we have favored the endorectal approach, which makes identification of any fistula and its subsequent closure very simple.

Postoperative care. Proper decisions as to the surgical choices and competent technical management of the lesion are only part of successful treatment of an imperforate anus. In the postoperative period, careful but vigorous and continuous dilatation of the reconstructed anus is essential to allow the collagen fibers to heal in such a way that some degree of elasticity of the anus results and an adequate, pliable anus that will be useful to the adult as well as to the infant is achieved. If the anus is allowed to heal with circumferential scarring, lifelong constipation problems with dilatation of the rectum and interference with the puborectalis sling function will result. Dilatation can begin somewhere between the second and third postoperative week and progress consistently over the next 2 weeks until the anus accepts a No. 14 or 15 Hegar dilator. At this point, the mother's small finger will usually fit into the anus and daily dilatations utilizing the mother's finger can begin. When the mother can successfully dilate the child's anus to the hilt of her little finger, she is instructed to progress to her index finger and then, depending on the size of the infant, to her middle finger. This provides serial dilatation on a daily basis and generally results over the course of the next 2 to 3 months in a soft, pliable, elastic anus. The frequency of dilatations is then decreased and careful assessment made to ensure that stricture formation does not occur. Finally, by approximately 4 to 5 months postoperatively, all dilatations can be stopped in most infants.

Toilet training. The final phase of successful continence acquisition is proper toilet training. Most toilet training has little basis in physiology, but for the child with an imperforate anus, proper toilet habits are essential. These must take advantage of the gastrocolic reflex. When food is placed in the stomach, the colon tends to contract massively, pushing stool into the rectal segment, as noted previously. This need to defecate can be overcome by voluntarily maintaining the initial involuntary contraction of the external anal sphincter until the internal sphincter relaxes and accommodates to the bolus of stool. As noted previously, that practice results in the rectal ampulla containing large amounts of stool and interferes with the functioning of the puborectalis sling. Although patients with normal anorectal mechanisms can usually function in this fashion because of the backup of the external sphincter function, children with imperforate anus will soil under these conditions because the puborectalis sling will either be left functionless by the dilatation of the rectal ampulla or will segment the stool, forcing the distal-most stool through the patulous anus. By training the child to take advantage of the postprandial gastrocolic reflex, the child will empty the rectal segment and, therefore, will not carry stool in the rectal ampulla. As a result, the puborectalis sling will be able to compress and kink the distal rectum, providing the continence mechanism the child requires.

The parents must be guided through the toilet training phase and be helped to discipline the child to use the commode after meals until this habit pattern is well established. They must thoroughly understand the anatomic reason for this requirement and the consequences of allowing the child to drift into less disciplined toilet habits.

Complications. Beginning with the colostomy, complications following the colostomy procedure are few. There used to be considerable difficulty with skin breakdown until the advent of Stomadhesive, a product that sticks well to the skin and protects it from the irritating effects of the liquid stool outflow of the colostomy. With carefully applied Stomadhesive and a collecting bag, colostomy care of the infant becomes relatively simple. Hemorrhage from the mucosa is due to abrasion of the sensitive mucosal surface and usually stops spontaneously or with a little pressure applied with gauze. Particularly if the bowel has become dilated and hypertrophied before the colostomy procedure, prolapse of the proximal segment may occur as the bowel shrinks down to a more normal size and becomes relatively too small for the fascial stoma. The prolapse usually can be controlled with a little pressure, and if it is not occurring too frequently, these episodes can be dealt with until such time as the child is ready for definitive repair. Stenosis of the colostomy has not been a major problem in our experience, although it is possible to make the stoma too small and leave the child with an inadequate opening.

Following definitive repair, whether by the perineal, sacroperineal, or abdominosacroperineal

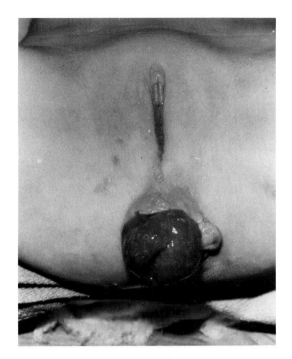

Fig. 10-59. Initial result of an abdominal sacroperineal pull-through procedure in which the bowel could not be anchored adequately to prevent prolapse. This is a common occurrence in the infant who has a poorly formed gluteal fold and a high anorectal atresia.

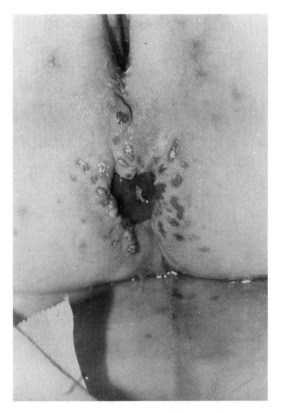

Fig. 10-60. Same infant as in Fig. 10-59 after secondary anoplasty. There is a more satisfactory gluteal crease and elimination of the prolapse. This child had hydrometrocolpos with rectovaginal and urethrovaginal fistulas and moderate sacral anomalies with deficiency of development of the pubococcygeus diaphragm. Nevertheless, she was able to achieve a reasonable degree of continence with careful toilet training.

approach, a significant problem is stenosis of the newly formed anus. This is usually best overcome by a carefully thought-out and controlled program of dilatations, as described previously. Constipation bordering on obstruction may occur in the early postoperative period before adequate dilatation of the stoma can be achieved. Overly vigorous and rapid dilatation of the stoma must be avoided to avoid injury to the fibers of the puborectalis sling. No more than one or two increases in size of the Hegar dilators should be achieved each week. The parents should be cautioned to ensure that the child is having a sizable stool each day and to utilize fruit juice, mineral oil, or even laxatives, if necessary, to keep the stool soft and to keep the child passing adequate amounts.

Particularly for the child with a high anorectal atresia, the repaired anus may not tuck into the gluteal fold well enough and may leave a complete or partial ring of mucosa pouting externally (Fig. 10-59). Such a ring usually leads to soiling, bleeding, and irritation. It is not unusual for extensive anorectal atresia repairs to require secondary tailoring of the perineal anoplasty to achieve a better-appearing and better-functioning

anus. Because the bowel is pulled through from such a high level, there is little fixation of the proximal neorectum; therefore, it is difficult to make the perineal skin tuck in as well at the initial pull-through procedure as one would like to have it. Once scarring fixes the neorectum to the pelvic structures, the rectum can be shortened and the perineal skin tucked further inside, forming a better gluteal crease (Fig. 10-60).

When the results of the initial pull-through procedure are less than satisfactory and there is mucosal pouting, complete prolapse of the rectum may occur, since inadequate support is being supplied to the distal rectum by the puborectalis sling under these circumstances.

Too-vigorous dilatations may lead to injury to the anastomosis with tearing loose of the rectoperineal suture line. Such injury may lead to sinus tracking or abscess formation in the perirectal tissue, which may require drainage of the abscess and may lead, in the long run, to additional scarring that interferes with the puborectalis function and increases the degree of anal stenosis.

Almost all of these complications can be avoided or at least handled appropriately and expeditiously if the surgical consultant provides the complete care that is needed for these lesions in terms of the correct procedure properly timed; a careful, considerate, and gentle but progressive program of postoperative dilatation; and appropriate advice to the parents regarding toilet training.

ABDOMINAL WALL DEFORMITIES
Omphalocele and gastroschisis

Omphalocele and gastroschisis, relatively common lesions of the abdominal wall in the newborn infant, are discussed together here in order to emphasize their differences, particularly those in clinical management. Much has been written in the literature concerning the embryology of each of these lesions, and over the years considerable argument has built up on both sides of the question as to whether or not they differ in etiology.[47] Generally, omphalocele has been seen as an arrest in development at the stage of herniation of the viscera through the as yet unformed ventral abdominal wall. Gastroschisis, on the other hand, has been explained as a failure of one of the components of formation of the abdominal

wall, allowing the viscera to herniate lateral to the normally formed umbilical cord. This explanation has always seemed a weak one and fails to account for the fact that the defect is almost invariably to the right of the cord.

Shaw's discussion of the problem regarding these entities[102] seems to make the most sense. He sees the omphalocele as a failure of formation of the umbilical ring with persistence of the membranous covering of the viscera and a true defect in formation of the abdominal wall. Gastroschisis, on the other hand, according to Shaw, is a rupture of the base of a normally forming umbilical ring and secondary evisceration of the intestines through the rupture. Shaw accounts for the fact that the defect is usually to the right of the cord by the fact that it is the right umbilical vein that atrophies, leaving a predominant left umbilical vein and the weakest point of the umbilical cord in the right superior region (Fig. 10-61). He emphasizes the facts that the defect is between the rectus muscles and that all the components of the abdominal wall are present.

Regardless of the acceptance or rejection of Shaw's theory, there are definite clinical differences between omphaloceles and gastroschisis. The major problem with the omphalocele has to do with its size and the deficient space within the peritoneal cavity. How much of a problem that is depends on the size of the omphalocele. Tiny omphaloceles are little more than glorified um-

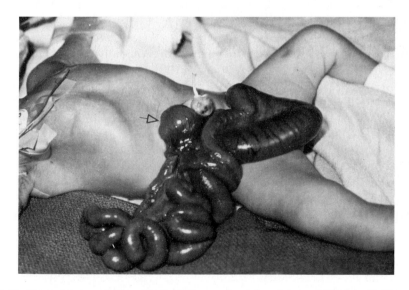

Fig. 10-61. Typical gastroschisis with the defect to the right of the umbilical cord. The stomach (arrow) is seen emerging from the defect.

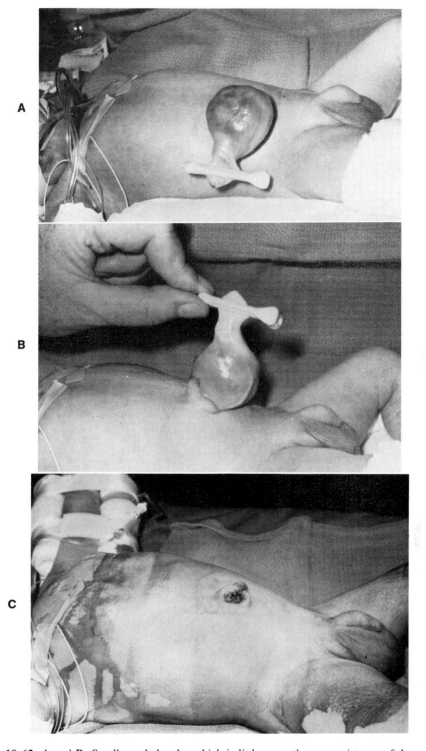

Fig. 10-62. A and **B,** Small omphalocele, which is little more than a persistence of the resolving herniation into the cord. It was easily fixed **(C)** in the neonatal period through a transumbilical approach that left little evidence of the incision after the reconstructed umbilicus had healed.

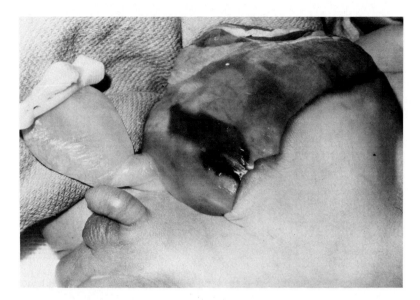

Fig. 10-63. A giant omphalocele that extends from the xyphoid to the pubis and involves most of the abdominal wall is a far more difficult entity to repair. Note that unlike the gastroschisis configuration, the umbilical cord comes off the omphalocele membranes. (From Filston, H. C., and Izant, R.: The surgical neonate: evaluation and care, New York, 1978, Appleton-Century-Crofts.)

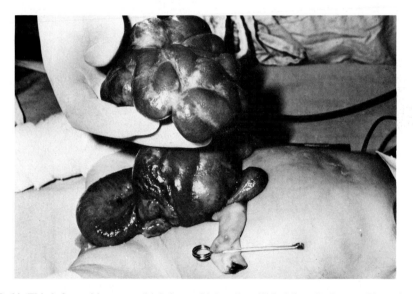

Fig. 10-64. This infant with gastroschisis has a thicker "peel" holding the loops of bowel adherent to one another. The increased difficulty in separating the loops of bowel may make primary closure more difficult. Again, note that the defect is to the right of the umbilical cord structures. (From Filston, H. C., and Izant, R.: The surgical neonate: evaluation and care, New York, 1978, Appleton-Century-Crofts.)

bilical hernias and can be repaired in simple one-stage operations with little morbidity and no mortality in a very short hospital course (Fig. 10-62). At the other extreme is the giant omphalocele that involves a deficit of the abdominal wall extending from the xyphoid to the suprapubic area and frequently from one anterior axillary line to the other (Fig. 10-63). There is little formation of the peritoneal cavity, and the liver occupies a major portion of the sac. Reduction of the viscera into the peritoneal cavity becomes extremely difficult because of the inability to reduce the liver beneath the costal margin. It may take multiple procedures and considerable time to achieve reduction in such lesions.

Gastroschisis lesions, on the other hand, are almost invariably minimally sized and have a well-formed peritoneal cavity. The primary concern in dealing with the child with gastroschisis is proper preoperative care. Unlike the omphalocele, in which the viscera are contained in a membrane and therefore subject to little in the way of evaporative loss of fluids or heat, the bowel in gastroschisis hangs free in the amniotic fluid and as a result sustains varying degrees of chemical injury, depending on the length of time during which the bowel is exposed to the amniotic fluid. When the evisceration occurs early in gestation, the bowel is thickened, edematous, foreshortened, and

covered with varying thicknesses of exudative "peel" (Fig. 10-64). When the rupture occurs later in gestation, there is less of the exudative peel as well as less edema and foreshortening; nevertheless, the child is born with the intestines exposed to the atmosphere. In either case, great amounts of heat and fluid are lost to the environment; and if the child is not managed properly, severe hypothermia and hypovolemia will result.

Preoperative care. As soon as gastroschisis is recognized, the bowel should be gently inspected; particularly, it should be ascertained that adequate room exists in the abdominal wall defect to allow the mesentery to pass through without strangulation. If this is not the case, the defect should be extended in the midline superiorly by placing a clamp beneath the abdominal wall in the midline and incising the full-thickness abdominal wall. If care is taken to ensure that the incision is directly in the midline, the amount of bleeding should be minimal and should be controlled with packing. The bowel should be gently elevated off the abdominal wall and loosely wrapped with a soft gauze roll saturated with saline solution. A small amount of compound iodine antiseptic can be added to the saline for antisepsis. The bowel should be wrapped in a turban-type wrap, which should then continue around the infant's trunk, coming back around the other flank

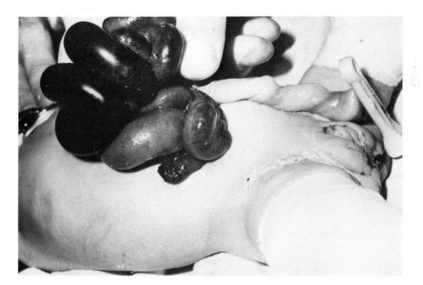

Fig. 10-65. This infant's bowel was not properly protected during transport and was allowed to kink at the gastroschisis defect. This led to vascular obstruction of the mesentery and ischemic necrosis of several loops of intestine.

and then enwrapping the intestines from side to side, making a double loop that will support the wrapped bowel on the abdominal wall and keep it from tilting over and kinking the mesentery (Fig. 10-65). This moist gauze wrap should then be followed by a dry wrap similarly applied and the entire wrapping then covered with a water-proof plastic film or sheeting to guard against heat and evaporative loss. The infant should be carefully maintained in an extra-warm isolette or under a well-functioning overhead warmer. Careful monitoring of the temperature should ensure that heat loss is not occurring despite the above efforts. This is one infant who would benefit from the placement of a well-functioning intravenous line prior to transport and the administration of at least twice his maintenance volume in balanced salt solution. The child will lose extracellular fluid from the exposed surface and replacement with hypotonic solutions usually used for maintenance in infants will result in severe electrolyte depletion as well as shifting of fluid along the diffusion gradient into the extravascular tissues. Urgent transport should be accomplished so that the child will benefit from the care affordable by those experienced in dealing with the lesion.

The transport of an infant with an omphalocele is nowhere near as urgent a problem as that with gastroschisis. The covering membrane protects the child from the losses noted under gastroschisis, and the major consideration is simply to cover the membrane with a protective layer of gauze

that may be impregnated with antiseptic ointment or petrolatum. As long as the membrane is intact, the child will be protected from abnormal losses. Since, unlike gastroschisis, omphalocele may be associated with other lesions,[100] ranging from multiple congenital anomalies with a chromosomal defect basis to the combined omphalocele-hypo-glycemia-macrosomia syndrome of the Beckwith-Weidemann syndrome,[6] thorough additional examination and evaluation of the child with an omphalocele should be undertaken. Gastroschisis is almost invariably an isolated defect, the only accompanying lesions being atresia secondary to bowel or mesenteric injury from the evisceration, the almost invariable presence of a nonrotation of the mesentery, and the frequent association of Meckel's diverticulum. The latter tends to confirm that gastroschisis is, in fact, a variant in the problem of failure of complete reduction of the herniation into the cord. Meckel's diverticulum represents a partial persistence of the omphalo-mesenteric duct to the yolk sac.

Medical versus surgical treatment. There is no medical therapy for the infant with gastroschisis or for the infant with a ruptured omphalocele in which the bowel is eviscerated but the membranes of the omphalocele sac are still identifiable. As soon as the child is stabilized, he should be taken to the operating room. As shown by Raffensperger and Jona,[86] primary closure can be achieved in a high number of instances when a combination of techniques is employed: evacuation

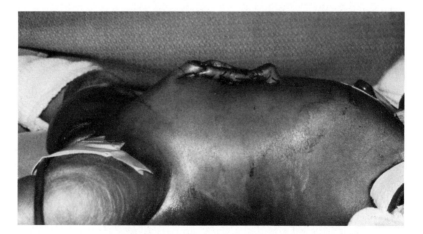

Fig. 10-66. This infant's gastroschisis was totally repaired in one procedure, utilizing saline wash-out of the meconium, stretching of the abdominal wall, and separation and distribution of the bowel loops throughout the peritoneal cavity.

of meconium, lysis of adhesions among the intestinal loops to allow spreading of the intestine throughout the peritoneal cavity, and stretching of the abdominal wall from the paraspinous area to the anterior defect (Fig. 10-66). If primary closure will result in too much pressure, interfering with excursion of the diaphragm, the use of a prosthetic pouch made of Silastic-covered Dacron (Silon) will allow a more gradual reduction of the viscera over the next several days (Fig. 10-67).

For the infant with an intact omphalocele, complete surgical repair is the ultimate goal. Nevertheless, one of the useful techniques, particularly for the very large or giant omphalocele, is the application of an antiseptic drying agent such as Mercurochrome, which will allow shrinkage of the omphalocele sac and overgrowth of the surrounding epidermis.[37] This may avoid the need

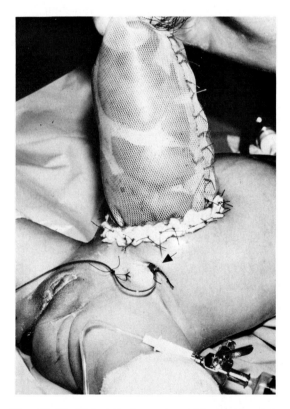

Fig. 10-67. This infant's gastroschisis could not be repaired by primary closure, and a Silon pouch technique was used. The left umbilical artery was transposed to a stab wound in the left lower quadrant of the abdomen and cannulated for postoperative blood gas monitoring (arrow). (From Filston, H. C., and Izant, R.: The surgical neonate: evaluation and care, New York, 1978, Appleton-Century-Crofts.)

for early surgery in an infant with a giant omphalocele, for whom early vigorous surgery may prove injurious to the fragile neonatal liver. As noted below, considerable manipulation of the liver may be necessary to achieve reduction in the giant omphalocele. On the other hand, for the child with a medium- to small-size omphalocele, the preferred therapy is early surgical closure.

Surgical options. As noted above, the goal for all of these is complete primary closure, which usually can be achieved in gastroschisis in one stage. When it is not achievable because the pressure would interfere with ventilation, short-term application of a prosthetic pouch followed by an aggressive program aimed at achieving complete closure of the defect within the first postoperative week should be employed.[2]

For the infant with an omphalocele, primary closure should be achieved whenever possible. However, even with medium-size defects, it may not be possible in one stage and a prosthetic pouch that allows gradual reduction of the viscera may be helpful.[99,101] Other options are skin closure over the omphalocele membrane with secondary repair of the ventral hernia and a similar technique using prosthetic sheeting beneath the skin to fill the fascial defect, followed by delayed secondary fascial reconstruction.

For the child with a giant omphalocele, the major hurdle to reconstruction will be the return of the liver to the intraperitoneal subcostal position that it should normally occupy. Because the liver has developed in the omphalocele sac unrestrained by the usual anatomic relationships, such as the costal structures, the diaphragm, and the vertebral column, the liver is often overly large and globular. It occupies such a large proportion of the omphalocele sac that staged reduction of a prosthetic sac is impossible. In addition, the peritoneal cavity is so poorly formed that the diaphragm frequently is partially eviscerated as a "mesentery" for the liver. Unless the subcostal fossa can be enlarged by stretching and the liver can be placed within it, even staged reduction of the intestines using a prosthetic pouch will be impossible. On the other hand, such rough handling of the liver and diaphragm in the immediate newborn period may lead to rupture of the liver capsule, resulting in exsanguinating hemorrhage. Painting the omphalocele membrane with a desiccating antiseptic solution will benefit the child by toughening the liver capsule so that it will better tolerate the manipulations required to place it beneath the costal margin. If this initial treatment achieves a complete epidermal ingrowth, closing the defect, considerably longer delay may be possible before the ventral defect is repaired. If, on the other hand, the epidermal ingrowth does not take place rapidly or infection or rupture of the omphalocele membrane begins to occur, surgery should be elected; the subcostal fossa is deepened by stretching the diaphragm, and the liver is manipulated into place within it. Care should be taken in this maneuver not to compress or kink the hepatic veins or the inferior vena cava. Once the liver is successfully manipulated into the subcostal fossa, a prosthetic pouch of Silon can be sewn to the edges of the defect and a gradual reduction of the intestines accomplished over the next several days (Fig. 10-68). Once the prosthetic pouch has been reduced to the point of being a flat membrane, the child is returned to the operating room and the prosthetic material imbricated on itself several times until the edges of the defect are apposed. Final closure is then achieved by direct suture of the abdominal wall.

Prognosis. With most of these lesions, surgery is successful and the child faces a normal future. Nevertheless, the giant omphalocele still presents one of the major challenges of pediatric surgery; and despite the multiplicity of approaches utilized, failure occasionally results.[113] The recent emphasis on primary closure of gastroschisis and the utilization of the prosthetic pouch for the medium-size omphalocele have vastly improved the survival for most of these children. Only a few years ago, mortality of 50% was being reported for gastroschisis, whereas over the last 5 years our survival rate has been 100%. Only about 20% fail initial primary closure, and these usually respond to the brief use of a prosthesis with complete closure being achieved secondarily a few days later.

Complications. The most immediate intraoperative complication is injury to the liver in attempts at repair of the giant omphalocele. Other complications are ischemic injury to the bowel in those infants with gastroschisis who have a small defect and compromise of the eviscerated mesentery. Infection is an ongoing risk until primary closure and healing have been obtained. On a long-term basis, the primary complication is intestinal obstruction from adhesions. Although nonrotation of the mesentery is usually present in these lesions, the volvulus and strangulation associated with malrotation are less likely to occur, because the configuration of nonrotation still leaves considerable spread of the base of the mesentery, albeit it is poorly attached. Also, adhesions probably help to fix the bowel, preventing volvulus. Thus, strangulating obstruction follow-

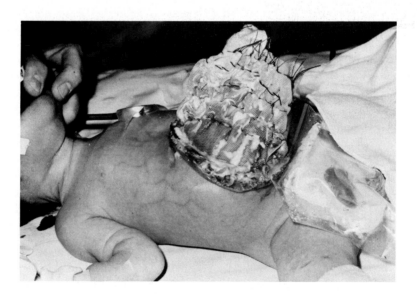

Fig. 10-68. Late stage in the reduction of a large prosthetic pouch placed for staged repair of a giant omphalocele. Note the several suture lines in the pouch, representing daily reduction of the abdominal viscera back into the peritoneal cavity. (From Filston, H. C., and Izant, R.: The surgical neonate: evaluation and care, New York, 1978, Appleton-Century-Crofts.)

Table 10-1. Complications of Meckel's diverticulum*

Complication	No.		Deaths
Hemorrhage	47		0
Intestinal obstruction	37		
Intussusception		(23)	
Bands and torsion		(14)	5
Diverticulitis (simulating appendicitis)	24		
Without perforation		(19)	
Perforation and peritonitis		(5)	1
Umbilical discharge	7		0
TOTAL	115		6 (5%)

*Reproduced with permission from Benson, C. D.: Surgical implications of Meckel's diverticulum, in the chapter The small intestine. In Ravitch, M. M., and others, editors: Pediatric surgery, ed. 3. Copyright © 1979 by Year Book Medical Publishers, Inc., Chicago.

ing these lesions is unusual but must be considered whenever the child has symptoms of bowel obstruction. Simple intestinal obstruction due to adhesions has approximately the same incidence for these lesions as it does with any other intraabdominal procedure.

Associated anomalies. Awareness of the anomalies associated with these lesions is important, particularly with the omphalocele. Gastroschisis is usually associated with nonrotation of the mesentery and Meckel's diverticulum. The diverticulum is not always removed at the time of initial surgery; in fact, we prefer not to add a procedure that could lead to anastomotic leakage. Whether one should electively return and remove the diverticulum is an unanswered question. Complications of the presence of Meckel's diverticulum include hemorrhage due to ulceration of the ileal mucosa adjacent to gastric mucosa in the diverticulum, perforation and inflammation of the diverticulum, and intussusception with the diverticulum acting as the leading point (Table 10-1).[10] Multiple associated midline defects may occasionally occur with an omphalocele, suggesting chromosomal abnormalities. In addition, the blood glucose level should be carefully monitored to identify hypoglycemia of the Beckwith-Weidemann syndrome.[6]

Absent abdominal wall musculature syndrome (prune belly)

A less common abdominal wall defect is that of the absent abdominal wall musculature syn-

drome. The etiology of this lesion is not well understood, and debate continues as to whether it represents failure of formation of the abdominal wall muscles or secondary atrophy. The most important aspect of this lesion is its associated anomalies in the genitourinary system, particularly those of obstructive uropathy with resultant hydronephrosis and renal parenchymal damage. This lesion occurs predominantly in male infants and is associated with undescended testicles and occasionally with hypospadias. The most striking finding may be the extensive elongation and dilatation of the ureters, with the ureters being several times the normal diameter and many times the normal length. Reconstructive procedures can reduce the ureters back toward normal size.[44] Early evaluation of these children by an experienced surgeon should be obtained to plan a long-term therapeutic program that will prevent additional damage to the kidneys. This entity is discussed more fully in Chapter 11 on urologic considerations of the newborn.

MASSES
Sacrococcygeal teratoma

Sacrococcygeal teratoma is the most common tumor *recognized* at birth.[90] Wilms' tumors and neuroblastomas, the more common tumors of childhood, are probably present in the newborn but are not recognized. The incidence is between 1 of 30,000 to 1 of 45,000 births. These lesions predominate in girls, and there is a significant incidence of twinning in the families.

Clinical presentation. When the sacrococcygeal teratoma presents as a large mass on the buttock, it is easily identified (Fig. 10-69). Occasionally, however, it may be either partially or completely intrapelvic and may be missed on the newborn exam. The intrapelvic sacrococcygeal teratoma may enlarge and present abdominally as a suprapubic mass. The lesion may be multilobulated and variably cystic. It arises from the coccyx and can generally be differentiated from the distal myelomeningoceles by the more caudal location of the lesion and the intact skin. It will occasionally be ruptured during delivery, or it may undergo breakdown of the epithelium in the early newborn period.

Treatment. Early excision is indicated, both for avoidance of complications and insurance against malignancy (Fig. 10-70). In our own experience, the incidence of malignancy has been low when the lesion is excised before the child is

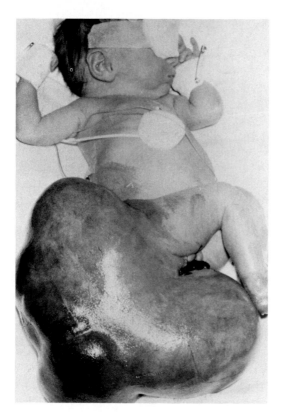

Fig. 10-69. Infant with a giant sacrococcygeal teratoma. The infant and tumor together weighed 4,200 g. and the infant postoperatively weighed 2,200 g. Note the meconium exuding from the anteroinferiorly displaced anus.

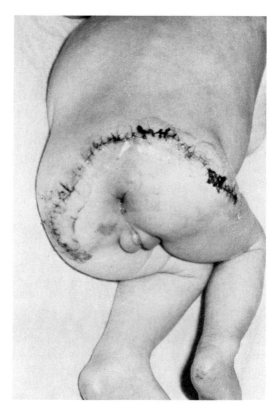

Fig. 10-70. Same infant as in Fig. 10-69 in the immediate postoperative period, showing good inversion of the anus with reasonably good anal tone.

1 month of age.[48] This low incidence of malignancy has been confirmed by most other authors, although a few cases of malignant consequences of the tumor have been reported even when the tumor was excised in the newborn period.[69] Complete excision of the lesion in continuity with the coccyx should be the goal, or the recurrence rate will be high. Recurrent lesions are often malignant. Recently, multimodal therapy has been tried for malignant lesions, but it is too early to evaluate results.

For the intrapelvic lesions, excision can often be accomplished through the usual sacrococcygeal incision; occasionally, however, a combined abdominal sacral approach will be necessary.

Complications. The giant sacrococcygeal teratoma may splay out the musculature of the pelvic diaphragm, so that the levator sling appears almost nonexistent. Infants in whom the anus is markedly patulous postoperatively have been observed. Careful dissection of the tumor using blunt dissection where possible to avoid injury to the pelvic nerves, to the bladder, and to the rectal continence mechanisms will usually result in return of function within 6 months following surgery (Fig. 10-71). Ultimately, constipation has been the one postoperative complication seen with any frequency, and it usually responds to conservative measures.

Cystic hygroma

Clinical presentation. Another tumor that may be recognized in the newborn period is the cystic hygroma (Fig. 10-72). This is a form of lymphangioma, usually presenting in the posterior triangle of the neck.[43] It frequently prevents the child from turning his head, which may lead to deformity of the cranium. Infection may develop in the static lymph. Furthermore, significant hemorrhage into the fluid may occur. Large lesions may compress the trachea. There are generally two varieties of this lesion, the more common being made up of large cysts. The less common lesion is a lymphangioma made up of small

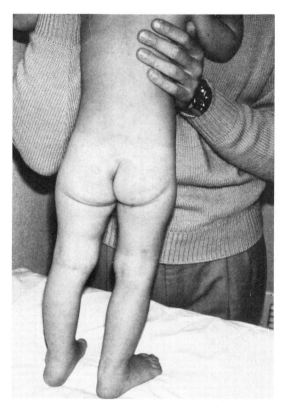

Fig. 10-71. Same child as in Fig. 10-69, 2 years following surgery. She is neurologically intact and is completely continent. There is no evidence of recurrence.

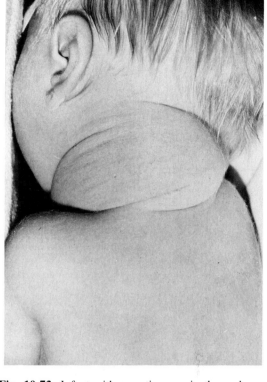

Fig. 10-72. Infant with a cystic mass in the neck representing a cystic hygroma. (From Filston, H. C., and Izant, R.: The surgical neonate: evaluation and care, New York, 1978, Appleton-Century-Crofts.)

grapelike clusters of abnormal lymph vessels; these lesions infiltrate throughout the normal tissues, enwrapping nerves and vessels and making complete excision difficult. Because of the high density of important anatomy in the neck, these latter lesions often cannot be completely excised without damage to normal structures. The cystic hygroma with large cysts is usually more easily removed. These lesions may extend into the mediastinum or may "dumbbell" into the axilla.

Medical versus surgical treatment. Delay in surgical excision will often lead to infection or airway obstruction. Infection may make subsequent surgery more difficult. Furthermore, children have been known to sustain severe, life-threatening hemorrhage into these lesions. Early excision is indicated for lesions that threaten the airway, are overly large, or have associated hemorrhage. Radiation therapy is contraindicated.[20,77]

Surgical options. Surgical options are partial or complete excision. Complete excision of the small grapelike clusters of enwrapping lymph tissue may cause damage to normal structures. For these lesions, partial excision may be preferable. Usually the remaining tissue will fibrose after frequent infections are controlled by antibiotics. Associated lesions are rare.

Ovarian lesions

Lesions of the ovary are rare in the newborn. Occasionally, an ovarian cyst will present either as a palpable mass on the newborn physical examination or as an acute abdominal condition due to torsion and necrosis (Fig. 10-73). One ovarian teratoma reported on obstructed the intestine and led to a proximal intestinal perforation.[97] Usually, ovarian lesions present beyond the newborn period.

Other tumors

Few other tumors present in the immediate newborn period. Occasionally a neuroblastoma or Wilms' tumor is palpated on newborn physical examination, but this is unusual. Obviously, these

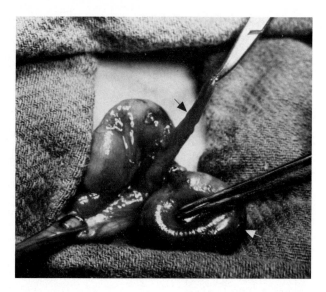

Fig. 10-73. Torsion and necrosis of an ovarian cyst (white arrow) has led to inflammation and adherence of the appendix to the cyst (black arrow).

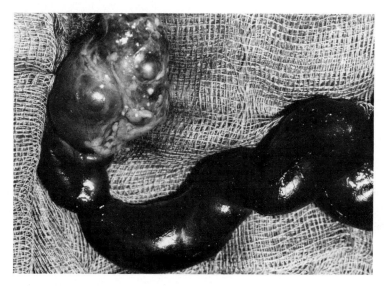

Fig. 10-74. Ureterovesical obstruction that led to a giant hydroureter and a dysplastic cystic kidney. The infant had a large abdominal mass.

tumors are present, however, so that careful evaluation of the abdomen on initial physical examination is important and any indication of a flank tumor should be thoroughly investigated. Certain renal anomalies such as obstructive uropathy at the ureteropelvic or ureterovesical junction can result in proximal dilatation with a hydroureter and/or hydronephrosis (Fig. 10-74). Multicystic or dysplastic kidneys may present as flank masses. The intravenous pyelogram usually goes far to-

ward differentiating these lesions from one another.

Hemangioma

Hemangiomas are discussed here and also in the section on the infant and toddler. Rarely is a hemangioma an obvious major problem in the immediate newborn period. However, with careful examination, several varieties of them may be discovered on the first examination. Common

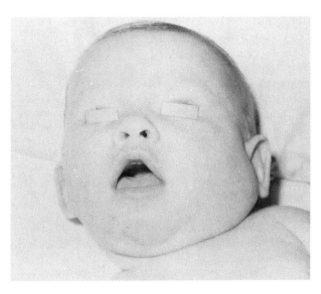

Fig. 10-75. Cavernous hemangioma occurring at the angle of the jaw, a common location for hemangiomas in infants.

locations for hemangiomas are about the face, particularly lateral to the eye, at the upper bridge of the nose, and at the angle of the jaw (Fig. 10-75). Tiny capillary hemangiomas are common on the upper lids of infants and are usually of little consequence.

Hemangiomas are generally described as being of two types: the superficial capillary hemangioma that involves primarily the skin and the deeper, cavernous hemangioma that extends into the subcutaneous tissues or may arise in any tissue or organ of the body. In reality, there is a vast array of vascular abnormalities that run the gamut from simple epidermal skin stains to aggressive, extensive angiomatous lesions of the deeper tissues and organs of the body.

In the immediate newborn period, what is usually found is a capillary hemangioma, and these need no immediate therapy. Their presence should be noted, and they should be carefully followed over the course of the first few well-baby visits. If rapid growth ensues, or if the location may subject a vital structure to functional impairment, early referral to a surgical specialist who is familiar with such lesions in children is indicated. The primary care physician must know that the surgeon to whom these children are referred is experienced in dealing with these lesions, for many of the lesions respond best with only expectant treatment. The surgeon who is unfamiliar with

such lesions may hasten to excise them unnecessarily and leave the child with a disfiguring scar or even functional impairment. This is not to say that there are not hemangiomas that require early excision, but they are the exception rather than the rule. In addition, large hemangiomas that involve normal tissues extensively may produce life-threatening hemorrhage if they are exposed surgically by someone unfamiliar with their potential for extensive infiltration and massive blood loss.

Lymphangioma

Lymphangiomas of the head and neck are included in the discussion on cystic hygroma. However, lymphangiomas may occur anywhere in the body, presenting as painless masses in the soft tissues of the extremities and trunk or even arising in the retroperitoneal area, presenting as tumor masses. Although most of the more superficial lesions will eventually present as asymptomatic masses, some of the deeper lesions, especially the retroperitoneal lesions, may initially present when infection supervenes. Thus, children being explored for acute abdominal conditions have been found to have infected retroperitoneal lymphangiomas.

Since the diagnosis can only be suspected from physical examination, and since differentiation from lipomas may be difficult, the initial lesion should probably be excised. This excision may be complete; because of the benign nature of the lesion, however, the surgeon must be careful not to invade normal tissue and do damage to surrounding structures in an inappropriate attempt to do a wide excision of a benign lesion. If lymphangiomatous tissue is left behind, a localized mass lesion may redevelop; often, however, subsequent infection and scarring will rid the patient of additional lymphangioma. Also, with the diagnosis confirmed, less aggressive therapy is warranted for recurrences.

If the lymphangioma initially presents with signs of infection, it should be treated with systemic antibiotics until the infection subsides or until progression to abscess formation forces incision and drainage. The latter is an unusual occurrence.

REFERENCES

1. Abrahamson, J., and Shandling, B.: Esophageal atresia in the underweight baby: a challenge, J. Pediatr. Surg. **7:**608, 1972.
2. Allen, R. G., and Wrenn, E. L., Jr.: Silon as a sac in the treatment of omphalocele and gastroschisis, J. Pediatr. Surg. **4:**3, 1969.
3. Ashcraft, K. W., and others: Early recognition and aggressive treatment of gastroesophageal reflux following repair of esophageal atresia, J. Pediatr. Surg. **12:**317, 1977.
4. Baran, E. M., and others: Foramen of Morgagni hernias in children, Surgery **62:**1076, 1967.
5. Barlow, B., and others: An experimental study of acute neonatal enterocolitis—the importance of breast milk, J. Pediatr. Surg. **9:**587, 1974.
6. Beckwith, J. B.: Extreme cytomegaly of the adrenal fetal cortex, omphalocele, hyperplasia of kidneys and pancreas, and Leydig-cell hyperplasia—another syndrome? Presented at the Annual Meeting of the Western Society for Pediatric Research, Los Angeles, November 11, 1963.
7. Bedard, P., Girvan, D. P., and Shandling, B.: Congenital H-type tracheoesophageal fistula, J. Pediatr. Surg. **9:**663, 1974.
8. Bell, M. J., and others: Neonatal necrotizing enterocolitis; therapeutic decisions based upon clinical staging, Ann. Surg. **187:**1, 1978.
9. Bell, M. J., and others: prepyloric gastric antral web: a puzzling epidemic, J. Pediatr. Surg. **13:**307, 1978.
10. Benson, C. D.: Surgical implications of Meckel's diverticulum. In Ravitch, M. M., and others, editors: Pediatric surgery, ed. 3, Chicago, 1979, Year Book Medical Publishers, Inc., p. 955.
11. Bill, A. H.: Malrotation of the intestine. In Ravitch, M. M., and others, editors: Pediatric surgery, ed. 3, Chicago, 1979, Year Book Medical Publishers, Inc.
12. Bishop, H. C., and Filston, H. C.: An inversion-ligation technique for incidental appendectomy, J. Pediatr. Surg. **8:**889, 1973.
13. Bishop, H. C., and Koop, C. E.: Management of meconium ileus: resection, Roux-en-Y anastomosis, and ileostomy irrigation with pancreatic enzymes, Ann. Surg. **145:**410, 1957.
14. Bishop, H. C., and Koop, C. E.: Acquired eventration of the diaphragm in infancy, Pediatrics **22:**1088, 1958.
15. Bray, P. F., and others: Childhood gastroesophageal reflux: neurologic and psychiatric syndromes mimicked, J.A.M.A. **237:**1342, 1977.
16. Brown, E. G., and Sweet, A. Y.: Preventing necrotizing enterocolitis in neonates, J.A.M.A. **240:**2452, 1978.
17. Burroughs, N., and Leape, L. L.: Laryngotracheoesophageal cleft: report of a case successfully treated and review of the literature, Pediatrics **53:**516, 1974.
18. Campbell, D. P., Vanhoutte, J. J., and Smith, E. I.: Partially obstructing antral web/a distinct clinical entity, J. Pediatr. Surg. **8:**723, 1973.
19. Carré, I. J.: A historical review of the clinical consequences of hiatal hernia (partial thoracic stomach) and gastroesophageal reflux. In Gellis, S. S., editor: Gastroesophageal reflux: report of the Seventy-sixth Ross Conference on Pediatric Research, Columbus, Ohio, 1979, Ross Laboratories, p. 4.
20. Chait, D., and others: Management of cystic hygromas, Surg. Gynecol. Obstet. **139:**55, 1974.
21. Clark, D. A.: Times of first void and first stool in 500 newborns, Pediatrics **60:**457, 1977.
22. Clatworthy, H. W., Howard, W. H. R., and Lloyd, J.: The meconium plug syndrome, Surgery **39:**131, 1956.
23. Collins, D. L., and others: A new approach to congenital posterolateral diaphragmatic hernia, J. Pediatr. Surg. **12:**149, 1977.
24. Coran, A. G.: Total intravenous feeding of infants and children without the use of a central venous catheter, Ann. Surg. **179:**445, 1974.
25. Cordonnier, J. K., and Izant, R. J., Jr.: Meconium ileus equivalent, Surgery **54:**667, 1963.
26. Davis, W. S., and Campbell, J. B.: Neonatal small left colon syndrome, Am. J. Dis. Child. **129:**1024, 1975.
27. Dibbins, A. W.: Neonatal diaphragmatic hernia: a physiologic challenge, Am. J. Surg. **131:**408, 1976.
28. Dibbins, A. W., and Weiner, E. J.: Mortality from neonatal diaphragmatic hernia, J. Pediatr. Surg. **9:**653, 1974.
29. Domres, B., Schweizer, P., and Flach, A.: Complete correction of malrotation, Z. Kinderchir. **20:**137, 1977. Abstract in J. Pediatr. Surg. **12:**1090, 1977.
30. Eigen, H., Lemen, R. J., and Waring, W. W.: Congenital lobar emphysema: long-term evaluation of surgically and conservatively treated children, Am. Rev. Respir. Dis. **113:**823, 1976.
31. Ellis, D. G., and Clatworthy, H. W.: The meconium plug syndrome revisited, J. Pediatr. Surg. **1:**54, 1966.
32. Filston, H. C., and Grant, J. P.: A safer system for percutaneous subclavian venous catheterization in newborn infants, J. Pediatr. Surg. **14:**564, 1979.
33. Filston, H. C., Johnson, D. G., and Crumrine, R. S.; Infant tracheostomy: a new look with a solution to the difficult cannulation problem, Am. J. Dis. Child. **132:**1172, 1978.
34. Fost, N. C., and Esterly, N. B.: Successful treatment of juvenile hemangiomas with prednisone, J. Pediatr. **72:**351, 1968.

35. Gans, S. L., and Berci, G.: Inside tracheoesophageal fistula: new endoscopic approaches, J. Pediatr. Surg. **8**:205, 1973.

36. German, J. C., and others: Prospective application of an index of neonatal necrotizing enterocolitis, J. Pediatr. Surg. **14**:364, 1979.

37. Grob, M.: Conservative treatment of exomphalos, Arch. Dis. Child. **38**:148, 1965.

38. Grosfeld, J. L., Boger, D., and Clatworthy, H. W., Jr.: Hemodynamic and manometric observations in experimental air-block syndrome, J. Pediatr. Surg. **6**:339, 1971.

39. Grosfeld, J. L., and others: Emergency thoracotomy for acquired bronchopleural fistula in the premature infant with respiratory distress, J. Pediatr. Surg. **15**:416, 1980.

40. Gross, R. E.: The surgery of infancy and childhood, Philadelphia, 1953, W. B. Saunders Co., p. 158.

41. Gross, S., and Melhorn, D.: Exchange transfusion with citrated whole blood for disseminated intravascular coagulation, J. Pediatr. **78**:415, 1971.

42. Haller, J. A., Jr., and others: Pulmonary and ductal hemodynamics in studies of simulated diaphragmatic hernia of fetal and newborn lambs, J. Pediatr. Surg. **11**:675, 1976.

43. Harkins, G. A., and Sabiston, D. C., Jr.: Lymphangioma in infancy and childhood, Surgery **47**:811, 1960.

44. Hendren, W. H.: A new approach to infants with severe obstructive uropathy: early complete reconstruction, J. Pediatr. Surg. **5**:184, 1970.

45. Hendren, W. H., and McKee, D. M.: Lobar emphysema of infancy, J. Pediatr. Surg. **1**:24, 1966.

46. Holschneider, A. M.: The problem of anorectal incontinence. In Rickham, P. P., Hecker, W. C., and Prevot, J., editors: Progress in pediatric surgery. Vol. 9. Anorectal malformations and associated diseases, Baltimore, 1976, University Park Press, p. 93.

47. Izant, R. J., Jr., Brown, E., and Rothmann, B. F.: Current embryology and treatment of gastroschisis and omphalocele, Arch. Surg. **93**:49, 1966.

48. Izant, R. J., Jr., and Filston, H. C.: Sacrococcygeal teratomas: analysis of forty-three cases, Am. J. Surg. **130**:617, 1975.

49. Johnson, D. G., Deaner, R. M., and Koop, C. E.: Diaphragmatic hernia in infancy: factors affecting the mortality rate, Surgery **62**:1082, 1967.

50. Johnson, D. G., and others: Evaluation of gastroesophageal reflux surgery in children, Pediatrics **59**:62, 1977.

51. Jones, D. S.: The origin of the vagi and the parasympathetic ganglion cells of the viscera of the chick, Anat. Rec. **82**:185, 1942.

52. Keith, H. H.: Congenital lobar emphysema, Pediatr. Ann. **6**:452, 1977.

53. Kennedy, J. H., and Rothmann, B. F.: The surgical treatment of congenital lobar emphysema, Surgery **121**:253, 1965.

54. Ketonen, P., and others: Surgical treatment of hernia through the foramen of Morgagni, Acta Chir. Scand. **141**:633, 1975.

55. Kiesewetter, W. B.: Imperforate anus. II. The rationale and technic of the sacroabdominoperineal operation, J. Pediatr. Surg. **2**:106, 1967.

56. Kim, S. H., and Hendren, W. H.: Endoscopic resection of obstructing airway lesions in children, J. Pediatr. Surg. **11**:431, 1976.

57. Kleinhaus, S., and others: Hirschsprung's disease—a survey of the members of the Surgical Section of the American Academy of Pediatrics, J. Pediatr. Surg. **14**:588, 1979.

58. Kock, N. G., Darle, N., and Dolevall, G.: Inhibition of intestinal motility in man by glucagon given intraportally, Gastroenterology **53**:88, 1967.

59. Koop, C. E., and Hamilton, J. P.: Atresia of the esophagus: increased survival with staged procedures in the poor-risk infant, Ann. Surg. **162**:389, 1965.

60. Kosloske, A. M.: Necrotizing enterocolitis in the neonate, Surg. Gynecol. Obstet. **148**:259, 1979.

61. Krasna, I. H., and others: Colonic stenosis following necrotizing enterocolitis of the newborn, J. Pediatr. Surg. **5**:200, 1970.

62. Ladd, W. E., and Gross, R. E.: Abdominal surgery in infancy and childhood, Philadelphia, 1941, W. B. Saunders Co., pp. 36, 62.

63. Leape, L. L.: Gastroesophageal reflux as a cause of sudden infant death syndrome. In Gellis, S. S., editor: Gastroesophageal reflux: report of the Seventy-sixth Ross Conference of Pediatric Research, Columbus, Ohio, 1979, Ross Laboratories, p. 30.

64. Lilly, J. R., and Randolph, J. G.: Total inversion of the appendix: experiences with incidental appendectomy in children, J. Pediatr. Surg. **3**:357, 1968.

65. Lindholm, C.: Prolonged endotracheal intubation, Acta Anaesthesiol. Scand. [Suppl.] **33**:1, 1969.

66. Lindsay, W. K.: Lips, tongue, and floor of the mouth. In Mustarde, J. C., editor: Plastic surgery in infancy and childhood, Philadelphia, 1971, W. B. Saunders Co., p. 122.

67. Lloyd, D. A., and Cywes, S.: Intestinal stenosis and enterocyst formation as late complications of neonatal necrotizing enterocolitis, J. Pediatr. Surg. **8**:479, 1973.

68. Louw, J. H., and Barnard, C. N.: Congenital intestinal atresia: observations on its origin, Lancet **2**:1065, 1955.

69. Mahour, G. H., and others: Sacrococcygeal teratoma: A 33-year experience, J. Pediatr. Surg. **10**:183, 1975.

70. Mansfield, P. B., and others: Pneumopericardium and pneumomediastinum in infants and children, J. Pediatr. Surg. **8**:691, 1973.

71. Martin, D. J.: Experiences with acute surgical conditions, Radiol. Clin. North Am. **13**:297, 1975.

72. Martin, L. W., and others: Hirschsprung's disease with skip area (segmental aganglionosis), J. Pediatr. Surg. **14**:686, 1979.

73. Miller, R. C., and Izant, R. J., Jr.: Sacrococcygeal perineal approach to imperforate anus, Am. J. Surg. **121**:62, 1971.

74. Moore, K. L.: The developing human, Philadelphia, W. B. Saunders Co., 1973.

75. Mustard, W. T., and others, editors: Pediatric surgery, ed. 2, Chicago, 1969, Year Book Medical Publishers, Inc.

76. Myers, N. A., and Aberdeen, E.: The esophagus. In Ravitch, M. M., and others, editors: Pediatric surgery, ed. 3, Chicago, 1979, Year Book Medical Publishers, Inc., pp. 461-464.

77. Ninh, T. N., and Ninh, T. X.: Cystic hygroma in children: a report of 126 cases, J. Pediatr. Surg. **9**:151, 1974.

78. Nixon, H. H.: Intestinal obstruction in the newborn, Arch. Dis. Child. **30**:13, 1955.

79. Nixon, H. H.: Surgical conditions in paediatrics, London, 1978, Butterworth and Co. (Publishers) Ltd., pp. 20, 263.

80. Noblett, H. R.: Treatment of uncomplicated meconium ileus by Gastrografin enema: a preliminary report, J. Pediatr. Surg. **4**:190, 1969.

81. Olivet, R. T., and others: Hemodynamics of congenital diaphragmatic hernia in lambs, J. Pediatr. Surg. **13**:231, 1978.

82. Olsen, L., and Grotte, G.: Congenital pyloric atresia: report of a familial occurrence, J. Pediatr. Surg. **11**:181, 1976.

83. O'Neill, J. A., Jr., and Holcomb, G. W.: Surgical experience with neonatal necrotizing enterocolitis (NNE), Ann. Surg. **189**:612, 1979.

84. Pettersson, G.: Inhibited separation of larynx and the upper part of trachea from oesophagus in a newborn: report of a case successfully operated upon, Acta Chir. Scand. **110**:250, 1955.

85. Philippart, A. I., Reed, J. Q., and Georgeson, K. E.: Neonatal small left colon syndrome, J. Pediatr. Surg. **10**:733, 1975.

86. Raffensperger, J. G., and Jona, J. Z.: Gastroschisis, Surg. Gynecol. Obstet. **138**:230, 1974.

87. Ramenofsky, M. L., and Raffensperger, J. G.: An abdomino-perineal-vaginal pull-through for definitive treatment of hydrometrocolpos, J. Pediatr. Surg. **6**:381, 1971.

88. Raphaely, R. C., and Downes, J. J., Jr.: Congenital diaphragmatic hernia: prediction of survival, J. Pediatr. Surg. **8**:815, 1973.

89. Ravitch, M. M.: Congenital malformations and neonatal problems of the respiratory tract. In Ravitch, M. M., and others, editors: Pediatric surgery, ed. 3, Chicago, 1979, Year Book Medical Publishers, Inc., pp. 523, 525.

90. Ravitch, M. M.: Sacrococcygeal teratoma. In Ravitch, M. M., and others, editors: Pediatric surgery, ed. 3, Chicago, 1979, Year Book Medical Publishers, Inc., p. 1119.

91. Richardson, J.: Pharmacologic studies of Hirschsprung's disease on a murine model, J. Pediatr. Surg. **10**:875, 1975.

92. Richardson, W. R., and Martin, L. W.: Pitfalls in the surgical management of incomplete duodenal diaphragm, J. Pediatr. Surg. **4**:303, 1969.

93. Rodgers, B. M., Rooks, J. J., and Talbert, J. L.: Pediatric tracheostomy: long-term evaluation, J. Pediatr. Surg. **14**:258, 1979.

94. Rogawski, M. A., and others: Hirschsprung's disease: absence of serotonergic neurons in the aganglionic colon, J. Pediatr. Surg. **13**:608, 1976.

95. Rowe, M. I., Buckner, D., and Clatworthy, H. W., Jr.: Wind sock web of the duodenum, Am. J. Surg. **116**:444, 1968.

96. Rowe, M. I., Seagram, G., and Weinberger, M.: Gastrografin induced hypertonicity: the pathogenesis of a neonatal hazard, Am. J. Surg. **125**:185, 1973.

97. Scholz, P. M., Key, L., and Filston, H. C.: Large ovarian cyst causing cecal perforation in a newborn infant, J. Pediatr. Surg., in press.

98. Schuster, M. M.: The riddle of the sphincters, Gastroenterology **69**:249, 1975.

99. Schuster, S. R.: A new method in the staged repair of large omphaloceles, Surg. Gynecol. Obstet. **125**:837, 1967.

100. Schuster, S. R.: Omphalocele, hernia, of the umbilical cord, and gastroschisis. In Ravitch, M. M., and others, editors: Pediatric surgery, ed. 3, Chicago, 1979, Year Book Medical Publishers, Inc., p. 784.

101. Seashore, J. H., MacNaughton, R. J., and Talbert, J. L.: Treatment of gastroschisis and omphalocele with biological dressings, J. Pediatr. Surg. **10**:9, 1975.

102. Shaw, A.: The myth of gastroschisis, J. Pediatr. Surg. **10**:235, 1975.

103. Shermeta, D. W., and others: Lower esophageal sphincter dysfunction in esophageal atresia: nocturnal regurgitation and aspiration pneumonia, J. Pediatr. Surg. **12**:871, 1977.

104. Shochat, S. J., and others: Congenital diaphragmatic hernia: new concept in management, Ann. Surg. **190**:332, 1979.

105. Skandalakis, J. E., and others: Anatomical complications of pancreatic surgery, Contemp. Surg. **15**:17, 1979.

106. Smith, E. D.: The identification and management of anorectal anomalies. In Rickham, P. P., Hecker, W. C., and Prevot, J., editors: Progress in pediatric surgery. Vol. 9. Anorectal malformations and associated diseases, Baltimore, 1976, University Park Press, p. 16.

107. Smith, E. I., Tunnell, W. P., and Williams, G. R.: A clinical evaluation of the surgical treatment of anorectal malformations (inperforate anus), Ann. Surg. **187**:583, 1978.

108. Snyder, W. H., Jr., and Greaney, E. M.: Congenital diaphragmatic hernia: 77 consecutive cases, Surgery **57**:576, 1965.

109. Stephens, F. D., and Smith, E. D.: Ano-rectal malformations in children, Chicago, 1971, Year Book Medical Publishers, Inc., pp. 239-247.

110. Stern, L. M., and others: Management of Pierre Robin syndrome in infancy by prolonged nasoesophageal intubation, Am. J. Dis. Child. **124**:78, 1972.

111. Stewart, D. R., Colodny, A. L., and Daggett, W. C.: Malrotation of the bowel in infants and children: a 15 year review, Surgery **79**:716, 1976.

112. Stewart, D. R., and others: Neonatal small left colon syndrome, Ann. Surg. **186**:741, 1977.

113. Stringel, G., and Filler, R. M.: Prognostic factors in omphalocele and gastroschisis, J. Pediatr. Surg. **14**:515, 1979.

114. Swenson, O., Rhinelander, H. F., and Diamond, I.: Hirschsprung's disease: new concepts in etiology—operative results in 34 patients, N. Engl. J. Med. **241**:551, 1949.

115. Tiffen, M. E., Chandler, L. R., and Faber, H. K.: Localized absence of ganglion cells of myenteric plexus in congenital megacolon, Am. J. Dis. Child. **59**:1071, 1940.

116. Touloukian, R. J., Aghajanian, G., and Roth, R. H.: Adrenergic hyperactivity in the aganglionic colon, J. Pediatr. Surg. **8**:191, 1973.

117. Touloukian, R. J., Morgenroth, V. H., III, and Roth, R. H.: Sympathetic neurotransmitter metabolism in Hirschsprung's disease, J. Pediatr. Surg. **10:**593, 1975.
118. Wagget, J., Bishop, H. C., and Koop, C. E.: Experience with Gastrografin enema in the treatment of meconium ileus, J. Pediatr. Surg. **5:**649, 1970.
119. Waterston, D. J., Bonham Carter, R. E., and Aberdeen, E.: Oesophageal atresia: tracheo-oesophageal fistula—a study of survival in 218 infants, Lancet **2:**819, 1962.
120. Wayne, E. R., and others: Eventration of the diaphragm, J. Pediatr. Surg. **9:**643, 1974.
121. Woolley, M. M., Gwinn, J. L., and Mares, A.: Congenital partial gastric antral obstruction: an elusive cause of abdominal pain and vomiting, Ann. Surg. **180:**265, 1974.
122. Woolf, R. M., Georgiade, N., and Pickrell, K. L.: Micrognathia and associated cleft palate (Pierre Robin syndrome), Plast. Reconstr. Surg. **26:**199, 1960.
123. Wrenn, E. L.: Tubular duplication of the small intestine, Surgery **52:**494, 1962.

CHAPTER 11

Urologic considerations

JOHN W. DUCKETT and HOWARD C. FILSTON

GENERAL CONSIDERATIONS

Between 10% and 15% of all neonatal deaths are attributable to gross congenital anomalies. Of autopsies performed in newborns or stillborns, 17% to 20% have one or more urologic anomalies, whereas only 0.8% of surviving neonates have a recognizable urologic abnormality.[22] Most abnormalities of the urologic system that are recognizable in the newborn infant are clearly visible or palpable, such as hypospadias or cryptorchidism. Oligohydramnios is most likely due to too little urine output by the fetus and accompanies the anephric state or severe renal dysplasia with obstruction (urethral valves). The fetus begins to urinate by the fourth month of intrauterine gestation and is making urine as early as the third month.[17]

At least half of the infants with neonatal ascites will have a urologic etiology for this condition. The usual cause is posterior urethral valves or other obstruction at the bladder outlet. Ascites may also result from a neurogenic bladder secondary to myelodysplasia.

A symptom that should lead to urologic evaluation is the failure of the infant to pass urine. Within the first 24 hours after birth, 94% of normal infants—including premature ones—void, and 100% do so within 48 hours. A dribbling urinary stream in a boy may indicate obstruction.[6,14]

Lesions of the urogenital system include the following:

Lesions that are visibly obvious
  Prune-belly syndrome
  Exstrophy of the bladder
  Exstrophy of the cloaca
  Epispadias
  Hypospadias
  Ambiguous genitalia
  Cryptorchidism
Obstructive lesions
  Hydronephrosis
  Multicystic kidney
  Large ureter or large bladder
Developmental lesions of the kidneys
  Horseshoe and ectopic kidneys
  Polycystic kidneys (infantile)
Acquired lesions
  Renal vein thrombosis
Tumors
  Wilms' tumor
  Mesoblastic nephroma (benign)
  Teratoma
  Neuroblastoma
Lesions of the female genital tract
  Hydrocolpos
  Ovarian cyst

Mass lesions of the kidney comprise 60% of abdominal masses in the newborn, whereas only 15% of abdominal masses are related to the gastrointestinal tract (duplications, biliary cysts, etc.).

Physical examination. A complete physical examination will identify many of the above lesions. The examination should include a careful evaluation of the abdomen with its wall relaxed. Bimanual examination may be productive. The flanks and suprapubic region should be carefully palpated. Tube decompression of the stomach and glucose water feeding by nipple may aid relaxation of the abdominal wall and enhance the ability to palpate the retroperitoneal organs. The umbilicus should be inspected for cord abnormalities, omphalomesenteric remnants, or a patent urachus.

Careful examination of the external genitalia and perineum may reveal abnormalities. Although the foreskin can rarely be retracted in the newborn male infant, its intactness circumferentially rules against hypospadias and epispadias. The straightness and ability of the penile shaft to be extended should be noted. The perineum of the female infant should be carefully and gently probed to confirm labial formation and patency, a normal urethral meatus, and an open hymenal ring.

Undescended testes in the newborn, especially the premature newborn, are of little significance. Scrotal masses, inflammation, or tenderness, however, should be investigated. Neonatal testicular torsion is a painless mass.

Findings on the general physical examination that may suggest urinary tract abnormalities include evidence of any anomalies of the VATER or VACTEL complex[3] (see Figs. 9-6 and 9-7), including vertebral, anal, tracheoesophageal, and renal anomalies or vertebral, anal, cardiac, tracheoesophageal, and limb anomalies, respectively. Thus, the presence of anomalies in any of these organs should indicate the need for a voiding cystogram and excretory urogram.

Laboratory and x-ray evaluations. Further evaluation of the urologic system should include urinalysis, urine culture and sensivitiy, and observation of voiding patterns. Ultrasonography or, occasionally, computerized tomography or a renal scan may be utilized in the evaluation, depending on the lesions found. Arteriography is generally reserved for evaluation of hypertension and, occasionally, unusual tumors. Venacavography is useful in the diagnosis of renal vein thrombosis to determine the degree to which the lesion is bilateral. The use of these entities is further discussed in this chapter under the discussions of the specific lesions and in subsequent chapters where appropriate.

Surgical consultation. Eventually, surgical consultation will be required. The choice of a consultant is extremely important. The surgeon must be experienced in dealing with *pediatric* urologic illness and must also have expertise in the overall management of the child patient. The primary care physician must be assured that the surgical consultant has the knowledge, experience, and interest to deal with the complexities of urogenital abnormalities in the pediatric age group. Most pediatric surgeons and urologists have not had specialized experience in pediatric

urology. However, there are a number in each specialty area who have, and their counsel should be sought. Often a phone call to a pediatric urologist will suffice in obtaining the most modern management. Petty competition and turf disputes are nonproductive.

EMBRYOLOGY AND ANATOMY OF THE UROGENITAL SYSTEM

Before embarking on a discussion of the individual lesions of the urogenital system, we will consider a brief outline of the embryology and anatomy of the system to enhance our understanding of the malformations and other abnormalities that occur.[17]

The initial pronephros evolves into the mesonephros, which matures into the wolffian body and forms the genital tract of the male. The distal-most part of the nephrogenic ridge becomes the metanephros, which matures into the permanent kidney. As the mesonephros evolves, it develops functioning glomeruli and collecting tubules. In the male, the mesonephric duct persists as the efferent ducts and paradidymis; in the female, small remnants of the mesonephric duct may persist as Gartner's duct and the paraoophoron. Anomalous ducts and openings can be explained by the persistence of embryologic ducts that usually disappear in the developmental process. The ureters develop as buds from the mesonephric duct and grow cephalad to meet the metanephric tissue, joining with the secretory units to form the collecting system. A failure of this union may be the cause of multicystic kidneys as well as malformations of the renal pelvis and ureters. Eventually the metanephros migrates cephalad, and the genital ridge migrates caudally (Fig. 11-1). Rotation and fusion deformities result from improper ascent of the kidneys.

The urogenital sinus and rectum develop as the cloaca is divided by a descending urorectal septum. The anterior allantoic portion eventually evolves into a bladder and urethra. The urachus will totally disappear except for a ligamentous remnant known as the middle umbilical ligament. Failures in this process may lead to persistence of cloacal-type hindgut anomalies and rectourinary fistulas. Exstrophy of the bladder and exstrophy of the cloaca are more extreme forms of anomalies of this embryologic evolution and are due to a persistent cloacal membrane into which mesoderm fails to migrate.

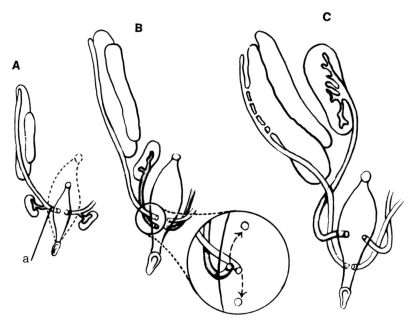

Fig. 11-1. Ureter and wolffian duct migration. **A,** Fifth week: common excretory duct *(a)* absorbed into the sinus. **B,** Seventh week: ureter migrates upward, wolffian duct migrates downward. **C,** Eighth week: adult positions assumed. (From Marshall, F. F.: Urol. Clin North Am. **5**(1):3, 1978.)

In the female the separate müllerian ducts fuse in their caudal aspect to form the upper two thirds of the vagina, with the more proximal aspects of the müllerian ducts developing into the fallopian tubes and the uterus. If the urorectal septum fails to descend, the vagina and uterus may be trifid or duplex.

The external genitalia are dependent on testosterone for their virilization in the male. If no testes are present, a normal female will develop. If, however, adrenal hyperplasia is present, a female will be virilized to varying degrees. Likewise, if there is localized androgen insensitivity, even in the presence of testes, no virilization will occur (testicular feminization).

With this embryologic background, we can now concentrate on the mature organ system, which consists normally of two retroperitoneal kidneys drained by individual ureters into a bladder that empties through a urethra. This basic anatomy is altered appropriately in the male and female, with the primary alteration being in the distal drainage system of the urethra, which is extended out the length of the penis in the male and ends at the verumontanum level in the female. Abnormalities may occur in any part of this system, and obstructive abnormalities in one part may affect the development of proximal parts.

• • •

The following discussions detail those abnormalities of the urogenital system that may be present in the neonate, beginning with those that are discoverable on the newborn physical examination or that may be indicated by symptoms or laboratory findings. Many of the latter and most internal anomalies may not be discovered until later infancy.

FLANK MASSES

A flank mass in the newborn is most likely a multicystic kidney or a hydronephrotic kidney. Differentiation between the two is often difficult. A lobulated mass is most likely multicystic. One that functions on delayed films is hydronephrotic. Rarely, bilateral masses will be infantile polycystic kidneys. A neonatal renal tumor may be a mesoblastic nephroma (benign) or Wilms' tumor (malignant) and show intrarenal distortion of the collecting system.

Renal tumors in the newborn and early infant age group are often mesoblastic variants of Wilms' tumor[5] (Fig. 11-2). These entities are associated

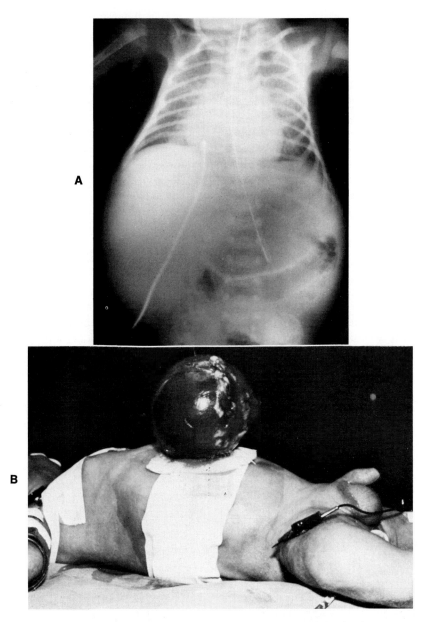

Fig. 11-2. A, Plain abdominal radiograph showing a large mass in the right flank of a premature newborn infant. **B,** The well-encapsulated, easily excised tumor is shown for size comparison to the infant following surgery. It proved to be a mesoblastic nephroma.

with a low level of malignancy and usually respond to surgical excision alone. They were probably responsible for the high curability of Wilms' tumor in infants under a year of age before the advent of multimodal therapy. With the advent of multimodal therapy consisting of surgery, radiation, and chemotherapy, the more malignant forms of Wilms' tumor are now also highly curable and have an overall survival rate approaching 90%.[7] However, unfavorable histology and wide-spread metastases are still associated with significant mortality. The best cures are obtained by a team approach consisting of knowledgeable surgeons, oncologists, and radiotherapists working under the guidelines established by the National Wilms' Tumor Study. This type of cooperative effort has led not only to increased cure of the tumors, but to a systematic withdrawal of unnecessary radiation and chemotherapy, avoiding the hazards associated with these entities.

Neuroblastoma of the suprarenal or paravertebral area will distort the collecting system from external pressure. Ultrasonography is often helpful in diagnosis, but arteriography is not usually necessary. The neuroblastomas presenting in the child under 1 year of age are also associated with a high cure rate if they are excised. Multimodal therapy is being studied in these entities, but the exact role and advantages of radiation and chemotherapy are not yet demonstrated. Again, a team approach under the guidelines of national protocols will provide optimal therapy and lead to the greatest accumulation of information on a long-term basis. Further discussion of these tumors can be found in Chapter 16 in the section on the infant and toddler.

HEMATURIA

Hematuria in the newborn is rare, but it is a prominent sign of several serious conditions that require immediate recognition and prompt and appropriate therapy. The most common of these is renal vein thrombosis.

Renal vein thrombosis

When a palpable flank mass is associated with hematuria in the newborn, renal vein thrombosis should be suspected.[4,11] The majority of patients with this entity are newborns less than 3 days of age, and almost all are infants under 1 month of age. The entity is seen commonly in infants of diabetic mothers and may be associated with severe diarrhea and dehydration. Occasionally, the thrombosis may have occurred antenatally. The thrombosis is thought to begin in the renal venules and to spread to the larger veins and the vena cava. There is almost always some degree of bilaterality. These infants may appear relatively asymptomatic except for their hematuria, or they may be severely ill with shock and vascular collapse. A coexisting coagulopathy may help to limit the extent of the thrombosis.

Evaluation. Evaluation of the urinary tract by intravenous pyelography may show decreased function on one or both sides (Fig. 11-3); since this is not an uncommon finding in the newborn period, however, it is a nonspecific finding. A

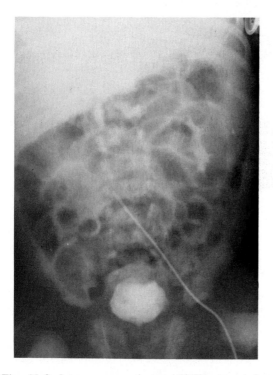

Fig. 11-3. Intravenous pyelogram (IVP) on an infant with a suspected renal vein thrombosis, showing nonfunction of the right kidney. Good function is noted on the left. A catheter is in place for subsequent venography. (Courtesy Donald Kirks, M.D., Durham, N.C.)

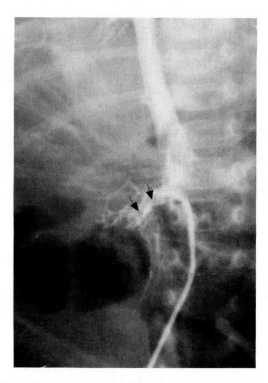

Fig. 11-4. Venacavography on the infant shown in Fig. 11-3, showing obstruction of the right renal vein with a thrombus present in the lumen, illustrated by the filling defect (arrows) within the dye-filled vein. (Courtesy Donald Kirks, M.D., Durham, N.C.)

rising blood urea nitrogen (BUN) level suggests the extent of renal dysfunction. Venacavography will confirm the diagnosis but is not always needed (Fig. 11-4).

Treatment. Treatment consists of supportive care with rehydration and maintenance of vascular volume. The use of antibiotics and anticoagulation is of questionable benefit. Considering the newborn immune deficient state, antibiotic coverage is probably warranted to prevent the damaged kidney from being a source of overwhelming sepsis.

Prognosis. Although there is significant mortality from this lesion, most infants recover and adequate renal function is preserved. Occasionally, when severe unilateral disease is present, nephrectomy may be needed; but conservative therapy is warranted initially (Fig. 11-5). A late complication is hypertension. Obviously, when both kidneys and the vena cava are extensively thrombosed, mortality is to be expected. Because of the small-vessel nature of the initial thrombus, thrombectomy is of little value.

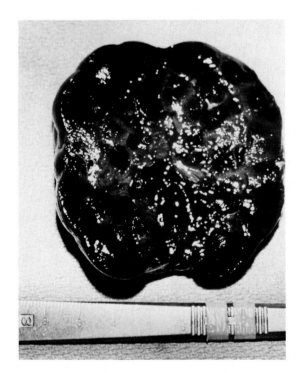

Fig. 11-5. Nephrectomy is not always necessary in renal vein thrombosis, but this extensively necrotic kidney was excised.

Renal artery thrombosis

Renal artery thrombosis usually presents with hematuria, proteinuria, and azotemia, but most important is the severe hypertension that may rapidly lead to congestive heart failure. Nonfunction on intravenous pyelogram (IVP) is common; but the kidney does not enlarge to a palpable mass, as it does with renal vein thrombosis.

Renal cortical necrosis

Renal cortical necrosis occurs in very sick infants with symptoms similar to renal vein thrombosis and usually is a fatal condition. Bilateral renal masses, hematuria, thrombocytopenia, anemia, and azotemia may be present.

NEONATAL ASCITES

The child born distended is likely to have ascites (Fig. 11-6). Some gastrointestinal lesions, such as meconium ileus due to cystic fibrosis or meconium peritonitis from in utero perforation and peritonitis, may produce ascites. It may also be associated with severe Rh incompatibility complicated by erythroblastosis fetalis, and hydrops. However, over half of the infants born with ascites will prove to have a urologic abnormality. The ascites usually results from extravasation of urine into the peritoneal cavity due to urinary tract perforation above a point of obstruction. This obstruction may be an anatomic one, such as urethral valves, or it may be a functional megacystis secondary to neurogenic bladder in a child with myelodysplasia (Fig. 11-7).

Evaluation. Evaluation should consist of a systematic workup of the urologic system, beginning with an attempted voiding cystourethrogram, followed by a prograde pyelogram. If the bladder cannot be successfully catheterized, urgent urologic consultation should be obtained to determine whether the child should have a perineal urethrostomy for further instrumentation and evaluation.

A definite perforation of the urinary tract may be identifiable, but frequently no such lesion is found. The ascites may gradually resolve. If the child has a myelomeningocele, a neurogenic bladder should be suspected.

Treatment and prognosis. Prolonged drainage of the bladder will usually achieve healing of any perforation. Other abnormalities, such as urethral valves, should be treated by appropriate reparative procedures.

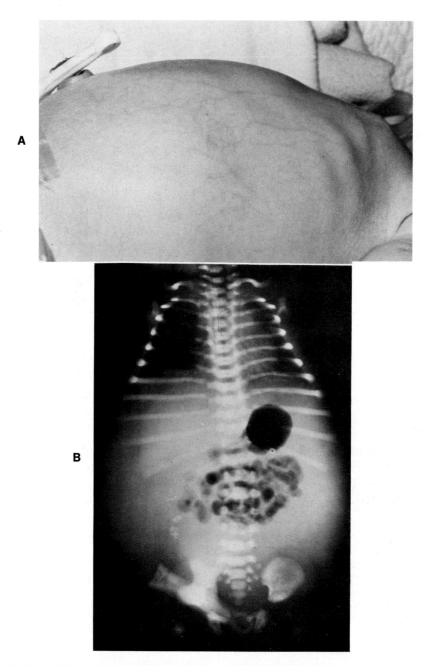

Fig. 11-6. A, This infant was born markedly distended—an unusual finding in gastrointestinal obstruction—and was subsequently demonstrated to have urinary ascites. **B,** Plain abdominal radiograph showing the abdominal gas pattern clustered toward the center as the gas-filled bowel floats in the ascitic fluid that completely surrounds it. (**B** from Filston, H. C., and Izant, R.: The surgical neonate: evaluation and care, New York, 1978, Appleton-Century-Crofts.)

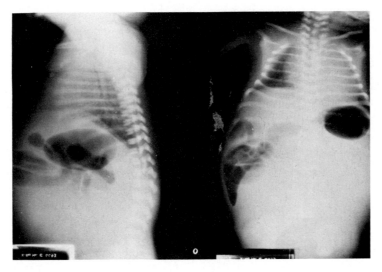

Fig. 11-7. Anteroposterior (AP) and lateral radiographs of the abdomen showing the bowel gas pushed up beneath the liver and diaphragm by a mass arising out of the pelvis, representing megacystis. Hydrometrocolpos would have a similar appearance in a female infant.

UMBILICAL ABNORMALITIES

Occasionally, the fact that the umbilicus is abnormal is obvious at the time of delivery; bowel can be seen extending into the base of the cord. Increased thickness of the cord may attract the obstetrician's attention. Most of the time, however, abnormalities of the urinary tract become manifest by the failure of the cord to desiccate and autoamputate in the normal fashion. In other instances, the base of the cord fails to heal and a sinus may be noticed (Fig. 11-8). This sinus may be an omphalomesenteric remnant, which is discussed earlier. On the other hand, it may represent a persistent urachal tract or vesicoumbilical fistula. As the cloacal septum separates the anterior urogenital compartment from the posterior gastrointestinal compartment, the initial formation of a combined bladder and allantoic tract is followed by maturation to the mature form of the bladder, with an extension called the urachus continuing to the umbilicus. This extension gradually atrophies and becomes ligamentous; and in the normal individual only a vestige, the middle umbilical ligament, remains. Persistence of a patent tract leads to urachal deformities, including urachal cysts and sinuses and wide-open vesicoumbilical fistulas. Urine noted passing through the sinus at the umbilicus is an immediate diagnostic clue. If a sinus is noted, it can be catheterized and contrast material injected into it. If the blad-

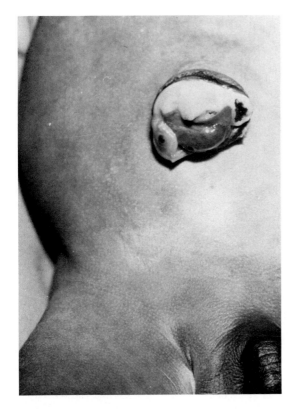

Fig. 11-8. Appearance of the umbilicus after the cord separates in an infant with a persistent urachus.

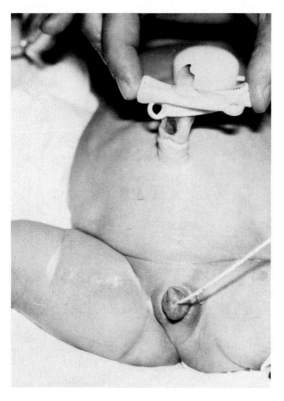

Fig. 11-9. A persistent urachus at the base of the cord in an infant with hydrometrocolpos with a urogenital sinus deformity, labial fusion, urethrovaginal, and rectovaginal fistulas.

der is outlined, the diagnosis is confirmed. Urachal cysts usually do not present in the immediate newborn period with abnormalities of the umbilicus, but subsequent to the newborn period with an enlarging inflamed mass due to abscess formation in the cyst. Cysts may be closed off with no communication to either the bladder or the umbilicus. Patency of the urachal remnant may be found in varying pathologic conditions, such as prune belly syndrome, or rarely with obstructive uropathy (Fig. 11-9). A urachal diverticulum is common with prune belly bladders.

Treatment. Treatment of a persistent urachus requires exploration of the umbilicus, dissection of the urachus back to the bladder wall, and excision and repair of the base of the tract (Fig. 11-10, *A*). A cosmetic closure will reestablish a normal-appearing umbilicus, and no scar need remain (Fig. 11-10, *B*). Umbilical cysts may require initial drainage followed by excision. If they present without abscess formation, primary excision of the cyst may be accomplished.

Prognosis. Results of surgery and long-term prognoses for children with these lesions are excellent if the lesions are managed appropriately by experienced surgeons.

A 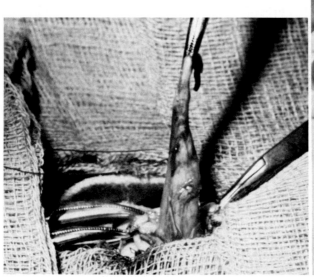   **B**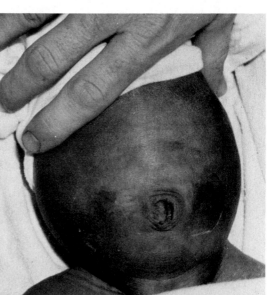

Fig. 11-10. A, Dissection of the urachal tract back to the bladder. This is then excised and the bladder wall oversewn to reinforce the closure. **B,** The appearance of the infant at the conclusion of the urachal surgery shows the reconstructed umbilicus with almost no evidence of the surgical procedure.

GENITAL, BLADDER, AND ABDOMINAL WALL ANOMALIES
Hypospadias

Hypospadias is a common urologic anomaly occurring in 1 of 150 live male births.[20] There is lack of tubularization of the urethra onto the phallus, with the most common defect being the glandular channeling. Three fourths of these anomalies are of the glandular or coronal type, many of which cause very little deformity. Surgical correction is generally warranted in these cases. Ten percent of the defects open on the penile shaft and 20% are found at the penoscrotal junction or along the scrotum and the perineum (Fig. 11-11). These are associated with chordee, which is a fibrous tethering of the ventral penis, causing a curvature with erection, and which must be repaired for sexual function (Fig. 11-12). Correction of the more severe problems has been best managed with a one-stage procedure using vascularized island flaps for the neourethra and moving the meatus out onto the glandular tip. Some of these children have associated hernias (8%), hydroceles (16%), or cryptorchidism (8%). Since very few have upper urinary tract anomalies, x-ray studies are not warranted unless symptoms of upper urinary tract problems are present.[12]

Exstrophy of the bladder and cloaca

When the infraumbilical mesenchyme fails to close in the cloacal membrane, the exstrophy and epispadias complex occurs. *Exstrophy of the bladder,* the common type of exstrophy, occurs in 1 of 30,000 births and has a 4-to-1 male predominance. The pubic bones fail to fuse, so that the symphysis is widely separated. The plate of bladder seen in the lower abdomen is the mucosa turned inside out like an everted orange peel (Fig. 11-13). The urethra is also splayed open, as is the glans penis. The orifices are located on the bladder plate among some polypoid mucosa. The upper tracts are almost always normal in pure exstrophy.

Cloacal exstrophy, the rarer but most severe form of exstrophy, is a complex of anomalies consisting of imperforate anus, a short colon segment, and an exstrophied ileocecal valve between two hemibladder exstrophies on the lower abdomen with an associated large omphalocele. The terminal ileum protrudes from the mass on the lower abdomen, but bowel obstruction is unusual (Fig. 11-14). Preservation of the blind-ending colon is vital for reconstruction. About 40% of the time there is an associated spinal dysraphism.

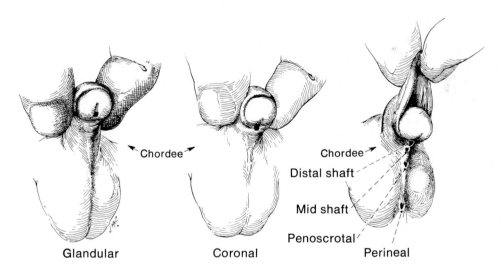

Fig. 11-11. Classification of hypospadias based on anatomic location of the urethral meatus. Associated chordee is best described in terms of its severity: mild, moderate, or severe. (From Belman, A. B.: The urethra. In Kelalis, P. P., King, L. R., and Belman, A. B., editors: Clinical pediatric urology, Philadelphia, 1976, W. B. Saunders Co., p. 577.)

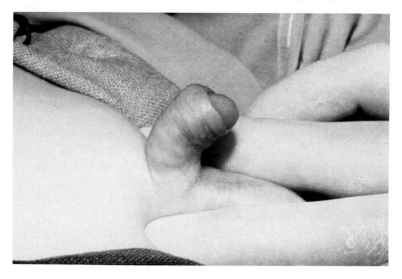

Fig. 11-12. Chordee and coronal hypospadias.

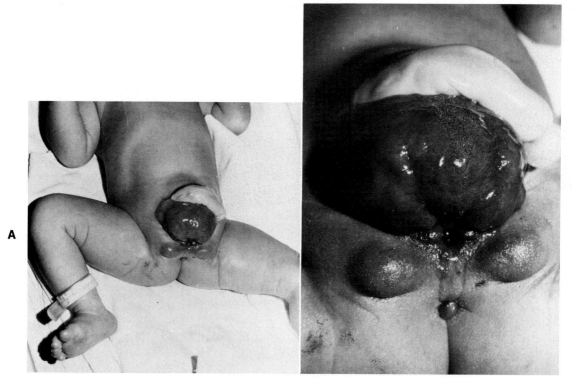

Fig. 11-13. A, Exstrophy of the bladder. **B,** Close-up of the infant in **A,** showing the everted bladder mucosa of the exstrophy, the epispadias, and the ill-defined scrotum. (From Filston, H. C., and Izant, R.: The surgical neonate: evaluation and care, New York, 1978, Appleton-Century-Crofts.)

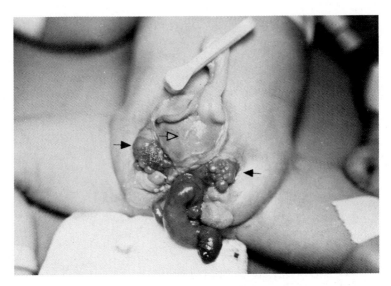

Fig. 11-14. Exstrophy of the cloaca. Scrotal sacs are noted on either side of the exenterated loop of intestine. The bladder mucosa is represented by the hypertrophied lateral areas (solid arrows), and there is a small omphalocele (open arrow).

Treatment. Until recently, surgical reconstruction of exstrophy of the bladder was most discouraging. However, newer surgical techniques have been developed, and in certain centers reconstruction can be done with adequate continence and preservation of normal upper tracts in 60% to 70% of selected cases. The current program is to turn in the bladder in the newborn period, bringing the symphysis together without an osteotomy by taking advantage of the "relaxing" hormone produced by the mother to soften the bony symphysis.[2] During the same procedure, penile lengthening is performed and the tethered urethral plate is divided. This procedure allows the bladder and the proximal urethra to drop back into the pelvis in a more normal position. Paraexstrophy skin pedical grafts are used to bridge the gap, creating a new urethra. No attempt is made during the first operation to gain continence. Secondary bladder neck reconstruction is accomplished when the child is about 3 to 4 years of age.

In cloacal exstrophy, a reasonable quality of life may be expected; thus, reconstructive efforts should be made. Preservation of the ileocecal segment and blind-ending colon are important aspects of the initial procedure, allowing construction of an end colostomy.

Epispadias

Pure epispadias is quite rare and is treated similarly to exstrophy of the bladder, with major reconstruction of the bladder neck area and plastic reconstruction of the urethra. Epispadias with exstrophy of the bladder is more common, and penile lengthening is deemed necessary for adequate sexual functioning in these children. Many young adults may be offered this surgical procedure if denied it in childhood. Patients with milder forms of epispadias who are continent will require less surgical reconstruction.

Other penile anomalies

The largest group of abnormalities of the penis are those associated with hypospadias. Nevertheless, other abnormalities ranging from agenesis to double phallus occur. The penis may present in a retroscrotal position. Agenesis is usually associated with hypogenitalism and anorchia and may be the result of primary testicular failure. Other anomalies are associated with defects in the pituitary hypothalmic axis, which controls gonadal development and function.

Less complex abnormalities affecting the penis are those of enlargement, duplication, penile torsion, chordee without hypospadias, and hemihypertrophy of the corpora cavernosa.

Prune-belly syndrome

Prune-belly syndrome, also known as abdominal muscle deficiency syndrome, is a triad of anomalies. First, it includes a wrinkled, flaccid abdominal wall with skeletal muscle deficiency

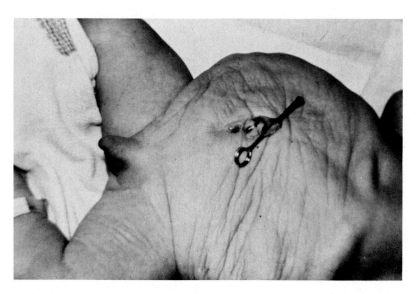

Fig. 11-15. Newborn infant with prune-belly syndrome. Note the obvious wrinkled abdominal wall through which the viscera can be seen.

and wrinkled abdominal skin that appears wizened like a prune[9] (Fig. 11-15). Second, there are typical urinary tract abnormalities with dilatation of the renal pelves, ureters, and bladder and various degrees of renal dysplasia. There is also a primary deficiency of the urinary tract smooth musculature. The third portion of the triad is bilateral undescended testes, usually intra-abdominal. Because of the large bladder, reflux, and large ureters, stasis of urine is the most serious problem. Once established, infection is difficult to eradicate. The diagnosis is relatively apparent in the classic presentation of the syndrome. However, some infants have an incomplete manifestation of the syndrome; they may have the typical urinary anomalies, yet their abdominal walls are firm without wrinkling and their testes are descended. These are called ''pseudoprunes'' and should be recognized as such so that their urinary tract anomalies may be managed like those of the prune belly syndrome and not as the simple obstructive uropathies with which they are frequently confused.

Treatment. Control of sepsis is the primary treatment in prune belly syndrome. Suppressive medication is started immediately on making the diagnosis. Surgical intervention may be needed at times; in general, however, reconstructive surgery is not necessary in the early stages. Temporary cutaneous vesicostomy, allowing a ''pop off'' system for the dilated urinary tract, is an effec-

tive way to control sepsis. As the child grows, there may be a relative obstruction at the membranous urethra, which will require surgical correction for better emptying. (Other problems occasionally associated with prune-belly syndrome are pectus excavatum, flared ribs, respiratory complications such as pneumonia, clubbed feet, malrotation, and megalourethra.) The undescended testes can be brought down into the scrotum.

Ambiguous genitalia or intersex problems

Few problems in the newborn infant cause as much consternation for the physician and the parents as do those in the intersex category. Careful evaluation of the genitalia should be a part of every newborn examination before the parents are told the sex of the child. Genital ambiguity makes the rightful assignment of gender an emergency in the neonatal period. If there is any ambiguity, immediate investigation should be undertaken so that a decision as to which sex to call the child can be made as quickly as possible. Consultation with physicians of any and all specialties with experience in this area should be obtained so that the best decision can be made. Procrastination because this is not a life-threatening matter cannot be tolerated, for the heartache and embarrassment suffered by the family in having to change the sex assignment later is considerable and can be easily avoided.

There are basically four determinants of sex:

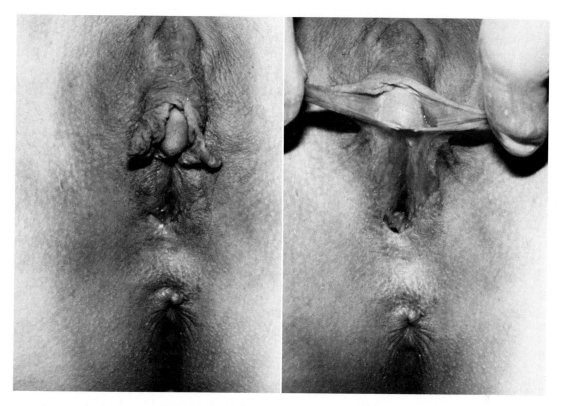

Fig. 11-16. Female child with ambiguous genitalia, hypertrophied clitoris, and fused labia secondary to the adrenal genital syndrome of the salt-wasting variety.

chromosomal or genetic sex, gonadal or hormonal sex, anatomic sex, and gender sex or the sex of rearing. In the normal case, all four coincide. When there is ambiguity of the genitalia, the primary consideration should be the adequacy of the phallus. If this is inadequate for sexual intercourse, it is best to rear the child as a female. It is far better to have an infertile female than an impotent male.

This does not imply that all infants with a phallus should be raised as males. Many female pseudohermaphrodites with adrenal hyperplasia have marked clitoral hypertrophy approaching that of a normal male phallus (Fig. 11-16). Nevertheless, these infants are gonadal females who are chromosomally normal; and with surgical correction of their external genitalia, they can be reared as normal females and function as normal females.[1] They can never function as normal, fertile males; therefore, if a phallus is present, the next step should always be to determine chromosomal and gonadal sex. Nonetheless, no infant with an inadequate phallus should be assigned the male gender. A small but adequate penis

with severe hypospadias and descended testes needs no further assessment. When the gonads are not palpable, however, no matter how virilized the genitalia, gender identity must be questioned.

Embryology of the genitalia. A brief discussion of the normal development of the gonads and external genitalia may be helpful in understanding some of the abnormalities that are seen. Components are the differentiation of the undifferentiated gonads, the development of male or female duct systems from the mesonephric and paramesonephric tubules, and the maturation of the external genitalia from the genital tubercle, genital folds, and genital swellings.

The gonad is undifferentiated until 6 weeks of gestation, at which time, if the Y chromosome is present, it will begin differentiating into a testis. The female gonad under the influence of the two X chromosomes differentiates later, at about 13 to 16 weeks of gestation.

Initially, both the mesonephric, or wolffian, duct system and the paramesonephric, or müllerian, duct system are present. If the testis develops under the Y chromosome influence, the wolffian duct matures into the epididymis, vas, and seminiferous tubules. In the absence of a testicle, the wolffian duct regresses and the müllerian duct develops into the fallopian tubes, uterus, and upper vagina. The testis provides testosterone, which influences development of the wolffian duct system, and also produces a müllerian-inhibiting substance.[8,16]

The external genitalia appear neuter until after 7 weeks of gestation, at which time the tubercle, genital folds, genital swellings, and urogenital sinus begin to differentiate. In the presence of testosterone, the urogenital sinus evolves into the prostate gland, the genital tubercle into the glans, and the genital folds into the urethra and shaft of the penis. The genital swellings become the scrotum. Without androgens, the female develops, with the urogenital sinus evolving into the lower vagina, the genital tubercle into the clitoris, the genital folds into the labia minora, and the genital swellings into the labia majora. Recognition of the common origin of the external genitalia is helpful in understanding the ease with which ambiguity may arise.

Etiology. The next most important aspect of dealing with the problem of ambiguous genitalia is to determine its etiology, at least to the extent of evaluating whether the cause is the *adrenal genital syndrome (congenital adrenal hyperplasia [CAH])*. This syndrome accounts for 70% of intersex problems and has life-threatening implications, because many of these children have a salt-wasting adrenal insufficiency. Until it can be ruled out, the child must be carefully monitored and supported with intravenous fluids so that dehydration and hyponatremia do not lead to collapse. These children are virilized females, the result of adrenal hormone effects on their genitalia. They may have varying degrees of masculinization of their external genitalia, but they are sex chromatin positive and are gonadal females. Chromatin determination of the buccal mucosa or of the white blood cells is, therefore, helpful. A 24-hour collection for urinary catecholamines as well as serum determination of androstenediol will determine the diagnosis of adrenal hyperplasia. A genitogram may be useful. These infants can be treated with appropriate steroids to correct their adrenal hyperplasia, and their ambiguous genitalia can be corrected surgically.

If one testis is descended and the other not palpable, *mixed gonadal dysgenesis (MGD)* is a possibility, and chromosomes will be helpful in determining this condition. If the phallus is miniscule, the female gender should be assigned. MGD is the second most common cause of intersex. A testis is present on one side and a streak gonad on the other, and the chromosomes are mixed XY and XO. A true hermaphrodite, with both XX and XY chromosomes and a normal testis palpable on one or both sides, is quite rare. An abdominal exploration and gonadal biopsy to demonstrate the ovotestis is necessary for the diagnosis of this condition.

Testicular feminization, a condition of androgen insensitivity, includes XY chromosomes, bilateral testes that are either descended or in the inguinal canal, and normal-appearing female genitalia. There is a short, blind-ending vagina with no female internal organs. Bilateral gonadectomy is indicated relatively early, since estrogen support at puberty is quite adequate in feminizing these children and the chance of gonadoblastoma is about 25% to 50% if the gonads remain.[21]

All abnormalities of sexual development are not associated with ambiguous genitalia. In *Klinefelter's syndrome,* in which a phenotypic male with normal male external genitalia has an XXY configuration, the extra X chromosome produces a positive buccal smear chromatin and degenerative effects in the testis. Gynecomastia may develop, and the body habitus may be eunuchoid; otherwise, the external genitalia develop in a normal male pattern. *Turner's syndrome,* that of a phenotypic female with a usually negative buccal smear chromatin, is caused by an XO chromosome complement. The major effect is on the ovaries, which are mere streaks; and there is a classic body habitus with a webbed neck. Nevertheless, these infants appear as normal females externally.

UPPER URINARY TRACT ANOMALIES

The following discussions deal with abnormalities of the urinary tract that are discoverable only when physical findings, urinary dysfunction, infection, or abnormal urinalysis have led to radiographic or endoscopic investigations. The demonstration of any one or more of these anomalies warrants expert pediatric urologic consultation to prevent further damage to the kidneys from obstruction or infection, the two major ravages of the urinary tract.

Renal agenesis

Fortunately, renal agenesis is a rare condition in infants; it presents with oligohydramnios, Potter facies, and skeletal anomalies such as clubbed feet. Pulmonary hypoplasia leads to pneumomediastinum and pneumothorax along with respiratory distress. The diagnosis is confirmed by the inability to palpate kidneys and by arteriography through the umbilical artery showing no renal arteries. Since the entity at present is uniformly fatal, its early identification avoids unnecessary surgical and resuscitative trauma to the child.

Renal hypoplasia

The general term *renal hypoplasia* includes *true hypoplasia* (which is a miniature kidney), poorly developed kidneys associated with gross reflux, and dysmorphic kidneys characterized by bizarre calyceal and parenchymal configurations such as in the prune-belly syndrome.

Solid dysplasia

Solid dysplasia is associated with ectopic ureters. There is production of urine in hypoplastic kidneys.

Cystic kidney disease
Multicystic kidney

Consisting of a uniform cluster of cysts without renal function, the multicystic kidney is the most common renal mass in the newborn (Fig. 11-17). The upper portion of the ureter is atretic. If the atretic segment extends down toward the bladder, there is a greater association with contralateral renal anomalies. If the palpable multicystic kidney is large, there is less chance of contralateral defects. Contralateral renal anomalies are more common when the multicystic kidney is small. This situation occurs in association with an imperforate anus, tracheoesophageal fistula, and other such conditions. The diagnosis is suspected on palpation because of the lumpy mass. Reflux into the atretic ureter is not unusual. Although a multicystic kidney is a benign condition, renal exploration is usually necessary, since absolute diagnostic criteria to rule out a tumor by ultrasound, pyelography, and arteriography are not available as yet. Removal of the nonfunctioning kidney may be achieved with very little morbidity through a small muscle-splitting flank incision.

Polycystic kidney

Infantile polycystic disease is suspected in an infant with large, smooth bilateral flank masses without a palpable bladder. Excretory urography shows a honeycombed, diffuse nephrographic phase with the collecting systems only vaguely delineated. Renal function is very poor, and oligohydramnios may have been present in the mother. This condition is autosomal recessive and is generally incompatible with life for more than a few weeks or months. The cut surface of these kidneys shows microscopic cysts with smooth renal contours. There may be associated portal fibrosis of the liver, making these children poor candidates for renal transplantation.

Cysts associated with obstruction

Potter[18] has described a type of cystic kidney associated with severe obstruction, usually due to urethral valves (Potter type IV). These kidneys have multiple cysts and function poorly. The diagnosis is pathologic and can be determined only by renal biopsy. Cystic dysplasia associated with unilateral reflux with valves occurs about 20% of the time with this condition and, in our experience, is mainly on the left side.

Anomalies of position
Simple malrotation

Incomplete rotation, rather than simple malrotation, is the proper designation, since after their

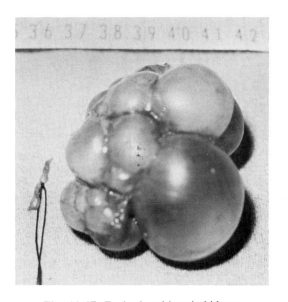

Fig. 11-17. Excised multicystic kidney.

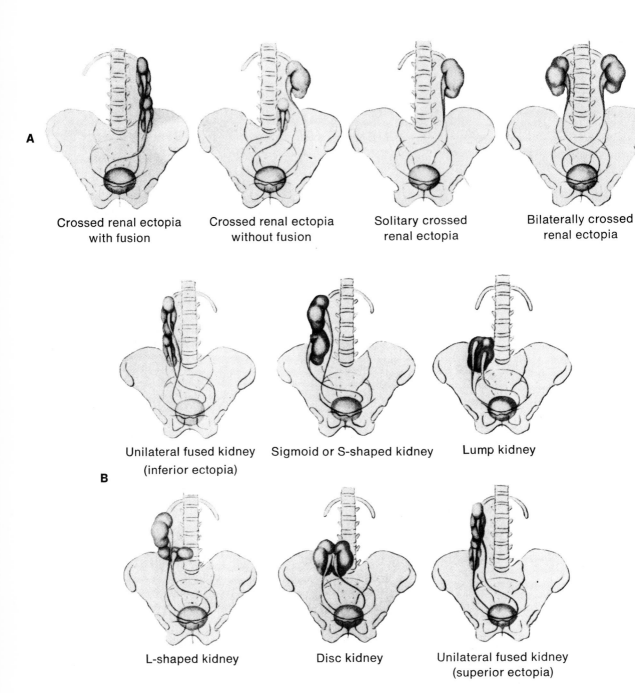

Fig. 11-18. A, Four types of crossed renal ectopia. **B,** Six forms of crossed renal ectopia with fusion. (From Perlmutter, A.: Anomalies of the upper urinary tract. In Hanson, J. H., and others, editors: Campbell's urology, Philadelphia, 1979, W. B. Saunders Co., pp. 1324-1325.)

formation the kidneys fail to undergo the 90-degree medial rotation that places the normal pelvis in the medial posterior position. In this anomaly, the pelvis exits the kidney anteriorly with the calyces pointing posteriorly. The kidneys may develop ureteropelvic junction obstruction because of the positioning of the ureter over the renal tissue.

Horseshoe kidney

Horseshoe kidney occurs because of inferior fusion of the two renal masses in the midline, so that each kidney remains incompletely rotated; the pelvis and ureters are anterior and lie over the renal isthmus. The kidneys are prone to ureteropelvic junction obstruction.

Crossed ectopia

It is possible for a renal segment to ascend on the side opposite the normal side, so that both kidneys are on the same side. Crossed fused ectopia is the more common presentation, with the lower pole portion of the fusion providing the ureter to the contralateral side of the fusion and the upper pole portion coming from the ipsilateral side (Fig. 11-18).

Pelvic ectopia

Fusion of both kidneys in the pelvic area forms a pancake kidney, a condition that in women may cause dystocia with childbirth. Unilateral pelvic kidneys may also exist; whenever there is absence of a kidney in the usual flank position, a search of the IVP is made for contrast medium in the pelvis. Obstruction of the ureteropelvic junction may be present with a pelvic kidney.

Hydronephrosis

Congenital ureteropelvic junction obstruction is the most common renal mass in children between the newborn period and 1 year of age.[13] Boys are more commonly affected (80% of cases), but the sex distribution is more equal after 1 year. The left side is more commonly affected (60% of cases) and bilateral obstruction is present in 5% of all cases but in 20% to 30% of those occurring in children under 1 year of age. In the infant, an abdominal mass is the most common presenting sign, whereas in the older child, pain is the primary complaint (80% of cases). A urinary infection (20% of cases) and vague gastrointestinal complaints may be the presenting signs.

Hematuria, especially with mild trauma, occurs in 15% to 20% of cases. In the more subtle obstructions, a urinary volume challenge with hydration and diuretics such as furosemide will sometimes reproduce the symptomatic pain and show the marked dilatation on the radiograph.

The pathologic findings at the ureteropelvic area are variable. Kinks and adhesions may produce stenosis. In many cases, no clear-cut intrinsic obstruction exists and the obstruction is functional. Aberrant accessory vessels to the lower pole are present in 30% of cases, whereas their usual incidence in only 10%. A ureteral kink over the accessory vessel is not an unusual finding. The radiograph shows compression of the collecting tubules in the medulla adjacent to the calyx, causing a "crescent sign." In the more severe lesions, there is a "rim sign" (Fig. 11-19) due to the contrast material providing a nephrogram effect before the dye reaches the collecting system. Delayed films are necessary to allow the contrast to reach the pelvis. In the infant with an extrarenal pelvis, a giant hydronephrosis may occupy almost the entire hemiabdomen (Fig. 11-20).

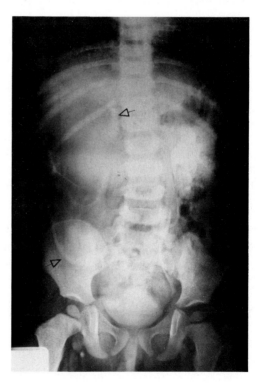

Fig. 11-19. Right hydronephrosis caused by a ureteropelvic junction obstruction, illustrating the "rim sign" (arrows) of giant hydronephrosis.

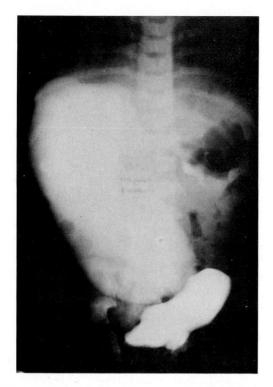

Fig. 11-20. IVP illustrating a right hydronephrotic kidney secondary to ureteropelvic obstruction.

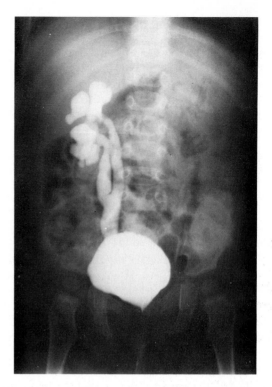

Fig. 11-21. Voiding cystourethrogram demonstrating duplication of the proximal right ureter with reflux.

Treatment and prognosis. A pyeloplasty is successful in over 90% of cases in reestablishing unrestricted flow to the bladder, even in the infant with poor visualization on the IVP and an enormous mass. Therefore, an attempt at surgical reconstruction should be made in all cases. Following relief of the obstruction, there is occasionally diuresis, which may last for several weeks or months, causing polydipsia and polyurea. The diuresis is caused by damage to the medullary concentrating mechanism and will improve with time.

Duplication of the ureter

Complete or incomplete duplication of the ureter may occur. The right side is affected twice as often as the left, and duplication is more common in females. A bifid ureter may join to form a Y ureter anywhere along the course of the ureter (Fig. 11-21). If the junction is in the midline, a "yo-yo" phenomenon may exist as the urine fails to progress effectively down to the bladder but churns back and forth in the upper segments. With complete duplication, the upper pole ureter enters the trigonal area at a level inferior to the lower pole ureter, which enters at a higher level and more laterally. Duplication of the ureters in itself is not considered an anomaly, but a variation of normal. Nevertheless, its presence may lead to complications. With two ureters coming through the hiatus of the bladder, a muscular weakness is more likely and the lower pole ureter may reflux. If the upper pole ureter is ectopic into the bladder neck area, there is likely to be an obstruction with dilatation or reflux into the upper pole segment during voiding when the bladder neck is open. Vesicoureteral reflux is more common with a duplex system; and although it will resolve spontaneously in many cases, it will require reimplantation surgery if it persists.

Ectopic ureter

In the embryogenesis of the ureter, the wolffian, or mesonephric, duct enters the urogenital sinus at the point of the verumontanum in the male to form the spermatic ducts and in the female it enters the sinus in the area of the urogenital tubercle. A ureteral bud comes from the mesonephric duct; and if it buds in the proper location, it will hit the nephrogenic bud in the center and form a normal kidney. However, if the ureteral bud is more cephalad or more caudad than usual, it is likely to influence the nephrogenic tissue in such a way that a less than adequate kidney or even a severe hypoplastic or dysplastic kidney is formed. Likewise, when the ureter is incorporated into the bladder, it will occupy an ectopic position either closer to the urethra or more laterally in the trigonal area. In the female, ectopic ureters may enter the urethra, the bladder neck, the introitus, the vagina, or, very rarely, the rectum. In the male, the bladder neck and proximal urethra are the common sites; but entrance into the ejaculatory duct, the vas deferens, or the seminal vesicle is possible. It is not embryologically possible in males for the ectopic ureters to be distal to the verumontanum. Therefore, there is no incontinence due to ectopia in the male infant.

Lateral ectopia in the bladder is associated with reflux and, in certain cases, poorly developed kidneys. The Stephens "bud theory"[15] postulates that the location on the mesonephric duct where the ureteral bud originates determines the quality of renal tissue induced by the ureter, so that certain small kidneys with reflux are congenital anomalies rather than a result of infection and reflux. The kidneys associated with more distal ureteral ectopia, such as into the bladder neck, urethra, seminal vesicles or vagina, may be associated with solid dysplasia or hypoplasia. In a girl, the symptom of constant wetness interspersed with normal voiding is a characteristic history for an ectopic ureter, either in the urethra distal to the sphincter mechanism or in the introitus or vagina. Locating these ectopic ureters is sometimes very difficult, but clinical suspicion is most important in their discovery.

Ectopic ureters are usually associated with a duplication coming from the upper pole segment. Single ureteral ectopia is rare and is usually found with a poorly functioning or a nonfunctioning renal segment with marked ectopia, such as to a seminal vesical or vagina. Bilateral single ureteral ectopia occurs mostly in females and is associated with a poorly formed bladder. Since the ureterovesical junction is important in proper trigonal development, which in turn contributes to development of the internal sphincter and bladder neck area, a deficient bladder neck and reduced bladder capacity may result from marked ectopia. The ureters are dilated and obstructed, and un-

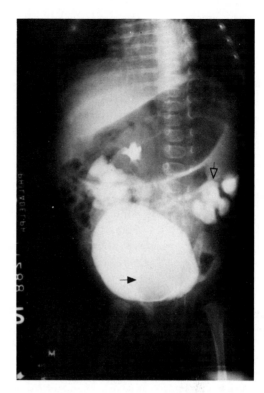

Fig. 11-22. Characteristic radiographic appearance of a ureterocele with a filling defect in the bladder (closed arrow) and the "drooping lily" appearance of the lower pole of the kidney (open arrow), caused by the poorly visualized upper lobe segment.

fortunately many of these children will require a urinary diversion.

Ureterocele

There are three types of ureteroceles. The acquired, or *adult type*, commonly seen as a "cobra head" defect of the distal ureter, may be associated with infection and stones. It is not seen in children. The *simple ureterocele* is a cystic dilatation of the distal end of the ureter in the usual position on the trigone. The *ectopic ureterocele*, with a large cystic dilatation prolapsing down into the urethra through the bladder neck, is the more common type. A ureterocele is more commonly seen with duplication of the ureters, with the upper pole segment associated with the ureterocele. The corresponding lower pole ureter frequently refluxes, or its orifice is drawn into the cystic dilatation in the bladder and is obstructed. Rarely, the ureterocele may prolapse through the bladder outlet, acting as an obstructing ball valve. Bilateral ureteroceles may occur.

A ureterocele has a very characteristic x-ray appearance on the IVP (Fig. 11-22). A filling defect is present as a negative shadow near the bladder neck area. The poorly visualized renal segment pushes the lower pole of the kidney down and out, giving a "drooping lily" appearance to the lower pole. Children usually have urinary infections or, rarely, obstructive symptoms. Surgical correction is variable for each case and may be complicated.

Megaureter

Megaureters and hydroureters have recently been classified by an international committee into obstructive megaureter; refluxing megaureter; and nonobstructing, nonrefluxing megaureter.[19] Each one of these divisions is subdivided into primary and secondary types. For instance, a refluxing megaureter may be of the primary type, due to a laterally positioned ureteral orifice, or it may be secondary to an outlet obstruction such as a urethral valve but with the ureteral orifice in a relatively normal position. The prune-belly syndrome ureter is considered nonobstructing and may be either refluxing or nonrefluxing. The prune-belly syndrome ureteral dilatation is due to a primary smooth musculature deficiency of the ureter itself. A megaureter associated with urethral valves may remain dilated even though distal obstruction is relieved. This classification based on etiology is helpful in determining the type of surgery required, if any, and in comparing results of therapy.

LOWER URINARY TRACT ANOMALIES
Bladder diverticula

In the past, most bladder diverticula were thought to be secondary to outlet obstructions such as urethral valves. Paraureteral diverticula occur at the ureteral hiatus, are usually associated with vesicoureteral reflux, and are not considered obstructing lesions. Some small paraureteral diverticula will resolve if the reflux ceases. Congenital bladder diverticula may also be found above and medial to the ureteral orifices on the posterior wall of the bladder. These diverticula may be single or multiple and require excision.

Bladder neck obstruction

Primary bladder neck obstruction is not considered an entity today. Secondary hypertrophy of the bladder neck musculature is seen in neuropathic bladder and with urethral valves, yet outlet obstruction in these cases is more functional than mechanical. In the past, many surgical procedures were done unnecessarily on the bladder neck on the basis of the erroneous concept that primary bladder neck obstruction was an entity.

Urethral obstruction (urethral valves)

The membranous urethra is divided into posterior and anterior segments. *Posterior urethral valves* course from the verumontanum distally toward the external sphincter, fusing anteriorly so that there is an obstructing oblique membrane with a posterior opening. The extent of the opening determines the severity of the obstruction. Chronic distension in utero leads to severe bladder thickening and results in obstruction at the ureterovesical junction and hydroureteronephrosis. If reflux is present, further damage is done to the developing kidneys. If reflux is unilateral, the side with the reflux suffers the greatest developmental dysplasia.

The diagnosis in the newborn is suggested by the finding of bilateral or unilateral flank masses and a distended, firm bladder. Although a dribbling stream is usual when valves are present, it is possible to have a respectable urinary stream and still have urethral valves with significant obstruction. These infants fail to thrive if the diagnosis is missed in the newborn period, and infection then frequently becomes the presenting problem. Most cases of urethral valve obstruction are now detected in the early months of life; a few, however, will escape notice until later years, when the damage is more severe and more difficult to manage. Because of the new instrumentation available in the last 10 years, primary ablation of the valves is now possible transurethrally or through a perineal urethrostomy destroying the attachment of the valves to the urethral wall.

A *congenital urethral membrane,* or congenital urethral stricture, is seen at the junction of the bulbous urethra and the membranous urethra at the point where the embryologic posterior and anterior urethras join. A congenital urethral stricture cannot occur in the bulbous or penile urethra. Although x-ray studies may suggest a narrowing in this area, spasm of the bulbocavernosus muscle is the usual cause.

An *anterior urethral valve* is really a diverticulum of the anterior urethra, whose distal lip creates a web and obstructs the outflow of urine. These entities are much rarer than posterior valves.

Megalourethra

Two types of megalourethras occur, although both are quite rare. The scaphoid type is more common and in over half the cases is associated with the prune-belly syndrome. There is a distinct chance of urosepsis occuring with investigation of the scaphoid megalourethra, since catheterization for x-ray studies through the contaminated dilated urethra will easily infect the urinary tract. The rarer, fusiform type of megalourethra is seen with severe prune-belly syndrome, imperforate anus, urethral atresia, and renal dysplasia. With voiding cystourethrography in boys, these lesions are seen in the proximal bulb.

Cystic dilatation of Cowper's gland duct

Cowper's glands drain by ducts into the posterior section of the cavernous urethra. Because of the course of the ducts, the glands do not cause obstructive problems but may be the cause of irritative symptoms or hematuria.

Valve of Guérin

A valve of Guérin is located in the dorsal urethra in the fossa navicularis and is very difficult to see radiologically, since this portion of the urethra is usually not filmed. The valve may form a small diverticulum that leads to urethral bleeding, particularly spotting of the diaper.

REFERENCES

1. Allen, T. D.: Reconstruction of the female with ambiguous genitalia. In Kelalis, P. P., King, L. R., and Belman, A. B., editors: Clinical pediatric urology, Philadelphia, 1976, W. B. Saunders Co., p. 1023.
2. Ansell, J. S.: Vesical exstrophy. In Glenn, J. F., editor: Urologic surgery, New York, 1975, Harper & Row, Publishers, Inc., p. 316.
3. Barnes, J. C., and Smith, W. L.: The VATER association, Radiology 126:445, 1978.
4. Belman, A. B.: Renal vein thrombosis. In Ravitch, M. M., and others, editors: Pediatric surgery, ed. 3, Chicago, 1979, Year Book Medical Publishers, Inc., p. 1178.
5. Bolande, R. P., Brough, A. J., and Izant, R. J., Jr.: Congenital mesoblastic nephroma of infancy, Pediatrics 40:272, 1967.
6. Clark, D. A.: Times of first void and first stool in 500 newborns, Pediatrics 60:457, 1977.
7. D'Angio, G. J., and others: The treatment of Wilms' tumor: results of the National Wilms' Tumor Study, Cancer 38:633, 1976.
8. Donahoe, P. K., and others: Müllerian inhibiting substance in human testes after birth, J. Pediatr. Surg. 12:323, 1977.
9. Duckett, J. W.: Prune belly syndrome. In Kelalis, P. P., King, L. R., and Belman, A. B., editors: Clinical pediatric urology, Philadelphia, 1976, W. B. Saunders Co., p. 615.
10. Duckett, J. W.: Epispadias, Urol. Clin. North Am. 5:107, 1978.
11. Duncan, R. E., Evans, A. T., and Martin, L. W.: Natural history and treatment of renal vein thrombosis in children, J. Pediatr. Surg. 12:639, 1977.
12. Jeffs, R. D.: Exstrophy. In Harrison, J. H., and others, editors: Campbell's urology, Philadelphia, 1979, W. B. Saunders Co., p. 1672.
13. Johnston, J. H., and others: Pelvic hydronephrosis in children: a review of 219 personal cases, J. Urol. 117:97, 1977.
14. Klaus, M. H., and Fanaroff, A. A.: Care of the high-risk neonate, Philadelphia, 1979, W. B. Saunders Co., p. 411.
15. Mackie, G. G.: Abnormalities of the ureteral bud, Urol. Clin. North Am. 5:161, 1978.
16. Marshall, F. F.: Vaginal abnormalities, Urol. Clin. North Am. 5:155, 1978.
17. Moore, K. L.: The developing human: clinically oriented embryology, Philadelphia, 1973, W. B. Saunders Co., pp. 198-238.
18. Potter, E. L.: Normal and abnormal development of the kidney, Chicago, 1972, Year Book Medical Publishers, Inc.
19. Smith, E. D., and others: Report of working party to establish an international nomenclature for the large ureter, Birth Defects 13(5):3, 1977.
20. Sweet, R. A., and others: Study of the incidence of hypospadias in Rochester, Minnesota, 1940-1970, and a case control comparison of possible etiologic factors, Mayo Clin. Proc. 49:52, 1974.
21. Wilson, J. D., and Walsh, P. C.: Disorders of sexual differentiation. In Harrison, J. H., and others, editors: Campbell's urology, Philadelphia, 1979, W. B. Saunders Co., p. 1484.
22. Woodard, J. R.: Neonatal and perinatal emergencies. In Harrison, J. H., and others, editors: Campbell's urology, Philadelphia, 1979, W. B. Saunders Co., p. 1855.

CHAPTER 12

Neurosurgical considerations

W. JERRY OAKES and ROBERT H. WILKINS

GENERAL CONSIDERATIONS

Diseases that primarily or secondarily affect the nervous system are of major concern to physicians who care for infants and children. This is true not only because the problems are associated with significant mortality but because the morbidity of even minor degrees of dysfunction of the brain or spinal cord can leave the patient incapacitated. Loss of fine motor control, vision, or hearing, or the development of paraplegia can clearly leave the patient unable to care for himself or to fully appreciate his environment. Lesions that primarily affect intelligence are equally, if not more, devastating to both the patient and the family. The recent decrease in the morbidity and mortality associated with both the investigation and surgical therapy of disorders of the brain and spinal cord has frequently forced parents to make difficult decisions regarding ''prophylactic surgery.'' In this situation, small lesions are diagnosed before the development of serious neurologic impairment. Parents are asked to allow a life-threatening operation to be performed while the child may still appear grossly normal. It is with such early procedures, however, that advances can be made. Early recognition and referral are the keys to continued improvement in both patient morbidity and mortality in neurosurgical diseases of the infant and child.

ABNORMAL SKULL CONFIGURATION

The neonatal skull demonstrates a remarkable degree of compliance. Changes in configuration associated with birth are common and are the result of adaptation of the skull as it passes through the birth canal. Although prominent at birth, these changes quickly disappear and the head resumes its normal configuration. Abnormal bony shapes that persist beyond the first week of life and show no tendency to correction should be investigated as to the cause of the abnormality. In the majority of cases, it is premature closure of one or more cranial sutures (craniosynostosis).

Routine examination for age. The brain of a full-term neonate weighs approximately 350 g. It is surrounded by pliable bones, which are joined to each other by fibrous connective tissue sutures (Fig. 12-1). At birth these junctions allow movement that one can appreciate by alternating the pressure on either side of the suture, noticing that

Throughout the writing of the four neurosurgical chapters in this text, numerous individuals have given unselfishly of their time and talents. Among those individuals are Robert Margulies, medical artist, who prepared the neurosurgical drawings; Faye Whitt, who carefully typed and retyped the text; and the Audiovisual Department of Duke University Medical Center, who prepared many of the illustrations. Our colleagues W. Cook, R. Kramer, B. Nashold, and G. Odom of the Division of Neurosurgery have kindly shared material on many of the patients depicted in the text. We believe this has allowed publication of the very best illustrative material available. Many of the high-quality neuroradiographic contrast studies would not have been possible without the expert assistance and support of our neuroradiology colleagues. Our thanks are also extended to the neurosurgical staff at The Hospital For Sick Children, Toronto, Canada, and The Hospital For Sick Children, Great Ormond Street, London, England, who inspired and taught one of us (W.J.O.) to care for infants and children with disease of the nervous system. During the time this text was being prepared, our families exercised patience and understanding to allow us the necessary time to complete this writing. This was clearly an unselfish act, since time once spent cannot be retrieved.

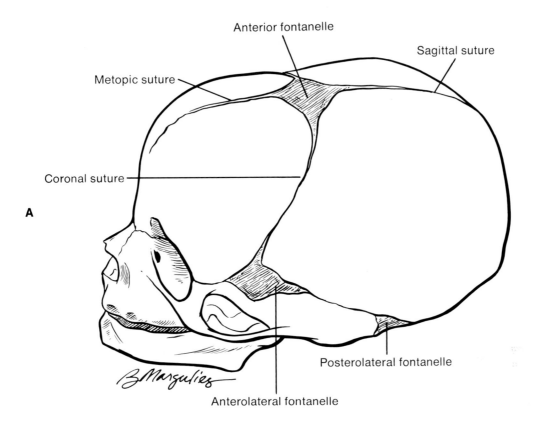

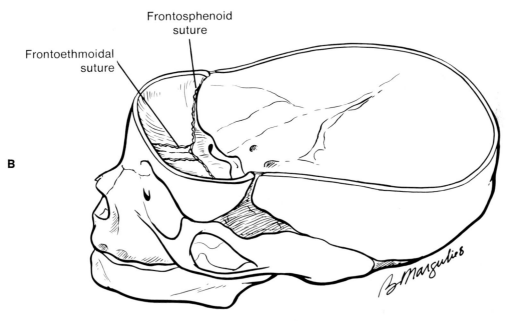

Fig. 12-1. A, External view of the infant's skull. **B,** Internal view of the infant's skull to show the position of the frontosphenoid and frontoethmoidal sutures.

movement of the adjacent bones is independent. This movement is most easily appreciated along the sagittal and coronal sutures. In addition, there are gaps in the bony protection that are readily palpable. The posterior fontanelle located in the midline at the junction of the parietal and occipital bones is usually easily felt at birth and remains open until the second or third month of life. The larger anterior fontanelle, also located in the midline at the junction of the parietal and frontal bones, frequently remains open until 18 months of age. Even though the head of a 2-year-old child may appear solid to palpation, this does not imply that the sutures are functionally fused. The vault sutures can quickly and easily be separated in response to increased intracranial pressure. The ability of the sutures to separate gradually decreases with age and is usually lost by the tenth year. It is the ability of the immature skull to enlarge that explains the low incidence of papilledema in infants. As the intracranial pressure begins to rise, the sutures separate and accommodate the rise in pressure by increased intracranial volume. Once the sutures do become functionally fused, this safeguard against increased intracranial pressure is lost. Functional fusion should not be confused with radiographic fusion, which does not normally take place until after the third decade.

Growth of the brain during the first 2 years of life occurs rapidly. By the child's second birthday, 70% of the adult brain weight has been obtained and the original brain weight has tripled.[33] Growth then continues more slowly until age 17 or 18, when full adult brain weight has been reached (Fig. 12-2). As the brain grows, the vault and base of the skull are induced to grow at a parallel rate. The growth of the skull is closely linked to the pressure of the underlying intracranial contents.

Skull shape may also be altered by positioning. If the infant's head is allowed to maintain a constant position, the dependent area will become flattened and the ipsilateral frontal area prominent. This condition is seen only in severely compromised infants with no head control and inadequate turning; if the head position is changed several times a day, it can be avoided.

Possible findings. When a suture prematurely closes over the developing brain, growth continues as long as other means of gaining intracranial volume are available.[17] Therefore, with closure of a single suture, the brain exerts pres-

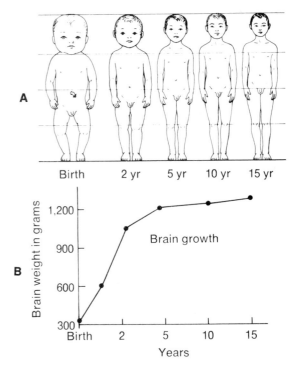

Fig. 12-2. A, Proportional drawings of the infant's and child's torso demonstrating that the head accounts for approximately 25% of the body length at birth and that with maturation this proportion decreases. **B,** Graph of brain weight versus age emphasizing the rapid growth that takes place during the first 2 years of life and the more gradual increase after that point. (**A** modified from Patten, B. M.: Human embryology, ed. 2, New York, 1953, McGraw-Hill Book Co.)

sure on the remaining open sutures and growth occurs in these directions.[2,33] With closure, growth is limited perpendicular to the involved suture and continues parallel to the suture. In the case of sagittal synostosis, growth is limited in the coronal plane and accelerated in the sagittal plane. The skull then takes on an elongated appearance (scaphocephaly or dolichocephaly), with narrowing of the biparietal diameter and elongation in a fronto-occipital direction. As the premature suture closure occurs, the suture loses its mobility and frequently develops a palpable ridge. The process of closure need not affect the entire suture simultaneously. Characteristically, the posterior portion of the sagittal suture is affected first and most severely. The closure process then spreads in both directions away from the original closure point. With involvement of the coronal suture, the lateral aspect of the suture is more commonly involved first. As the closure spreads, it can then

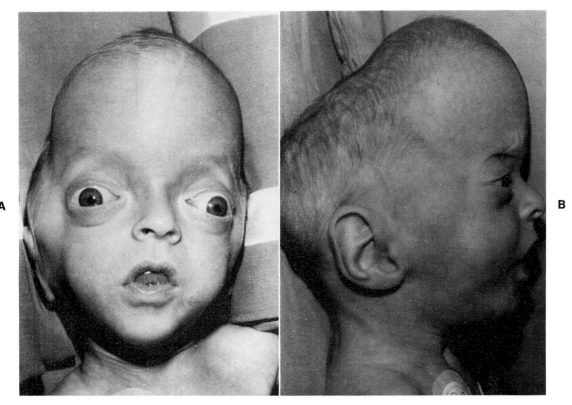

Fig. 12-3. A, Frontal view of an infant with Crouzon's syndrome. The orbits are hypoplastic and shallow, with the eyes appearing proptotic. The palate is highly arched, resulting in significant obstruction to nasal breathing. Venous engorgement of the scalp and forehead is indicative of increased intracranial pressure. A prominent temporal bulge is present bilaterally. **B,** Lateral view demonstrating the shallow orbit and midface hypoplasia. The posterior cranial vault shows marked restriction of growth, with compensatory expansion of the brain occurring through the open anterior fontanelle. Despite this compensation, the infant has bilateral papilledema.

involve the squamosal, frontosphenoidal, and even the frontoethmoidal sutures.[23,42] The anterior fontanelle may remain open, as well as the more medial aspect of the coronal suture itself.

The premature closure process may involve the facial sutures, as well as the vault and skull base.[48] Crouzon's, Apert's, and Carpenter's syndromes are examples of various degrees of facial involvement with bicoronal synostosis. One hallmark of all these syndromes is midface hypoplasia (Fig. 12-3). The maxillas appear recessed and the orbits hypoplastic. The excessively arched hard palate may result in nasal obstruction and necessitate mouth breathing.

It is commonly believed that when only a single suture is affected, the brain is not severely damaged by taking on the configuration necessary to fit within the deformed skull. As the number of sutures involved increases, the probability of

significant restriction of brain growth increases. Elevated intracranial pressure, papilledema, optic atrophy, and mental retardation can all occur if the condition is left untreated.[1,43] In addition, if the orbits are hypoplastic, the corneas may dry and develop exposure keratitis because of the exophthalmos and inability of the lids to adequately close and moisten the anterior aspects of the globes. In cases of multiple suture involvement with evidence of exposure keratitis or increased intracranial pressure, prompt surgical attention is necessary.

Suture closure may also occur in response to an underlying brain abnormality. If the entire brain is retarded in its development, the skull growth will be similarly retarded (secondary microcrania). The vault will maintain a normal configuration, but the face-to-skull ratio and body-to-skull ratio will be abnormal (Fig. 12-4). Rather than being generalized, the retarded brain development may be focal and may result in a localized lack of vault expansion. In this condition the sutures over the atrophic brain stop growing and fuse in advance of the sutures on the normal side. Other causes of abnormal skull configuration include pathologic expansion, either generally or focally. With hydrocephalus, the entire vault expands at an accelerated rate, causing alteration of the face-to-vault ratio. The expansion may also be local and result in bulging and thinning of the overlying bone (Fig. 12-5). This is most commonly seen with arachnoid cysts and superficially placed neoplasms. Chronic subdural hematomas sometimes

cause frontal bossing and a squared-off appearance of the skull.

The most common cause of an abnormal head shape at birth is the presence of extracranial hemorrhage as a result of the neonate's passage through the birth canal. A cephalohematoma is the accumulation of blood between one of the bones of the calvarium and its pericranium. These hemorrhages are limited by the cranial sutures and are associated with skull fractures in 25% of cases.[35] In the vast majority of cases, no treatment is needed and the cephalohematoma will simply reabsorb over a period of days or weeks. Rarely, the cephalohematoma will calcify or be-

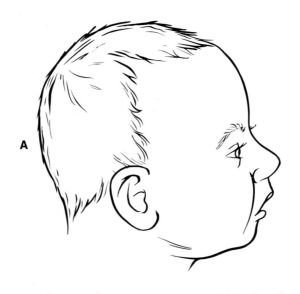

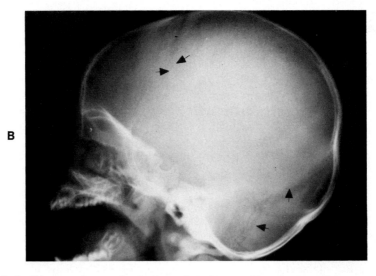

Fig. 12-4. A, Primary microcrania. **B,** Lateral skull x-ray film shows vault sutures to be patent, eliminating diffuse craniosynostosis as a cause of the microcrania.

come infected. Additional causes of abnormal head shape include leptomeningeal cysts and neoplasms of the scalp and skull.

Common occurrences. Isolated sagittal synostosis is the most common form of craniosynostosis. The condition comprises more than 50% of most surgical series and has a male predominance of 4 to 1. Rarely, it has been thought to have been inherited as an autosomal dominant trait. Most cases, however, demonstrate a sporadic occurrence. The diagnosis of this type of craniosynostosis as well as others can be made at birth. The characteristic appearance is that of an elongated narrow skull, frequently with a palpable ridge or keel over the fused sagittal suture. The posterior aspect of the head may take on a bullet-like appearance and protrude over the posterior fossa. The term for this skull deformity is scaphocephaly or dolichocephaly (Fig. 12-6). This condition is only rarely associated with other congenital anomalies either intracranially or outside the nervous system.

The coronal is the next most commonly involved suture. When unilateral and bilateral cases

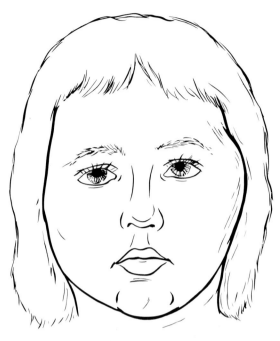

Fig. 12-5. Left temporal prominence secondary to expanding middle fossa mass.

Craniosynostosis

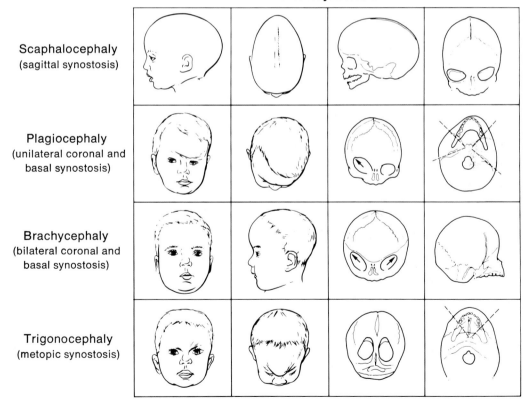

Scaphalocephaly
(sagittal synostosis)

Plagiocephaly
(unilateral coronal and basal synostosis)

Brachycephaly
(bilateral coronal and basal synostosis)

Trigonocephaly
(metopic synostosis)

Fig. 12-6. Clinical and radiographic appearance of patients with the most common forms of craniosynostosis.

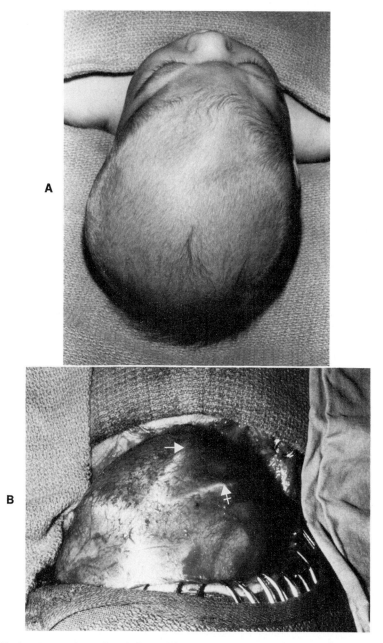

Fig. 12-7. A, Vertex view of an infant with multiple suture involvement from craniosynostosis. There is a left parietal bulge and synostosis of the metopic suture and both coronal sutures. **B,** Intra-operative photograph of the vertex confirming the displacement of the metopic suture (→) to the right and anterior displacement of the right coronal suture (↦).

are grouped together, they make up 30% to 35% of surgical series. The condition is somewhat more common in female infants, with a predominance of 3 to 2. Unilateral involvement is characterized by flattening of the supraorbital ridge on the involved side (Fig. 12-6). The anterior fossa is shortened and narrowed. The sphenoid ridge has a particularly high attachment to the inner aspect of the skull. The inner aspect of the ridge itself will deeply crease the underlying dura separating the frontal and temporal lobes. The angle created between the sphenoid and petrous ridge is decreased, emphasizing the involvement of the basal sutures. This appearance is termed plagiocephaly. Bilateral coronal synostosis results in anterior displacement of the anterior fontanelle. The entire forehead is broad, and the fronto-occipital skull diameter is decreased. This appearance is termed brachycephaly. As the base of the skull and face become more involved, the restriction of growth of the orbits and midface becomes more prominent. Crouzon's syndrome is a dominantly inherited trait in which bilateral coronal synostosis is associated with midface hypoplasia. Apert's syndrome, also an autosomal dominant trait, is characterized by brachycephaly, midface hypoplasia, syndactyly, and widening of the distal phalanx of the thumb and great toe. When both coronal sutures as well as the basal sutures are involved, restriction of brain growth may be quite significant and careful evaluation for the presence of increased intracranial pressure should be undertaken.

Trigonocephaly is the deformity that results when the metopic suture is prematurely fused in utero. The forehead has a beaked appearance, there is a palpable vertical ridge in the midforehead, and the distance between the orbits may be decreased (hypotelorism). This is an unusual form of craniosynostosis and makes up less than 5% of cases.

The lambdoid suture is rarely involved by itself, but when this does happen, the occiput on the involved side becomes flattened.

The remainder of cases are composed of combinations of premature suture closure (Fig. 12-7). In general, the greater the number of sutures involved, the more likely there is to be significant restriction of brain growth. Evidence of increased intracranial pressure is not unusual. The ultimate involvement is to have all sutures involved equally and simultaneously. In this case the vault may

have a normal appearance but fail to grow. These children develop microcrania because of the inability of the developing brain to gain intracranial volume. This primary microcrania must be differentiated from secondary microcrania, wherein the skull fails to grow because of retarded brain growth, because primary microcrania demands immediate attention and surgery whereas secondary microcrania does not. Differentiation can usually be done simply by obtaining x-ray films of the skull to determine if the sutures are fused and if there is evidence of increased intracranial pressure. With primary microcrania, both entities should be present.

Evaluation. In all cases of primary premature closure of cranial sutures, the process is present at birth and is clinically apparent. If any doubt exists as to whether an unusual head shape is the result of skull molding from passage through the birth canal or the result of craniosynostosis, good-quality skull films can readily differentiate the two conditions. Oblique views may be necessary to define the coronal sutures clearly; otherwise, routine skull radiographs are diagnostic. They also provide an objective basis on which to judge subsequent therapy. When multiple sutures are involved and increased intracranial pressure is suspected, a computerized tomographic (CT) scan of the brain will document ventricular size, establish the presence of periventricular lucency (associated with acutely raised intracranial pressure), and reveal associated intracranial congenital anomalies that influence treatment and prognosis. Certainly, not every patient with craniosynostosis needs a CT brain scan prior to surgical correction. Isolated sagittal synostosis can safely be repaired with no more than routine skull x-ray examination as a diagnostic evaluation.

Cases of secondary suture closure occurring after birth are unusual. Causes of secondary craniosynostosis include a fracture across a suture, hypophosphatemia, neonatal hyperthyroidism, iatrogenic hyperthyroidism, and sudden reduction of the intracranial volume, causing the bones of the vault to overlap. This latter situation is most commonly encountered following a successful shunting procedure for hydrocephalus, with marked reduction of the ventricular volume and overlapping of the vault sutures.

Referral. The diagnosis and initial evaluation of craniosynostosis can easily be made by any knowledgeable practitioner. Doubtful cases are usually easily sorted out by examination of the skull films. Once a diagnosis has been established, the intracranial tension and the state of the corneas need to be assessed. If the anterior fontanelle is thought to be tense or there is other evidence of increased intracranial pressure, referral takes on a more urgent disposition. It is our view that in the presence of extreme exophthalmos with drying of the corneas, immediate referral to the nearest center equipped to deal with this situation is indicated. With evidence of increased intracranial pressure, referral should not be delayed but is not urgent. The majority of patients can be evaluated electively, allowing a more deliberate evaluation. Evaluation should not be delayed, however, to see if the condition "corrects itself." Rather, cases of craniosynostosis should be evaluated by a neurosurgeon knowledgeable in the field. Surgery within the first 4 to 6 weeks after birth is desirable, and the referral should be within that time frame.[13,33] The ideal time for surgery is before the sixth postdelivery week, because much of the expansion of the skull takes place in the first few months of life. If the majority of brain growth has already taken place, little effect will be seen from simple craniectomy, since this procedure relies heavily on brain growth to reshape the skull. More involved cranial reconstructive procedures can be performed for severely affected children when they reach 7 to 10 years of age. Older children who have escaped medical attention can certainly be seen and evaluated and the parents counseled as to possible cosmetic improvement that could be obtained. They may also receive genetic counseling as regards the particular condition.

Medical versus surgical treatment. Currently there is no effective medical therapy for craniosynostosis. The decision is, therefore, between no specific therapy and surgical intervention. In the presence of increased intracranial pressure or exposure keratitis, little doubt exists; if full supportive measures are to be used for the child, surgery must be considered. When the cosmetic appearance of the child is the primary indication for the procedure, many other factors must be evaluated. The degree of improvement that could reasonably be expected from the procedure is balanced against the risk of the procedure. Generally, the older the infant, the less the anticipated improvement in appearance from a simple craniectomy. Fortunately, mortality and morbidity

figures for simple craniectomies are quite low. Mortality of much less than 1% and serious morbidity of less than 5% are standard in most centers.[43]

Surgical options. Surgically, two broad groups of procedures are available. The first group involves simple excision of the prematurely fused suture, followed by a series of maneuvers to delay subsequent bony reunion. In addition the pericranium adjacent to the involved suture is widely resected, since a significant proportion of the bony regeneration capabilities is derived from the pericranium. In addition to resection of the pericranium, the craniectomy edges may be lined with Silastic sheeting to retard the regrowth of bone in the craniectomy site. These procedures are recommended in the first few weeks and months of life, when the developing brain can reshape the skull as unrestricted growth occurs.

The second group of procedures involves release of bony structures, followed by intraoperative correction of the deformity. With these procedures, there is little to no reliance on the growing brain to mediate the correction. The amount of correction necessary is estimated before surgery. At the time of surgery, the detached bony structures are reshaped and repositioned to the full degree of desired correction. Since these procedures do not rely on brain growth to reshape the skull, they may be performed in children after the rapid phase of brain growth.[23] The indication for this major type of reconstruction is the desire of the patient or family for cosmetic improvement and social acceptability, and the procedures are done in conjunction with a plastic surgeon experienced in major craniofacial reconstruction.[9,31,37] The types of defects involved include hypertelorism, hypotelorism, midface and orbital hypoplasia, and orbital asymmetry. The procedures involve a bifrontal craniotomy with extradural dissection to the sphenoid wing. Some procedures can be performed without mobilization of the dura over the cribiform plate, thereby preserving the sense of smell. Dural tears created by mobilization are then repaired, usually with a pericranial graft. The orbits and maxillas are freed by osteotomy and then moved into the desired position. They are then held in place with wires and a series of bone grafts[49] (Fig. 12-8).

Postoperative course. Following linear craniectomy, infants are able to feed within 6 to 12 hours. Hyperpyrexia and irritability are frequent

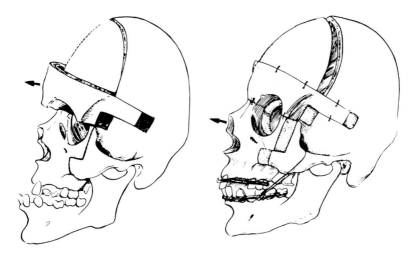

Fig. 12-8. Diagram of midface and bifrontal advancement. Bone grafts are placed behind the advanced supraorbital ridge and midface to maintain the forward position. (From Epstein, F. J., and others: Radical one-stage correction of craniofacial anomalies, J. Neurosurg. **42:**522, 1975.)

within the first hours. Careful attention is always paid to any elevated temperature that persists for longer than 36 hours. Antipyretic medications and surface cooling are employed to prevent the occurrence of febrile seizures. Blood transfusion is usually necessary either during or after this type of procedure, and no operation should be begun without the availability of adequate blood replacement.

Because serosanguineous fluid frequently accumulates under the skin flap, some surgeons employ drains or aspirate the wound. Neither of these procedures is employed in our hospital, and the rate of healing does not appear to be affected. Wound infection is also borne in mind, especially after the implantation of a foreign body. Fortunately, this is quite unusual. However, if it does occur, the wound must be reopened and the Silastic sheeting removed.

The infants are held and nourished as usual, with no protective apparatus for the head. Typically, patients are discharged on the third or fourth postoperative day with instructions to the parents to return on the seventh day for stitch removal and wound inspection. As the complexity and length of the surgery increase, so do the serious complications. Patients undergoing craniofacial reconstruction are best managed postoperatively in a neurosurgical intensive care unit. Fluid and electrolytes as well as transfusion requirements need frequent adjustment. Cerebrospinal fluid rhinorrhea, meningitis, wound infection, sub-

dural hematoma, and cerebral edema can all occur following this type of procedure. Bone graft infection is a particularly feared complication requiring debridement and, frequently, removal of segments of the infected bone. Postoperative recovery is usually complete within 10 to 14 days, barring any serious complications.

Prognosis. Cosmetic improvement is usually substantial but may not be fully appreciated for several months. Postoperative x-ray films will frequently show continued separation of the craniectomy edges several months following the procedure. Occasionally, coronal synostosis treated by linear craniectomy may need revision in early childhood if a full cosmetic improvement has not been realized with the initial procedure. The secondary procedure involves enlarging the orbit and anterior fossa, forcing the lateral aspect of the supraorbital ridge forward, and holding it in an advanced position with a bone graft.[23]

Important aspects of follow-up. Follow-up of uncomplicated cases is mainly to assess the success of the procedure. Major complications are quite unusual. Rarely, a dural tear will go unrecognized and present as a leptomeningeal cyst months after the procedure. Late-onset infections are rare but possible. The initial postoperative visit is made at 6 weeks; then, further visits are at the discretion of the referring physician. When multiple sutures are involved, a much closer and protracted follow-up period is necessary.

CONGENITAL ENCEPHALOCELE

Cranium bifidum, like spina bifida, represents a spectrum of diseases ranging from simple cranium bifidum, wherein there is normal brain development and lack of midline bone formation, to anencephaly, wherein skin, bone, and dura mater of the vault are absent or only partially formed. In anencephaly, the cerebral hemispheres are absent or severely dysmorphic, but the brain stem and cerebellum are usually present. Between these two extremes lie cerebral meningoceles, in which the meninges alone protrude through a bony cranial defect, and encephaloceles, in which brain tissue herniates with the leptomeninges.

Routine examination for age. The examination of the neonate's nervous system is limited in the number of parameters that can be assessed. Each variable that can be measured and characterized, therefore, takes on increased importance. In each case the vital signs (pulse, blood pressure, respirations, and temperature) should be assessed and recorded carefully. Not only is the respiratory pattern and rate important, but the muscles involved are also noted. This may be the simplest method of recognizing a paraplegic or quadraplegic neonate with diaphragmatic breathing and no intercostal muscle function. The undisturbed infant is then simply observed for its posture, the position of its extremities, and the presence and distribution of spontaneous motion. Reflex spinal movement is easily confused with purposeful movement; and for that reason, care must be taken in interpreting any movement that is not spontaneous. The infant's resistance to motion or muscular tone is assessed in the extremities and trunk. Responses to multiple external stimuli (light, sound, pain, and sudden change in position) should also be tested and the reaction recorded.

Possible findings. The diagnosis of most encephaloceles is obvious at birth. Small sessile lesions may not be noticed initially, and basal lesions projecting into the orbit, nasal cavity, or pharynx may escape attention into adult life (Fig. 12-9). The typical vault lesion is frequently pedunculated and located in or near the midline of the occiput. The lesion may be covered by full-thickness skin, epithelialized meninges, or, simply, exposed arachnoid. Pressure on the encephalocele reduces its size and is associated with a corresponding increase in intracranial tension felt over the anterior fontanelle. Extension of cerebral

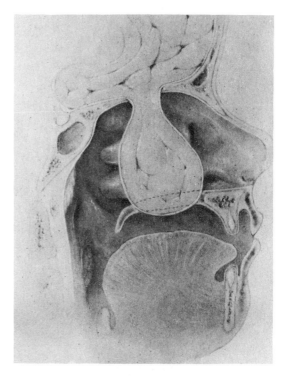

Fig. 12-9. Diagrammatic midsagittal section of an infant with a large encephalocele protruding into the nasal cavity. (From Matson, D. D.: Neurosurgery of infancy and childhood, ed. 2, 1969. Courtesy Charles C Thomas, Publisher, Springfield, Ill.)

tissue into the lesion can be appreciated by gentle palpation and transillumination. Frequently, a capillary hemangioma will surround the base of the lesion either totally or partially. Excessive hair may be present at the base of the lesion as well. The size of the sac does not correspond with the presence or absence of cerebral tissue. Large sacs may contain no brain tissue, whereas small sacs may be completely filled. In general, the more pedunculated the neck of the sac, the less likely it is to contain brain tissue. Infants with occipital encephaloceles and microcephaly with an abrupt posterior slope to the forehead are usually found to have a significant quantity of brain tissue present in the encephalocele (Fig. 12-10).

Results of the initial examination of the nervous system immediately after birth are characteristically normal.[51] This is true whether the lesion represents a cerebral meningocele or an encephalocele with a large quantity of brain tissue in the sac.

Common occurrences. The typical lesion is a

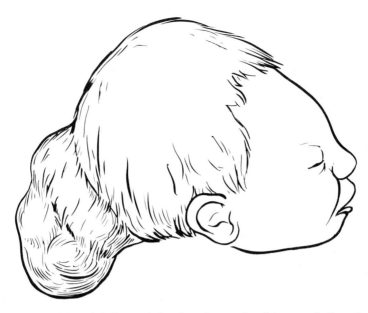

Fig. 12-10. Neonate with occipital encephalocele, microcrania of the true skull, and abrupt posterior slope of the forehead, implying that the encephalocele contains a significant quantity of brain tissue.

pedunculated occipital mass that projects from the skull in or near the midline. Occipital and parieto-occipital lesions make up 90% of congenital encephaloceles seen in North America. The brain within the encephalocele may be the posterior portion of the occipital lobes, the cerebellum, the brain stem, or a combination of these structures. Recently, it has been recognized that frontal and basal lesions have a particularly high rate of occurrence in Southeast Asia.[47] Although they are rare in North America, frontal and basal encephaloceles take on an exaggerated clinical importance because of their benign nature and excellent prognosis. When the lesions project anteriorly into the region of the glabella or inner canthus, they may be associated with hypertelorism and a cystic swelling at the base of the nose. Those that present in the orbit, either through the superior orbital fissure or the frontoethmoidal suture, may present with exophthalmos or decreased visual acuity.[40] Occasionally, lesions presenting in the nose or pharynx are confused with nasal polyps and are biopsied. Consideration of this diagnosis with all intranasal masses and appropriate evaluation performed preoperatively should prevent such an occurrence. Rarely, basal lesions are seen in association with a cleft lip or palate.

Evaluation. Once the neonate has received a complete clinical assessment, x-ray films of the skull should be obtained. Basal encephaloceles in the older infant and child may also require tomography to define the bony defect accurately. This procedure is not usually necessary with lesions over the vertex. Following skull films, a CT scan of the brain may help to evaluate the extent of brain tissue herniation objectively. Sagittal projections of the CT brain scan may be quite helpful in this assessment. In addition, associated structural anomalies and secondary phenomena, including hydrocephalus, agenesis of the corpus callosum, Chiari malformation, Dandy-Walker cyst, and holoprosencephaly, can be evaluated. The CT brain scan can also give a clear picture of the bony defect. Rarely, angiography may be indicated to establish the relationship of the lesion to the major venous sinuses or to verify the extent of the brain herniation. Pneumoencephalography and ventriculography add little of practical importance that cannot be obtained from one of the other diagnostic studies.

Referral. Lesions not completely covered by epithelium are at high risk of rupture and should be evaluated urgently. Once rupture has occurred, there exists a risk of meningitis that increases with time. Meningitis in the immature central nervous system is a particularly dreaded problem and should be avoided by early surgical intervention in those cases selected for therapy. Lesions that are completely skin covered can be dealt with in a less urgent fashion. Many authors, however, think that clinically obvious encephaloceles are so emotionally upsetting to the parents and disfiguring to the child that every effort should be made to repair the lesion before the family takes the child home. Basal lesions presenting as nasal and pharyngeal masses or with exophthalmos without evidence of meningitis are elective in their referral and evaluation. All lesions, no matter what their size, should be evaluated by a neurosurgeon experienced in congenital anomalies, because the size of the lesion does not correlate with the extent of cerebral herniation or the eventual prognosis.

Medical versus surgical treatment. As with other structural congenital anomalies, there is no medical therapy available for the primary defect. There is also no surgical procedure that can return the dysmorphic brain to proper function. Therefore, the goals of surgery include (1) closing open skin defects to prevent infection and drying of viable brain tissue, (2) allowing ease of handling of the infant by parents and nursing staff without fear of causing rupture of a tenuous encephalocele sac, (3) giving a more accurate assessment of the portion and extent of the brain that is dysmorphic, and (4) opening cerebrospinal fluid (CSF) pathways in an attempt to avoid shunting procedures for hydrocephalus. Surgery is not intended to improve neurologic function but to maintain it at its preoperative level. Repair is recommended in the vast majority of patients. If large quantities of vital brain tissue are contained within the sac, hydrocephalus is present, and other major congenital anomalies exist, the lesion may be left unrepaired. If the child survives the first few months of life and nursing or custodial care is compromised by the lesion, the need for surgical excision should be reevaluated.

Surgical options. With occipital lesions, preparations are made for posterior fossa exploration. The skin over the encephalocele is dissected free on both sides and is held laterally. Extradural attachments from the dura to the bony defect are divided. The dura is then opened, and the intradural contents are inspected. Adhesions between the brain tissue and dura are divided. These are found to be particularly dense at the site of the

bony constriction. Dysmorphic, nonfunctional tissue is amputated. Viable, healthy-appearing tissue is retained and replaced within the skull.[3] A watertight dural closure is made, and the skin is approximated over the lesion. Adequate skin coverage is rarely a problem. No attempt is made at the time of primary repair to perform a cranioplasty. If the lesion is found to be infratentorial, a posterior fossa exploration is carried out with the idea of reestablishing CSF pathways by lysis of adhesions. If hydrocephalus remains uncontrolled, a ventriculoperitoneal or ventriculoatrial shunt may be necessary at a later date.

Anterior and basal lesions are approached through a frontal craniotomy with intradural inspection and repair of the dural defect. Herniated portions of the orbital surface of the frontal lobes are amputated. No attempt is made to dissect the dural sac from the orbit or nasopharynx; it is simply disconnected from the subarachnoid space through a watertight dural closure. A small portion of the craniotomy bone flap may be used to fill the bony defect at the base of the skull. Hydrocephalus is rarely a problem with lesions in the frontal and basal areas.

Postoperative course. Following surgical excision of the typical posteriorly placed lesion, over half of the pateints will develop hydrocephalus and require shunting. CSF-cutaneous fistula can be avoided by a watertight dural repair and early placement of a ventriculoperitoneal or ventriculoatrial shunt when hydrocephalus becomes apparent. The presence of hydrocephalus is evaluated with serial head circumference measurements and estimation of the tension of the anterior fontanelle. Ultrasound and CT brain scanning are also used postoperatively to evaluate ventricular size. Postoperative hemorrhage and wound infection are unusual if there has been no preoperative rupture of the encephalocele sac. Without the development of hydrocephalus, a 7- to 10-day hospital stay can be expected. The development of hydrocephalus usually doubles this figure.

Prognosis. The prognosis is clearly associated with several factors[27,32,34]: the location of the lesion, the extent and character of the brain herniation, the development of hydrocephalus, and the occurrence of meningitis. With the presence of brain herniation into posterior lesions, follow-up has shown that most of these children have retarded motor and intellectual function. In addition, more than 50% will require shunting for hydrocephalus. Lesions located in the parietal area tend to have the outlook determined largely by location.[32] The closer the lesion occurs to the anterior fontanelle, the more serious the associated cerebral malformations and the worse the prognosis. Lesions involving the frontal and basal areas, however, are usually associated with normal intelligence and motor development. Hydrocephalus is rarely seen with encephaloceles in these locations.

Important aspects of follow-up. The most important aspect of early follow-up is to ensure that ventricular pressure is normal. Irritability, anterior fontanelle tension, and head circumference measurements are evaluated; and when the question of increased intracranial pressure arises, a repeat CT brain scan or ultrasound study of the head is performed. In the older child with a repaired frontal encephalocele and hypertelorism, improvement of the cosmetic appearance is a major challenge of reconstructive surgery. Psychologic assessment of intellectual function is not accurate in young infants and should be deferred until the child reaches 2½ to 3 years of age. At that time a more meaningful assessment can be made of intellectual function. Genetic counseling for further pregnancies is an important aspect of the total care of the patient and the family. Subsequent siblings run an increased risk of having spinal or cranial dysrhaphism. Depending on the geographic area, this incidence ranges from 2% to 5%.[7] Screening of further pregnancies with alphafetoprotein determinations in the maternal serum and amniotic fluid and by ultrasound examination of the fetus is advised. This information is important whether or not therapeutic abortion is considered. If the parents elect to bring the child with a known encephalocele to term, the delivery should take place in an institution equipped for immediate repair of the dysraphic anomaly.

Complications. Long-term complications from posterior encephaloceles are rare. If problems do arise, they are usually related to the management of hydrocephalus or to the intrinsic intellectual and motor deficits for which therapy is supportive. Infants with anterior and basal encephaloceles may develop CSF rhinorrhea postoperatively. If meningitis occurs, particularly if it is caused by *Streptococcus pneumoniae* or *Hemophilus influenzae,* the infant should be further evaluated for CSF rhinorrhea. Complaints of watery

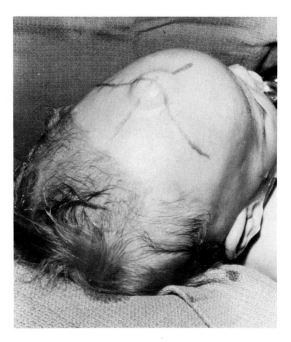

Fig. 12-11. Inclusion dermoid cyst of the anterior fontanelle.

nasal discharge or persistent nighttime cough should raise this possibility.

Other, less common lesions. Certainly, not every swelling over the scalp in a neonate or child is an encephalocele. Mobile elliptical masses that are midline and that lie over the anterior fontanelle are frequently found to be dermoid inclusion cysts (Fig. 12-11). The infant is clinically normal, as are his skull x-ray films. Complete surgical excision is advised and is rarely associated with intraoperative or postoperative problems. Hemangiomas may occur over the scalp and may attain tremendous size. Neither dermoid inclusion cysts nor scalp hemangiomas fluctuate in size with time or body position. If fluctuation occurs, it suggests communication between the lesion and the subarachnoid space or the cerebral vasculature. Dermoid sinus tracts occur primarily over the occiput and may be associated with a hairy tuft in the mouth of the tract and a surrounding capillary nevus in the skin (Fig. 12-12). These tracts may on occasion discharge material onto the skin and may be associated with a subcutaneous dermoid cyst. They are of importance because they may be associated with intracranial dermoid tumors and may be a source of repeated bouts of meningitis. Sinus pericranii can also be confused with a small sessile encephalocele. These lesions are

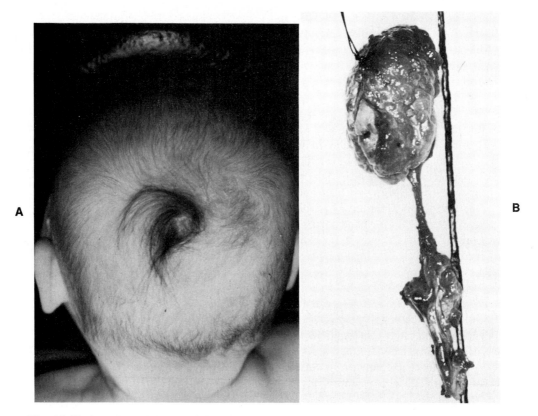

Fig. 12-12. A, Infant with an occipital dermal sinus tract. The lesion is accentuated by the surrounding hirsutism and capillary hemangioma. **B,** Excised subcutaneous occipital dermoid tumor and dermal sinus tract. A cutaneous opening and small ellipse of surrounding skin are included in the specimen. The dermal sinus tract extended within the dura but was not associated with an intracranial tumor.

cystic outpouchings of the cerebral venous system but are more likely to be somewhat away from the midline. Additional differential diagnoses include parietal foraminas and cystic hygromas of the scalp.

Simple cranium bifidum in which no meninges or nervous tissue protrude through the bony defect can safely be followed as long as there is adequate skin coverage and the defect is not so large as to represent a threat of trauma to the underlying brain. If there is concern about the extent of the bony defect, a cranioplasty can be performed. However, it should be delayed, if possible, until the child is through the rapid growth phase of the skull, or until age 3 to 4 years.

MYELOMENINGOCELE AND ASSOCIATED ABNORMALITIES

Of the nonlethal developmental anomalies of the central nervous system that are apparent at birth, myelomeningoceles are the most common,

occurring in approximately two neonates in every thousand live births.[35] These unfortunate infants have a portion of their malformed spinal cord appear on or near the skin surface. Although the most obvious element of their problem is apparent at birth, the developmental anomaly is not confined to the spine and spinal cord but has frequent and important associated manifestations in other parts of the central nervous system. Their management is controversial and continues to be a major challenge to pediatric neurosurgeons.

Routine examination for age. The neurologic examination of the neonate requires time and patience. Before the examination is begun, the patient's temperature should be normalized. Lengthy transportation will frequently result in a cold neonate whose reactions and movements are sluggish. Inaccurate and misleading information will be generated if the infant is examined in suboptimal conditions.

The patient is completely undressed in a warm

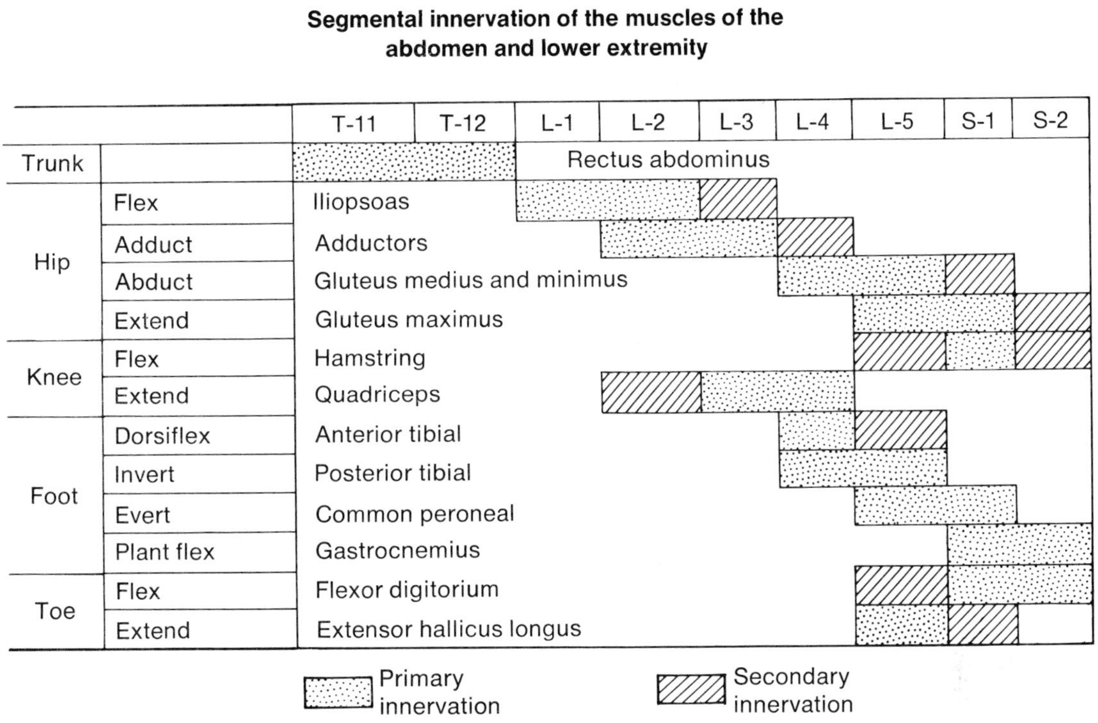

**Segmental innervation of the muscles of the
abdomen and lower extremity**

			T-11	T-12	L-1	L-2	L-3	L-4	L-5	S-1	S-2
Trunk			Rectus abdominus								
Hip	Flex	Iliopsoas			P	P	S				
	Adduct	Adductors				P	P	S			
	Abduct	Gluteus medius and minimus						P	P	S	
	Extend	Gluteus maximus							P	P	S
Knee	Flex	Hamstring							S	P	S
	Extend	Quadriceps				S	P	P			
Foot	Dorsiflex	Anterior tibial						P	S		
	Invert	Posterior tibial						P	P		
	Evert	Common peroneal							P	P	
	Plant flex	Gastrocnemius								P	P
Toe	Flex	Flexor digitorium							S	P	S
	Extend	Extensor hallicus longus							P	P	S

Primary innervation   Secondary innervation

Fig. 12-13

room and observed in both the prone and supine positions. The posture and position of the extremities are noted and recorded. Muscular imbalance may be manifested by an abnormal resting position of the involved extremity.[30] Contractures and joint dislocations may be present if the muscular imbalance has been long standing and severe.

Spontaneous motor activity will be seen in the vigorous neonate at the hip, knee, ankle, and toe joints. Movement of the legs will frequently alternate from side to side and be synchronized with arm and facial movements. The presence of spontaneous motor activity can be confirmed, and strength can be graded by resistance to stretch of specific muscle groups. Response to painful stimulation as a method of testing motor function should be avoided, since reflex spinal movement is easily confused with spontaneous motor activity. The movements of the lower extremities should be analyzed by muscle group and recorded as being present +, absent −, or questionable ±. The sepcific segmental innervation of the muscles of the lower extremities can be seen in Fig. 12-13.

Sensation should be tested in response to pinprick stimulation that is slowly moved from an area of presumed diminished sensation to an area

of normal sensation. As a first approximation, the sacral dermatomes should be tested, followed by the lower lumbar and, finally, the upper lumbar areas (Fig. 12-14). The fact that normal response to a noxious stimulus applied to an extremity may be delayed by several seconds necessitates that the examiner wait 15 to 30 seconds between stimulations and that the neonate be calmed during that period. Facial grimacing or crying should be the end point sought, not reflex withdrawal of the extremity. The motor and sensory examination of the upper extremities is conducted in a similar manner to that of the lower extremities. Anal sphincter tone and the anal wink reflex should both be assessed. In the remaining portion of the neurologic examination, attention is directed to the head, with an estimation of the intracranial tension and measurement of the circumference. The pupils should be circular and equal in size and have a brisk response to light. Spontaneous extraocular movements are normally conjugate and full. The gag and suck responses as well as the Moro reflex should be tested. Careful attention to the inspection and palpation of the spine is an important aspect of the examination of every neonate. The detailed neurologic examination is not

Sensory dermatomes of the infant

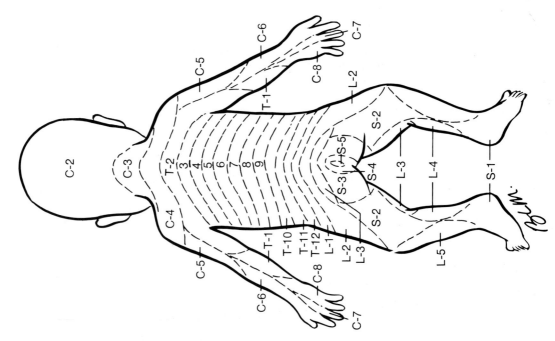

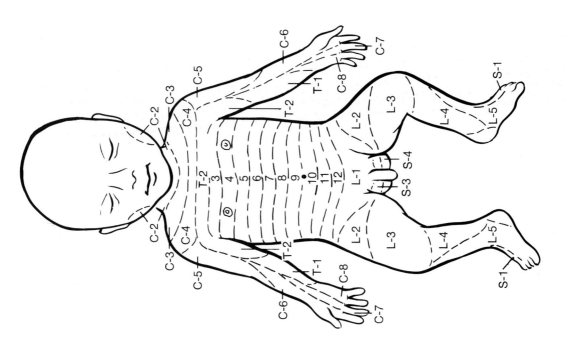

Fig. 12-14

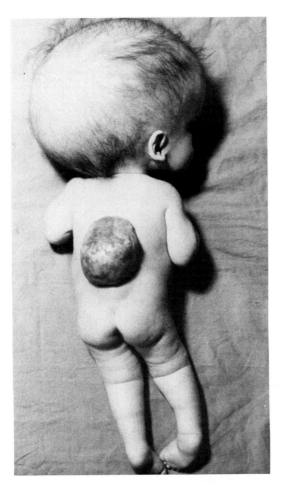

Fig. 12-15. Six-month-old infant with untreated thoracolumbar myelomeningocele and severe hydrocephalus.

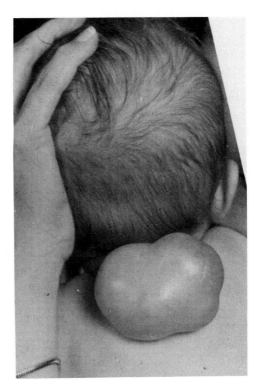

Fig. 12-16. High thoracic meningocele. The infant is neurologically intact. (Courtesy G. L. Odom, M.D., Durham, N.C.)

performed in isolation; rather, it is an integral part of the general physical examination.

Possible findings. The diagnosis of a myelomeningocele is usually obvious at the time of birth. The lesions are characteristically located in the caudal third of the spine and are frequently seen to be on a broad sessile base oriented vertically (Fig. 12-15). In the center of the lesion is an elliptical neural placode that may be covered by various amounts of granulation tissue or epithelium. The placode is the surface presentation of the malformed spinal cord and should be kept moist with sterile saline sponges and protected from trauma. At the upper end of the placode is the central canal, which may be seen to release spinal fluid periodically. The placode represents the malformed portion of the spinal cord that is not fused dorsally. Frequently surrounding the neural placode is a transparent arachnoidal membrane. With time, the placode will develop superficial suppuration and the arachnoid will become opaque. Surrounding the delicate transparent membrane is epithelium that has grown over the underlying leptomeninges. This partial-thickness skin is an effective barrier to infection and may be used to cover the lesion at the time of the surgical repair. Adjacent to the epithelialized leptomeninges is full-thickness skin frequently associated with excessive hair or a capillary hemangioma. A rough determination of the quantity of neural tissue within the sac may be made by transillumination or by gentle palpation. Rather than being sessile, the lesion may be pedunculated and have a rather narrow constricted base. This is usually an encouraging sign, indicating a limited amount of nervous tissue that is dysmorphic and displaced into the cystic malformation. Pedunculated lesions in the cervical and upper thoracic areas may represent true meningoceles with ballooning of the leptomeninges through a dorsal mesodermal defect without spinal cord involvement (Fig. 12-16). These infants are characteristically neurologically intact with a low incidence of hydrocephalus and associated anomalies. Hamartomas, dermoids, and teratomas found over the spine may be mistaken for myelomeningoceles.[50] They are usually not associated with neurologic abnormalities, and routine x-ray examination of the spine will not show the characteristic changes of spina bifida cystica (myelomeningocele).

Physiologically, myelomeningoceles may be seen to affect the function of either the upper or lower motor neurons.[45,46] With primary involvement of the lower motor neuron, either as a result of the dysmorphic process or as a result of a secondary injury to the exposed neural placode, the muscles innervated by the abnormal neural segment will demonstrate atrophy or hypoplasia and will be flaccid to manipulation.[46] Lesions with incomplete involvement of the lower extremity may demonstrate a muscular imbalance about a joint with an abnormal resting posture. The knee may demonstrate extension without the ability to flex, and the feet may have normal dorsiflexion and inversion as well as weakness of plantar flexion and eversion. The specific posture of the extremity is dependent on the level of the lesion. If dorsal fusion fails to occur somewhat cephalad to the conus medullaris, the neonate may develop evidence of an upper motor neuron lesion and will have spastic lower extremities without evidence of atrophy or hypoplasia. Movement secondary to reflex spinal activity may be easily provoked by external stimulation. The motion will frequently alternate from one leg to the other and may even take on a complex character. Following withdrawal of the stimulus, however, movement will quickly subside. Associated spinal lesions (syringomyelia and diastematomyelia) and intracranial lesions should be sought as alternative explanations for spastic paraplegia.* A third alternative is for the lesion to be mixed, with elements of both upper and lower motor neuron involvement. The involvement of the lower extremities need not be symmetric, nor must the sensory level correspond to the motor level. The examination should be judged on the factual information available and not on the predicted or expected findings from knowledge of the level and extent of the spinal lesion.

When involved, the anus is patulous and the anal wink is lost. With crying, the perineum will

lose its slight concave appearance and become flattened while the rectum may actually prolapse slightly. The bladder may be distended, and urination will be by overflow incontinence. Abdominal pressure or the Valsalva maneuver will frequently yield small amounts of urine.

Careful attention is paid to the examination of the head for the presence of hydrocephalus. This is present in 25% of cases at the time of birth.[35] The maximum head circumference is measured, and the tension of the anterior fontanelle is assessed. The fundi should be carefully searched for the presence of chorioretinitis or congenital abnormalities of the optic nerve. The lower cranial nerves should be evaluated by watching the infant feed and specifically by checking the gag reflex. Aspiration or nasal regurgitation of feedings may be the first manifestation of a symptomatic Chiari malformation and may herald respiratory distress or arrest.[22] Alterations of extraocular movements are common and should be documented. The complete spine is carefully palpated and examined for the presence of kyphosis, scoliosis, and other bony anomalies, which may be present at some distance from the actual myelomeningocele sac. Other organ systems are then surveyed for the presence of other congenital anomalies.

Common occurrences. In addition to the neurologic deficit that results from the dysmorphic spinal cord, there are almost always associated anomalies of the remainder of the central nervous system, most of which can be classified under the heading type II Chiari malformation.[14,39] This particular group of malformations has many features, only a few of which will be summarized here. Hydrocephalus is present in the large majority of cases. This is particularly true in infants with lumbar or thoracolumbar meningomyeloceles; 75% to 90% of such infants will have demonstrable hydrocephalus in the newborn period.[28] The incidence of hydrocephalus decreases to approximately 50% when the lesion is located purely in the sacral area.[25] The hydrocephalus is usually on the basis of aqueductal stenosis or forking.

Virtually any area of the brain can be associated with the dysmorphic process. The cerebral mantle may show abnormal neuronal migration patterns with polymicrogyria and heterotopia of gray matter. There may be agenesis of the corpus callosum, and the massa intermedia may be partic-

---

*See references 4, 11, 19, 21, and 38.

ularly large. The falx and tentorium are almost always hypoplastic with a low attachment of the tentorium to the skull. The quadrigeminal plate may be fused and have a beaklike posterior projection. The cervicomedullary junction may be kinked or elongated to take on an S configuration, while the exiting cervical nerve roots will take a cephalad course before their dural exit. The fourth ventricle is caudally displaced, frequently extending into the upper portion of the cervical spinal canal. The inferior portion of the cerebellar vermis will follow the caudally displaced fourth ventricle and lie in the upper cervical spine. The displaced cerebellum will become gliotic and have a smooth, uniform surface with loss of the fine superficial vascular network. The extent to which each of these is present varies with the individual case.

The etiology of the anomalies seen in spina bifida cystica (myelomeningocele) is unknown, but any explanation that is offered must be able to explain all of the frequently found features. The current theories can generally be divided into two groups, those postulating an arrest of the development of the neural tube and those postulating a reopening.[8] A more recent idea is that the neuroectodermal changes are only secondary to a primary mesodermal developmental anomaly.[29]

Evaluation. Following a detailed history and physical examination, x-ray films of the spine, skull, and chest are taken. Spinal radiographs help to determine the extent of the dorsal bony defect and the presence of associated defects of the anterior aspects of the spine, including the vertebral bodies and discs. Hemivertebrae and congenital bony fusions are frequently found. Skull films are important to establish the presence of suture separation as an indication of hydrocephalus and to reveal any other congenital bony deformity of the skull (Fig. 12-17). The chest film is to add assurance that no major intrathoracic congenital anomaly is left undiagnosed before a decision is made regarding the appropriate therapy. A CT scan of the brain will establish the ventricular size and the presence of any large structural congenital anomaly within the brain. Evaluation of the presence or degree of polymicrogyria and cerebral heteropia, which would be helpful in making a decision regarding therapy, cannot currently be done accurately with CT scans. Intravenous pyelography and myelography are not routinely performed before consideration of repair of the myelomeningocele. If electromyographic (EMG) facilities are readily available, these can provide supportive evidence to further establish the functional spinal segments. Somatosensory-evoked potentials can be used both preoperatively and intraoperatively to determine the presence of spinal nerve root function.[12,41]

Referral. These neonates should be quickly referred to the nearest center equipped to deal with a myelomeningocele patient. The referral

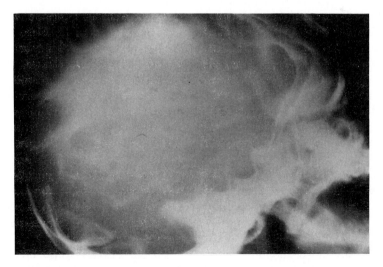

Fig. 12-17. Skull film of a neonate with widely separated coronal and lambdoid sutures indicating increased intracranial pressure and craniolacunia (lückenschädel). Craniolacunia is commonly seen in neonates with myelodysplasia and is resolved over a period of weeks to months.

should be made as soon after birth as possible, since closure of exposed myelomeningoceles should be done within 24 hours after birth to minimize the risk of meningitis.[30] Many major centers have now developed teams of health care professionals prepared to care for these patients, and this approach appears to maximize the patient's chance of obtaining independent function in society. The teams are usually composed of a pediatrician, an orthopedist, a urologist, a physical therapist, a social worker, nursing staff, and a neurosurgeon. The decision regarding therapy should be carefully assessed in the medical group caring for the patient before the parents are counseled. Receiving conflicting information and advice from several medical specialists on a complicated congenital anomaly may cause the parents to feel stress to their emotional and intellectual limits. It is best that no opinion regarding operability be given until a careful and complete assessment is made.

Medical versus surgical treatment. The decision making surrounding the treatment of a patient with a myelomeningocele can be difficult and emotionally taxing to all concerned. Little debate exists that every effort should be made to support the neonate with a low-lying lesion who has normal function of the lower extremities. In the presence of a wide-based thoracolumbar lesion and total paraplegia, congenital hydrocephalus, and serious associated congenital anomalies outside the nervous system, many physicians would not recommend active treatment. The difficulty, then, lies between these two extremes. There is no simple formula that can be applied blindly to arrive at a decision. Factors that are positive include preoperative evidence of muscle function at or below the L-3 level (which is necessary to maintain ambulation in adult life), presence of an anal wink or anal sphincter tone, and a concerned family who had intelligently evaluated the situation and agreed to accept the challenge of caring for a handicapped child. Negative factors include total paraplegia with bowel and bladder incontinence; the presence of severe congenital hydrocephalus; the presence of congenital scoliosis or kyphosis; a broad-based, poorly epithelized lesion (making early repair lengthy and technically difficult); evidence of a severe birth injury or intraventricular hemorrhage; and associated major congenital anomalies in other organ sys-

tems. The difficulty then is deciding with the family if full surgical support is advisable for their particular child.[5,18,27,44] Patients who do not have initial repair should periodically have this decision reviewed with consideration given to repair of the myelomeningocele sac and cerebrospinal fluid shunting to facilitate nursing care.

Surgical options. The actual repair of the malformation is done with the patient under a general anesthetic with the abdomen hanging free between supports under the chest and pelvis. The procedure is begun by making an elliptical incision around the neural placode. The incision is placed at the edge of the epithelized leptomeninges, and a dissection plane is created between the superficial epithelial layer and the underlying leptomeninges. The dissection is continued extradurally to the point of emergence of the dural sac through the lumbodorsal fascial defect. An intradural inspection is then made, and the placode is freed from any attachments to the surrounding leptomeninges. These are usually especially well developed at the vertical extremes of the neural placode. Once the placode is free, with the use of magnification, it is gently trimmed of granulation tissue and residual epithelium and is replaced within the dura. The spinal cord immediately cephalad to the placode may be enlarged, usually indicating segmental hydromyelia. The arachnoidal edges of the placode are then approximated with fine sutures. This procedure reconstructs the spinal cord into a tube surrounded by arachnoid. Almost always, there is then ample dura to create a watertight closure without constricting the intradural contents. Flaps fashioned from the lumbodorsal fascia to cover the defect further ensure a watertight closure. Redundant skin is trimmed away, and a cosmetic closure is then accomplished with two layers of fine sutures. An attempt should be made to keep the axis of the skin closure vertical in anticipation of subsequent spinal procedures to stabilize a scoliotic or kyphotic spine. In unusual cases, where adequate skin coverage is not available locally, various rotation flaps or other plastic surgical procedures may be used to ensure skin coverage of the area of the repair. A moisture-resistant bandage is then applied over the closure.

Postoperative course. Following surgery, the neonate is nursed prone on a frame designed to allow drainage of urine and feces away from the wound. This position is maintained until the sutures are removed on the seventh postoperative day. As soon as the patient recovers sufficiently from the anesthetic, the neurologic examination is repeated and compared with the preoperative examination to determine if further neurologic compromise has occurred during the surgical repair. All future decisions regarding alteration of function are based on this examination. It should, therefore, be as precise as possible. During the first few days after surgery, careful attention is given to the anterior fontanelle tension and the head circumference measurements. The CT brain scan or ultrasound determination of ventricular size can be carried out to assess the development of hydrocephalus. Every effort is made to prevent the CSF pressure from rising to the point that cerebrospinal fluid leaks from the site of the spinal repair. A ventriculoperitoneal shunt should be placed before the intracranial pressure rises to this level.

Wound infection with meningitis and ventriculitis is a serious complication. If infection occurs, the chances of mental retardation are significantly increased.[24] If any question of infection exists, spinal fluid should be obtained and proved to be sterile before consideration is given to placement of a shunt. No intravenous punctures are made in the scalp before the insertion of the CSF shunt. This maximizes the cleanliness and sterility of the potential surgical site. Casting of any orthopedic foot deformities is delayed until the back wound is healed and the neonate is being nursed and handled in the usual manner. If hydrocephalus does not develop, the patient is usually discharged 10 to 14 days after the spinal surgery. If a shunt does prove necessary, discharge is delayed for an additional 7 to 10 days. Prior to discharge, measurement of somatosensory evoked responses or an EMG (or both) is repeated to act as a further baseline for follow-up examination.

Prognosis. Recent long-term follow-up studies of aggressively treated myelodysplastics indicate that the majority (60% to 90%) will be alive by age 7 years. Those who are intellectually normal continue to do well, whereas those who are subnormal appear to die at an accelerated rate.[44] The cause of death within the first 6 months is predominantly central nervous system infection and progressive hydrocephalus. After 6 months of age, chronic urinary tract infection, renal failure, and complications from shunt therapy are the primary causes of death. The outlook for these children is currently much brighter than in the past, and there is cause for guarded optimism as the therapy for this condition continues to improve.

Important aspects of follow-up. Follow-up of a myelomeningocele patient must be frequent and extensive. It is fair to say that the initial repair is the beginning of a close association between surgeon, patient, and family. To facilitate interdisciplinary consultation, a multispecialty clinic can streamline and improve the patient's care.

From the neurologic standpoint, during the first 6 to 12 months after early repair of a myelomeningocele, the primary problem is maintenance of normal ventricular pressure. Since the majority of these infants have already had a ventriculoperitoneal shunt placed, it is important to ensure the continued function of the shunt. Anterior fontanelle tension and head circumference are monitored; and when questions arise, a repeat CT brain scan or ultrasound examination is performed. Those patients who have not required immediate shunting following the myelomeningocele repair should be watched with special regard to the development of hydrocephalus. Their follow-up, as with the shunted patients, includes physical examination for the assessment of intracranial hypertension and regularly scheduled CT brain scans or ultrasound studies of the head to determine ventricular size.

There may be further deterioration of neurologic function of the lower extremities. With worsening of the motor or sensory examination in the lower extremities, reinvestigation of the spinal lesion is indicated. Associated spinal anomalies not previously diagnosed, including diastematomyelia or syringomyelia, may be responsible.[4,11,19,21] Development of a spastic paraparesis, with stretching of the corticospinal fibers serving leg function, may be secondary to unrecognized hydrocephalus. These fibers pass the greatest distance over the expanded lateral ventricles and tend to be selectively involved with severe hydrocephalus. The development of respiratory stridor not associated with acute inflammation of the respiratory tract is a particularly difficult development.[6,16,22] In its early stages this syndrome consists of respiratory stridor, loss of gag reflex, poor feeding, and frequent aspiration, which can be quickly followed by respiratory embarrassment and death within hours. These symptoms are believed to occur primarily as a response to medullary compression by the caudally displaced cerebellar vermis in the type II Chiari malformation. The syndrome is currently managed by posterior fossa decompression and cervical laminectomy to the level of the most caudally displaced cerebellar tissue. A dural graft is then sewn into place to further decompress the neural structures. Results in advanced cases are poor, but if the syndrome is recognized early and treated aggressively, full recovery of medullary function can be seen.

The emotional outlay of the parents of a child with myelodysplasia is enormous. Constant encouragement is helpful and necessary for them.

Genetic counseling is an important aspect of follow-up. Subsequent siblings of the patient have approximately a twenty-five–fold increase in the incidence of neural tube closure deficits (myelomeningocele, encephalocele, or anencephaly).[26] In recent years this fact has taken on more importance, since alphafetoprotein has been shown to be an effective maternal serum marker for the presence of a fetus with an open dysrhaphic syndrome. Maternal screening of serum-alphafetoprotein between the sixteenth and twentieth weeks of gestation combined with ultrasound examination of the fetus can now accurately identify more than 80% of women who will eventually deliver an affected fetus.[15,20] If these mothers then have amniocentesis with substantiation of elevated levels of alphafetoprotein in the amniotic fluid, therapeutic abortion can be discussed. In those cases where the fetus is known to have a repairable defect and abortion is not desired, the mother should have the delivery performed in a hospital where immediate repair can be accomplished.

Other, less common lesions. If the cystic leptomeningeal outpouching contains no nervous tissue, the lesion is known as a meningocele. Characteristically, these infants are neurologically intact and associated neurologic abnormalities are unusual. Repair of meningoceles is similar to that of myelomeningoceles. The prognosis is excellent, and follow-up may be much less extensive. Meningoceles may also project anteriorly or laterally through the spine and sacrum and present as cystic swellings in the posterior mediastinum or pelvis.[52]

VASCULAR DISORDERS; TRAUMA

The discussions on vascular disorders and trauma, including problems ranging from birth through the teenage years, are included in Chapter 27 in the section on the teenager.

REFERENCES

1. Anderson, B., and Woodhall, B.: Visual loss in primary skull deformities, Trans. Am. Acad. Ophthalmol. Otolaryngol. **57:**497, 1953.
2. Anderson, F. M., and Geiger, L.: Craniosynostosis: a survey of 204 cases, J. Neurosurg. **22:**229, 1965.
3. Barrow, N., and Simpson, S. A.: Cranium bifidum, investigation, prognosis and management, Aust. Paediatr. J. **2:**20, 1966.
4. Batnitzky, S., and others: Meningocele and syringohydromyelia, Radiology **120:**351, 1976.
5. Black, P. M.: Selective treatment of infants with myelomeningocele, Neurosurgery **5:**334, 1979.
6. Bluestone, C. D., Delerme, A. N., and Samuelson, G. H.: Airway obstruction due to vocal cord paralysis in infants with hydrocephalus and meningomyelocele, Ann. Otol. Rhinol. Laryngol. **81:**778, 1972.
7. Blyth, H., and Carter, C.: A guide to genetic prognosis in paediatrics, Dev. Med. Child Neurol. [Suppl.] **18:**14, 1969.
8. Brocklehurst, G.: The pathogenesis of spina bifida: a study of the relationship between observation, hypothesis, and surgical incentive, Dev. Med. Child Neurol. **13:**147, 1971.
9. Converse, J. M., and others: Craniofacial surgery, Clin. Plast. Surg. **1:**499, 1974.
10. Davis, G. H., Jr., and Alexander, E., Jr.: Congenital nasofrontal encephalomeningoceles and teratomas, J. Neurosurg. **16:**365, 1959.
11. Day, A. L., and others: Communicating hydromyelia, Surg. Neurol. **7:**157, 1977.
12. Duckworth, T., and others: Somatosensory evoked cortical responses in children with spinal bifida, Dev. Med. Child Neurol. **18:**19, 1976.
13. Edgerton, M. T., and others: The feasibility of craniofacial osteotomies in infants and young children, Scand. J. Plast. Reconstr. Surg. **8:**164, 1974.
14. Emery, J. L., and MacKenzie, N.: Medullo-cervical dislocation deformity (Chiari II deformity) related to neurospinal dysraphism (meningomyelocele), Brain **96:**155, 1973.
15. Ferguson-Smith, M. A., and others: Avoidance of anencephalic and spina bifida births by maternal serum-alphafetoprotein screening, Lancet **1:**1330, 1978.
16. Fitzsimmons, J. S.: Laryngeal stridor and respiratory obstruction associated with myelomeningocele, Dev. Med. Child Neurol. **15:**533, 1973.
17. Foltz, E. L., and others: Craniosynostosis, J. Neurosurg. **43:**48, 1975.
18. Forrest, D. M.: Spina bifida: some problems in management, Proc. R. Soc. Med. **70:**233, 1977.

19. Guthkelch, A. N.: Diastematomyelia with median septum, Brain **97:**729, 1974.
20. Haddow, J. E., and Macri, J. N.: Prenatal screening for neural tube defects, J.A.M.A. **242:**515, 1979.
21. Hall, P. V., and others: Meningomyelocele and progressive hydromyelia: progressive paresis in myelodysplasia, J. Neurosurg. **43:**457, 1975.
22. Hoffman, H. J., Hendrick, E. B., and Humphreys, R. P.: Manifestations and management of Arnold-Chiari malformation in patients with myelomeningocele, Child's Brain **1:**255, 1975.
23. Hoffman, H. J., and Mohr, G.: Lateral canthal advancement of the supraorbital margin, J. Neurosurg. **45:**376, 1976.
24. Hunt, I. M., and Holmes, A. E.: Factors relating to intelligence in treated cases of spina bifida cystica, Am. J. Dis. Child. **130:**823, 1976.
25. Lorber, J.: Systematic ventriculographic studies in infants born with meningomyelocele and encephalocele: the incidence and development of hydrocephalus, Arch. Dis. Child. **36:**381, 1961.
26. Lorber, J.: The family history of spina bifida cystica, Pediatrics **35:**589, 1965.
27. Lorber, J.: The prognosis of occipital encephalocele, Dev. Med. Child Neurol. [Suppl.] **13:**75, 1966.
28. Lorber, J.: Ethical problems in the management of myelomeningocele and hydrocephalus, J. R. Coll. Physicians Lond. **10:**47, 1975.
29. Marin-Padilla, M.: Clinical and experimental rachischisis. In Vinken, P. J., and Bruyn, G. W., editors: Handbook of clinical neurology. Vol. 32. Congenital malformations of the spine and spinal cord, Amsterdam, 1978, North Holland Publishing Co.
30. Matson, D. D.: Neurosurgery of infancy and childhood, ed. 2, Springfield, Ill., 1969, Charles C Thomas, Publisher.
31. Matthews, D. N.: Experiences in major craniofacial surgery, Plast. Reconstr. Surg. **59:**163, 1977.
32. McLaurin, R. L.: Parietal cephaloceles, Neurology **14:**764, 1974.
33. McLaurin, R. L., and Matson, D. D.: Importance of early surgical treatment of craniosynostosis, Pediatrics **10:**637, 1952.
34. Mealey, J., Jr., Dzenitis, A. J., and Hockey, A. A.: The prognosis of encephaloceles, J. Neurosurg. **32:**209, 1970.
35. Milhorat, T. H.: Pediatric neurosurgery, Philadelphia, 1978, F. A. Davis Co.
36. Moss, M. L.: Functional anatomy of cranial synostosis, Child's Brain **1:**22, 1975.
37. Munro, I. R.: Orbito-cranio-facial surgery: the team approach, Plast. Reconstr. Surg. **55:**170, 1975.
38. Odake, G., Yamaki, T., and Naruse, S.: Neurenteric cyst with meningomyelocele, J. Neurosurg. **45:**352, 1976.
39. Peach, B.: The Arnold-Chiari malformation, Arch. Neurol. **12:**613, 1965.
40. Pollock, J. A., Newton, T. H., and Hoyt, W. F.: Transsphenoidal and transethmoidal encephaloceles, Radiology **90:**442, 1968.
41. Reigel, D. H., and others: Intra-operative evoked potential studies of newborn infants with myelomeningocele, Dev. Med. Child Neurol. [Suppl.] **37:**42, 1976.
42. Seeger, J. F., and Gabrielsen, T. O.: Premature closure of the frontosphenoidal suture in synostosis of the coronal suture, Radiology **101:**631, 1971.
43. Shillito, J., and Matson, D. D.: Craniosynostosis: a review of 519 surgical patients, Pediatrics **41:**829, 1968.
44. Shurtleff, D. V., and others: Myelodysplasia: decision for death or disability, N. Engl. J. Med. **291:**1105, 1974.
45. The spinal cord in spina bifida (editorial): Lancet **2:**830, 1973.
46. Stark, G. D., and Drummond, M.: The spinal cord lesion in myelomeningocele, Dev. Med. Child. Neurol. [Suppl.] **25:**1, 1971.
47. Suwanwela, C., and Hongsaprabhas, C.: Fronto-ethmoidal encephalomeningocele, J. Neurosurg. **25:**172, 1966.
48. Tessier, P.: Relationship of craniostenoses to craniofacial dysostoses, and to faciostenoses, Plast. Reconstr. Surg. **48:**224, 1971.
49. Tessier, P.: Experiences in the treatment of orbital hypertelorism, Plast. Reconstr. Surg. **53:**1, 1974.
50. Tibbs, P. A., and others: Midline hamartomas masquerading as meningomyeloceles or teratomas in the newborn infant, J. Pediatr. **89:**928, 1979.
51. Whatmore, W. J.: Sincipital encephalomeningoceles, Br. J. Surg. **60:**261, 1973.
52. Wilkins, R. H., and Odom, G. L.: Anterior and lateral spinal meningoceles. In Vinken, P. J., and Bruyn, G. W., editors: Handbook of clinical neurology, vol. 32, Amsterdam, 1978, North Holland Publishing Co.

CHAPTER 13

Orthopedic considerations

ROBERT J. RUDERMAN and PETER W. WHITFIELD

GENERAL CONSIDERATIONS

The management of neonatal musculoskeletal disease is based on a simple precept: early recognition of physical impairment and prompt institution of treatment afford the best opportunity for correcting congenital abnormalities or lessening the degree of disability. Yet, the matter is complicated by several seeming contradictions. On the one hand, the most obvious and dramatic of identifiable defects may be of little early significance; indeed, these defects may be perfectly compatible with long-term survival, good general health, and even excellent function. On the other hand, an obvious structural defect may herald a covert syndrome or association of abnormalities that is of life-threatening proportions.

Defects of morphogenesis

Defects of morphogenesis occur in as many as 1 in 20 newborns.[4] Approximately 40% of these defects may be considered deformities; that is, abnormalities that are produced by fetal constraint that aberrantly molds otherwise normal tissue. They may range from variations in "attitude," which are easily correctable by passive manipulation, to contracture deformities, which may fail to respond to passive manipulation and will require casting or surgical correction. Sixty percent of identifiable defects are true malformations of genetic or teratologic origin. These anomalies result from intrinsic problems in developing embryonic tissue and as a rule will not respond to passive manipulation or subsequent attempts at molding. They may be very difficult to treat functionally and cosmetically. Recognizing this distinction between deformity and malformation is essential in appreciating which of the abnormalities identified in the newborn nursery demand immediate attention and referral and provides a basis for understanding prognosis and treatment.

The common denominator in all forms of neonatal deformation is probably fetal constraint (Fig. 13-1). This constraint has three possible causes: (1) uterine compression, which might result from increased tone, a large fetus, or oligohydramnios; (2) intrauterine compression, as with multiple fetuses, bicornuate uterus, or uterine fibroids; or (3) extrauterine compression from elevation of abdominal tone, excessive lumbar lordosis, or a small pelvis. The orthopedic evaluation thus begins with a review of the antenatal history, since certain patterns of deformation can be predicted in particular clinical situations. One example of a predictable pattern of deformation is the well-known oligohydramnios tetrad of diminished size for gestational age, compressed face, limb deformity, and lung hypoplasia; another is the fourteenfold increase in the incidence of congenital dislocation of the hip and genu recurvatum or dislocation known to be associated with the breech position.

EXAMINATION

In order for the physician to cope with the above complexities, it is mandatory that an orderly and thorough musculoskeletal examination be per-

We would like to acknowledge Mrs. Dee Staples for her assistance in preparation of the manuscript for the four orthopedic chapters in this text; Judith G. Ruderman, Ph.D., for her editorial assistance; and Herman Grossman, M.D., and the Pediatric Radiology staff at Duke University Medical Center for their kindness in allowing us to utilize their excellent pediatric radiology teaching collection, from which many of our case examples are drawn.

166

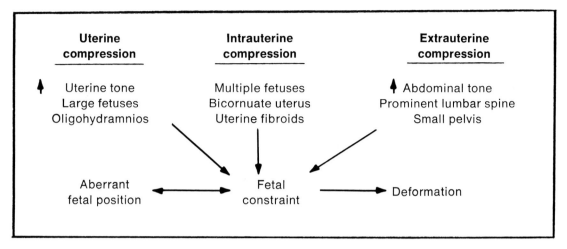

Fig. 13-1. Fetal constraint seems to be the central feature of most forms of neonatal deformation. (Adapted from Clarren, S. K., and Smith, D. W.: Pediatr. Clin. North Am. **24:**666, 1977.)

formed on every newborn child and be repeated on multiple subsequent occasions.

A thorough orthopedic examination can easily be integrated into the routine newborn evaluation and requires no special equipment. As background, one should be familiar with the normal developmental sequence and remember such details as the fact that the spine does not assume its normal adult configuration until the upright posture is achieved later in life. Normal cervical lordosis does not occur until the child can hold his head up; and lumbar lordosis does not appear until sitting and, subsequently, standing are mastered. In addition, the normal development of axial rotation of the limbs during fetal development within the confines of intrauterine life accounts for shapes and ranges of motion of the extremities that are unique for this period of life.

The physical examination[20] begins, as always, with observation, in this case, of the unclothed, warm infant during both rest and activity. Crude reflex activity may be misinterpreted as active muscle power if the movement is observed during physical stimulation by the examiner. The physician should then fold the infant into the position of greatest comfort, which is the uterine position. This maneuver has a marked tranquilizing effect and is of particular use in beginning the examination of a crying child. Also, it yields insight regarding the origin of deformations and provides an expectation of what position and range of motion can be considered normal for this individual infant. The child is observed for failure of movement, swelling, obvious pain, redness, and local warmth, any of which might suggest paralysis, birth injury, pyarthrosis, or osteomyelitis. All skin folds must be inspected carefully, and it should be determined that the skin will move freely over underlying tissue. Constriction bands may be hidden in an obese child.

With the child supine, the *neck, chest,* and *shoulders* are examined. The infant's lack of head control makes visualization of the neck easy despite the overlap of fatty chin folds and the chest. The examiner's hand is placed behind the back, and the infant's head is allowed to fall gently back into extension, making the shoulders and thorax prominent. The neck is inspected for asymmetry, webbing, torticollis, and for the short neck of the Klippel-Feil syndrome. However, congenital fibromuscular torticollis may not be apparent on the initial examination. It is not at all unusual for the newborn to have a normal range of motion, with the classic tender, olive-shaped mass not appearing until the fourth to eight week of life. It is useful to extend the head rapidly enough to elicit a startle response. The resultant thrashing of the arms will give information as to the state of muscle control of the upper extremities. Lack of motion may mean fracture, infection, or paralysis.

The *chest, clavicle, neck,* and *shoulders* are then palpated in order and the range of motion for each part tested. The neck should be rotated and flexed from side to side as well as carried through flexion and extension. Range of motion of the shoulders is tested by allowing the infant to grasp a finger and then carrying the arm through internal and external rotation. One wants to feel equal resistance to motion in either direction. Absence of this resistance, particularly as one brings the arm into internal rotation, may be the only evidence of paralysis or pain (in this instance, weakness of the external rotators of the humerus) and will help to establish the diagnosis of birth injury or infection. The physician then examines the remainder of the upper extremity, inspecting and palpating each part and joint individually in the search for swelling or deformity. Comparison of one side with the other is made so that hypoplasia or hyperplasia is detected. Traumatic dislocation of the shoulder or elbow is rare in the newborn, and gross deformity may well represent epiphyseal separation.

The *elbow* is often flexed in the fetal position, and the normal newborn elbow will not fully extend for several weeks. Persistent limitation suggests joint deformity, and one should suspect arthrogryposis. If swelling and deformity occur, one must remember that dislocation is rare. Crepitation may indicate a fracture through the epiphysis, and the presence of warmth may be the only evidence of infection.

The *forearm* is a common site for gross deformities or limb deficiencies. In addition to palpating both bones of the forearm, one needs to test the range of pronation and supination; limitation of rotation suggests radial-ulnar synostosis. The frequency of occurrence of this abnormality in Klinefelter's syndrome needs to be remembered.

The *hand* is one of the most commonly affected areas for isolated abnormalities as well as for syndrome components. *Digits* obviously have to be counted. Malpositions and particularly overlap of the digits may indicate an associated chromosomal trisomy or other variation. Contractures such as clinodactyly (lateral curvature, commonly of the fifth digit) or camptodactyly (flexion contracture at the proximal interphalangeal [PIP] and metacarpophalangeal [MP] joints) should be observed. The *thumb* at birth is normally held flexed into the palm; active extension should be observed during the Moro response, and the thumb should be checked for full passive extension. Like torticollis, congenital trigger thumb often presents later in infancy.

The child is now turned prone onto the examiner's hands, and the *hips* and *spine* are allowed to relax and flex. The dorsum of the infant is examined for symmetry and gross contour. As the child is lifted, his attempts at spinal extension and hip extension with kicking will help exclude pyarthrosis, birth injury, or paralysis. The back is inspected for dimples, folds, hairy patches, and fatty masses, all of which may be clues to occult spinal dysraphism. The buttocks, groin, and gluteal areas are inspected for contour and symmetry of subcutaneous folds. Deeper or more numerous folds may indicate shortening of the thigh and upward dislocation of the hip; absent folds may suggest genetic abnormality. However, minor asymmetries are quite common in the normal child and are, therefore, the least reliable sign of congenital hip dislocation (CDH). With the child in this position, the ischial tuberosities are palpated and the relationship of the greater tuberosity of the femur determined in relation to them: one is seeking apparent shortening of the femur. The buttocks are palpated for prominences in the posterior acetabular region.

The child is again turned supine and similar inspection accomplished in the groin and peri-

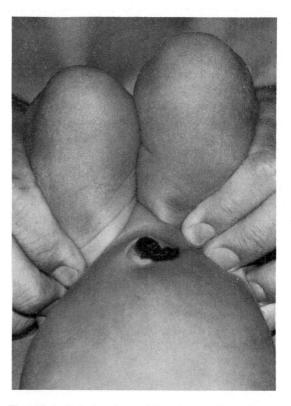

Fig. 13-2. Relative femoral length may be estimated by Galeazzi's or Allis' sign. In CDH, the proximal femur on the affected side is posterior and superior to the acetabulum. The affected leg appears short.

neum. In the average infant, the fatty thighs will obscure the perineum when the legs are extended and at neutral abduction. Any asymmetry or widening of the perineum or apparent deepening of the groin cleft may indicate upward and outward displacement of one or both hips.

The child is turned toward the side. The level of the trochanter, which should fall below an imaginary line drawn between the anterosuperior iliac spine and the ischial tuberosity, is determined. A more cephalad position of the trochanter may indicate CDH or coxa vara. This portion of the examination should be accomplished on a firm surface, because the child's hips and knees are then flexed to 90 degrees and the level of the knee

observed for Galeazzi's or Allis' sign (Fig. 13-2). The knees should be at the same level; shortening may mean limb length discrepancy or upward displacement of the hip.

One then tests the range of motion of the hips. Flexion contracture is normal in the newborn for several weeks, and absence of this contracture may be an important indicator of CDH. Although relative limitation of abduction may represent nothing more than the result of intrauterine position, it is also one of the most significant indicators of CDH. If the other clinical findings are not present, careful reexamination is imperative.

At this point, one performs the Ortolani and Barlow tests of hip stability. These tests are de-

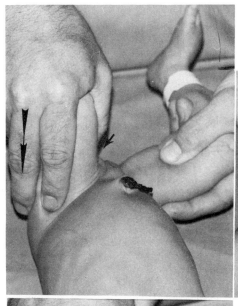
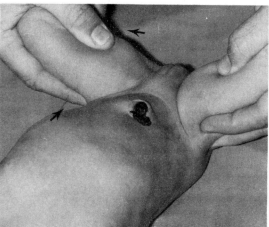
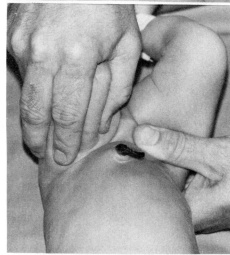

Fig. 13-3. Tests of hip stability. In the Barlow maneuver (**A**) instability is demonstrated by dislocating the hip. While the pelvis is stabilized with the opposite hand, the thigh is abducted and gentle pressure is exerted posteriorly. The femoral head may be felt to slip out of the acetabulum. One may then relocate the joint, using the Ortolani maneuver (**B**). The abducted thigh is gently lifted forward as the long finger applies pressure over the greater trochanter. As the femoral head is guided over the limbus of the acetabulum, relocation is felt but not heard. An alternative method of stabilizing the pelvis (**C**) is to place the fingers over the sacrum and the thumb on the pubic symphysis.

signed to provoke hip dislocation and then allow the examiner to palpate the dislocation and subsequent relocation (Fig. 13-3). Results of the tests are often positive only in "typical" CDH and are not necessarily positive in the teratologic hip. Even in the typical situation, positive results are usually confined to the newborn infant and may not persist beyond the first several weeks. At a later age, the absence of the Ortolani sensation of reduction does not indicate that a hip cannot be dislocated but that it may *be* dislocated and cannot be relocated!

One then proceeds to review the remainder of the lower extremities, seeking swelling, deformity, pain, and paralysis, in the same manner as with the upper extremities. At the *knees,* the presence and size of the patellas should be determined. Genu recurvatum and dislocation are a spectrum of abnormalities commonly seen in breech constraint with full knee extension. Deficiencies of one or another portion of the tibial or fibular side of the legs are common, and it should be recalled that fibular deficiencies or deficiencies of the lateral portion of the foot are commonly associated with such hip abnormalities as proximal femoral focal deficiency.

Bowing of the infant *tibia* is normal, and tibial torsion is commonly present though also commonly overdiagnosed. Strictly speaking, the term *tibial torsion* refers to the relationship of the bicondylar axis of the distal femur or the axis of flexion of the knee to the bimalleolar axis of the ankle. This relationship may be difficult to define.[24] One good indicator is the so-called thigh-foot angle (Fig. 13-4), which is measured with the infant prone and the knee flexed; one simply observes the long axis of the foot relative to the long axis of the thigh. Normally the bimalleolar axis or the long axis of the foot is rotated 20 degrees externally in relation to the proximal extremity. This relationship may be very easily miscalculated, and clinical significance should be attached only with caution.

The *foot* is the skeletal part most frequently affected by positional abnormalities. When examining the foot, one needs to examine the portions of the foot and their motion separately and in relationship to each other. The heel and hindfoot should be stabilized with the thumb and index finger of one hand while the forefoot and midfoot are manipulated with the opposite hand. The hindfoot should be at neutral and slight valgus. Motion

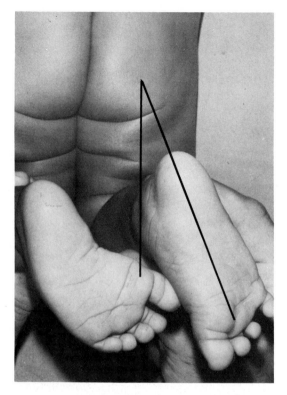

Fig. 13-4. Tibial torsion may be estimated by the angle formed by the intersection of the long axis of the foot and the long axis of the thigh.

of the fat pad of the heel in the pudgy infant foot may mask a fixed contracture of the ankle and lead to confusion of such a fixed abnormality as the true clubfoot with a more minor abnormality of the forefoot alone. It should be noted, as well, that all infants have "fat feet," not "flat feet." The fat pad over the abductor hallucis is always prominent in the infant and masks the normal longitudinal arch. In examining the motion of the forefoot, one observes the sole of the foot and bisects the heel along the long axis of the foot with a hypothetical line that should fall at the second toe or at the second interdigital web space. If the line falls more laterally than this, it is an indication of metatarsus adductus. Finally, the *digits* are inspected and variations noted, as with the hand. Overlapping of the toes is more common (from uterine constraint) than overlapping of the fingers but may also be an indicator of chromosomal abnormality. Even small abnormalities such as an overlapping fifth toe may be of later significance in shoeing and should be carefully evaluated and documented.

Skeletal evaluation. To this point, we have

emphasized focal abnormalities of the musculo-skeletal system as possible indicators of systemic abnormalities. The converse holds true as well. For example, the child with an imperforate anus or tracheoesophageal fistula needs careful evaluation for a spinal abnormality (VATER complex). As each individual part is inspected and examined, the overall configuration and symmetry of the skeleton and body must be considered.

Skeletal dysplasias are rare entities and are difficult to delineate, but accurate diagnosis is exceedingly important if one is to identify hidden defects and provide an accurate prognosis of physical and intellectual function and appropriate genetic counseling. In most instances the practitioner must rely on the variety of atlases and compendiums[3] available for the identification of syndromes as well as on referral to a birth defect center for identification and subsequent treatment. However, several simple measures can be performed during the routine examination that will help categorize the abnormalities.[8] After establishing the age of onset, associated abnormalities, and family history, one should pay attention to the head circumference, which will be enlarged in a number of conditions. The most notable of these is *achondroplasia,* which is the most common form of short-limb dwarfism. The head circumference is normal in several other syndromes, such as *spondyloepiphyseal dysplasia congenita,* that are commonly mistaken for achondroplasia. The chest circumference should be measured as well, since a diminished measurement will suggest *asphyxiating thoracic dysplasia* or one of the other skeletal dysplasias that are associated with severe respiratory distress and limited survival. Measurement of the lower body segment is useful until the child is almost 10 years of age; however, the head and trunk are disproportionately large in relationship to the lower extremities.

Another measure of the relative length of the limbs and trunk may be obtained by measuring the so called AF/AT ratio. The distance from the anterosuperior iliac spine to the tibial tuberosity is the AT distance, and the distance from the anterosuperior iliac spine to the tip of the long finger with the arm extended and held at the thigh is the AF distance. The normal ratio for all age groups is between 0.4 and 0.65; in infancy this ratio is in the lower ranges with the number increasing with age as the lower extremities increase in relative length. If the limbs are

relatively short, the arm will not extend a normal length down the thigh, and this ratio will be decreased; it might, for example, be as low as 0.3 in achondroplasia. In the short-trunk dwarfing syndromes, the ratio is increased.

These simple measures will allow one to group the abnormality and proceed with more detailed investigation of one of the many dysplastic syndromes. The reader is referred to Feingold's article "Clinical Evaluation of the Child with Skeletal Dysplasia,"[8] for tables that will help categorize this information, as well as to Goldberg's article, "Orthopaedic Aspects of Bone Dysplasias."[9] Despite the complexity of the classification of these disorders and the pleomorphic expression of these conditions, in the well-defined skeletal dysplasias, the site and nature of the orthopedic abnormalities are reasonably constant.

SPECIFIC ORTHOPEDIC ABNORMALITIES
Brachial plexus palsy

Most authors indicate that the incidence of brachial plexus stretch injury is decreasing as obstetric practice improves; but when careful examination is carried out in the newborn nursery, many more minor or transient instances of this injury are noted than are usually reported in major series. The mechanism of injury is traction that forcefully distracts the head and neck from the shoulder girdle and upper extremity. The infants involved are often larger than average and the delivery difficult. Forced lateral flexion of the head and neck seems to be the particularly harmful maneuver and can occur in both vertex and breech deliveries.[2]

The injuries are most commonly classified according to the components of the brachial plexus involved. The C5-6 lesion (Erb-Duchenne) involves paralysis of the shoulder abductors, external rotators, the elbow flexors, and perhaps the supinator. Sensory deficit is usually limited to the upper outer arm. The C8-T1 (Klumpke) lesion is characterized by loss of the wrist and finger flexors and intrinsic musculature of the hand. Sympathetic denervation with concomitant Horner's syndrome may occur. Sensation is often normal in this condition. The mixed lesion has multiple components and often total paralysis and extensive sensory loss of the entire upper extremity.

In addition to the above anatomic classification, a neurophysiologic classification based on the extent of the lesion can be made, as with any other nerve injury. Where the injury is mild, without disruption of the continuity of the nerve and without axonal death, complete recovery can be anticipated in a relatively short period of time. In a moderate lesion, the nerve remains in continuity but significant intraneural hemorrhage and edema occur, axonal disruption takes place, and axonal death occurs. Significant intraneural fibrosis may result. Recovery depends on axonal regrowth over the entire length of the nerve, and recovery of function will be slow and often incomplete, particularly in the more distally innervated muscles. In severe lesions with complete disruption of the nerve trunk, prognosis is poor, particularly if the disruption takes place at the level of the neural foramen, with avulsion of the nerve trunk from the spinal cord itself.

Examination and clinical findings. The arm is held motionless at the side with the elbow extended and the entire extremity internally rotated (Fig. 13-5). The forearm will usually be pronated and the wrist flexed. During a Moro response, the affected arm fails to respond. If the lower nerve roots are involved, the grasp reflex will be lost. Horner's sign, characterized by enophthalmus, myosis, and ptosis, may be seen and indicates a poor prognosis. If the lesion is quite proximal and nerve roots have been avulsed directly from the cord, transient hematomyelia may occur, with the weakness and hyperreflexia of upper motor neural lesions occurring in the other extremities. This condition is usually transient. There may be tenderness and swelling about the shoulder or in the supraclavicular region, complicating the differential diagnosis, which includes fractured clavicle, separation of the upper humeral epiphysis, and fracture of the humeral shaft, all of which may coexist with a brachial plexus injury. Infection must be ruled out. Usually, infection develops over several days rather than being present immediately following birth.

Referral. Where pediatric orthopedic consultation is readily available, it should be obtained immediately. The majority of these lesions will resolve during the first 72 hours. If recovery is not evident by this time, referral is indicated and becomes mandatory when paresis persists beyond 6 weeks. The neurologic examination is highly subjective, and failure to obtain early consultation deprives the consulting specialist of the op-

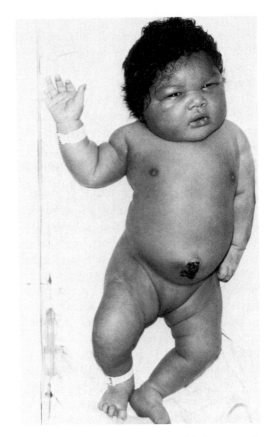

Fig. 13-5. Brachial plexus injury. This large newborn daughter of a diabetic mother had a difficult delivery. The affected arm is held at the side, the elbow is extended, and the arm is internally rotated.

portunity to form a longitudinal impression of the condition and makes it difficult for this person to formulate an accurate prognosis and treatment plan.

Treatment. The initial treatment is directed at making the child comfortable and maintaining range of motion. The importance of avoiding fixed contractures, if possible, cannot be overemphasized; but often, over the course of months and years, these are inevitable. The common practice of pinning the extremity to the bed sheet in the abducted and externally rotated position may prove dangerous if the infant struggles against the fixed position or if the child is lifted inadvertently. Rigid orthoses are difficult to maintain and are probably unnecessary in the newborn period, where range of motion exercises can be accomplished by the parent with each diaper change. If contracture is seen to be developing, splinting should be initiated and the splint removed three or four times a day for range of motion exercises.

Prognosis. Most lesions that are going to recover will probably do so within the first 3 to 6 months. These lesions probably constitute the majority of injuries when one takes into account those that are so mild that they are often missed. Resolution of more severe cases may continue over a period of as long as 18 months to 2 years[29]; this is not a matter of further recovery, however, but one of the strengthening of intact musculature with time. Little can be done to affect the neurologic recovery. To date, attempts at surgical repair have not been successful. If no recovery is evident, even in the more proximal muscles, by 1 year, the lesion can be considered permanent.

Important aspects of follow-up: late surgical correction. Recent improvements in neurologic surgery, primarily the application of microsurgical techniques and increasing success with nerve grafting, have led many authors to reconsider surgical treatment of brachial plexus lesions in the older population (To date, no significant series has been reported in newborn infants.)

Late treatment of brachial plexus palsies is directed at releasing contracture and regaining range of motion. In the most common form of this condition—a lesion of the upper trunk, or Erb's palsy—the major deformity will be internal rotation and adduction contracture. In this instance, reconstructive procedures may be undertaken with the child as young as 18 months of age or, more commonly, around 3 years of age. The longer these procedures are delayed, the more likely it is that secondary osseous changes will result.[12] In the older patient (Fig. 13-6), osteotomies of the humerus or forearm bones may be necessary. If significant weakness of the deltoid muscle exists, transfers can be performed to provide abduction. The postoperative management consists of casting in the corrected position for a period of 3 to 6 weeks, followed by slow and gentle resumption of range of motion until healing has completely ensued. Splinting will need to be maintained for as long as 3 months while range of motion is regained under careful supervision by the physical therapist. Night splinting should probably be continued for at least 6 to 12 months, or indefinitely if the tendency to contracture persists.

With spotty or more distal involvement, the surgical procedure will vary with the specific deformity. In general, the same pattern holds: lengthening of contracted musculature and transfer of functioning musculature in an attempt to balance

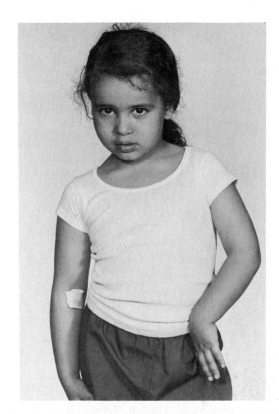

Fig. 13-6. Brachial plexus injury. In the untreated child, the typical posture persists: the arm is internally rotated, the forearm pronated, and the wrist flexed.

strength about the affected joint. A similar postoperative regimen should be followed.

Although a large number of patients who have never been treated are now leading normal lives, they still experience a certain cosmetic and functional loss. There is really no excuse for nontreatment.

Congenital constriction bands (Streeter's dysplasia)

Circular grooves and constriction bands can occur anywhere along the extremity and occasionally will involve the trunk.[13] They will range from shallow grooves that are of little clinical significance to severe constriction that results in autoamputation in utero (Fig. 13-7). Multiple bands are not uncommonly present with this form of dysplasia, and multiple absent digits or partial amputations can also occur. These constrictions are almost certainly not the result of amniotic bands but are probably some form of primary defect in embryogenesis. There is no hereditary or genetic component.

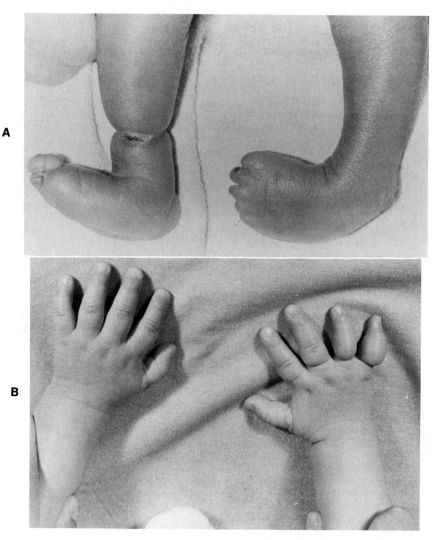

Fig. 13-7. Streeter's dysplasia. **A,** Severe involvement in the newborn has led to autoamputation of multiple toes. **B,** In this child the bands of the index and long finger of the right hand are minor, but the edema and swelling of the ring and little fingers are evident.

Treatment. The treatment will vary with the degree of severity. Milder grooves can be followed until the child is between 6 months and 2 years of age, when treatment is made easier by growth of the neurovascular structures. These grooves are generally managed with staged Z-plasties down to normal tissue. In general, circumferential repair is necessary; but for purposes of safety, only 180 degrees of the arc will be managed on any one occasion. In more severe instances, where circulatory embarrassment of the distal segment is evident, the procedure may be emergent and performed in the immediate neonatal period. Despite adherence of the constricting groove to the periosteum, often the neurovascular structures are not involved, so that function of the distal part can be preserved. Where autoamputation has occurred, syndactyly of the most acral portions of the remaining digits—generally involving only the skin—is often seen. Small bridges may be separated by ligation with a suture in the newborn nursery, but more extensive procedures may be required in subsequent months.

Congenital dislocation of the hip[5]

Many think of CDH as the quintessential pediatric orthopedic problem of the newborn, occurring in 1 or 2 of every 1,000 births. Early diagnosis and treatment lead to excellent results, but detection on the newborn exam can be difficult. If the diagnosis is missed, significant disability will result.

There are at least two main types of congenital dislocation. Those associated with multiple congenital anomalies, systemic abnormalities, or neuromuscular disease are referred to as *teratologic*. When they are associated with neuromuscular difficulties, these dislocations may be easy to locate but maintaining reduction may be difficult. In other conditions, such as arthrogryposis, the dislocation occurs before birth, and contracture and secondary structural abnormality have already developed. Thus, the usual signs of hip instability in the newborn are absent, and the hip cannot be located. The physical findings are those usually associated with congenital dislocated hip in later infancy and early childhood. By and large, teratologic hips are not responsive to nonsurgical measures; they require early referral and will be complex, long-term orthopedic problems.

The majority of dislocated hips fall into the category referred to as *typical*. This category includes several variations: (1) the so-called dysplastic hip, in which dislocation is not known to have occurred, but in which abnormal development of the acetabulum occurs secondarily; (2) lax and unstable subluxed hips; (3) hips that are dislocatable with provocative maneuvers; and (4) hips that are identified initially in the dislocated position.

A variety of genetic and environmental determinants have been identified as being important in the etiology of CDH. There is a clear family predisposition, and the recurrence risk is approximately 3% to 5% in subsequent siblings. In addition, the frequency is much higher in female infants, a fact that may relate to response to maternal hormonal variations. There is at least a fivefold increase in incidence in infants presenting in the breech position, whether or not they are actually delivered in that position. Careful screening of all newborns for CDH is mandatory, but attention to these high-risk factors will enable one to focus particularly on those most likely to be affected.

Evaluation. The emphasis is on early diagnosis. We have already discussed the examination of the newborn's hip, but several features need to be repeated and emphasized. The diagnosis of congenital dislocation in the newborn period is entirely clinical. The absence of ossification of the proximal femur and acetabular components and the frequently transient nature of the dislocation make radiographs highly unreliable in this period. The classic findings of femoral shortening, asymmetric skin creases, hip clicks, and limited abduction may all be misleading, and the examination in the newborn period may be entirely normal with the exception of the palpable sensation of relocating and dislocating the unstable hip. Once having experienced and identified this sensation, the examiner finds it to be rather distinctive; unfortunately, the individual practitioner who is unfamiliar with it may miss it.

Treatment. Once a diagnosis had been made, therapy should be instituted rapidly; taking a few days to confirm the diagnosis, however, will not be harmful. The newborn infant may have significant relative joint laxity for 3 to 10 days following birth, and there is no question that a certain number of dislocatable hips correct spontaneously, even in the absence of treatment. Of course, repeated dislocations of the hip for purposes of demonstrating the physical finding will, in and of themselves, make contracture and stabilization difficult and should be limited to those occasions that are definitely necessary.

The treatment consists of maintaining the hip in the abducted and flexed position, which can be accomplished in a variety of ways. Diapers have no real place in the management of true dislocation of the hip but are occasionally useful as a temporizing measure while an orthotic device is being obtained or in those few children in whom the examination itself is indeterminant. While heavy diapering may achieve wide abduction, the requisite flexion often is lacking.

Wide abduction in the frog leg position is usually not necessary to stabilize the hip. Extremes of position seem to impair blood supply to the capital femoral epiphysis. Furthermore, the widely abducted hip may continue to point in a direction superior to the acetabulum. Flexion is what allows the head and neck of the femur to align with the triradiate cartilage. If appropriate alignment can be maintained, reduction should be achieved and maintained.

A multitude of pillows, splints and devices have been utilized successfully (Fig. 13-8). The device we have found most useful is the Pavlik harness,[22] which not only maintains the desired position, but encourages spontaneous reduction and allows

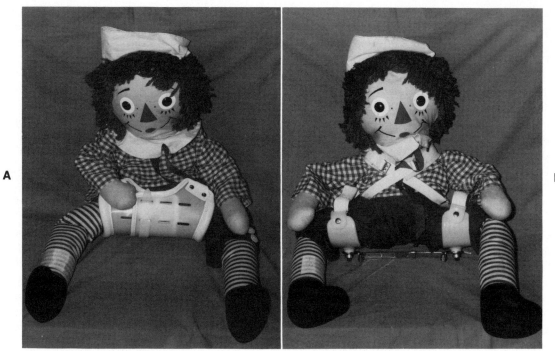

Fig. 13-8. Multiple devices are available for treating congenital dislocation of the hip. **A,** Modification of the Craig splint. **B,** Ilfeld splint.

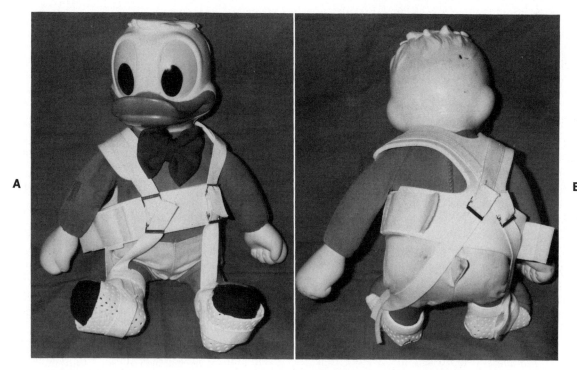

Fig. 13-9. Anterior **(A)** and posterior **(B)** views of the Pavlik harness. This device seems so simple that it could be utilized by anyone. Proper positioning, however, is necessary for this harness to be effective.

Treatment Scheme for CDH

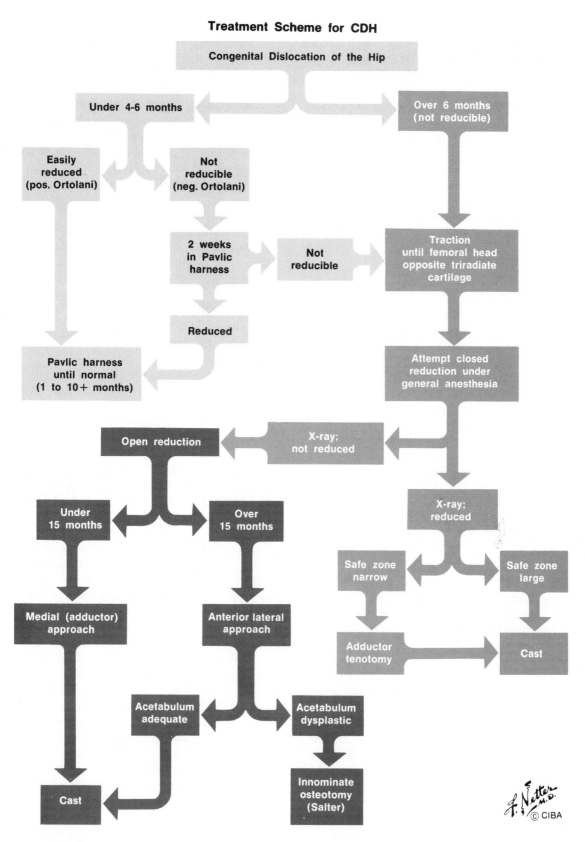

Fig. 13-10. Flow sheet for the management of CDH. (From Hensinger, R. N.: Clin. Symp. **31**(1): 30, 1979. © Copyright 1979 CIBA Pharmaceutical Co., Division of CIBA-GEIGY Corp. Reprinted with permission from Clinical Symposia, illustrated by Frank Netter, M.D. All rights reserved.)

physiologic movement of the hip. The harness can be fitted in the immediate neonatal period (Fig. 13-9). It consists of a shoulder and abdominal harness that serve as suspension and of leg stirrups that are connected to the abdominal harness by anterior and posterior belts. The posterior belts are adjusted to prevent full adduction of the hips and to encourage active abduction. This abduction will occur both in the prone position and by the normal muscular activity and force of gravity when the infant is supine. The anterior straps are adjusted to maintain the requisite flexion, which should be at least 90 degrees. Once the harness is applied, the position is checked radiographically.

The orthosis is worn full time. Reasonable hygiene without removal of the harness is possible. If the parents find hygiene difficult to manage, however, periodic bathing with the orthosis removed can be accomplished but should be performed only with specially trained medical personnel holding the hip in the reduced position. The hip may be reduced on the initial examination and simply maintained by the orthosis. Certain hips will not be reduced initially but should be reduced within the first 1 to 2 weeks of treatment with the Pavlik device. The hip is then maintained in the orthosis full time for at least 6 weeks, at which point periodic removal for bathing and dressing is allowable. Treatment, however, will probably be continued for approximately 3 months.

With this treatment protocol, more than 65% to 80% of all hips will be successfully reduced and stabilized. The vast majority of these will subsequently develop normally, but a small percentage may evidence inadequate development of the acetabulum in later life. For this reason, continued observation for at least several years may be necessary and some children will require secondary reconstructive hip procedures.

The apparent simplicity of the initial forms of treatment should not imply that they should be undertaken by the average practitioner. When misapplied, these devices can be harmful. The management of CDH in the early months of life is a continual decision-making process in which the treatment modalities need to be adjusted at each of several stages (Fig. 13-10). Reasonable experience will be required to achieve consistently good results, and even many orthopaedists will recommend referral to a pediatric orthopaedic center at this stage.

In those few children in whom satisfactory reduction is not accomplished, manipulative reduction with the patient under general anesthesia is the next step. In order to facilitate reduction and to reduce the incidence of avascular necrosis, a period of prereduction traction is required. Skin traction is utilized in the newborn period, but occasionally skeletal traction through a distal femoral or proximal tibial pin is required. Either technique requires hospitalization; only in very special circumstances can it be accomplished at home. Use of a body cast or special frame against which traction can be applied may be necessary. The traction period will vary from a few days to as long as 2 to 3 weeks. Traction is maintained until the femoral head can be brought distally at least opposite and often below the acetabular level. Adduction contracture will have been stretched out in the Pavlik harness or in traction; on occasion, however, persistent contracture requires surgical release.

Once it has been established that the femoral head can be brought easily opposite the acetabulum as a result of the preliminary use of either the Pavlik harness or traction, it is safe to proceed with attempted closed reduction. General anesthesia is required, so that the maneuver need not be forced and so that once reduction is obtained, a satisfactory cast can be applied (these results are impossible in an awake or agitated infant). If a manipulative reduction is accomplished, an arthrogram is performed in the operating room to establish that the reduction is complete and concentric. If reduction requires a forced or extreme position, or if the arthrogram suggests inadequate reduction, an open reduction is indicated. After closed reduction, redislocation can occur in the cast; but this occurrence suggests that the initial reduction was incomplete, unstable, or both.

Postoperatively, the child should be comfortable. Pain suggests possible impending vascular problems; and if pain occurs, the cast may need to be removed. Once reduced, the hips are maintained in plaster for a minimum period of 6 to 12 weeks. During the later stages of treatment, one may replace the cast with a Pavlik harness to maintain stability yet allow some motion. The potential problem of acetabular dysplasia still exists, but for the most part secondary procedures are not required.

In the child under the age of 6 to 9 months, closed techniques, if instituted early, will usually succeed. Nevertheless, some children will rapidly develop contracture about the hip or other anatomic factors will intervene, and open surgical reduction will be required. Surgery may be elected at the time of unsuccessful closed reduction.

Postoperative care. Most of the treatment of CDH in the newborn period can be accomplished on an ambulatory basis. Hospitalization, if required, may last anywhere from a few days to a few weeks, depending on the course of treatment elected and the success at each stage. Once the usual postoperative problems are surmounted, the particular problems of aftercare relate to management of the body cast. In an infant this usually means perineal hygiene. Before the child is discharged from the hospital, the parents should be instructed in routine cast care, careful inspection of visible portions of the skin for areas of irritation or breakdown, and the dangers of inserting any foreign objects or materials beneath the cast. Perineal hygiene is often facilitated by nursing the child on a suspended frame with a cutout hole, beneath which a bedpan can be placed. Use of plastic wrap about the edges of the cast will protect it from soiling. These casts cannot be changed without risks of redislocation, and parental cooperation is required.

Complications and follow-up. Long-term problems can develop, even with successful reduction. Avascular necrosis may require little or no therapy; but when it is severe, it can significantly compromise the result. Early, satisfactory reduction should ensure normal acetabular development; on occasion, however, later reconstructive procedures are necessary. Acetabular reconstruction is almost never performed in a child younger than the age of 18 months. As long as progress in acetabular development is observed, intervention may be delayed until the child reaches the age of 3 or 4 years.

Congenital limb deficiencies

Congenital limb deficiencies are discussed in more detail in Chapter 18 in the section on the infant and toddler because, in most instances, treatment is begun at that age. They are mentioned here because the limb deficiencies are, by and large, obvious abnormalities noted at birth. Three points should be made in the context of the newborn nursery:

1. There is a high association of visceral anomalies with many of the limb deficiencies; the primary care physician needs to be aware of the constellation of abnormalities so that careful medical evaluation can be undertaken and appropriate diagnostic and therapeutic measures instituted.
2. The long-term functional outcome in many of the partial deficiencies is reasonably predictable, and familiarity with this outcome will help provide the family with at least some prognostic guidelines.
3. While therapeutic measures for limb deficiencies are relatively unusual in the immediate newborn period, some of the distal abnormalities such as an associated clubfoot or vertical talus may require immediate care.

The long-term goal is to allow the child to pass through normal growth and developmental sequences. Thus, surgical attention to certain defects or prosthetic fitting should be accomplished far earlier than one might otherwise imagine. Early referral to a multidisciplinary pediatric amputee facility is mandatory.

Congenital trigger thumb

Trigger thumb is often unrecognized at birth because of the normal thumb-in-palm posture of the newborn child. In fact, it may not be recognized until the child is 18 to 36 months of age, when the parents will notice inability to extend the interphalangeal joint of the thumb during certain activities. If care is taken in the newborn examination to extend the thumb and interphalangeal joints passively to their full extent, this condition should be diagnosed at or shortly after birth. The disorder consists of fusiform swelling of the flexor pollicis longus in its fibro-osseous canal, which becomes too wide for the annular ligament at the metacarpal head. This nodular enlargement of the tendon can often be palpated at the base of the thumb but may be difficult to separate from the sesamoid bones.

Treatment. In a significant percentage of these children, the condition will either resolve spontaneously or will respond to manipulation or splinting. Surgical treatment should, therefore, be deferred until the child reaches the age of 3 to 6 months. The surgical procedure consists of a transverse incision at the base of the thumb, with a longitudinal incision of the annular ligament, which will then re-form in an elongated manner so that adequate room is allowed for full flexion and extension. The nodular swelling of the tendon is resolved with release of the constriction.

Permanent deformity of the articular or osseous

structures does not result unless surgical release is unduly delayed. In the absence of intraoperative problems, complete resolution with a normal functional result is anticipated. The operative exposure is limited, and the procedure can be performed easily in an ambulatory surgical facility.

Postoperative care. Motion is encouraged as soon as initial wound healing is accomplished. Postoperative care is minimal.

ABNORMALITIES OF THE FEET

In no other part of the musculoskeletal system are the effects of fetal constraint more evident and the need for distinction between deformation and malformation more important than in the feet. The heel is normally in neutral, and most newborn children can dorsiflex the feet to the anterior aspect of the tibia. Variations include increased or fixed plantar flexion, described as equinus; increased dorsiflexion, known as cal-

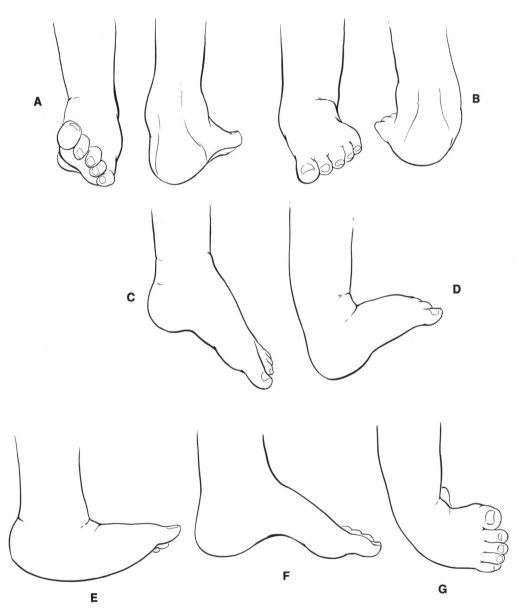

Fig. 13-11. Terminology of foot position and deformity. **A,** Varus. **B,** Valgus. **C,** Equinus. **D,** Calcaneus. **E,** Rocker bottom (congenital convex pes planus or vertical talus). **F,** Cavus. **G,** Clubfoot (congenital talipes equinovarus).

caneus; medial and lateral deviations from the midline, known as varus and valgus; and supination and pronation as they occur in the upper extremity. These terms are applied separately to the hindfoot, midfoot, and forefoot; using combinations of these descriptive terms, one can accurately relate the appearance of the foot (Fig. 13-11). All foot deformities are not "equinovarus," and all children with abnormal feet are not "clubfooted."

Metatarsus adductus (varus)

The most common congenital deformity of the foot is deviation of the forefoot at the level of the tarsometatarsal joints. Some authors distinguish between the purely adducted forefoot and the varus forefoot by the degree of inversion or supination, but this distinction seems artificial. The incidence of metatarsus adductus has been estimated to be 1 in 1,000 births, but it often seems to be more frequent. There is an increased incidence in siblings of affected infants (1 in 20 births). This genetic influence in a condition that is thought by most to be a purely positional deformity is not well understood, although, obviously, subsequent siblings have the same parental risk factors for fetal constraint.

In metatarsus adductus, the hindfoot is in neutral or valgus and the deviation takes place at the base of the metatarsals. There is a prominent fifth metatarsal and a convex lateral border of the foot. The medial border of the foot is concave, and in severe cases there may be a deep crease along the medial arch. The first ray may be the most widely deviated, and there is often a wide separation between the first and second toes. The degree of severity varies greatly. Some feet maintain this posture at rest but are highly flexible. These feet can be passively overcorrected when the hindfoot is stabilized, a finger is placed at the level of the cuboid behind the fifth metatarsal, and the foot is stressed laterally. Other feet are rigid and cannot be corrected, even to neutral. This deformity is distinguished from a true clubfoot by the absence of contracture in the hindfoot and midfoot; also, the talar head is well covered by the navicular bone, and a sinus tarsi is readily palpable. In metatarsus adductus, the hindfoot is normally aligned and mobile. Full dorsiflexion and plantar flexion at the ankle can be achieved (Fig. 13-12, *A*).

The same basic positional forces that produce internal tibial torsion and excessive rotation of the foot in relationship to the ankle produce metatarsus adductus. Thus, all these deformities often coexist, accentuating the clinical appearance of inturning and in-toeing.

The fact that there is no known increase in other organ abnormalities in this condition underlines the concept of metatarsus adductus as a positional deformity rather than a true limb bud malformation; there is, however, an increased incidence of congenital hip dysplasia. Every child under treatment for metatarsus adductus should have careful and repeated examination of the hip.

Treatment. The prognosis is excellent for the vast majority of children with metatarsus adductus, and correction can be achieved with relatively simple conservative measures. At least a fourth and perhaps as many as half of the affected children have mild, flexible deformities that are corrected either spontaneously or can be corrected with manipulation. Sleeping prone with the internally rotated lower extremities tucked beneath the child tends to perpetuate the deformity, and discouraging this position can be corrective in the mild case. For manipulations to be successful, the parents must be carefully instructed to stabilize the hindfoot with the thumb and index finger while stressing the forefoot into the correct position (Fig. 13-12, *B*). Otherwise, the tendency is to grasp the entire foot, which externally rotates the leg and has little effect on the site of deformity. The presence of a grandmother who has the time to spend in a rocking chair rubbing and manipulating baby's feet is a good prognostic sign!

Severe, rigid cases will not respond to simple measures, and a full course of cast correction is necessary. The pitfall here is to continue to observe the child for spontaneous correction while what is an initially mild to moderate deformity becomes more severe and increasingly resistant to correction. Ideally, treatment should be initiated in the newborn nursery but can be delayed for as long as 6 weeks, depending on the availability of referral sources and the parents' ability to cope with the situation.

When formal treatment of metatarsus adductus is initiated, it is in the form of a long leg cast, quite similar to that which is applied for clubfeet. The cast is carried above the flexed knee in order to control rotation and maintain corrective forces. The total period of casting will range from 3 weeks to 3 months, depending on the patient's age at the time of cast application and the severity of

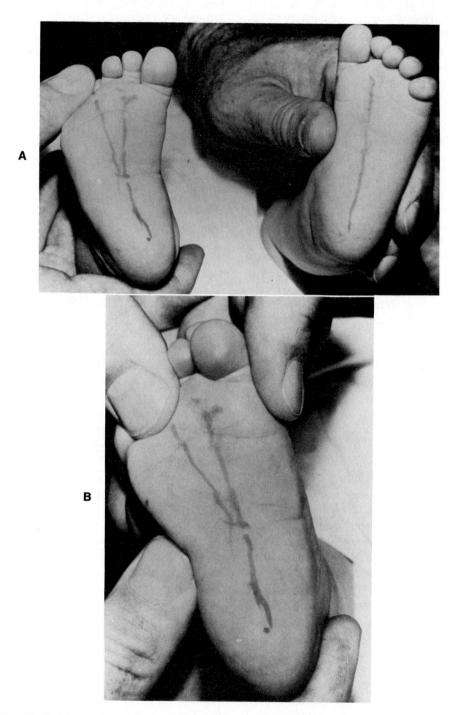

Fig. 13-12. Metatarsus adductus. **A,** A line that bisects the heel should fall at about the second toe or the second to third web space (right). In metatarsus adductus (left), the line intersects one of the lateral toes. **B,** Correction of the deformity is accomplished by stabilizing the hindfoot with the thumb and index finger and stressing the foot into abduction.

the deformity. The cast is changed initially at 1- to 3-week intervals and later (in the somewhat older child) as infrequently as once a month. In the later stages of treatment, the cast may be below the knee.

A serious complication that can occur with cast therapy is vascular embarrassment from constriction or overcorrection. The cast is removed immediately if there is any question about the capillary refill or warmth of the foot, or if there is excessive swelling or discoloration. Even in a well-molded cast, an active infant can wiggle his foot. If the toes change their position in relation to the end of the cast, the cast should be removed immediately, since it will no longer be functional in this malposition. In addition, skin compressive problems may occur.

Casts are often removed by a variety of cast saws or scissors but there is a danger of skin injury with a saw. We routinely have the parents soak the cast off the day before the return clinic appointment. Soaking is not only safe, but when it is employed the night before, it allows the skin some time to recover before a new cast is applied. The addition of 1 tablespoon of vinegar per gallon of water makes removal easier. The softened cast is then unwound or cut with nurses' scissors.

In the neglected case, or in the small percentage of resistant cases, surgery may be necessary. The results are generally better with early surgery, but a conservative course should always be tried first and surgery postponed until the child is between 3 and 6 months of age. In the younger child (below the age of 24 months) the procedure consists of a soft tissue release of all the tarsometatarsal joints, followed by a 6- to 12-week period of casting. Then, out-flared shoes may be used to help hold the position. More often, some form of rigid night splinting is employed. Soft tissue releases can be utilized in a child as old as 6 or 7 years, but they are much less satisfactory at that age. In the child beyond the age of 18 to 24 months, one may need to consider bony procedures in the form of midfoot osteotomies or osteotomies at the base of the metatarsals, to gain correction.

Postoperative care. The postoperative care for an osteotomy is approximately the same as for soft tissue release. Should surgery become necessary, the total hospital stay may be only a few days. All subsequent care, including pin removal, can be accomplished on an outpatient basis.

Clubfoot

The term *clubfoot* is often used in a general sense to cover almost any equinovarus deformity of the foot, whether it is congenital or acquired. In this text, we will use *clubfoot* only in reference to true congenital malformations with primary abnormalities in the development of the foot, ankle, and leg (Fig. 13-13). Clubfeet are common, occurring as often as 1 in 1,000 live births. When clubfeet occur as isolated abnormalities, the genetic pattern is multifactorial and the recurrence risk for subsequent siblings is approximately 5%. Not infrequently, clubfeet are associated with any number of other organ abnormalities. Among the more common musculoskeletal conditions that are associated with clubfeet are arthrogryposis multiplex congenita, myelodysplasia, congenital myopathies, many of the dwarfing syndromes, and several chromosomal abnormalities. In addition, there is an increased incidence of subluxation or dislocation of the hips. It is important to identify these associated conditions, not only because the general prognosis is altered, but because the feet in these conditions are often resistant to therapy.

Clubfeet come in all degrees of severity. The common denominator is equinus and varus of the hindfoot, with marked supination and varus of the forefoot. The malposition is fixed and cannot be corrected with passive manipulation. Often, the skin of the hindfoot is mobile and gives a false sensation of motion of the ankle joint. The more rigid, severely affected feet are marked by a deep crease on the medial and posterior aspect of the ankle joint, just above the heel, and by a deep transverse crease at the level of the instep. The body of the talus is rotated in relation to the ankle joint in three planes, the neck of the talus is malformed, and the talar head points more medially than normal. However, the navicular is even further displaced medially, often abutting the medial malleolus. The head of the talus, despite its medial direction, is uncovered laterally and is palpable on the lateral aspect of the foot. The navicular cannot be reduced over the head of the talus, and the normal depression at the site of the sinus tarsi cannot be obtained. The lateral malleolus is prominent and posterior.

The calf musculature is contracted, and the entire calf is small, underlining the primary limb bud deficiency. Indeed, electron microscopy and histochemistry of calf muscles in clubfeet are abnormal.[15] Regardless of the method of treatment,

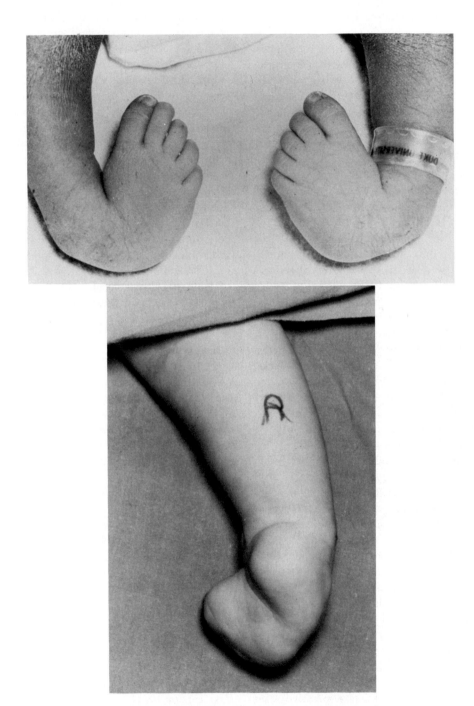

Fig. 13-13. Clinical appearance of true talipes equinovarus (clubfoot).

the foot will always be small and the calf thin; it is important to review this certain outcome with the parents when discussing the long range prognosis.

There is still much discussion regarding the pathology and etiology of clubfeet, but all would agree that it is a generalized problem of the entire distal extremity, involving the bones, the joints, the ligaments, and the musculature.

Evaluation and referral. Because the infant's centers of ossification are not well developed, radiographs of an infant with clubfoot are not terribly useful for routine diagnostic purposes. Clubfeet should be evident clinically, and referral to an orthopedist is mandatory. Treatment should be initiated as soon as feasible, given the child's general condition.

Medical versus surgical treatment. In the past it was thought that the majority of clubfeet could be corrected in plaster, although it might take several years of continuous casting. Most orthopedists now find such a prolonged period of casting unacceptable, and the end results do not warrant the effort. The true clubfoot or, at least, all those deformities that are more than the very mildest, will not respond to casting and surgery will become necessary. Given these objections,

surgery is now performed early and aggressively, even in the neonatal period, but more usually when the child is about 3 months of age. The benefit of initial casting lies in stretching the soft tissues and preventing progression of the deformity, both of which will make surgical correction easier.

Surgical options. The surgical procedure required is an extensive one,[10] since all the tendinous structures on the posterior medial side of the ankle will need to be lengthened at the level of the medial malleolus. The ankle joint, itself, is extensively released to allow the talus to derotate. Additional ankle and forefoot releases are usually required. In the older child or more resistant foot, osteotomies may become necessary.

Postoperative care and follow-up. The aftercare is similar to that described for metatarsus adductus and includes a postoperative period of 3 months of casting and prolonged postoperative splinting. However, once the child is out of full-time plaster casts, special shoeing will usually not be necessary.

In the moderate to severe problem, the need for one or more secondary reconstructive procedures is the rule rather than the exception.

Prognosis. Despite generally satisfactory surgical results and the description of the surgical

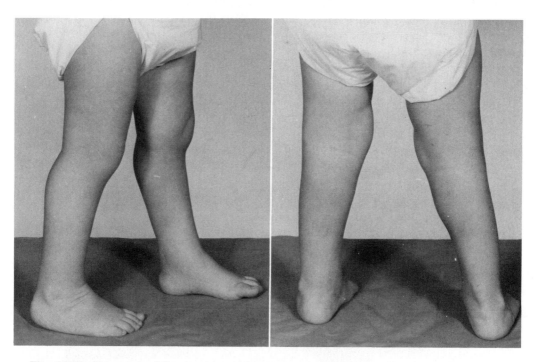

Fig. 13-14. Six months following corrective surgery for bilateral clubfeet. The goal of surgery is not to restore the foot to "normal" but to produce a plantigrade foot that will be painless and functional throughout the child's life.

procedure as "total correction," several limitations need to be understood at the outset. The goal of surgery is a plantigrade foot that will be painless and functional throughout the child's life and that will fit in standard shoes (Fig. 13-14). This is not to say that the basic deficiencies in musculature and development of the bony structures can be overcome or that the foot will ever be "normal." The foot will be small, the calf will be thin, and a certain degree of postoperative stiffness will result. This end result will vary with the severity of the initial problem. Nevertheless, if the condition is an isolated one, a very good functional result can be expected; the child should be able to run and play with his peers, albeit without the same facility. The parents can be reassured that their child will not be grotesquely deformed or "crippled."

Calcaneovalgus

The range of dorsiflexion of the newborn's foot is markedly increased in comparison with that of an adult. In many children in the nursery, the dorsum of the foot can be approximated to the anterior aspect of the tibia. This posture is more frequent in firstborn children of young mothers; presumably, it is secondary to increased uterine constraint from stronger uterine and abdominal musculature. When the deformity is severe enough that the foot cannot be passively manipulated into or maintained in the corrected equinovarus position, the child must have a short period of casting to achieve full range of motion and prevent permanent contracture or resistant deformity. Surgery is rarely necessary.

Calcaneovalgus should not be confused with vertical talus—it is important that this differential diagnosis be made. In addition, it is necessary to demonstrate active plantar flexion of the feet, because such a neuromuscular condition as spinal dysraphism, in which the lower sacral elements are involved, will produce a similar deformity.

Vertical talus

As mentioned earlier, all newborns have "fat feet," not "flat feet," and the usual varieties of flat feet are not discernible at birth. Flatfoot carried to its extreme has the appearance of a truly convex plantar surface ("rocker bottom") (Fig. 13-15). When this deformity is rigid and the talus plantar flexed, it is known as congenital convex pes valgus or vertical talus. The primary disorder appears to be a teratologic dislocation of the talonavicular joint.[25] The talus is fixed in plantar flexion and becomes prominent on the plantar, medial aspect of the foot. The navicular bone and the midfoot are dislocated dorsally, locking the forefoot in a dorsiflexed and valgus position. The long toe extensors, the anterior tibial muscle, and the peroneal muscles may all become markedly contracted. Even in the newborn, the marked plantar flexion of the talus (which may lie parallel to the long axis of the tibia) is evident radiographically. This is in contradistinction to positional calcaneovalgus, wherein both the talus and the calcaneus are dorsiflexed and mobile with stress.

As with clubfeet, vertical tali show a marked association with other abnormalities. Chromosomal abnormalities, in particular, should be sought.

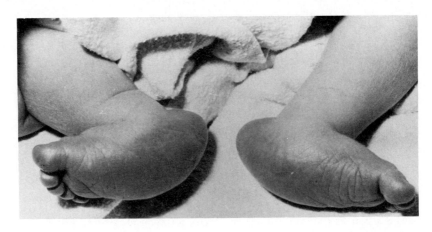

Fig. 13-15. Rocker bottom appearance of congenital convex pes valgus (vertical talus).

Treatment. Treatment should be initiated immediately. The long-term prognosis is limited, and conservative measures are almost invariably unsuccessful. Again, as with clubfeet, early casting has its merits in preparation and improvement of the results of surgical procedures. The goal of surgery is to obtain a plantigrade foot. The true vertical talus of more than the most minimal severity will always result in a small and stiff (but functional) foot. The surgical procedure is directed at extensive soft tissue release, reduction of the talonavicular joint, dorsiflexion of the talus, and reconstruction of the supporting structures of the longitudinal arch. The surgical correction is often held by percutaneous pins that will be incorporated in or held beneath the postoperative cast and are removed approximately 6 weeks after surgery.

Postoperative care. In general, postoperative care is the same as that outlined for clubfeet.

Other abnormalities of the feet

The list of other congenital abnormalities that affect the foot is seemingly endless: any combination of the primary positions of varus, valgus, equinus, and calcaneus can occur in association with additions or deletions of various parts. A number of other conditions that may be of great importance, such as tarsal coalition, may be present but not evident at birth. The management of these important other conditions that present later in life is discussed in later sections of this text.

Two other, not uncommon deformities are congenital curly toes and overlapping or underlapping toes. Overlapping is most common in the fifth toe and may be a familial problem. Obviously, an overlapping toe presents no difficulty to the newborn; later, however, it may be a significant consideration in shoeing. Simple strapping or taping of the toe in the corrected position is all that is reasonable in the newborn. Not infrequently, taping fails and some form of surgical release or the creation of a surgical syndactyly between adjacent toes becomes necessary to maintain correction.

Minor abnormalities of the feet are important because they may interfere with shoeing later. If the condition is an isolated one rather than a symptom of a more generalized neuromuscular disorder, the parents can anticipate a good functional result, even in severe conditions requiring multiple operations. We expect the child to be not only mobile but also ambulatory; certainly, we expect the child to be able to participate in all the forms of social interaction that define success in life. The primary care physician should also understand that the child who fails to meet major motor milestones is probably delayed for some reason other than the foot deformity. Even children with severe clubfeet will stand and walk at the appropriate time.

FRACTURES AND BIRTH INJURIES

As obstetric care continues to improve, the incidence of musculoskeletal injury decreases. Yet, fetal anoxia, urgent delivery, and abnormal presentation or abnormal fetuses continue to produce a significant number of such injuries.

Multiple fractures may ensue if the fetus itself is mechanically unable to conform to the birth canal, as in *arthrogryposis multiplex congenita,* wherein the elbows or knees are fixed in rigid extension. This diagnosis is usually self-evident. Fortunately, the list of generalized conditions that will produce multiple fractures in the newborn is small. *Osteogenesis imperfecta* has such a wide range of expression that the typical clinical features may not be present and the possibility of *hypophosphatasia, cystinosis,* or *pyknodysostosis* should be considered. *Rickets* has been described in the newborn period in children of rachitic mothers and, on occasion, in premature infants who received inadequate calcium or phosphorus intake during long stays in the intensive care nursery. In the older child, abuse and neglect must always be considered in any instance of multiple fractures.

More typically, we are faced with isolated injuries that occur in the setting of difficult or prolonged delivery. The most common injuries are fractures of the clavicle and humeral shaft, followed by fractures of the femoral shaft and traumatic fracture separations of the proximal and distal humerus at the shoulder and elbow, respectively, and of the capital femoral epiphysis and distal femoral epiphysis.[17] Fractures of the more distal portions of the extremity below the elbow and knee are quite rare. Fracture of the tibial shaft in the newborn is almost invariably pathologic, and a diagnosis of *congenital pseudoarthrosis of the tibia,* perhaps associated with neurofibromatosis, should be considered.

The diagnosis of a fracture is often easy in the presence of deformity, crepitus, and pain; but it may also be entirely asymptomatic or, rather, may present as pseudoparalysis.

FRACTURES OF THE LONG BONES

Clavicle fracture is the most common injury. It may be diagnosed only on routine chest x-ray examination and in some series is reported as occurring in as high as 2% of all deliveries. An asymptomatic fracture can be ignored; it will unite without any specific therapy and with an excellent cosmetic and functional result as growth and development remodel the fracture site (Fig. 13-16). If the fracture is grossly unstable and displaced, a small roll beneath the shoulder while the patient is lying in the prone position will abduct the shoulders and align the fracture. Occasionally, a soft wrap is applied in a figure-of-eight manner. Union should ensue within 10 days to 2 weeks.

In the symptomatic instance, particularly when the presenting symptom is diminished function of the upper extremity, isolated clavicle fracture must be distinguished, if possible, from brachial plexus palsy. These two injuries may coexist, and it may be impossible to define residual neurologic deficit until after the fracture has united and become painless. Pseudoparalysis, local swelling, and pain are also symptoms of neonatal osteomyelitis. Clavicle fracture and osteomyelitis should be distinguishable radiographically by the presence of lucency with mixed sclerosis in the instance of osteomyelitis; and, of course, the possibility of pathologic fracture should be considered. Congenital pseudarthrosis of the clavicle always occurs on the right side and is painless.

Fractures of the humerus are the next most common injuries. These usually occur in the middle third of the bone and may be associated with a radial nerve palsy, which would be expected to resolve within 6 to 8 weeks. Again, the coexistence of clavicular fractures, humeral fractures, and obstetric brachial plexus injuries must be remembered and unraveled through time and continued observation. Treatment consists of flexing the elbow and wrapping the arm to the side in a Velpeau bandage. Union can be expected within 2 weeks. Almost any degreee of angulation will be remodeled, and an excellent functional result should ensue.

Traumatic fracture separations of either the proximal or distal humeral epiphysis are not common but are important in that they will present as swollen, painful joints and may be difficult to distinguish from pyarthrosis. Because the ends of the bones are cartilaginous and radiolucent, x-ray films may suggest dislocation; but a traumatic dislocation of an otherwise normal joint in the newborn almost never occurs. Aspiration of the joint may be required to distinguish these conditions, and arthrography is useful.[8] Often, the nature of the injury is not apparent until callus begins to appear. At this point, further immobilization is probably unnecessary. When the diagno-

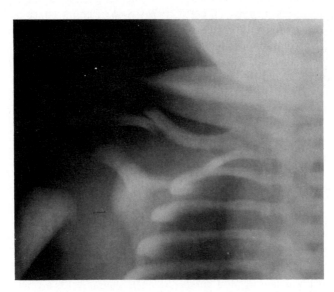

Fig. 13-16. Clavicle fracture, the most common newborn injury of the long bones. The fracture invariably unites, and one anticipates an excellent cosmetic and functional result, even with significant displacement of the fracture fragments.

sis is made at birth, reduction should be accomplished and the part splinted. The prognosis is excellent in these fractures, but limitation of motion may occur with elbow fractures.

Femoral shaft fractures, when they do occur as an obstetric injury, usually are in the middle third of the bone and somewhat transverse in orientation. These can be managed with manual longitudinal traction and immobilization. The use of splints or plaster spica casts depends on the size of the child and the degree of displacement of the fracture. Again, the capacity for remodeling is so great that much angular deformity can be accepted; however, gross displacement and shortening should be avoided to prevent subsequent limb length discrepancy.

Fracture separation of the femoral epiphyses does occur. The distal femoral epiphysis is ossified at birth; therefore, the radiographic diagnosis can usually be made, although often this injury is not apparent until the healing phase has already ensued. In the proximal femoral epiphysis, pseudoparalysis, pain, and swelling again make the diagnostic differentiation from pyarthrosis difficult. In addition, the shortening of the femoral shaft suggests congenital hip dysplasia. Since the proximal femur will be entirely cartilaginous, routine x-ray films may be misleading. Reduction of this fracture occurs as the hip is held in abduction, medial rotation, and extension and not in flexion, abduction, and external rotation, the position that reduces a dislocated hip. However, arthrography may be necessary to distinguish between these two entities. Avascular necrosis is not a complication of this injury, since the vascular supply of the cartilaginous anlage remains with the head. With satisfactory reduction, the prognosis is excellent; but residual coxa vara has been reported in instances where the injury was not detected until the healing phase.

The use of traction in management of lower extremity fractures is discussed in detail in subsequent sections of this text. It should be noted that most of these injuries do not require longitudinal traction for a prolonged period of time, and overhead or Bryant's traction should never be used because of the potential catastrophic complications of vascular embarrassment.

MUSCULOSKELETAL INFECTION

The general principles of management of osteomyelitis and pyarthrosis are outlined in more detail in subsequent sections of this text. Twenty percent of all cases of acute hematogenous osteomyelitis will occur in children under the age of 1; and it even occurs in the newborn nursery, often in association with maternal mastitis or endometritis. Variations in the vascular anatomy in infantile bone and its response to infection may account for several important differences in the presentation of these diseases in the newborn.[11]

The organisms involved, in order of frequency of report, are *Staphylococcus aureus, Streptococcus,* and *Hemophilus influenzae.* However, there have recently been increasing numbers of reports of non–group A beta-hemolytic streptococcal osteomyelitis and pyarthrosis. In contrast to the difficulty encountered in managing this organism in meningitis, the reports, to date, of management of this organism in osseous and joint infections indicate a satisfactory response to standard antibiotics and routine clinical measures.

Clinical presentation. While the newborn infant may present with both the typical picture of localized inflammation—erythema, warmth, swelling, and tenderness—and the systemic findings of septicemia, the peculiarity of the disease in the newborn period is the frequent absence of well-localized symptoms. Not uncommonly, the infant is afebrile, and even the nonspecific findings of irritability and poor feeding may be minimal. If there are local signs, the swelling may be quite diffuse and the entire extremity edematous, with no areas of increased redness or heat (Fig. 13-17). Only the most careful digital palpation may reveal an increase in tenderness over the metaphyseal region. The only abnormality may be pseudoparalysis, making infection difficult to distinguish from a fracture or neurologic injury. Radiographs will be useful in this instance. Pathologic fracture does occur in the newborn period, but by this point the gross changes of osteomyelitis are usually evident. The paralysis of obstetric brachial plexus injury should be immediately evident at the time of birth and most profound in the immediate postpartum period. This weakness should improve during subsequent hours to days, and any progressive loss of function during this period should make one concerned about infection. A needle aspiration of the area in question should be performed to establish a diagnosis as well as to make an appropriate identification of the organism.

Unique pathophysiology. Two important

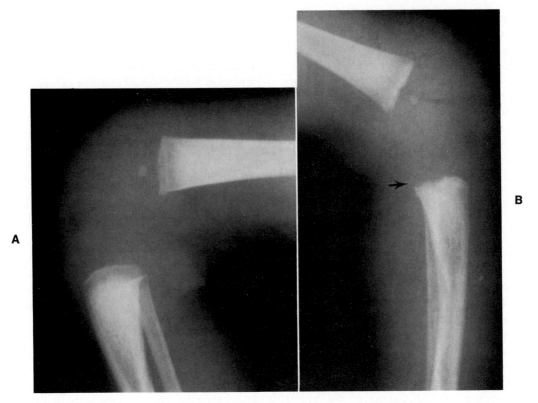

Fig. 13-17. Neonatal osteomyelitis. The only local sign of infection in this premature neonate was diffuse swelling and mild edema of the entire extremity. The radiograph (**A**) showed only periarticular osteoporosis. One week later (**B**) erosion and irregularity of the proximal tibial metaphysis is evident.

variations in infantile osseous anatomy account for important variations in the presentation and management of these diseases in the newborn period. Beyond the age of 8 to 12 months, the vascular arcades of the metaphysis end on the metaphyseal side of the physeal plate, accounting for the propensity for localization in the metaphysis in acute hematogenous infection after infancy. The physis serves as an effective barrier to the infection, which subsequently will decompress itself subperiosteally. Because of the physeal barrier, direct extension to the joint is unusual except for those joints in which the metaphysis is intra-articular, specifically, the shoulder, hip, and ankle. In the newborn and until the age of 8 months, there are direct vascular connections across the physeal area and into the epiphysis, and true epiphyseal osteomyelitis is not unusual. Associated pyarthrosis is more common and can affect any joint.

A second variation is that the cortical bone in the metaphyseal region of infantile bone is less compact than in older childhood, and the periosteum is more loosely attached. Thus, the cortex serves as less of a barrier to advancing infection, which may more easily decompress into the subperiosteal region. For this reason, surgical decompression of the metaphysis is rarely necessary in this age group.

Treatment. Given the variations noted above and the importance of maintaining adequate hydration in the septic infant, the general principles of management of osteomyelitis and pyarthrosis in this age group do not vary from those of older children. Immobilization is instituted immediately to relieve symptoms, assist in control of infection, and prevent pathologic fracture. Parenteral antibiotic therapy is instituted, and surgical drainage is reserved for either those instances in which adequate medical management has failed to control local or systemic symptoms or those anatomic areas (particularly the hip) where local findings cannot be evaluated adequately. The potential for catastrophic results is so great in pyarthrosis that even a short delay in the institution of surgical treatment is contraindicated.

ABNORMALITIES OF THE UPPER EXTREMITY

Positional variations of the upper extremity are seen much less commonly than in the lower extremity. Indeed, there are no major problems in the upper extremity that are felt to be the result of intrauterine constraint. On the other hand, any teratologic factor that has its effect in the first trimester—when the limb buds are undergoing their primary formation—can result in failure of differentiation, segmentation, or rotation and result in significant upper extremity abnormalities. Because the upper and lower limbs of the embryo develop at slightly different times, major anomalies may be seen in either the upper or lower extremity without necessarily coexisting with concomitant deformities in the other extremities. Because multiple organ systems are developing in parallel, the abnormalities of the upper extremity may be the visible harbingers of major problems in other organ systems.[23]

Camptodactyly

Camptodactyly, which literally translates as "bent finger," refers to a flexion contracture, particularly at the PIP joint. The little finger is most commonly affected, followed by the ring finger and, less frequently, by the long and index fingers. Camptodactyly is to be distinguished from lateral curvature or clinodactyly. The condition may be hereditary, with a dominant mode of inheritance.

There are all degrees of severity of camptodactyly. A mild contracture, which is passively correctable when first detected, may respond to splinting. More commonly, multiple structures are involved, including shortening of the superficialis tendons, skin contracture, ligamentous contracture, and even joint deformity, and surgical correction is required.

Mild contractures of 30 degrees or less are perfectly compatible with excellent function; but if the contracture is progressive, it becomes significantly disabling. Surgical correction is an extremely difficult and sophisticated procedure and should be attempted only by an experienced hand surgeon. Prolonged splinting may be necessary, even after surgical release. Surgical correction is usually deferred until such time as the structures

of the finger are large enough to make the procedure practical. Some residual deformity is to be expected.

Congenital dislocation of the radial head

Dislocation of the radial head occurs as an isolated deformity; in any condition with hyperlaxity of the joints and frequent dislocations; and in other, more complex anomalies of the upper extremity. Dislocation should be suspected whenever the normal neonate elbow flexion contracture fails to disappear after the first several weeks of life. The proximal radius is not ossified until well after birth, but dislocation can be recognized radiographically if the shaft of the radius is not opposite the capitellum.

Other than limitations of motion, the symptoms in the young child are mild. One can reduce the radial head at birth; but it is difficult to maintain the reduction, even with operative procedures. Resection of the radial head, the definitive treatment, is usually deferred until skeletal growth has been completed, because the short proximal radius may lead to secondary abnormalities in the distal radial ulnar articulation.

Polydactyly

The presence of extra digits, or portions thereof, is a common congenital variation and may be familial. As with most structural defects, a dominant mode of inheritance is most common. The extra digits are usually along the ulnar border of the hand and may involve varying degrees of fusion with the adjacent digit. Small skin tags can be ligated in the newborn nursery and require no further care; more extensive skin bridges and the presence of other shared structures require more complex surgical procedures. While separation of a simple skin bridge may present few problems, the identification and division of shared neurovascular structures or joint structures, with reconstruction of a stable configuration, is technically demanding.

Treatment is usually deferred until the involved structures reach adequate size, although it certainly should be accomplished well before the child reaches school age, when the extra digits might present a social problem. Three years seems to be a popular age for surgery; whenever possible, however, amputation of extra parts should be planned to precede the period of maximal Oedipal concerns. Hospitalization will be brief, and the degree of aftercare, though varying with the extent of the surgical procedure, may be minimal.

Radial clubhand

Radial clubhand properly should be included within the group of limb deficiencies discussed elsewhere in this chapter. However, because of its frequency and its significant associated visceral anomalies, it will be considered separately. The deficiency is limited to the radial side of the extremity and thus is considered to be a paraxial hemimelia. It may be either terminal, with complete absence of all elements of the radial side of the forearm and first ray (thumb), or intercalary, with a normal hand. The absence of the radius may be partial or complete, and the involvement of the thumb may range from complete absence to hypoplasia of the intrinsic musculature. When partial absence of the radius occurs, it is usually the distal portion. The ulna is shortened and curved, and the hand is radially deviated. In severe cases, the angle of the hand and the long axis of the forearm may be greater than 90 degrees (Fig. 13-18). The muscles, nerves, blood vessels, and bones of the radial aspect of the hand and wrist are involved, and a great variety of anatomic varia-

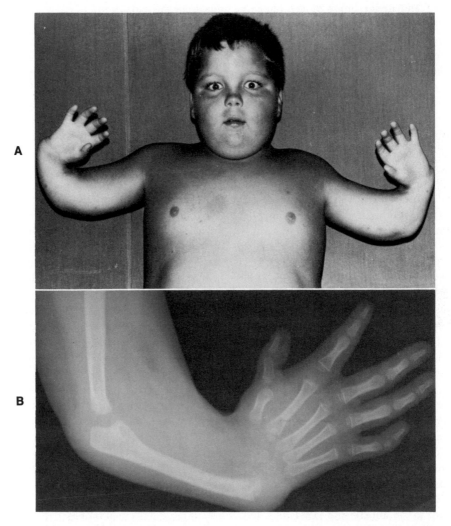

Fig. 13-18. Clinical (**A**) and radiographic (**B**) appearance of a child with bilateral radial clubhand. During infancy, this child had thrombocytopenia, which resolved spontaneously. In the thrombocytopenia–absent radius syndrome, the extremity defect is always bilateral and there is always complete absence of the radius. The thumbs are always present but may be hypoplastic, as in this case.

tions is possible, including absence of shoulder musculature.

Associated anomalies. Other abnormalities frequently associated with clubhands include cleft lip and cleft palate, clubfeet, hydrocephalus, rib anomalies, lung aplasia, and hemivertebra. The association of anomalies known as the VATER syndrome[21] should be kept in mind; this includes vertebral anomalies (most commonly, midthoracic hemivertebrae), esophageal atresia, tracheoesophageal fistula, anal atresia, and radial anomalies. Heart and renal abnormalities are also common. The association with congenital heart disease, particularly septal defects, is well known and is described as the heart-hand or Holt-Oram syndrome.[14] Associated hematologic abnormalities are also well recognized and are important to consider.[18] In the thrombocytopenia–absent radius (TAR) syndrome, the radius is always completely absent bilaterally, and the thumb is always present, if often hypoplastic. In Fanconi's syndrome, with pancytopenia and anemia as well as late development of malignancy, the thumbs are always absent.

Treatment. Obviously, the presence of these other major anomalies will greatly affect the treatment plan and the ultimate prognosis. The other defects may not be evident at birth but should be sought when the obvious skeletal abnormality is noted. The initial treatment begins immediately following birth and consists of passive stretching exercises, range of motion exercises and splinting. The goal is maintenance of range of motion and prevention of more severe deformity and contracture. Surgery of one form or another is almost always required, and the first stages can begin when the child is as young as 3 to 6 months of age if there are no contraindications. The thrombocytopenia of the TAR syndrome will usually resolve spontaneously, without specific therapy, within the first 12 months of life. Surgery should be deferred at least until that time.

The surgical approach consists of the lengthening of contracted structures, which may include Z-plasty or even grafting of the skin of the radial side of the hand, and centralization of the hand over the ulna.

In cases of bilateral anomalies, particularly those in which the elbow does not have a normal range of motion, the shortened, curved forearm with radial deviation of the hands may be necessary in order for the child to function in the midline and to bring his hands to the face and body for activities of daily living. In these instances, rigid centralization of the carpus over the ulna is contraindicated because it may actually impair function. In the case of unilateral deformity, or the instance in which the elbow has a good range of motion and where the thumb is close to normal, the loss of the mobility at the wrist will be overcome by using the good contralateral hand as well as the elbow and thumb and fingers of the affected side. In this latter instance, rigid stabilization provides a much superior cosmetic result that will be worth the loss of function. If there is any question, a period of preoperative casting may establish the functional costs of the superior cosmetic result.

The decision to reconstruct the thumb will depend on the degree of hypoplasia. The small thumb may be reinforced with bone graft and tendon transfer, but the severely hypoplastic "floating thumb" might best be amputated. Consideration should be given to pollicization of the index finger, particularly in the case of bilateral deformity. The multiplicity and complexity of the surgical possibilities make it clear that early referral to a pediatric orthopedic hand surgeon is indicated in this condition.

Radial ulnar synostosis

Varying degrees of osseous union may occur between the proximal radius and ulna. The forearm is usually in midposition or in some degree of pronation and is fixed. The lack of rotation is evident in the newborn child. The several anatomic variations depend on the extent of the osseous bridging and the presence or absence of the proximal radius, as well as on the dislocation of the proximal radius. The condition may be familial, and most reported families demonstrate a dominant mode of inheritance. The synostosis may be bilateral. There is an increased incidence of congenital synostosis in Klinefelter's syndrome, and this association should be considered whenever this diagnosis is made.

Because of the marked mobility at the shoulder joint, even in the case of bilateral deformity, functional impairment is often negligible. Therefore, the only time that a surgical procedure is indicated is when the forearm is fixed in a nonfunctional position, such as maximal pronation. In such an instance, a rotational osteotomy to a more functional position would be indicated.

Syndactyly

Webbing of two or more digits of the hand may occur as an isolated problem and is frequently familial. All modes of inheritance have been described; and, most commonly, the trait is dominant. There is tremendous variation in the clinical presentation, and anomalies of the other structures of the hand may be associated. Typically, the ring and long fingers are joined, but any combination can occur and all four fingers may be affected (Fig. 13-19). The shared tissue may be only a skin web, but one may find bony fusion of the distal phalanx or even complete juncture of all bony structures, with shared neurovascular bundles. Particularly severe syndactyly, with true mitten hands, occurs in Apert's syndrome or in the variation of this condition described by Carpenter, wherein polydactyly is associated with the syndactyly.

Treatment. No immediate measures are necessary. Referral to a surgeon experienced in pediatric hand problems can be accomplished at the family's convenience but should occur within the first few months of life. If the digits are of unequal length, separation may be undertaken in the child as young as 5 to 9 months of age to prevent secondary deformities. In the more complex problem, skin grafting is always required and ultimate function will depend on the degree of stability and involvement of the joints as well as on the nature of shared neurovascular structures. This is particularly so in the extreme cases seen in Apert's syndrome. When more than two digits are involved, multiple procedures may be required, since only one side of a finger can be safely released at any single surgical procedure. If adequate skin and subcutaneous tissue are available to construct a wide and deep web and adequate coverage can be obtained on the other fingers, correction may be permanent. However, in the more severe cases and in those instances where coverage is marginal, contractures may recur and late operative revisions may be necessary.

Other, less common abnormalities
Congenital absence of the ulna

Congenital absence of the ulna occurs, but much less frequently than that of the radius. One or more of the ulnar border digits may be absent as well. There are several variations of development of the elbow joint associated with this anomaly, and this variation greatly affects the ultimate prognosis. Elbow joint abnormalities range from complete fusion of the radiohumeral joint to an apparently normal elbow joint at birth. Even in the ostensibly normal elbow, the radius may dislocate as a result of tethering of the distal radius and continued growth proximally. Early treatment consists of splinting to prevent further contracture. Later, proximal osteotomy of the radius combined, perhaps, with fusion to the remnant of the proximal ulna will create a one-bone forearm. As with surgery for radial clubhand, postoperative casting will be extensive and prolonged. Postoperative splinting will be necessary, at least at night, during continued growth and development.

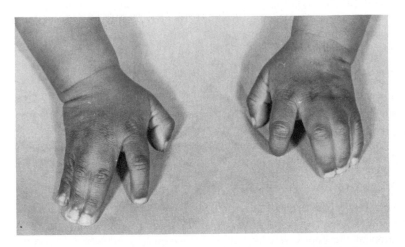

Fig. 13-19. Bilateral syndactyly involving the long, ring, and little fingers.

Congenital pseudarthrosis of the clavicle

Congenital pseudarthrosis of the clavicle is less common than its counterpart in the tibia and is less frequently associated with neurofibromatosis. Deficiencies in the central one third of the clavicle are often overlooked at birth. The pseudarthrosis always occurs on the right side and may be related to the right-left variation in embryology of the great vessels. The pseudarthrosis is often asymptomatic; if pain or instability is a problem, however, surgical fixation and bone grafting, though difficult, can be undertaken. This condition is to be distinguished from *cleidocranial dysostosis,* in which there is subtotal or complete absence of the clavicle, usually bilaterally, and the shoulders can be adducted to the midline. The skull changes in cleidocranial dysostosis are typical, and anomalous or absent musculature about the shoulder is common. Patients adapt to this anomaly quite well, and no treatment is indicated.

Gigantism

Gigantism of one or more digits is usually associated with neurofibromatosis, arteriovenous fistulas, or other vasculolymphatic hamartomatous lesions. Treatment includes excision of the involved tissues where possible and shortening of the bone or epiphysiodesis in an attempt to reduce the digit to the size of the uninvolved fingers.

Madelung's deformity

Madelung's deformity is a congenital, hereditary condition that becomes apparent only with growth and development. The basic abnormality is maldevelopment of the volar, ulnar aspect of the distal radial epiphysis, which leads to subsequent deformity, curvature of the radius, prominence of the distal ulna, and limitation of motion of the wrist, particularly in pronation and supination. The function of the hand itself is rarely affected. Pain is uncommon; but should it occur, or if one desires cosmetic or functional improvement, resection of the distal ulna and osteotomy of the distal radius will be useful. Surgery is usually deferred until the completion of skeletal growth. The distal radial physis does not close until the late teenage years.

ARTHROGRYPOSIS MULTIPLEX CONGENITA

The term *arthrogryposis* translates as "curved joint" and is used to describe a congenital syndrome in which there are multiple rigid, usually symmetric joint contractures at birth.[7] The condition is not progressive and is not hereditary. Many diverse conditions that exhibit joint contractures have been lumped together under the diagnosis of arthrogryposis, but one should restrict this diagnosis to those children who have involvement of at least two limbs and five major joints. Contractures become worse at the peripheral portions of the limb, and there is relative sparing of the proximal joints and trunk. Other paralytic disorders must be ruled out.

Clinical presentation. The usual pattern is of internal rotation of the shoulders with extended elbows and pronated forearms (Fig. 13-20). Flexion at the wrist may be accompanied by curling

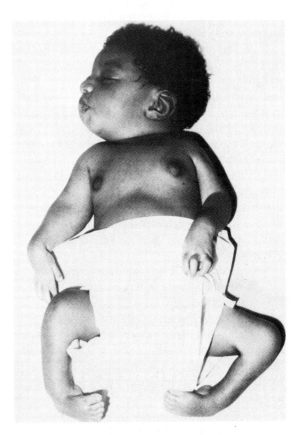

Fig. 13-20. Arthrogryposis multiplex congenita. There is internal rotation of the shoulders and pronation and extension contracture of the forearms. Wrist flexion, curling of the fingers and thumb, and palm deformity are common. The child shows hip and knee flexion contractures, and there are bilateral clubfoot deformities. The knees illustrate the typically enlarged joints with loss of normal skin flexion creases.

of the fingers, and the thumb may be fixed in the palm. The lower extremities are usually flexed, abducted, and externally rotated at the hips. The knees may be flexed or extended; when flexed there may be webbing in the popliteal space. Frequently there are severe clubfoot deformities. Scoliosis is common. The head is usually not involved with contractures, but the facies are often expressionless and have been described as "wooden doll"–or "Pinocchio"–like.

The joints themselves are diffusely enlarged. The surrounding skin and subcutaneous tissues may be thickened and may have a somewhat indurated feel. Skin webs may be present, and there is usually loss of the normal skin flexion creases. Muscles are severely atrophic. The deep tendon reflexes will not be detectable in the affected limbs. The rigid limb deformities at birth often lead to difficulties with delivery, and multiple fractures may result.

It is important to remember that intellectual function is not altered in arthrogryposis.

Etiology. Adams, Denny-Brown, and Pearson[1] have divided arthrogryposis into two basic groups: the so-called neuropathic and myopathic forms. Many authors believe that the "myopathic" forms are actually some form of congenital muscular dystrophy or one of the "benign" congenital myopathies. In that group, the distal muscles may be larger than the proximal ones, the contractures are less rigid, and the underlying disease should be distinguishable on electromyography and muscle biopsy, which should include electron microscopy.

The neuropathic form of arthrogryposis is by far the more frequent. In this condition, the muscles are replaced by fat and connective tissue, but no diagnostic findings are evident on biopsy. Autopsy studies have shown a reduction in the number of anterior horn cells. It is not uncommon for mothers of arthrogrypotic children to recall reduced fetal movement during pregnancy, and this observation has led many investigators to attempt to reproduce this condition with methods that produce fetal paralysis. An arthrogrypotic-like syndrome can be produced in chick embryos by injecting curare, and similar changes have been created in other animals with a variety of teratologic and toxic agents.[6] This experimentation has lent credence to the concept that an intrauterine insult that results in loss of anterior horn cells

and subsequent loss of fetal movement is the underlying basis of the joint contractures and muscular atrophy.

• • •

When this condition is confronted in the newborn, several generalizations can be made for the parents:

1. It is likely that the trunk will be relatively spared, and this will be an asset.
2. As a rule, intelligence will be normal; indeed, some individuals report that these patients as a group are more intelligent than the norm.
3. In most cases, children with arthrogryposis will be able to walk.
4. There is no significant recurrence risk for subsequent siblings.

One should recognize that the condition has been present for a long time, that it is more than simple muscular atrophy, and that there are thick, fibrotic, periarticular contractures.

Treatment. Treatment in the newborn period has two main goals. First, one must avoid the development of any further postural contractures. Second, serial manipulation and casting of contractures that are already present are begun in an attempt to minimize the deformity and in preparation for subsequent surgical correction. The contractures will not respond to physical therapy or splinting, nor will they respond well to surgical measures that are not directed at release of these joint structures. In the ensuing weeks and months, a general plan of surgical and orthotic management can be outlined, with the goal being to eliminate lower extremity deformities and provide a stable base for ambulation by the time the child is 2 years of age. The desired end point is a stable hip and straight knee over a plantigrade foot. Fortunately, joint instability is not the problem it is in other paralytic conditions; but joint stiffness, of course, is. As a rule, the range of motion that can be restored surgically will not increase from that which is present at birth. The aim is to change the arc of motion into a functional range. Subsequently, attempts can be made to supply muscle power for those activities that will afford the child independence in self-care and daily activities.

The surgical procedure selected will, of course, depend on the joints involved and the deformity present. Clubfeet are common and are severely resistant to correction, often requiring multiple procedures. In the younger child, surgery is limited to soft tissue release, as it is with all other joints, and prolonged postoperative bracing will be required. Such extensive procedures as complete talectomy or, in the older child, osteotomy and fusion may be required.

For the most part, osteotomies are performed as the child approaches skeletal maturity. If one must be performed earlier than that, it is done with the expectation of recurrence of deformity and the need for repeated procedures. The knee is always released before correction of hip deformity because it is almost impossible to prevent recurrent hip flexion contracture when the knee is flexed. The hips are frequently dislocated, but this is not as disabling a problem as severe hip contracture. It will not interfere with ambulation, nor does it necessarily become painful. Closed methods never succeed in the management of dislocated hips in arthrogryposis, and surgical procedures are always required.

The problem is somewhat more complex in the upper extremity than in the lower extremity. In the upper extremity, motion and dexterity are more important than stability, which is the primary aim in the lower extremity. As a rule, upper extremity surgical procedures are performed in the child at a later age than those in the lower extremity. Because one cannot improve the overall range of motion but can only change the arc, one must carefully plan anything that will alter the position of the upper extremities. The child will need to be able to reach his perineum for personal hygiene but will also need to be able to bring both hands together in the midline for two-handed activity as well as bring one hand to the mouth for feeding. The combined motions of all joints must be considered, and surgical releases and/or muscle transfers undertaken with great care by an experienced surgeon.

With regard to the spine, the trunk is often spared but there is a high incidence of congenital scoliosis; in addition, the deformities about the hip lead to pelvic obliquity and secondary scoliotic problems. If one combines all these aspects, probably 25% of children with arthrogryposis will have scoliosis that requires treatment. Bracing can be attempted, but the curve may progress, even at a young age, and early fusion may become necessary.

In summary, arthrogryposis is a nonprogressive but severe and disabling condition. The sparing of the intellect usually means that with proper motivation, satisfactory adaptation and functional results can be achieved. The general principles of management of each joint affected by this condition are similar to those used to manage isolated abnormalities, but the treatment plan must always be more radical, and the need for subsequent bracing and orthotic management is much greater.

REFERENCES

1. Adams, R. C., Denny-Brown, D., and Pearson, C. M.: Diseases of muscle: a study in pathology, ed. 2, New York, 1962, Harper & Row, Publishers, Inc.
2. Adler, J. B., and Patterson, R. L.: Erb's palsy: long-term results of treatment in eighty-eight cases, J. Bone Joint Surg. **49A:**1052, 1967.
3. Bergsma, D.: Birth defects compendium: ed. 2, New York, 1979, Alan R. Liss, Inc.
4. Claven, S. K., and Smith, D. W.: Congenital deformities, Pediatr. Clin. North Am. **24**(4):665, 1977.
5. Coleman, S. S.: Congenital dysplasia and dislocation of the hip, St. Louis, 1978, The C. V. Mosby Co.
6. Drachman, D. B., and Coulombie, A. J.: Experimental clubfoot and arthrogryposis multiplex congenita, Lancet **2:**523, 1962.
7. Drummond, D. S., Siller, T. N., and Cruess, R. L.: Management of arthrogryposis multiplex congenita. In American Academy of Orthopaedic Surgeons: Instructional course lectures, vol. 23, St. Louis, 1974, The C. V. Mosby Co., p. 79.
8. Feingold, M.: Clinical evaluation of the child with skeletal dysplasia, Orthop. Clin. North Am. **7**(2):291, 1976.
9. Goldberg, M. J.: Orthopaedic aspects of bone dysplasias, Orthop. Clin. North Am. **7**(2):445, 1976.
10. Goldner, J. L.: Congenital talipes equinovarus—fifteen years of surgical treatment, Curr. Pract. Orthop. Surg. **4:**61, 1969.
11. Green, W. T., and Shannon, J. A.: Osteomyelitis of infants: a disease different from osteomyelitis of older children, Arch. Surg. **32:**462, 1936.
12. Green, W. T., and Tachdjian, M. O.: Correction of residual deformities of the shoulder in obstetrical palsy, J. Bone Joint Surg. **45A:**1544, 1963.
13. Gupta, M. L.: Congenital annular defects of the extremities and trunk, J. Bone Joint Surg. **45A:**571, 1963.
14. Holt, S. M., and Oram, S.: Familial heart disease with skeletal malformations, Br. Heart J. **22:**236, 1960.
15. Isaacs, H., and others: The muscles in clubfoot—a histological, histochemical and electron microscopic study, J. Bone Joint Surg. **59B:**465, 1977.
16. Lovell, W. W., and Winter, R. B., editors: Pediatric orthopaedics, Philadelphia, 1978, J. B. Lippincott Co.
17. Madsen, E. T.: Fractures of the extremities in the newborn, Acta Obstet. Gynecol. Scand. **34:**41, 1955.
18. McKusick, V.: A comparison between fanconi anemia and radius-platelet hypoplasia (RPH), the clinical of birth

defects. Part 3. Limb malformations, Birth Defects **5**(3): 194, 1969.

19. Moe, J. H., and others: Scoliosis and other spinal deformities, Philadelphia, 1978, W. B. Saunders Co.

20. The orthopaedic examination of the newborn, American Academy of Orthopedic Surgery Instructional Sound-Slide Program No. 514, Chicago, 1972.

21. Quan, L., and Smith, D. W.: The VATER association: vertebral defects, anal atresia, T-E fistula with esophageal atresia, radial and renal dysplasia: a spectrum of associated defects, J. Pediatr. **82:**104, 1973.

22. Ramsey, P. L., Lasser, S., and MacEwen, G. D.: Congenital dislocation of the hip: use of the Pavlik harness in the child during the first six months of life, J. Bone Joint Surg. **58A:**1000, 1976.

23. Rang, M.: Children's fractures, Philadelphia, 1974, J. B. Lippincott Co.

24. Staheli, L. T.: Torsional deformity, Pediatr. Clin. North Am. **24**(4):799, 1977.

25. Tachdjian, M. O.: Congenital convex pes valgus, Ortho. Clin. North Am. **3:**133, 1972.

26. Tachdjian, M. O.: Pediatric orthopaedics, Philadelphia, 1972, W. B. Saunders Co.

27. Temtany, S. A., and McKusick, V.: The genetics of hand malformations, Birth Defects **19**(3), 1978.

28. Trueta, J.: The normal vascular anatomy of the human femoral head during growth, J. Bone Joint Surg. **39B:**358, 1957.

29. Wickstrom, J.: Birth injuries of the brachial plexus, J. Bone Joint Surg. **42A:**1448, 1960.

The infant and toddler

CHAPTER 14

General considerations

HOWARD C. FILSTON

It is at the first well-baby visit that a careful check on the physical examination performed in the newborn should be accomplished. Anomalies and tumors that may have been inapparent or missed during the initial newborn examination can now be identified. Particular attention should be paid during this examination to the neck, the heart, the abdomen, the genitalia, and the anorectal area.

SURGICALLY ORIENTED EXAMINATION
The neck

The most common lesion to be discovered during the well-baby examination that was inapparent in the newborn period is that of *muscular torticollis*. Many think that this lesion is not present in the newborn period and is a result of injury to the sternocleidomastoid muscle during delivery.[2,4] An inordinate number of these children are born by breech presentation.[3] Others believe that it is the presence of the torticollis and its effect on the infant's head and neck that lead to inability of the head to engage and, therefore, to the high number of breech presentations. Nevertheless, it is often at the 4- to 6-week well-baby visit that torticollis is appreciated and that the sternocleidomastoid "tumor" can be palpated (Fig. 14-1). Management of this lesion is discussed in Chapter 18.

Other entities that may be appreciated in the neck at this time are the sinuses and fistulas from the second branchial cleft. This lesion usually presents along the midportion of the anterior aspect of the sternocleidomastoid muscle and may be identified as a small pit that intermittently drains clear or mucoid secretions.[5] Cartilaginous remnants of the second branchial arch may be present in the same areas. Cysts originating from branchial structures usually present later in childhood or in adulthood,[5,7] and cysts originating from the first branchial cleft are much less common than those of second origin.[7] Lymphangiomas, cystic hygromas, and hemangiomas that were occult during the newborn examination may become apparent at this time. Thyroglossal duct remnant lesions may first make their appearance in this age group, although they more frequently present in the child over 2 years of age.

The abdomen

Abdominal examination is again important in this age group. In the asymptomatic patient, tumors of renal and adrenal origin may be palpable and anomalies of the genitourinary system identified. Hepatic tumors may be signaled by marked hepatomegaly, and cystic lesions of the mesentery and ovaries together with duplications of the intestine present as masses that are cystic and highly mobile.

The heart

The heart should be examined carefully at this time for murmurs that may have been inapparent in the immediate newborn period. That is particularly likely to be the case if a ventricular septal defect is present. Although most asymptomatic murmurs are of little consequence, note should be made of them and the child evaluated over the ensuing months for any evidence of cyanosis or fatigue. Eventually, an electrocardiogram and chest x-ray films should be obtained and a cardiology consultation sought, especially if the child is to undergo anesthesia for a surgical procedure.

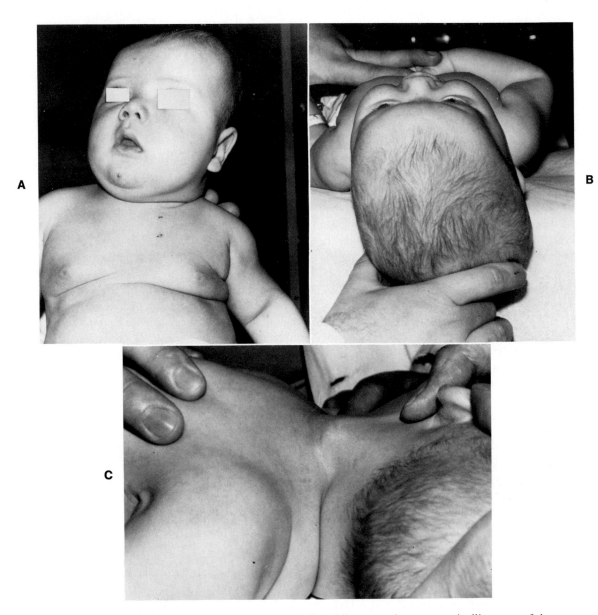

Fig. 14-1. A, Marked facial asymmetry and skull molding secondary to a torticollis tumor of the left side of the sternocleidomastoid muscle. In **B,** the molding and obliquity of the anteroposterior (AP) diameter of the skull is seen when the face is placed in the straightforward position. **C** shows the tight sternocleidomastoid muscle on the left side with the visible and palpable ''tumor.''

The rectum

Although in the small infant a careful rectal examination may be difficult to perform in the immediate newborn period, it should be the intent of the primary care physician to achieve such an examination at some time in the child's early life. If it is postponed during the newborn physical examination, it should be accomplished whenever the anatomic size allows it. Only by this means can pelvic sacrococcygeal teratoma and anterior myelomeningocele be discovered. Although both of these lesions are rare, they must be detected early. This is particularly true of the intrapelvic sacrococcygeal teratoma, because the longer this lesion is left untreated beyond the age of 1 month, the greater the propensity for malignancy.[1,6]

The genitalia

Evaluation of the genitalia should be undertaken at this time. In the male infant, the position of the testicles should be carefully ascertained and any hernias that may have become apparent noted. A hydrocele noted on the newborn examination should be followed carefully over the next 6 months, and a hydrocele inapparent on the newborn examination that develops subsequently should be considered a hernia.

In the female infant, careful evaluation of the vaginal introitus and the rest of the vulvar area for cysts or prolapse of the urethra should be performed.

The extremities

Finally, the extremities should again be carefully examined and the joint range of motion ascertained. Particularly, the ability to fully "frog leg" the hips should be demonstrated and any questions investigated.

REFERENCES

1. Izant, R. J., Jr., and Filston, H. C.: Sacrococcygeal teratomas: analysis of forty-three cases, Am. J. Surg. **130:** 617, 1975.
2. Kiesewetter, W. B., and others: Neonatal torticollis, J.A.M.A. **157:**1281, 1955.
3. Ling, C. M.: The influence of age on the results of open sternomastoid tenotomy in muscular torticollis, Clin. Orthop. **116:**142, 1976.
4. Mickelson, M. R., Cooper, R. R., and Ponseti, I. V.: Ultrastructure of the sternocleidomastoid muscle in muscular torticollis, Clin. Orthop. **110:**11, 1975.
5. Moore, K. L.: The developing human: clinically oriented embryology, Philadelphia, 1973, W. B. Saunders Co., pp. 136-166.
6. Ravitch, M. M.: Sacrococcygeal teratoma. In Ravitch, M. M., and others, editors: Pediatric Surgery, Chicago, 1979, ed. 3, Year Book Medical Publishers, Inc., p. 1117.
7. Telander, R. L., and Deane, S. A.: Thyroglossal and branchial cleft cysts and sinuses, Surg. Clin. North Am. **57:** 779, 1977.

CHAPTER 15

Specific problems

HOWARD C. FILSTON

VOMITING
Nonbilious vomiting

Although many babies are "spitters," frank vomiting of significant portions of a feeding should be considered a sign of either esophageal dysfunction or intestinal obstruction. The two most common causes of vomiting of nonbilious material relate to pharyngeal and esophageal dysmotility, which occasionally may be associated with minimally brain-damaged infants and with dysfunction of the gastroesophageal junction in gastroesophageal reflux.[32] The latter is becoming increasingly recognized, not only as a cause of vomiting in the infant, but also in association with such problems as failure to thrive, chronic aspiration, and abnormal positioning (opisthotonos, Sandifer's syndrome)[13,15,34]; it may even play a role in sudden infant death syndrome.[41] Furthermore, chronic gastroesophageal reflux may lead to esophagitis and subsequent stricture formation.

When the child's vomiting is persistent and is accompanied by failure to gain weight or a decrease in the volume and number of stools, further investigation is warranted. Beginning at about 2½ weeks of life and running through to about 3 months of life, pyloric stenosis is a common cause of such vomiting. Classically associated with first-born male infants, it occurs in both sexes and without regard to birth order. Its management is discussed further in the material on acute abdominal emergencies.

Bilious vomiting

Bilious vomiting should also be considered a sign of mechanical obstruction of the gastrointestinal tract. Although bilious vomiting may be associated with sepsis and occasionally with severe congestive heart failure, it is most often the primary sign of upper gastrointestinal obstruction. The obstruction obviously must be beyond the entrance of the common duct into the duodenum to present with bilious vomiting. Although in the immediate newborn period duodenal atresia and an annular pancreas may be the cause of bilious vomiting, once the patency of the gastrointestinal tract has been demonstrated, bilious vomiting almost invariably represents an acute obstruction of the gastrointestinal tract. The most likely cause of such an obstruction is volvulus due to malrotation of the mesentery. The threat of strangulation obstruction resulting in necrosis of the entire small intestine is ever present in this entity. Bilious vomiting should, therefore, always be looked on as an emergency situation requiring immediate demonstration of the patency of the gastrointestinal tract and normal configuration of the mesentery. If patency cannot be demonstrated, emergency surgery must be performed to avoid extensive bowel loss.

SUBGLOTTIC STENOSIS FROM INTUBATION INJURY

As more and smaller infants have been successfully managed through the respiratory difficulties of the newborn period, complications of therapeutic intervention for support of respiratory function in the infant have become a problem. It was recognized early that the cuffed endotracheal tubes utilized for adults often caused pressure necrosis of the infant's airway, and these were soon abandoned. However, they were replaced with tightly fitting plastic endotracheal

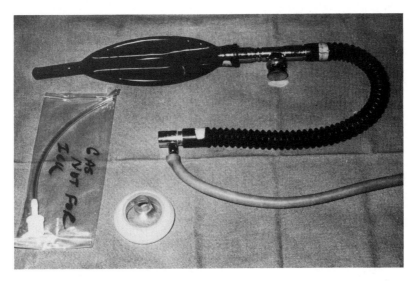

Fig. 15-1. Equipment used for airway management in infants includes a small mask, a bag with an adjustable "pop off" for pressure release, and an inlet tubing for high-flow oxygen intake entering as close as possible to the endotracheal tube. In the sterile package is an uncuffed straight plastic tube with an appropriately sized connector of the type recommended for use in infants.

tubes, some of which caused considerable tissue reaction. The size tube selected often was one that would fit snugly through the infant's larynx; the anatomic difference in the infant's airway, which makes the cricoid or subglottic area narrower than the laryngeal opening itself, unlike in the adult,[33] was not realized. Consequently, until a few years ago when this fact was widely appreciated, many infants who were managed for neonatal ventilatory problems with endotracheal intubation developed severe subglottic stenosis, often requiring a secondary tracheostomy and prolonged and often frustrating attempts to reopen the proximal airway.[45]

The recent use of plastic endotracheal tubes of low tissue reactivity sized to fit loosely through the infant's airway has all but eliminated this problem despite prolonged periods of endotracheal intubation in the tiniest infants (Fig. 15-1). Nonetheless, there still are considerable numbers of infants who have subglottic damage from intubation injury. Additional infants have intubations with inappropriate (type or size) tubes for other reasons than neonatal respiratory problems, and the subglottic stenosis that they develop may defy the most knowledgeable and extensive attempts at treatment.

Clinical presentation. These infants may show signs of acute airway obstruction at the time of attempted extubation, or they may develop it insidiously over the course of several months as increasing tidal volumes required by growth of the infant make the narrowed airway inadequate. Mild cases may present with inspiratory stridor, but severe cases usually present with acute obstructive airway symptoms immediately on removal of the endotracheal tube.

Evaluation. Evaluation for the mildly symptomatic patient should include lateral airway films followed by bronchoscopy and laryngoscopy utilizing the optical telescopic infant endoscope. Obviously, for the child who has acute airway obstruction, emergency reintubation must precede these diagnostic procedures. Rarely is an emergency tracheostomy necessary, since translaryngeal intubation can usually be accomplished even in severe subglottic stenosis.

Medical versus surgical treatment. There is no medical therapy for subglottic stenosis, since it is a scar resulting from compression ischemia to the mucosa and underlying structures of the trachea. The necrotic tissues heal with the formation of granulation tissue, which is replaced by fibroblasts and collagen, forming a narrowing scar at the level of the compression.

Surgical options. Surgical therapy has involved a combination of careful excision of the scar in small segments, often followed by the use of intraluminal stents.[35,52] Usually, a tracheostomy has been required to maintain safe airway control while the stenosis is being treated. Additional aids to reconstruction are dilatation of the narrowed area and the injection of steroids directly into the scarred tissue.[51] Successful therapy may take months to years to accomplish, during which time the child must be managed with a tracheostomy. If the parents can be taught to manage the tracheostomy and its potential complications, the child may be managed at home between surgical procedures.

Despite all efforts, some of these children are not reparable in the infant age group and may have to await subsequent excision of the scarred area of the trachea and reconstruction, which is more likely to be successful later in childhood.

• • •

These surgical procedures are difficult ones; special equipment and experience is required to carry through a highly individualized therapeutic program. A few centers around the country have been particularly successful in dealing with these children, and the primary care physician should seek out such expert help when presented with a patient with such problems.

This problem is extremely serious, damaging, and costly; its prevention through proper airway management and the use of properly selected and sized intubation equipment is mandatory.

ACUTE ABDOMINAL EMERGENCIES
Malrotation

The most dire emergency in the infant age group is that of malrotation. This anomaly relates to the attachment of the mesentery to the posterior peritoneal wall. As the embryo develops, the gastrointestinal tract elongates faster than the embryo, and therefore loops out into a ventral herniation, sometimes called a herniation into the cord.[49] At approximately 12 weeks of gestation, the gastrointestinal tract, having formed in this herniated position, returns to the peritoneal cavity. By this time, the body wall is further developed and only the ventral defect exists. The gastrointestinal tract, as it returns to the peritoneal cavity, undergoes two separate 270-degree rotations: one of the proximal bowel, involving primarily the duodenum, and one of the distal bowel, involving primarily the colon.[8] The proximal bowel, beginning at the distal esophagus, undergoes rotation as follows: The stomach flops over to the left side (this is not part of the rotation). Beginning at the pylorus, the duodenum rotates 270 degrees counterclock-

wise, with the junction of the duodenum and the jejunum coming to a point well up behind the stomach in the mid–left upper quadrant. There, it attaches firmly to the posterior peritoneum by peritoneal folds known as the ligament of Treitz. The colon, beginning at the upper rectum, rotates 270 degrees counterclockwise, forming the sigmoid, descending colon, transverse colon, and ascending colon, with the ileocecal junction coming to rest and being attached to the posterior peritoneum well into the right lower quadrant.

These two rotations effectively spread the base of the small bowel mesentery, that is, the broad folds carrying the superior mesenteric artery to the jejunum and ileum, across the longest distance measurable in a rectangle: the diagonal across the two corners. This broad attachment of the mesentery ensures that the vital superior mesenteric artery cannot be strangled by twisting (volvulus) of the mesenteric base.

Malrotation may exist in any degree, but in its most severe form, both the proximal and distal 270-degree counterclockwise rotations are incomplete, the duodenal loop ending to the right of or just overlying the spine and the "pseudo ligament of Treitz" being in the mid–upper abdomen, overlying the origin of the superior mesenteric artery. Concomitantly, the transverse colon and ascending colon rotation are incomplete and the cecum frequently turns back on itself, coming to rest in the right upper quadrant. The two points of fixation (ligament of Treitz and the ileocecal area) are superimposed on one another and overlie the base of the superior mesenteric artery. Thus, the previously broad-based mesentery now arises from a single point, like an oriental fan, and can easily undergo volvulus or rotation, usually clockwise, around the base of the superior mesenteric artery, leading to strangulation obstruction of first the venous and then the arterial supply to the entire small intestine. Ischemic necrosis and death of the entire small intestine, including the ascending colon and transverse colon, may ensue, since this is the part of the intestine supplied by the superior mesenteric artery.

Lesser degrees of malrotation may exist anatomically, but these are rarely provable short of laparotomy. Therefore, the identification of any degree of malrotation should suggest ischemic necrosis of the intestine and urgent surgery should be accomplished.

Malrotation is rarely symptomatic unless volvulus has already occurred. It is, therefore, best to consider that volvulus has ensued when a child has symptoms of upper gastrointestinal obstruction and a malrotation is identified. Asymptomatic cases of malrotation have occasionally been identified in the newborn period when x-ray studies were obtained for other purposes. Delay in treatment may be warranted in the asymptomatic patient if other illnesses preclude safe surgery. The malrotation can then be corrected when these preexisting conditions are eliminated.

The importance of malrotation cannot be overemphasized; it is the most serious and most frequent cause of intestinal obstruction seen in the nursery. It greatly outnumbers all other causes of small bowel obstruction.

Hypertrophic pyloric stenosis

A more frequent but less serious entity causing obstruction in the infant-toddler age group is hypertrophic pyloric stenosis. As noted previously, this entity has classically been associated with firstborn male infants; but it can occur in both sexes and in any birth order. It rarely presents before the child is 2½ weeks of age and is frequently found in children between the ages of 3 weeks and 2 months. It should be suspected

in any child who has persistent vomiting of nonbilious material, especially if the child shows failure to thrive and a decrease in the volume and number of stools.

Careful physical examination will identify most cases of hypertrophic pyloric stenosis. In the suspect infant, a nasogastric tube should be passed and the gastric contents emptied and noted. The tube should be left in place for frequent aspiration during examination, because these babies cry and are massive air swallowers. It is almost impossible to feel a small pyloric "tumor" under a massively dilated, air-filled stomach. It would be like trying to feel an olive through an inflated balloon.

Once the stomach is emptied, the pyloric tumor is easily palpable. It is best felt by lying the infant with the head to the examiner's left. The examiner's right hand should grasp the infant's feet and ankles and gently rock them back and forth over the abdomen. This maneuver releases the strain on the rectus muscle and makes abdominal palpation easier. The examiner's left hand should then come down over the xiphoid and carefully and gently palpate the edge of the liver (Fig. 15-2). The liver should be retracted and the epi-

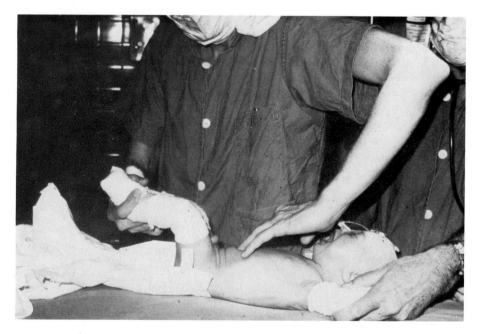

Fig. 15-2. Successful palpation of the hypertrophic pyloric mass of pyloric stenosis requires that the infant's stomach be decompressed with a nasogastric tube, that the stretch be relieved from the rectus muscle by gently moving the lower extremities up and down, and that the examiner's left hand gently palpate over the edge of the liver into the epigastrium, with the examiner's fingers rolling in a craniocaudal motion, seeking the transversely oriented "olive tumor."

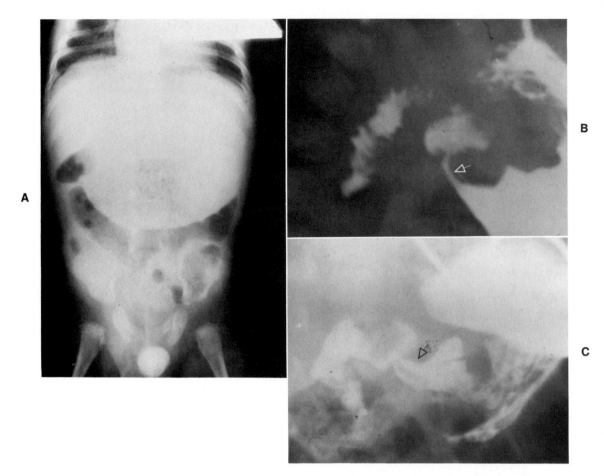

Fig. 15-3. **A,** Plain abdominal radiograph of an infant with hypertrophic pyloric stenosis showing the overfilled stomach with its greater curvature outlined by the gas-filled lumen of the tranverse colon. **B,** Total reliance on the upper gastrointestinal contrast study may mislead the surgeon into operating for a nonexistent hypertrophic pyloric stenosis. This view shows a narrowed pylorus (arrow) in a case of pylorospasm. **C,** A subsequent view shows relaxation and widening of the area (arrow).

gastrium gently palpated. Relaxation of the abdominal wall is enhanced by feeding the child sugar water or formula during the examination. (Having an assistant during the examination is helpful.) Gentle probing of the epigastrium, with the examiner's fingers rocking in a craniocaudal direction, will often suffice to engage the small pyloric tumor. The examination should be gentle, and progress should be slow. Rapid, firm pressure in the epigastrium will be countered by resistance from the infant, and the tumor will not be appreciated.

If a typical tumor is palpable, radiologic examination is unnecessary and the child can be referred to a surgeon for further evaluation and treatment. Upper gastrointestinal evaluation should be

performed when significant obstruction is suspected but the lesion is not palpable. Doing so will expedite referral, but the surgeon who performs surgery for pyloric stenosis on the basis of the x-ray film alone is risking a surgical procedure that may prove unnecessary. The tumor should be palpated in all cases where pyloric stenosis is the primary diagnosis. Esophageal reflux and esophageal dysmotility problems may be associated with pylorospasm and may appear similar to pyloric stenosis on upper gastrointestinal radiographs (Fig. 15-3). If the tumor is not palpable on the initial examination, reexamination at frequent intervals is warranted. The child should be carefully observed for signs of dehydration and malnutrition. Early referral to an experienced

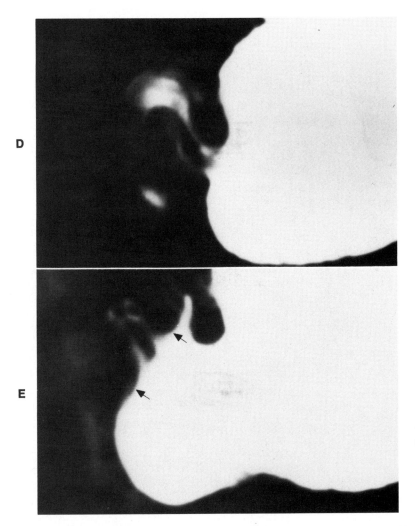

Fig. 15-3, cont'd. D, Another example of narrowing of the pylorus with "railroad tracking." **E,** A "mass effect" of a pyloric "tumor" impinging on the distal antrum (arrows) is suggested. This child had an obstruction of the pylorus and proximal duodenum by an enlarging choledochal cyst.

Continued.

pediatric surgeon will often expedite treatment and avoid the ravages of malnutrition and dehydration that were so common in these children in the past.

When pyloric stenosis is the disease entity encountered, the parents can be reassured that this is one of the "happy" lesions of childhood. Although any illness in a child is difficult to accept, at least this one is almost overwhelmingly associated with a successful surgical procedure, a short hospital stay, and a lifelong cure.

Intussusception

The third of the common gastrointestinal lesions in the infant-toddler period is that of intussusception, perhaps the most difficult one to diagnose.

It classically occurs in the otherwise healthy child between 3 months and 2 years of age, although it frequently occurs beyond this period. Occasional cases are seen in children younger than 3 months of age.[66,70] This is the age group of the so-called idiopathic intussusception, in which no anatomic leading point is identifiable. Actually, almost all of these cases are associated with an anatomic leading point, that is, the hypertrophied Peyer's patch. Beyond the age of 2 years, idiopathic intussusception continues to occur but the incidence of other anatomic leading points such as intussuscepted Meckel's diverticulum and polyps becomes more frequent.[60]

Clinical presentation. Symptoms of intussusception are commonly described as those of intes-

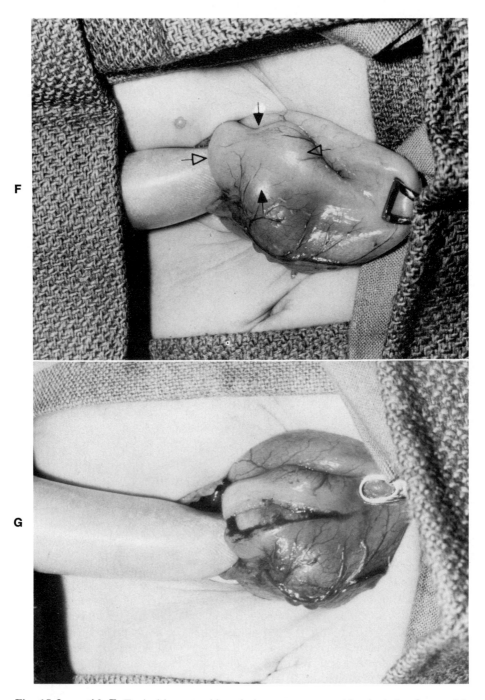

Fig. 15-3, cont'd. F, Typical hypertrophic pyloric tumor supported by the index finger of the operating surgeon. The linear extent is represented by the open arrows and the width by the closed arrows. **G,** Completed pyloromyotomy showing the fracture of the muscle layers of the hypertrophied pylorus down to the mucosa with the incision extending well up onto the antral surface. (**B** and **C** courtesy Donald Kirks, M.D., Durham, N.C. **F** and **G** from Filston, H. C., and Izant, R.: The surgical neonate: evaluation and care, New York, 1978, Appleton-Century-Crofts.)

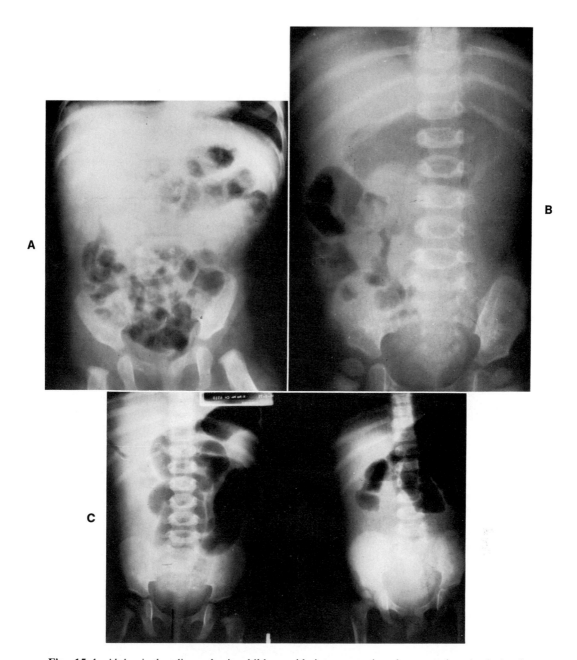

Fig. 15-4. Abdominal radiographs in children with intussusception demonstrating the lack of specificity of findings for this entity and emphasizing the need for performing barium enema studies when appropriate symptoms are present in the age group at risk. **C** is suggestive of intussusception in that there is a sparsity of bowel gas on the right side of the abdomen.

tinal obstruction associated with bloody stools. Classically, therefore, one would see bilious vomiting, abdominal distention, and currant jelly–like stools. However, bloody stools occur in only 30% to 50% of patients. Blatant signs of intestinal obstruction, such as bilious vomiting and distention, are late signs in intussusception. In order to diagnose this entity early, when treatment may be successful and bowel loss and death avoided, the subtle signs of early intussusception must be appreciated. The typical case is one of a healthy infant who suddenly begins having discomfort. Often the only sign is that of irritability in an otherwise healthy child. When the parents are good historians, they can often pinpoint the exact time that the infant began having symptoms, such as on awakening from his afternoon nap. Questioning them about intermittency of the pain must be done carefully. The question, ''Does the pain come and go?'' may not register with them if the symptoms have continued over a 6- or 8-hour period. The fact that the child's symptoms seem worse for a few minutes, then better for a few minutes, especially if they are associated with drawing-up of the knees, is highly suggestive of the crampy pain associated with intussusception.

Evaluation. Physical examination early in the course of intussusception may be unrewarding, since the abdomen is usually soft and no peritoneal signs are present. Frequently, with careful examination, a sausagelike mass may be appreciated. One must be willing to do barium enemas in the face of minimal symptoms in this age group in order to diagnose the lesion early in its course. At this stage, abdominal films usually are nonspecific (Fig. 15-4). Occasionally, the intussusceptum can be seen in an air-filled colon, but this event cannot be totally relied on.

Medical versus surgical treatment. Hydrostatic barium enema reduction, rather than surgical correction, should be attempted whenever the diagnosis of intussusception is made and peritonitis in not present. Obviously, known perforation of the gastrointestinal tract would be a contraindication to hydrostatic reduction; but duration of symptoms is not a contraindication, nor is the presence of obstructive signs on the plain abdom-

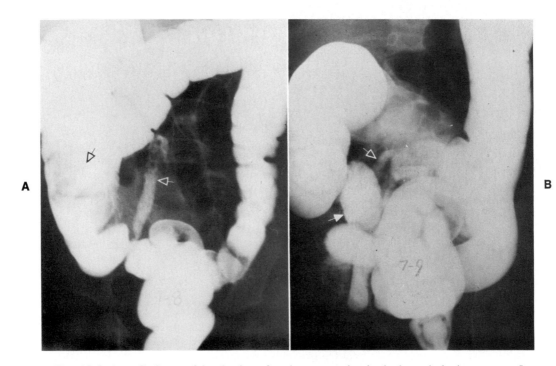

Fig. 15-5. A to **C,** Successful reduction of an intussusception by hydrostatic barium enema. In **A,** the intussusceptum is reduced only to the cecum (open black arrow) and the filling of the appendix, indicated by the open white arrow, could be mistaken for filling of the distal ileum. In **B,** the intussusceptum is completely reduced and the closed white arrow indicates filling of the distal ileum. The open white arrow again indicates the filled appendix originally seen in **A.**

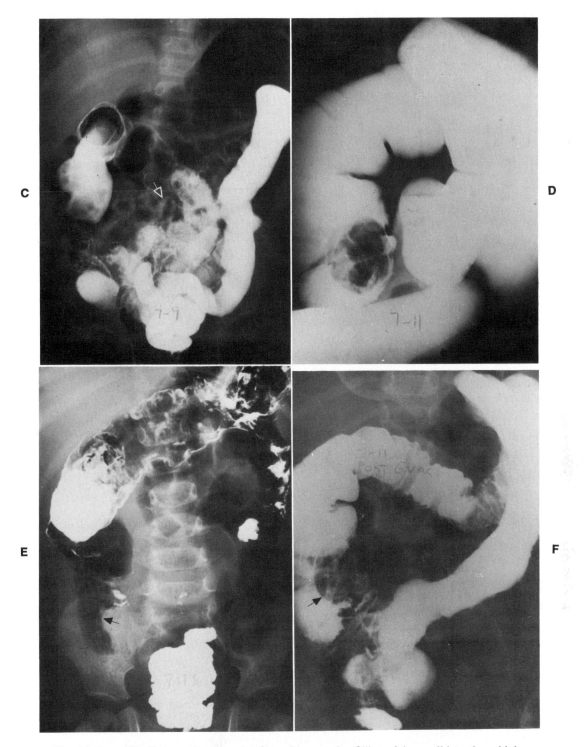

Fig. 15-5, cont'd. C shows the emptying film with extensive filling of the small intestine with barium. The open white arrow again indicates the appendix. **D** to **F,** Unsuccessful reduction of an intussusceptum by hydrostatic barium enema. **D** shows the intussusceptum reduced to the cecum with no filling of small bowel. Despite repeated attempts and prolonged pressure, **E** still reveals a filling defect in the distal cecum with no filling of the small intestine. The arrows in **E** and **F,** the emptying film, show the persistence of the intussusceptum at the ileocecal area.

inal films, although this idea is controversial.[58,60] Careful attention to the technique of the procedure is important, however. A pressure balloon should never be used in the rectum, since it is the most common cause of perforation of the rectum. It may slip out of the confined pelvic space into the upper rectum, expanding rapidly and tearing the rectum. The height of the barium column should be carefully controlled and kept between 30 to 36 inches; undue manipulation of the mass is contraindicated. Several attempts may be made to reduce the mass with periods of evacuation between. However, if two good pressure columns are held for 10 minutes and the mass fails to reduce, hydrostatic reduction should be abandoned.

Successful reduction is recognized by the free reflux of barium well into multiple small bowel loops (Fig. 15-5). Entry into the distal ileum alone may be associated with persistent ileoileal intussusception and a recurrence of the ileocolic intussusception on discontinuance of the hydrostatic pressure.

If successful reduction is accomplished by barium enema, recurrence is probably no more common than with reduction by surgical manipulation. Follow-up x-ray films should be obtained over the next day or so to ensure that the intussusception has not recurred. Obviously, the child's clinical course must be followed carefully, as

well. Repeated immediate recurrences of the intussusception should lead to surgical correction, but repeated episodes of intussusception at significant intervals of weeks or months should not be considered a contraindication to attempting subsequent hydrostatic reductions. It is probably unlikely that a significant anatomic leading point can be completely reduced.[20]

Prognosis. Intussusception, when diagnosed early, can be a benign lesion amenable to hydrostatic or surgical therapy. Bowel loss is unusual under these circumstances. On the other hand, when the diagnosis is missed for several days, severe intestinal obstruction and strangulated gangrenous necrosis of the bowel may occur; and this entity, with its ensuing sepsis, may be lethal.

Other abdominal emergencies

Appendicitis is fortunately rare in this age group[26,55]: fortunately, because it is so unlikely to be diagnosed before perforation and peritonitis occur. Although it cannot be completely discounted in the etiology of the acute abdominal condition, of equal importance are such entities as perforation of an inflamed Meckel's diverticulum and closed loop obstructions and volvulus around persistent omphalomesenteric remnants.[49]

Meckel's diverticulum is said to occur in approximately 2% of the population and is symp-

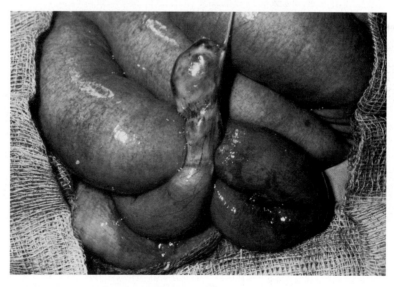

Fig. 15-6. Meckel's diverticulum. This inflamed diverticulum has adhered to a loop of bowel in such a way that a second loop of bowel has herniated beneath the diverticulum, causing a closed loop obstruction.

tomatic in 25% of those who have it. Common consequences of Meckel's diverticulum include inflammation, perforation, ulceration with bleeding, and intussusception.[7] The inflamed diverticulum may present with the symptoms of appendicitis, or it may adhere to an adjacent loop of bowel, leading to internal herniation of a third loop with resultant obstruction and possibly strangulation necrosis (Fig. 15-6). The history is that of a fairly rapid progression of an abdominal illness similar to appendicitis, including fever, leukocytosis, abdominal pain, and peritoneal signs. The child usually presents a clear-cut picture of having an acute abdominal condition and often undergoes surgery for appendicitis. In our experience, Meckel's diverticulitis is so frequent in this age group that we frequently make the preoperative diagnosis of Meckel's diverticulitis, rather than appendicitis. The complications of a persistent *omphalomesenteric duct* are discussed in the next section.

UMBILICAL LESIONS: OMPHALOMESENTERIC DUCT REMNANTS, PERSISTENT URACHAL REMNANTS, AND HERNIAS

The embryo is nourished by a yolk sac that is a diverticulum off of the primitive gastrointestinal tract.[49] This yolk sac functions as a source of nutrients for the child until the placental circulation is well established. Subsequent to good placental function, the yolk sac and its stalk should atrophy. Persistence may take varying forms, including persistence of the entire duct out into the cord, persistence of the duct as a patent fistula from the small bowel to the umbilicus, persistence of the ligamentous attachment between the small bowel and the umbilical area with or without the development of cysts within the remnant, and persistence of a diverticulum at the site of the omphalomesenteric duct, which is Meckel's diverticulum.

The most serious consequence of the persistence of an *omphalomesenteric duct remnant* when it is ligamentous is volvulus of a loop of intestine with strangulation obstruction around the ligamentous remnant (Fig. 15-7). As in the case of Meckel's diverticulitis, this lesion presents as an acute abdominal condition including peritonitis. It can be suspected by the accompanying picture of small bowel obstruction, although such obstruction may also be present in long-standing appendicitis or diverticulitis.

When either a persistent omphalomesenteric duct or a patent urachus is present, the umbilical stump fails to heal and frank drainage of bowel

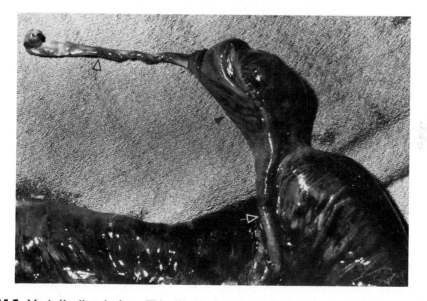

Fig. 15-7. Meckel's diverticulum. This diverticulum had a ligamentous omphalomesenteric duct remnant extending to the umbilicus, around which a loop of ileum underwent volvulus, producing a strangulation obstruction. The ligamentous remnant is illustrated by the open black arrow, Meckel's diverticulum by the closed black arrow, and the vitelline vessel supplying Meckel's diverticulum and the omphalomesenteric remnant by the open white arrow.

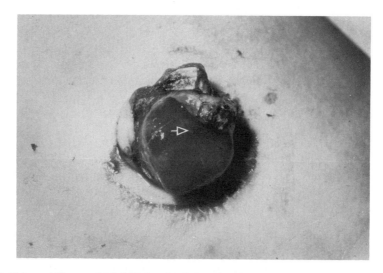

Fig. 15-8. This umbilicus, which failed to heal, has the appearance of mucosa. The arrow points to a fistula tract representing the lumen of a persistent omphalomesenteric duct remnant. (From Filston, H. C., and Izant, R.: The surgical neonate: evaluation and care, New York, 1978, Appleton-Century-Crofts.)

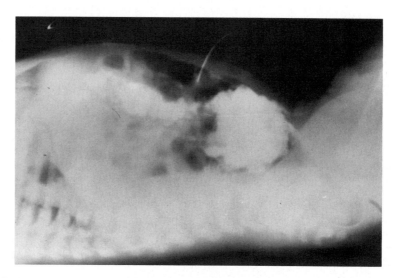

Fig. 15-9. Contrast injection of the fistula tract seen in Fig. 15-8 reveals communication with the intestinal tract, confirming an omphalomesenteric duct remnant. The radiopaque catheter can be seen entering the fistula tract at the umbilicus.

contents or urine may be noted. The differential diagnosis is that of a granuloma persisting at the umbilical site. Careful inspection may reveal a lumen in the granulation tissue, indicating a patent fistula to the bladder or the bowel (Fig. 15-8). This finding can be confirmed by inserting a small plastic catheter, injecting radiopaque dye, and obtaining an x-ray film (Fig. 15-9). When only granulation tissue is apparent and no sinus tract

can be identified, thorough cauterization of the granulation tissue, removing it down below the epithelial surface, will allow healing of the epithelium over the area. If this maneuver fails, further workup for a persistent embryologic remnant is indicated.

Urachal remnants may be completely patent from the bladder to the umbilical area, or they may present as cysts, frequently becoming in-

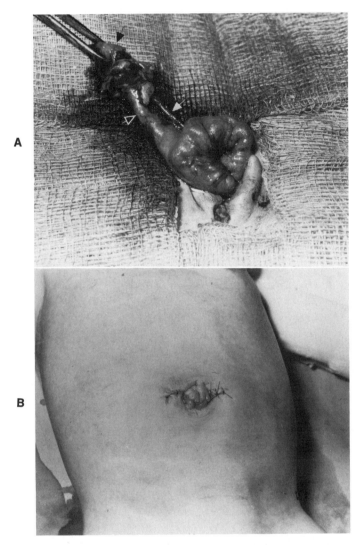

Fig. 15-10. A, Persistent omphalomesenteric duct remnant (open white arrow) extending to the umbilicus (black arrow) from the loop of ileum. The vitelline vessel is illustrated by the closed white arrow. **B,** An excellent cosmetic result is achieved by reconstructing the umbilicus following the excision.

fected and presenting as abscesses between the umbilicus and the suprapubic area. Such cysts, when infected, should be initially drained and then completely excised. A patent urachus or an omphalomesenteric remnant can be removed through an incision incorporating the umbilical remnant. The latter can then be closed and the umbilicus reconstructed in such a fashion that the operative site is completely hidden in the umbilical folds (Fig. 15-10).

Umbilical hernias represent persistent defects in the linea alba at the point of entry of the umbilical vessels. Failure of closure in this area is common, particularly in black children. Except in the infrequent event of incarceration of bowel loops within the umbilical hernia, urgent treatment is unnecessary. Most of these hernias can be observed over the course of 2 to 3 years and the degree of closure evaluated. If the child has shown no evidence of closure of a significant defect by the age of 2 years, herniorrhaphy should be accomplished any time thereafter. For many children over the age of 2, the umbilical hernia becomes a source of emotional concern as other children tease them about it. If that becomes a problem, earlier surgery is probably warranted.

On the other hand, a closing defect can be watched through the entire childhood years if progress is being made in closure without surgery. These defects should all be repaired before pregnancy or before extensive participation in athletics in either sex.

Although it is noted that umbilical hernias rarely become incarcerated, when they do, it often leads to ischemic necrosis of the bowel. Even when reduction can be accomplished by manual manipulation, recurrence of the incarceration is common. Therefore, incarceration should be an indication for early surgical repair of the defect.

Other lesions occur in the linea alba and are known as ventral hernias or epiploceles. These are usually defects in the linea alba between the xiphoid and the umbilicus; and since the falciform ligament is attached in this area, only preperitoneal fat herniates through the defect. The lesion usually presents as a small tender lump in the midline, which may on occasion be quite painful and tender. If the lesion is symptomatic, it can be repaired in early infancy; or repair can be postposed until later childhood, when it can be done with the child under local anesthesia, if desired.

CONSTIPATION (HIRSCHSPRUNG'S DISEASE)

Constipation occurring in early infancy should always raise the question of Hirschsprung's disease or aganglionic megacolon. Most infants are not constipated. Occasionally, one finds that when the child goes home, the parents mix the formula incorrectly, causing constipation. Other reasons for constipation exist, but Hirschsprung's disease should always be considered a possibility in the early infancy period when constipation is a problem. As noted in Chapter 10 in the section on the newborn, 95% of normal infants will pass meconium within the first 24 hours in the nursery and will continue to establish a normal stool pattern. These infants continue to have a normal stool pattern as they leave the hospital and go home. The child who fails to pass meconium normally in the hospital or who, early in infancy, develops constipation is a candidate for a thorough workup for Hirschsprung's disease. The importance of this workup cannot be overemphasized, since Hirschsprung's disease is a common lesion occurring several times more frequently than all of the congenital atresias put together.

Evaluation. Evaluation of the infant for Hirsch-

sprung's disease should consist of a careful physical examination, with the examiner noting distention of the abdomen and whether stool can be palpated in the colonic loops. Rectal examination will frequently confirm the absence of stool in the rectum, although this sign of Hirschsprung's disease is less reliable in this age group. Plain films of the abdomen will show dilated loops of bowel, and these will probably be colonic loops.

It must be recognized that the identification of Hirschsprung's disease cannot be made with certainty on plain films in the child under 2 years of age. Any suggestion of Hirschsprung's disease or obstructed loops on the plain films should lead to a barium enema study performed by a knowledgeable radiologist. The common location for the transition zone in Hirschsprung's disease is in the sigmoid colon or upper rectum, and the best views for evaluating this are the postevacuation films of the barium enema (see Fig. 10-34). Water-soluble contrast media should not be used for contrast studies of infants suspected of having Hirschsprung's disease. They may give a false-negative picture, since the infant may empty the irritating material. Retention of the barium is an important sign of Hirschsprung's disease.

If a clear-cut transition zone cannot be identified, the infant should be observed without stimulation for 24 hours and follow-up films obtained. Prolonged failure to empty the barium is a sign of Hirschsprung's disease and should lead to rectal biopsy if a transition zone cannot be identified (see Fig. 10-35).

Interpretation of a rectal biopsy may be a difficult procedure, especially for a pathologist who is not experienced with Hirschsprung's disease. Ganglion cells typically have large nuclei with inclusion bodies and heavily staining cytoplasm. They are classically "kite shaped" (Fig. 15-11). Other large cells with large nuclei may be misidentified as ganglion cells. When true ganglion cells are identified, Hirschsprung's disease is ruled out. However, the absence of ganglion cells in one or two sections of the rectal biopsy does not prove that Hirschsprung's disease is present, because ganglion cells are scattered throughout the myenteric plexus and every section may not contain a ganglion cell. Therefore, it is necessary that the pathologist make several major "steps" through the tissue and then make several sections of each step. After as many as 20 to 40 sections with no ganglion cells have been examined, the

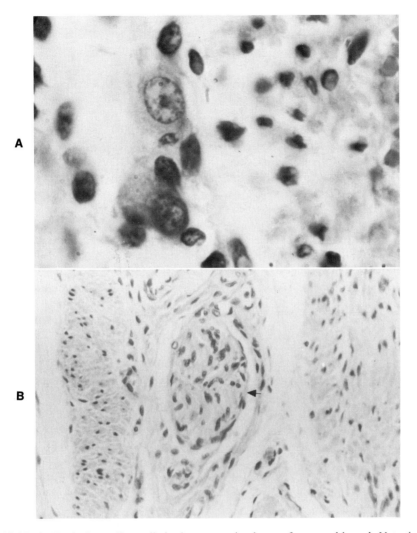

Fig. 15-11. A, Typical ganglion cells in the myenteric plexus of a normal bowel. Note their "kite shape" and their large nuclei with distinct nuclear material and prominent stippled cytoplasm. **B,** Myenteric plexus of a child with Hirschsprung's disease with absence of ganglion cells and a hypertrophied nerve bundle (arrow).

diagnosis of Hirschsprung's disease can be confirmed.

Even with this careful histopathologic treatment, mistakes are still occasionally made. Therefore, it is difficult to understand the enthusiasm for suction mucosal biopsies or punch biopsies, which give the pathologist minimal tissue with which to work.[17,62] These superficial or mucosal biopsies depend on identification of ganglion cells in the submucous plexus of Meissner, an identification that is more difficult to make for most pathologists than is that of Auerbach's plexus. We have, therefore, continued to prefer full-thickness rectal biopsy for the diagnosis of Hirsch-

sprung's disease, as do the majority of pediatric surgeons.[38]

Mucosal suction biopsies may be a reasonable screening mechanism, since they can be done easily, without anesthesia. If definite ganglion cells are seen, no further biopsy is necessary; but if the ganglion cells are not found in the suction biopsy specimen, a full-thickness biopsy should be obtained. Because this diagnosis can be difficult for even the most experienced pathologist, it is difficult to condone the practice of performing such biopsies in isolated medical facilities where the pathologist has little experience and rarely sees these lesions.

Medical versus surgical treatment. As noted in Chapter 10, some individuals occasionally try to tide the infant through with colonic washouts; but the risk of pseudomembranous enterocolitis is so great that doing so subjects the child to a potential hazard. Once the diagnosis is confirmed by either the classic findings on barium enema study or by rectal biopsy, the child should have a colostomy carefully placed in the ganglion-containing bowel just proximal to the transition zone and the presence of ganglion cells in the colostomy site should be confirmed by frozen section. A loop colostomy with all layers of the abdominal wall carefully sutured to the bowel to prevent herniation of the small bowel around the colostomy will provide the child with good colonic functioning during the ensuing months prior to definitive therapy (see Fig. 10-37). Care of the colostomy is discussed in Chapter 7 in the section on general considerations.

Surgical options. After the dilated and hypertrophied proximal bowel has had a chance to tone up and shrink back to normal size, a process that usually requires 3 to 4 months of colostomy diversion, the definitive surgical procedure can be accomplished. We have generally preferred to have the child be 9 to 12 months of age and 18 to 20 pounds in weight, because at this size the pelvic dissection, which is the most important part of the procedure, is relatively easily accomplished. Doing the procedure with the child at a younger age and a smaller size is possible, however, and is indicated if the child has any complications of the colostomy that would make earlier surgery preferable.

Three surgical procedures and their modifications have been the common ones performed in the United States for Hirschsprung's disease. The general principles and techniques are discussed primarily to give the primary care physician some understanding of the concepts on which the operations are based and to provide the physician with the knowledge necessary to evaluate any complications that occur postoperatively. The principle on which all the operations are based is that the problem of Hirschsprung's disease will be eliminated if ganglion-containing colon can be anastomosed to the rectum within 1 cm of the anus. This procedure brings functioning ganglionated bowel, with its coordinated peristalsis, down to a level from which it can propel stool through the anus, while it still leaves the entire anal sphincter mechanism intact and functioning. It has been shown that 1 cm of aganglionic rectum can be left circumferentially without resulting in persistent symptoms of Hirschsprung's disease. Therefore, that is the goal of all of the surgical procedures.

The Swenson procedure was the first to solve satisfactorily the problem of a low anastomosis accomplished deep in the pelvis. It was devised by Swenson in 1948,[65] and it is the procedure against which all others have been measured. Because of complications with the Swenson procedure, the Duhamel procedure was devised and popularized in the late 1950s and early 1960s.[19,46] A large number of American pediatric surgeons still favor this operation today. The most popular procedure for Hirschsprung's disease in the United States today is the Boley modification of the Soave procedure.[12] This operation is an endorectal pull-through procedure in which the mucosa is stripped from the aganglionic rectal segment and the normal bowel, containing ganglion cells, is pulled through this muscular tunnel to the anal level. Each of these procedures works well in experienced hands. Nevertheless, each has its unique complications, which are discussed in Chapter 20 in the section on the child from 2 to 12.

Postoperative care. The postoperative care of these patients should be in the hands of a surgeon who has done the procedure and who is experienced in the care required for each of these major procedures. Careful anorectal dilatations are essential to achieve softening of the anastomosis and to give some elastic quality to it. Without such careful postoperative dilatations, a circumferential strictured scar will result and the child's anorectal function will be impaired.

Prognosis. Generally, children who are otherwise normal will have a good result from the definitive procedures for Hirschsprung's disease, and their subsequent bowel functioning will be normal.[36] Particularly with the Swenson and Soave procedures, there may be some early problem with the frequency of bowel movements because the pulled-through colonic segment acts more as a propelling conduit than a rectal reservoir and may evacuate small amounts of stool very frequently. This complication may cause considerable difficulty with the perianal skin, and adequate therapy will be necessary until the child's new rectum accommodates and heals completely.

Important aspects of follow-up. The important aspects of follow-up for each of the major procedures are discussed in Chapter 20.

• • •

The infant who does not have Hirschsprung's disease but is constipated may have an anal fissure. The child may have a hard stool and tear the anal mucosa and develop a fissure. Subsequently, bowel movements are painful and the child withholds his stool, leading to dehydration of the contents and further constipation. Treatment of such infants consists of a good stool softener, which must usually be mineral oil, and sitz baths to heal the fissure. Healing may take some time to accomplish. Other stool softeners commonly used in adults are often ineffective in children. Many pediatricians object to the use of mineral oil because of the risk of lipoid pneumonia from aspiration; but if the mineral oil is always given well before bed or nap time, that is, immediately after arising from overnight sleep or a nap, this problem can be avoided.

More extensive discussion of constipation will be found in Chapter 20.

BLEEDING

Bleeding episodes in this age group fall essentially into two categories: those associated with other symptoms and those unassociated with other symptoms. Upper gastrointestinal hemorrhage in this age group is rare inasmuch as those lesions that cause upper gastrointestinal bleeding later in childhood have not had time to develop to the point of causing hemorrhage. Occasionally, a child in this age group will develop hemorrhage from a peptic ulcer or develop hemorrhagic gastritis during the course of a serious illness, but for the asymptomatic child at home in this age group to have upper gastrointestinal bleeding is unusual. Lesions such as arteriovenous malformations or hemangiomas of the bowel could lead to such bleeding at this age.

Lower gastrointestinal bleeding in the asymptomatic child in this age group is most likely to be associated with constipation and either anal fissure formation or some irritation of the rectal mucosa. Occasionally, ulcerative colitis or granulomatosis disease of the bowel develops; but again, it is most unusual. Large-volume asymptomatic bleeding wherein the blood is clearly mixed with stool rather than streaked on it is likely to be due to Meckel's diverticulum, and bleeding from Meckel's diverticulum does occur at this age. Furthermore, juvenile polyps will sometimes lead to considerable lower gastrointestinal hemorrhage.

The lesion that must always be thought of, however, when rectal bleeding, especially of dark blood with clots, is seen in the asymptomatic or relatively asymptomatic child is intussusception. As noted earlier, the symptoms of intussusception may be minimal, especially early in the disease.

An accurate impression of the extent and type of bleeding is important. When the blood is clearly streaked on the stool rather than mixed thoroughly with it, the site of bleeding is most likely lower in the bowel in the area of the rectum or anus and a fissure or irritated rectal mucosa should be suspected along with the possibility of a low-lying polyp.

Occasionally, children in this age group will develop inflammatory bowel disease, the main manifestation of which may be rectal bleeding. Chronic anemia is usually associated with this condition, and the diagnosis is usually made after other, more acute lesions have been ruled out.

ABDOMINAL MASSES

Every primary care physician caring for children must develop the technique for abdominal examination to the point of expertise. It is unfortunately the rule rather than the exception that children with intra-abdominal and retroperitoneal masses have been examined repeatedly by otherwise knowledgeable and capable physicians and the masses obviously missed. Furthermore, a consistent, thoughtful approach to abdominal examination is essential in the diagnosis of acute inflammatory conditions related to the gastrointestinal tract and peritoneal cavity.

Abnormalities of the urinary tract, several major malignant tumors, and some less common benign lesions present in the infant-toddler age group as silent abdominal masses. The best opportunity for early diagnosis of major intra-abdominal and retroperitoneal malignancies occurs at the initial and follow-up well-baby visits. The two most common malignant tumors are neuroblastoma arising in either the suprarenal gland or in the paraspinous ganglia and Wilms' tumor arising in the kidney itself. These masses are retroperitoneal, may be of any size, and are relatively

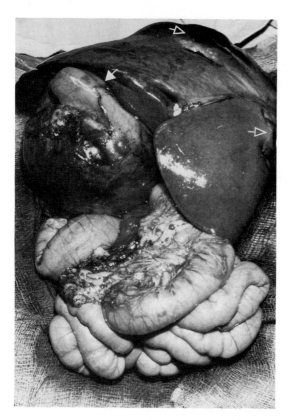

Fig. 15-12. Hepatoblastoma infiltrating extensively through both lobes of the liver. The almost unrecognizable gallbladder is seen embedded in the tumor mass (closed white arrow), and positive biopsy sites are noted in both lobes of the liver (open white arrows).

fixed. Either may cross the midline when the increase in size is great enough. The next most common abdominal malignancies are hepatoblastoma and hepatocarcinoma. Hepatocarcinoma becomes less common in the child over 2 years of age and then has a secondary incidence in adolescence. Hepatoblastoma almost always presents in a child under the age of 2 years (Fig. 15-12). Other asymptomatic causes of hepatomegaly are benign hamartomas, including hemangioendothelioma, and some of the storage diseases. Hepatomegaly should always be thoroughly investigated.

Benign masses usually present in the asymptomatic patient and are intra-abdominal. They are most often mobile and frequently can be pushed from one quadrant of the abdomen to another (see Fig. 10-44). All are unusual, but the most likely to be found are either mesenteric cysts or duplications. These are difficult to dif-

ferentiate from one another prior to surgery. They may become symptomatic before they are discovered on physical examination if they lead to intestinal obstruction. Mesenteric cysts can lead to volvulus of a portion of the mesentery or to adhesive obstructions secondary to inflammation. Duplications may become inflamed, may be the lead point of the volvulus, or may be the beginning point of an intussusception (see Fig. 10-45).

Intravenous pyelography is essential to the differentiation of retroperitoneal masses. Usually the anomalies of the urinary tract can be clearly differentiated from the retroperitoneal malignant tumors. When the mass is secondary to obstructive uropathy, hydroureter and hydronephrosis will be clearly evident. Dysplastic or multicystic kidneys, however, may show no function whatsoever on the pyelogram, a finding that supports the likelihood of a retroperitoneal mass being a dysplastic kidney. Occasionally, some contrast is apparent on the films and makes differentiation from Wilms' tumor difficult when the tumor is large with a very splayed-out caliceal system. In the past, final diagnosis had to await surgical exploration; but today, modern radiologic techniques such as ultrasound and computerized tomographic (CT) scanning may prove highly accurate in differentiating these entities.

The most common abdominal mass found in this age group is the hypertrophic pyloric tumor of pyloric stenosis, which is rarely discovered in an asymptomatic patient. Usually it is only found after being carefully sought in a child with nonbilious vomiting, as discussed previously.

Hematuria is an infrequent finding in infants unless a clear-cut urinary tract infection is present. It is occasionally noted after trauma and may lead to the discovery of a retroperitoneal mass. Hematuria developing in a child after minimal trauma has occurred should raise suspicions that a major anomaly or tumor is present in the kidney. Such underlying abnormalities are found in 10% to 25% of patients with injured kidneys and are particularly likely to be present when the injury seems more minor than the degree of damage indicated.[48,54]

JAUNDICE

Jaundice arising after an anicteric newborn period, or increasing jaundice after the newborn physiologic jaundice seemingly has ebbed, should

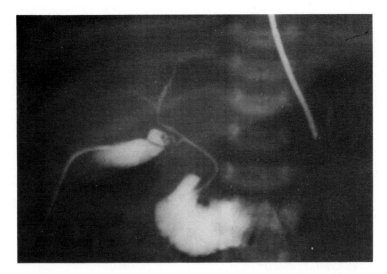

Fig. 15-13. Intraoperative cholangiogram showing a hypoplastic but intact extrahepatic biliary tree in a jaundiced patient. No further surgery other than a liver biopsy is indicated.

immediately suggest biliary atresia. Although the differential diagnosis of jaundice in this age group is considerable and includes the TORCH* infections, various hematologic conditions, storage diseases of the liver, and sepsis,[4,68] most infants developing jaundice in this age group will have some variant of the spectrum ranging from giant cell or neonatal hepatitis to outright biliary atresia.[9] Present thinking views these lesions as differing manifestations of an underlying inflammatory lesion that Landing[40] has termed ''infantile obstructive cholangiopathy.'' Early thorough evaluation and subsequent surgical exploration, when indicated, for suspected biliary atresia are essential today, since the evolution of the Kasai procedure (hepatoportoenterostomy) has brought new hope to these infants.[3,36,43]

Evaluation. Evaluation consists of eliminating infectious and metabolic reasons for the jaundice followed by early surgical exploration. To date, no tests reliably differentiate the intrahepatic cholestatic and hepatitic phases of this disease from the extrahepatic biliary destructive phases. If surgery is to be successful, it must be performed before the child is 12 weeks of age; and it would appear that earlier exploration generates improved results.[3,36,43]

Surgical options. Once the decision for surgery has been made, the procedure should be performed by someone with extensive knowledge of the hepatobiliary tree in the infant. The techniques are a balance between seeking out the etiology and finding any intact duct systems while at the same time avoiding injury to the minute remnants of the biliary tree so that a functioning reconstructive procedure can be accomplished. The procedure, therefore, consists of exploring the abdomen, observing the liver, and seeking out the gallbladder. If one is present, a cholecystostomy tube is placed and contrast material injected for cholangiography. These films are studied, and the extent of intactness or atresia of the biliary tree is observed. If a patent biliary tree is demonstrated, no further surgery is performed; the liver is biopsied and the procedure concluded (Fig. 15-13). Occasionally, an intact extrahepatic biliary tree will be noted but retrograde filling of the intrahepatic branches cannot be achieved on the intraoperative cholangiogram (Fig. 15-14). Often these cases merit leaving the cholecystostomy tube in place and repeating the studies in the radiology department with the patient awake. Better films can be obtained and more concentrated dye used. If repeated cholangiograms fail to demonstrate a connection between the intrahepatic and extrahepatic biliary tree and no bile is present in the extrahepatic tree, reexploration is warranted.

*Toxoplasmosis, rubella, cytomegalovirus, and herpes.

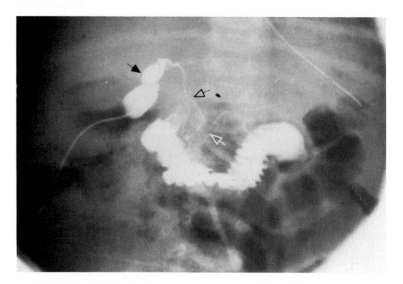

Fig. 15-14. Intraoperative cholangiogram in a jaundiced patient showing an intact gallbladder (closed black arrow), a tiny hypoplastic common duct (open black arrow), and an equally tiny pancreatic duct (open white arrow) with good flow of contrast into the duodenum.

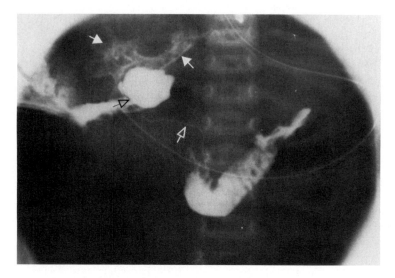

Fig. 15-15. Intraoperative cholangiogram obtained at reexploration 2 weeks following a "gall-bladder Kasai" in which the distal gallbladder was anastomosed to the porta hepatis, showing a hypoplastic common duct (open white arrow) carrying dye freely into the duodenum. The open black arrow indicates the gallbladder and the closed white arrows indicate reflux of dye into the biliary system within the liver.

When either no gallbladder or an atretic remnant is found, the gallbladder is traced to the common duct and the portahepatis carefully explored for any remnants of the biliary ducts. The distal-most areas are explored first, so that the most distal intact duct can be identified and damage to the more proximal structures avoided. However, the dissection should continue all the way into the substance of the liver if no patent ducts are found. At any point that a patent duct is found, a modified Roux-en-Y bowel loop is brought up and sutured to the area of the patent duct. If no duct is found patent prior to incision into the hilum of the liver, this step is taken and the excised piece of hilum sent for frozen section. It has generally been thought that microscopic ducts of 150 μ diam-

Table 15-1. Results of portoenterostomy in 43 patients, 1972-1978*

Extended bile drainage	29
Alive—no jaundice	(16)
Dead—unrelated, no jaundice	(2)
(Improved prognosis—18; 42%)	
Alive—jaundiced	(5)
Dead—jaundiced	(6)
Temporary or no bile drainage	14
Alive—liver failure	(4)
Dead—liver failure	(10)

*Modified from Altman, R. P.: Ann. Surg. **188**:351, 1978.

eter must be present for the Kasai procedure to be successful.[31] However, we have had children whose jaundice cleared when the diameter of the ducts was less than 100 μ. If there are ducts approaching 50 μ, it is probably worthwhile to attempt the procedure.

Finally, the ideal procedure can be achieved when the gallbladder, cystic duct, and distal common duct are present with free flow into the duodenum but the atresia affects the common hepatic duct. The hilum of the liver can be incised; and if adequately sized microscopic ducts are present, the gallbladder can be sewn to the hilum of the liver, providing a "gallbladder Kasai," which provides drainage to the duodenum but leaves intact the sphincter mechanism of the distal common duct (Fig. 15-15). The incidence of postoperative cholangitis is lower in these patients.[42]

Complications. The major complication of the Kasai procedure is postoperative cholangitis, originally thought to be due to stasis and foodstuff rising up the Roux-en-Y limb. Several modifications of the procedure have been proposed that vent the Roux-en-Y limb in various ways. These modifications have served to lessen the incidence of ascending cholangitis but have not totally eliminated it.[29,30] Much of the reason for the cholangitis is probably the minute size of the intrahepatic ducts causing stasis within the liver itself. Episodes of cholangitis should be treated vigorously with intravenous antibiotics covering a broad spectrum of bowel flora organisms. Anerobic organisms may be involved.

Prognosis. Table 15-1 provides a reasonable summary of what can be expected from the hepatobiliary procedures. Although the jaundice will clear in only 50% of patients postoperatively and only half of these will have good health over the long term, it is still a significant improvement

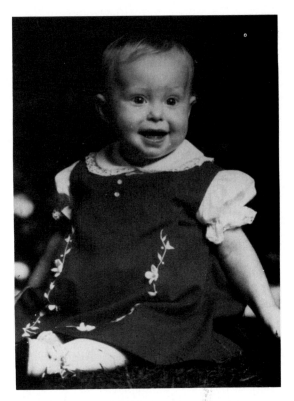

Fig. 15-16. The child whose intraoperative cholangiograms are shown in Figs. 15-14 and 15-15 at 1 year of age. She is free of jaundice and shows only minimal hepatic dysfunction.

over the pre-Kasai days of treatment of biliary atresia, when essentially 100% of patients with this entity died[2] (Fig. 15-16).

GASTROESOPHAGEAL REFLUX

Insufficiency of the gastroesophageal antireflux sphincter mechanism is becoming an increasingly recognized problem in infancy. Long denied as a significant entity in the United States, it has been recognized frequently in Europe; and recent articles in the American literature have pointed out its significance in the American population as well.* Gastroesophageal reflux is being recognized as a cause of recurrent tracheobronchitis and as an etiological factor in many cases of asthma. The relationship of sudden infant death syndrome to laryngobronchial spasm caused by nighttime gastroesophageal reflux has also been considered.[41]

Clinical presentation. The clinical manifesta-

*See references 15, 22, 26, 44, and 57.

tions of gastroesophogeal reflux are protean and range from straightforward evidence of regurgitation and aspiration to the insidious symptoms of opisthotonic posturing, finger clubbing, and mental aberrations.[13,28]

The presence of hiatus hernia is inconsequential from the clinical standpoint, although most patients with hiatus hernia will have reflux. Hiatus hernia need not be present for gastroesophageal reflux to occur. On the other hand, the presence of hiatus hernia without gastroesophageal reflux is of little clinical significance unless herniation and volvulus of the stomach should occur. Nevertheless, hiatus hernia is associated with gastroesophageal reflux in a significant percentage of cases.[22]

Gastroesophageal reflux should be thought of in the differential diagnosis of a wide variety of newborn and infant abnormalities, particularly those related to chronic or recurrent respiratory disease, frequent vomiting, or failure to thrive.

Evaluation. Confirming the diagnosis may be difficult because routine cine-esophagography may fail to demonstrate the reflux. It must be remembered that the child's gastroesophageal junction must prevent reflux 24 hours a day and that the barium examination is only a small part of that period. Even when it is performed by an expe-

rienced and interested pediatric radiologist, and even when the so-called water siphon overfilling of the stomach is performed, not all patients who have significant gastroesophageal reflux will demonstrate the abnormality.[47] Various manometric and pH studies of the actual sphincteric area have been developed by those who have led the way in recognizing the frequency of this lesion. These involve the placement of tubes in the esophagus for monitoring pressure or for pH analysis. A far greater diagnostic success rate is possible with these methods.[11]

Referral. A child thought to have gastroesophageal reflux should be referred to a center where experienced personnel can evaluate him for this lesion.

Medical versus surgical treatment. Once the diagnosis is confirmed, a trial of medical therapy involving positioning the child in the antireflux position 24 hours a day; giving small, frequent feedings; and withholding feedings before prolonged sleep periods is indicated. Satisfactory positioning of the infant in an antireflux posture requires the child to be prone on a board elevated 45 degrees (Fig. 15-17). The child is held in place by a large peg padded with diapers, which he straddles. Attempts to elevate the child in an infant seat or crib usually are unsuccessful because the child slouches

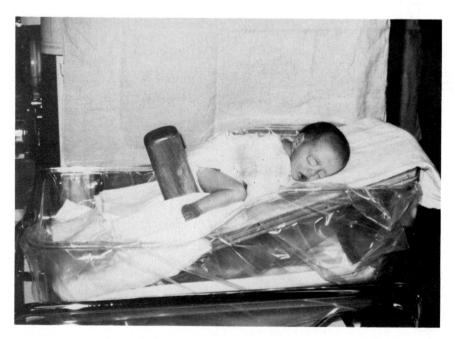

Fig. 15-17. This infant is positioned on an antireflux board to discourage gastroesophageal reflux and aspiration. This treatment may result in correction of the deformity.

down into the lower part of the seat and overcomes the attempt at elevation. Because a large percentage of infants with this lesion can be treated medically, it is worth the effort to maintain the proper position in the hope of avoiding surgery.

Surgery is indicated for children with complications of gastroesophageal reflux such as esophageal stricture or severe hemorrhage; for those with a significant hiatus hernia with gastric herniation, particularly if it is accompanied by gastric volvulus; and for those in whom the reflux remains uncorrected after several months of medical therapy. Surgery is also indicated for children who continue to have aspiration problems in the antireflux position. Children over a year of age are less likely to respond to nonsurgical therapy than infants receiving treatment earlier in life.[14,16]

Surgical options. The surgical procedures that have been advocated for the correction of this lesion have evolved over many years, beginning with those that were directed primarily at correcting the hiatus hernia by repairing the crura of the diaphragm. These procedures generally fail to prevent gastroesophageal reflux, and more specific antireflux procedures have been developed. The most successful has been the Nissen fundoplication, which involves wrapping the fundus of the stomach around the distal esophagus, holding a sizable segment of the esophagus below the diaphragm, and providing a valvelike mechanism created by the fundic wrap.[21,57] Dilatation of the fundus causes pressure against the distal esophagus, preventing reflux (Fig. 15-18). This procedure ends up with a configuration very similar to that of an inflated Foley balloon.

It should be noted that some pediatric surgeons with extensive experience with this lesion have advocated the simple Boerema procedure for treating gastroesophageal reflux in the infant.[34] This is a simple anterior gastropexy in which the stomach is sutured to the anterior abdominal wall in such a way as to stretch out the abdominal esophagus and the lesser curvature of the stomach, enhancing the angle of His. Others have not found this simple procedure to be adequate in most instances.

Postoperative course. The postoperative course

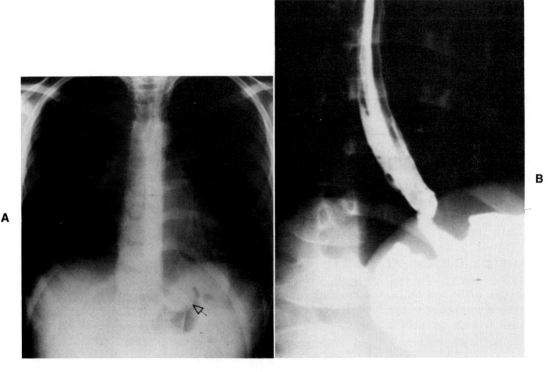

Fig. 15-18. A, Plain abdominal radiograph showing the mass effect in the gastric air bubble of the Nissen fundoplication (arrow). **B,** Enwrapment of the distal esophagus by the fundus of the stomach in the Nissen antireflux fundoplication. (Courtesy Donald Kirks, M.D., Durham, N.C.)

is generally benign. The major complication of the procedure in experienced hands has been the gas-bloat syndrome. Following a successful antireflux procedure with the Nissen fundoplication, many children cannot regurgitate air or vomit and the result may be marked gastric distention with symptoms of pain and dumping. The problem is generally self-limited, with adaptation occurring over the course of the few months following surgery. Many surgeons place a gastrostomy tube at the time of the antireflux procedure to allow a ''pop off'' valve for the stomach. This is generally a good idea, particularly for smaller infants.

Considerable judgment is required regarding how tight to wrap the fundus about the distal esophagus; it is possible to wrap it too tightly, thus interfering with normal swallowing, and also to fail to wrap it tightly enough, thus failing to prevent reflux. Nonetheless, the overall prognosis following surgery is excellent; most children have a good result with prevention of the previous complications of gastroesophageal reflux.[26]

Important aspects of follow-up. Obviously, the important aspects of follow-up are to reevaluate the success of the repair at any time that evidence of gastroesophageal reflux returns. Persistent failure to thrive, persistent asthma, or recurrence of any other preoperative symptoms should lead to reevaluation of the distal esophageal sphincter function.

CYSTIC MASSES

Numerous benign masses make their appearance in the infant-toddler age group, and these same lesions may be initially found in the older child as well. The common lesions are cysts of various types such as dermoids and epidermoids, thyroglossal duct cysts, and branchial cleft remnants. In addition, hemangiomas and lymphangiomas may be found almost anywhere in the body.

Often the diagnosis is suggested by the location of the lesion. Thyroglossal duct cysts occur close to the midline of the neck near and below the hyoid bone. Above the hyoid, midline masses may be sublingual thyroid, submental lymph nodes, or plunging ranulas. Superficial cystic lesions in this area of the neck are usually epidermoid cysts filled with sebaceous material.

The thyroglossal duct cyst can sometimes be differentiated from the others by the fact that it

rises with protrusion of the tongue. This maneuver and evaluation of the movement of the thyroglossal duct cyst may not be easily accomplished in the young infant, however. Although ultrasound will demonstrate the cystic nature of the lesions and fluorescent scanning may show the presence of thyroid tissue in them,[10] often final differentiation must await surgical exploration. Although it has frequently been suggested that thyroid scanning should be done in any patient suspected of having a thyroglossal duct cyst to be sure that the cyst does not represent the only thyroid tissue in the patient,[64] we believe that scanning represents unnecessary exposure of the patient to radioactive material as well as an unnecessary expense. The incidence of thyroglossal duct cysts containing the only thyroid tissue is low, and the patient can be screened before and after surgery for thyroid function. Either way, the cyst should be excised and, if necessary, long-term thyroid replacement provided.

Branchial cleft cysts and the sinus remnants of the second branchial cleft present along the anterior border of the sternocleidomastoid muscle, usually in the middle to lower portion. The sinus or fistula openings are more common in the infant age group, the cysts becoming more common in later childhood and adolescence and into adulthood.[23,67] When a sinus opening is present, the

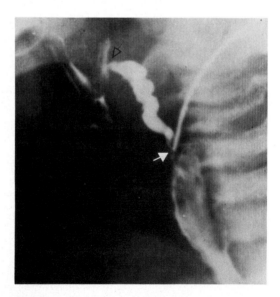

Fig. 15-19. Injection of a branchial cleft sinus (white arrow) shows cephalad tracking of the dye and entry into the hypopharynx and the tonsillar fossa (open black arrow).

tract usually extends upward in the neck through the bifurcation of the carotid artery and on to the tonsillar fossa (Fig. 15-19). All of these lesions have a significant risk of becoming infected, and it is primarily for this reason that excision is warranted whenever the diagnosis is made.

Remnants of the first branchial cleft present in the area at the angle of the jaw, often in relation to the seventh nerve.[23] Fistulas of first branchial origin are extremely rare and usually connect to the external auditory canal. The tiny skin pits that present in the preauricular area have been confused with first branchial sinuses but are, in fact, ectodermal remnants left by the enfoldings of the skin in the formation of the auricle and usually extend as a sausagelike mass of tiny cysts, ending at the anterior-most cartilage of the ear.[23,63] They do not enter the external auditory canal.

Ranulas are mucoceles formed by obstruction of the salivary glands.[56] They most commonly present in the immediate sublingual area and appear similar to the nictitating membrane of the frog. When the ranula extends down through the tissues of the floor of the mouth and presents in the neck, it is called a plunging ranula.[59] These are usually thought to be due to obstruction of the duct from the sublingual salivary gland and require excision of the gland in continuity with the cyst and duct for certain cure.

The most common location for *dermoid cysts* in the child is at the lateral aspect of the eyebrow. Cystlike tumors presenting here may be very solid in consistency, and tangential skull films may show erosion of the outer table of the bone. Although these lesions must be differentiated from the metastases of neuroblastoma that may occur in the zygoma and other areas of the maxilla, the characteristic location at the outer edge of the eyebrow makes diagnosis of the dermoid cyst fairly certain.[39]

The most common lesion occurring in the neck of an infant is *acute suppurative lymphadenitis* in the cervical glands. In the past, these lesions were usually due to streptococcal organisms; in recent studies, however, staphylococcus has been responsible in over one third of the cases cultured, and the organism is frequently resistant to penicillin.[6] Treatment consists of antibiotic coverage and incision and drainage of the abscessed node when indicated. Tumors in the lymph nodes of the neck in the infant-toddler age group are extremely rare. These lesions are covered more extensively in Chapter 20.

Hemangiomas and *lymphangiomas* may occur anywhere in the body (Fig. 15-20). Lymphangiomas that do not present in the immediate newborn period as large saclike cystic hygromas may develop clinical size in the infant-toddler age group and present as submandibular or posterior cervical masses. Their first presentation may occasionally be that of infection. Other frequent locations for lymphangiomas are the axillary area and the dorsal trunk.

Hemangiomas may be primarily capillary, cav-

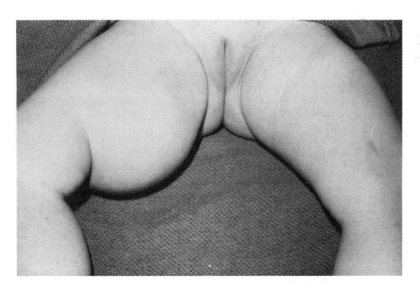

Fig. 15-20. Large lymphangioma of the right thigh.

ernous, or a mixture of the two. When a capillary component is present, it helps in making the diagnosis, since the spiderlike entwinings of the capillary blood vessels are obvious in the skin. When the lesion is primarily of a cavernous nature, a bluish hue may be noted through the skin. These cystic masses are usually discrete, but they often involve tissues deeper and at wider locations than what is palpably obvious. Although the incidence of frank malignancy in vascular tumors in infancy is low, the hemangiomas as a group vary considerably in their rate of growth and in the degree of local agressiveness. With rapid growth, they may be extremely disfiguring; and if they involve structures such as the eyelid or the external auditory canal, rapid growth may lead to functional impairment such as amblyopia and decreased auditory acuity. Most hemangiomas go through a growth spurt during infancy; then, after the child is a year or so of age, they begin to slow down and gradually recede. If the child can be tided through these months and years, usually an excellent cosmetic result can be obtained.

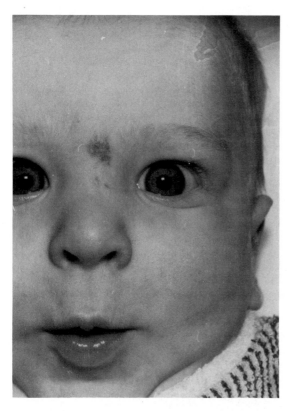

Fig. 15-21. Typical small capillary hemangioma of the face, which is usually best treated nonsurgically.

This is particularly true for the small lesions on the face that would require skin grafting for replacement (Fig. 15-21). Nevertheless, careful follow-up of these lesions must be provided by someone knowledgeable as to their course and variations, and that individual must provide the parents with constant reassurance that they are doing the right thing in postponing surgery. Other lesions found in childhood are lipomas, fibromas, and occasional sarcomatous tumors.

BREAST LESIONS

Hypertrophy of the newborn breast is a common finding and is thought to be due to the transplacental estrogen effects from the mother. These hypertrophied subareolar masses usually recede over the course of the next weeks or months. Occasionally, they may persist throughout childhood. More commonly, the child, either in infancy or early childhood, will develop a unilateral hypertrophy of the subareolar tissue. This is an end-organ effect due to the child's own normal serum estrogen levels. It rarely indicates any endocrine imbalance, particularly when it is unilateral.[61] It does not represent precocious puberty. When other effects of hormonal imbalance such as hair growth, areolar and labial pigmentation, and external genitalia hypertrophy are evident, further evaluation is warranted. Infections in the breasts of infants are rare, and tumors are extremely uncommon.

HERNIAS AND HYDROCELES

Hernias and hydroceles make up the most common problems of a surgical nature that occur in the infant.

Hernias are extremely common and tend to be somewhat familial. The hernia may be present at birth, particularly in the premature infant. Understanding of the anatomy is essential to an understanding of the array of findings that may be present. In the developing fetus, a patent processus vaginalis testis is present. This is a diverticulum of peritoneum similar to a finger on a glove, which extends through the internal ring, down the inguinal canal through the external ring, and on into the scrotum, blending with the tunica albuginea about the testicle. Normally, the tunica vaginalis closes and atrophies late in gestation. Although it may fail to close in the full-term baby, the incidence of patent processus is obviously higher in the premature infant who is born at the time of closure or before the closure would normally take place. Frequently, the patency is only a potential one, with the walls of the tunica being in apposition to each other. In a sense, this situation is similar to that of the plastic trash can liner that comes in a box and is difficult to open when it is first removed. The space is present, but finding the opening may be difficult.

This type of adherence of the walls is present in most hernias; thus, they are not apparent at birth. Exactly what causes them to open is never well defined, but it may be the continual or acute straining that goes with coughing or straining at stool. Nonetheless, once the processus opens, it usually fills with peritoneal fluid and remains open. Loops of bowel are then pushed in and out of the sac; and in response to this trauma, the sac thickens and enlarges.

As long as the bowel is easily reduced, only a simple hernia exists. When the bowel becomes caught in the sac, it is said to be incarcerated. With incarceration, air is pushed through the lumen of the bowel into the incarcerated loop but has trouble exiting from it. Edema of the wall further traps the bowel loop within the hernia sac; and, in time, first lymphatic and then venous obstruction occur at the internal ring. If this situation is allowed to persist for a considerable period of time, vascular compromise to the loop of bowel occurs. This compromise of the bowel has been greatly overemphasized in comparison with the vascular compromise that occurs to the testicle with incarceration. The internal ring in the child is less than 1 cm in diameter, and the fragile structures of the cord vessels must pass through it. When this tight ring is occupied by a loop of intestine, the blood supply to the testicle is likely to be compromised long before any obstruction to the vascular supply to or from the intestinal loop occurs. Thus, preservation of the testicle becomes a primary concern in dealing with the incarcerated hernia.

Hydroceles should be seen as different-shaped hernias. A hydrocele in a child should be considered a hernia. Generally, it represents a narrow tract residual of the tunica vaginalis testis, often less than 1 mm in diameter. This tract then opens out into a large sac at the level of the testicle, although this sac may be present along the cord itself. The connection to the peritoneal cavity allows peritoneal fluid to exit from the peritoneum and travel down into the hydrocele sac. Thus,

treatment of the hydrocele primarily requires suture ligation of the tract at the level of the internal ring, which is the exact procedure accomplished for herniorrhapy in the infant. Hydroceles can occur in infant girls as well and are known as hydroceles of the canal of Nuck.

Since hydroceles are hernias, most should be operated on when they are discovered. One exception to this is the hydrocele present at birth. This hydrocele may represent fluid caught in the tunica vaginalis testis prior to birth. The usual late gestational closure of the upper processus may have occurred, and with time the fluid may be reabsorbed. Thus, if the hydrocele is present at birth and over the course of weeks or months does not increase in size but gradually grows smaller, it can be observed without surgery. However, at any time that the hydrocele is noted to increase in size, connection with the peritoneal cavity is proved and herniorrhapy should be accomplished.

A typical history for a child with a hydrocele is that the hydrocele is a small one that is soft and easily expressible for a period of weeks or months. Gradually the hydrocele may increase in size and become firm. Also, occasionally this increase in size takes place suddenly, within the space of a few hours, and may be accompanied by discomfort or a bluish discoloration. Such instances are often misdiagnosed as incarcerated hernias.

Careful examination demonstrating the absence of a mass at the level of the internal ring and transillumination showing that the entire mass is transilluminable will go far toward confirming the hydrocele. Careful rectal examination may demonstrate the presence of an incarcerated loop of bowel in a hernia sac, differentiating it from a long hydrocele sac.

The anatomic configuration of a hydrocele has not been widely appreciated. It is, however, a recurring anatomic theme in the body, being similar to the cardioesophageal junction or gastroesophageal sphincter and also to the ureterovesical junction. As the hydrocele fills with fluid, it tends to shut off its own tract.

Referral and treatment. Since hernias in this age group are highly likely to become incarcerated because of the small tight, intact internal ring, surgery for them should be considered at least as urgent, if not more so, than for hernias first noticed in the older age groups. The tiny infant whom many primary care physicians hesitate to refer for surgery is just the patient in whom the hernia is likely to become incarcerated insidiously and in whom the obstruction to the blood supply to the testicle may occur early in the course of the incarceration, with loss of the testicle resulting. Although repair of a hernia should be considered a reasonably urgent problem in any age group, the older child often is more vocal about such problems and the likelihood of the incarceration being missed long enough to lead to testicular or gastrointestinal strangulation is lessened.

In most children's centers that have given any thought to the problem today, hernia surgery can be accomplished on an outpatient basis in a day surgery setting. This fact is particularly important for the older infant and for the infant of any age who is still breastfeeding. It eliminates the problems of separation from the mother and assures continuance of the breastfeeding program. It lessens the anxieties for the child in the toddler age group and also eliminates much of the disruption for the family as a whole.

Hernia surgery in the young infant should certainly be accomplished only by surgeons and anesthesiologists who are quite familiar with the care of the young child. Hernia surgery in the infant is a delicate procedure, and the risks of injury to cord structures or weakening of the abdominal wall musculature by inexperienced or occasional child surgeons is considerable. Every child need not be referred to a major center for hernia surgery, but the primary care physician should be assured that the child will obtain first-rate anesthesia management by an experienced anesthesiologist and that the surgeon is trained in and experienced in this type of surgery in very young children.

Postoperative care and follow-up. The postoperative care and follow-up after hernia surgery in infancy should be minimal. Usually, buried absorbable sutures are used and the wound is covered with a plastic coating to facilitate bathing and eliminate the problems of stool and urine coming in direct contact with the wound. Since there are no sutures to remove, the follow-up by the surgeon can be delayed, if necessary, and the likelihood of complications should be extremely low. The wound needs protection against direct trauma only during the 2 to 3 weeks of initial healing. The child may be bathed immediately, and activities need not be restricted. There is no risk of disrupting a repair by straining, coughing, or crying, since there is no repair involved in the usual infant herniorrhaphy.

Complications. Complications of the procedure other than the problems of wound infection involve damage to the cord structures; and the most common complication is that a retractile testicle will be pulled up into the healing herniorrhaphy wound and scarred to it, so that the testicle will no longer descend into the scrotum. The surgeon should be aware of this problem; and if the testicle is poorly attached to the scrotum, an orchidopexy of some type should be accomplished.

When an infant's hernia has been incarcerated, even though it may have been reduced prior to the surgical procedure, atrophy of the testicle may follow due to strangulation of the cord structures, as noted above. This condition may be noted by gradual disappearance of the testicle from the scrotum or may be indicated merely by the failure of the testicle on that side to grow. It is important to make these observations so that an unnecessary exploration for the undescended testicle does not result some years later. In addition, it must be appreciated that incarceration is an intestinal obstruction. Even though the incarcerated loop is not ischemic, hypovolemia and generalized hypoperfusion may result in serious organ injury throughout the body.

The incidence of recurrence after a properly done herniorrhaphy should approach zero. These hernias are indirect congenital ones representing persistence of the processus vaginalis testis; and if they are properly dissected free and ligated high at the internal ring, there is little reason for recurrence. However, in a child with chronic straining, such as a child with cystic fibrosis, the possibility of pushing more peritoneum out through the internal ring exists. It is only in such children that recurrent hernias are usually seen. A recurrent hernia in an otherwise normal child usually represents a failure of the initial surgery. Children in whom two to three herniorrhaphies were performed by inexperienced surgeons have been found on reexploration to have virginal sacs that had never been dissected free and ligated (Fig. 15-22).

• • •

All in all, hernia surgery in childhood can be a pleasant, thoughtful, meticulous operation in which the family's convenience as well as the child's safety are taken into consideration. It should be accomplished with relatively little trauma to the child and little disruption of the family's activities. Ideally, it should be accomplished on

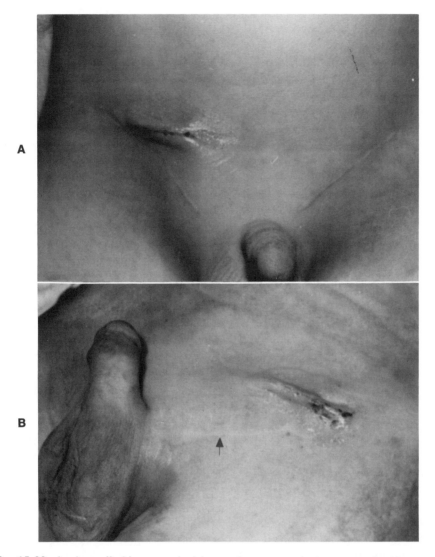

Fig. 15-22. A, A small skin crease incision made transversely is compared with two previous oblique incisions for herniorrhaphies. Failure of the previous surgery was due to lack of identification, proper dissection, and high ligation of the hernia sac. **B,** This infant had five previous procedures for inguinal hernia with multiple recurrences. The hernia sacs had been ligated distal to the external ring, leaving a sizable segment of hernia sac within the inguinal canal. Note the cosmetically unattractive oblique suture line with scarring from the large skin sutures that had been placed (arrow). The tiny transverse incision in the skin crease with subcuticular catgut closure and collodion dressing will leave an almost imperceptible scar.

a day surgery basis with the child returning home that evening. The success rate should approach 100%.

BURNS

Although major burns occur in all age groups, a distinctive form of burn injury first occurs in the infant-toddler age group and is discussed here. Resuscitation of major burns for the older child is discussed in Chapter 20.

The typical burn of the infant-toddler age group is that of the splash burn with hot water or hot coffee. The typical history is that the parent either has placed a tea kettle, coffee pot, or pan of boiling water on the stove or has just transferred such a utensil to the counter or kitchen table. The toddler, either ambulating independently or in a walker, reaches up and pulls the utensil over. The hot liquid splashes over the table onto the child's head, face, neck, trunk, shoulders, and arms. On the face, trunk, and extremities where the hot liquid is exposed to the air, cooling occurs rapidly and usually a blistered medium second-degree burn results. However, in the folds of the infant's neck, the heat is retained and a deeper second- or third-degree burn may result.

The calculated extent of this burn is usually under 15%. Such a burn in an older child or adult could usually be treated on an outpatient basis. This approach may be disastrous in the infant-toddler age group, however, because the infant sustaining such an injury may develop a severe ileus and fail to take in adequate amounts of fluid to replace that lost through the burn wound. Therefore, when the extent of the burn approaches 10% or greater, the child should be hospitalized and treated with intravenous fluid resuscitation. If vomiting ensues, nasogastric tube decompression should be added. Usually, only a moderate amount of fluid beyond maintenance requirements is needed; but this does prevent the child from developing the severe dehydration that often occurs when the child is sent home without this precaution. Only a day or two in the hospital is required, and advantage can be taken of this time to begin therapy for the local burn wound, which can usually be successfully treated without the need for skin grafting.

The following therapeutic regimen has been found to be highly efficient and efficacious in dealing with such wounds. It is a regimen that is applicable to any minor burn regardless of its extent and location.

Local care of the blistered second-degree burn wound. This treatment regimen is applicable to the blistered second-degree burn. It would be unsuccessful in the management of a second-degree burn so deep as to involve the dermis all the way to the rete pegs and, thus, the areas of subcutaneous fat surrounding the rete pegs. Such a deep second-degree burn should be treated as a third-degree burn, with topical antiseptic ointment or initial excision and grafting.

A blistered second-degree burn is a wound of minimal to moderate depth, very similar to a donor site of a skin graft. The epidermis and superficial layers of the dermis are raised from the underlying dermal tissue by destruction of intracellular bridges and elevation of the injured tissue by the ensuing transudate. If the blisters are debrided under sterile conditions, the dermal base is washed gently with an antiseptic solution such as povi-

done-iodine, and fine-mesh gauze soaked in povidone-iodine is applied to the wound, held in place by dry sterile gauze wraps, and allowed to dry and stick to the wound, contamination of the local burn wound will be prevented and healing of the epithelium will occur over the course of 10 days to 2 weeks. Twenty-four hours after application of the dressing, the bulky dry gauze can be removed down to the fine-mesh gauze and the fine-mesh gauze dried to the site with a warm-air hair dryer or cast dryer.

If the fine-mesh gauze has raised up off the site, additional povidone-iodine solution may be applied and the gauze smoothed back over the site and dried in place. Once initial drying and adhesion of the gauze takes place, frequent inspection of the site is necessary to ensure that it remains dry and that the fine-mesh gauze remains tightly applied to the site. If no wetting of the gauze occurs in 24 hours, it can be assumed that the gauze is adequately dry and adherent.

If persistent wetting of the gauze occurs, especially if the moist area has an exudative appearance, the depth of the burn has probably been misjudged and a deeper second-degree burn with exposure of some subcutaneous tissue is allowing liquefaction of the injured fat to prevent adherence of the gauze to the burn wound site. This regimen should be abandoned if that situation occurs.

Although this approach to management of the blistered second-degree burn is easily accomplished in the hospital, it is equally successful as a management regimen for more minor burns that can be managed on an outpatient basis. The local burn wound is treated as discussed above, and the patient is sent home with instructions for the parents to remove the bulky gauze on the following day and apply additional antiseptic solution to the fine-mesh gauze and dry it in place with a hair dryer. They are instructed to check it repeatedly throughout the course of the following 24-hour period and to provide additional solution and drying as needed. Once it is dry, it should be checked again by the physician to ensure that all areas of the burn wound are dry and that the fine-mesh gauze is adherent throughout.

As the epithelium grows back from the dermal base and from the epithelial margins, the fine-mesh gauze will be lifted from the burn wound site and eventually will fall off. A healed, intact epidermal surface will be found beneath.

The ease of this therapeutic regimen and its relative inexpensiveness as far as the costs of dressings and dressing changes makes it widely applicable to the blistered second-degree burn of any extent.

FOREIGN BODY ASPIRATION*

Aspiration of foreign materials into the airway is a common problem in young children. The tendency of many children to explore their environments by licking, tasting, and ingesting objects leads to frequent swallowing of small objects and less frequently, but in still significant numbers, to aspiration. Total obstruction of the airway is fortunately uncommon. Partial obstruction with varying degrees of respiratory distress is the usual presenting feature. Retrieval of these objects is a major undertaking and may lead to serious complications and even to death.

Discussion

Safe management of young children who have aspirated objects requires early recognition; a well-prepared plan for intraoperative management by the endoscopist and anesthesiologist; bronchoscopic instruments capable of providing an adequate airway evaluation for an endoscopist experienced in the care of infants; knowledge, skill, and imaginative instrumentation techniques for retrieval of the foreign objects; and a competent nursing facility for postoperative airway support.

---

*From Filston, H. C.: Foreign body aspiration in children—recognition and safe management, N.C. Med. J. **40**:79, 1979 (North Carolina Medical Society).

Recognition

Foreign body aspiration is easily recognized when airway obstruction is acute and essentially complete. When obstruction is partial or segmental in the tracheobronchial tree, symptoms may range from the fairly acute onset of dyspnea, cough, stridor, and progressive respiratory failure to a slower, more insidious development of segmental pneumonia which persists after seemingly adequate therapy. Foreign body aspiration should be considered in the differential diagnosis of persistent pneumonias. Any child presenting with the acute onset of dyspnea should be suspected of having aspirated. A careful history of ingestions or mouthing of objects should be obtained. If the history is positive and the child is symptomatic, airway evaluation is mandatory. In the absence of a positive history, the young child with acute onset of dyspnea and coughing should be suspected of having aspirated a foreign object.

The chest roentgenogram gives important clues. The most common finding when partial obstruction of a major bronchus is present is hyperaeration on the ipsilateral side. This may be hard to appreciate on inspiratory films, but is usually clearly demonstrated when inspiratory and expiratory films are obtained concomitantly (Fig. 15-23). The failure of the partially obstructed lobe to collapse may be more easily demonstrated in uncooperative infants by obtaining lateral decubitus views. A normal lung will show decreased volume when it is the lower side of a decubitus view, according to Grossman.* Most aspirated objects will be vegetable material such as nuts or beans, which are not radiopaque, although an occasional one will be directly visible on the chest radiograph.

---

*Grossman, H.: Personal communication, 1978.

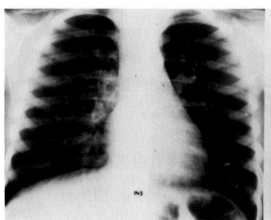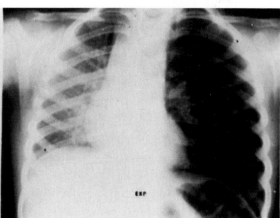

Fig. 15-23. Inspiratory and expiratory films of an infant with a foreign body in the left main stem bronchus. Although the inspiratory films appear normal, the expiratory films show the failure of the left lung to collapse, illustrating partial obstruction of the left main stem bronchus. (From Filston, H. C.: N.C. Med. J. **40**:79, 1979; courtesy Herman Grossman, M.D., Durham, N.C.)

Bronchoscopy

Recently Ward and Benumof[69] reported three cases of foreign body removal with serious complications and emphasized the importance of pre-bronchoscopic planning between the surgeon and the anesthesiologist. Assurance of a well-controlled airway with continuous ability to ventilate the child is mandatory. Muscle relaxants should be relied upon to insure relaxation during the maneuvers and to avoid undue trauma to the respiratory tract. Temperature, heart rate, blood pressure, and EKG should be carefully monitored.

Significant advances have been made in bronchoscopy of infants and children with the recent advent of the optical telescopic bronchoscopes, which range from 3-mm outer diameters to adult sizes and allow successful procedures in the tiniest prematures.[24] The outer bronchoscopic sheath permits dependable airway control and ventilation and imaginative instrumentation. The inner rod lens telescope, with its surrounding fiberoptic light bundles, provides a large, well-illuminated clear field of view so that segmental bronchi can be clearly visualized in the tiny infant (Fig. 15-24).

Removal of the foreign body

The usual approach to a foreign body has been to pass a grasping forceps through the bronchoscope. In infants this usually obstructs the view when old-style bronchoscopes are used. Foreign bodies made of vegetable matter are frequently broken, and smaller segments may then be dispersed throughout the tracheobronchial tree.

We prefer to pass a Fogarty balloon catheter (4 Fr) through the instrument channel of the telescopic bronchoscope. The catheter occupies only a small part of the visualized field and can be carefully threaded beyond the object. The balloon is then inflated and used to deliver the foreign body into the lumen (Fig. 15-25). The entire bronchoscope is then slowly removed. Good ventilation and paralysis must be maintained so that immediate reintubation can be done. Usually, the object is easily removed, but if lost it can be recaptured with ease.

If removal is unsuccessful with the balloon catheter, the Dormia stone basket may be used. It, too, can pass through the instrumenting channel of the telescopic bronchoscope. The foreign body is manipulated into the open wires of the basket and the wires then tightened about it. Again, the entire instrumenting unit is removed.

Reevaluation

Once the foreign body is removed, bronchoscopy should be repeated to search for other foreign objects and to assess damage to the airway. We have then usu-

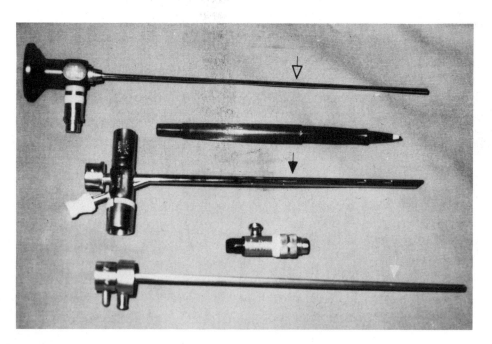

Fig. 15-24. Hopkins rod lens telescopic system in the 2.7-mm size for the newborn infant. The open black arrow indicates the rod lens telescope, the closed black arrow the standard infant bronchoscope sheath, and the white arrow the protective sheath for the telescope, which allows defogging of the lens and instrumentation. A standard felt-tipped pen is included in the picture for size comparison. (From Filston, H. C.: N.C. Med. J. **40:**79, 1979.)

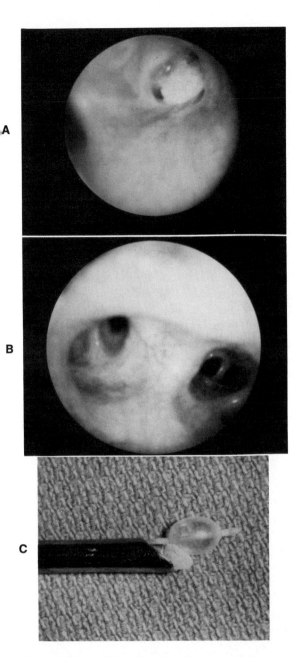

Fig. 15-25. A, View through the telescopic bronchoscope of a foreign body (aquarium pebble) lodged in
the right main stem bronchus of an infant. **B,** Appearance of the right main stem bronchus with some of the
segmental bronchioles visible after removal of the foreign body. Note the hemorrhagic appearance of the
mucosa. **C,** The method of removal of the foreign body
is illustrated with the inflated Fogarty balloon. After
the pebble has been extracted from the right main stem
bronchus and lodged in the tip of the bronchoscope,
the entire bronchoscope is removed with the pebble
and inflated balloon. (From Filston, H. C.: N.C. Med.
J. **40:**79, 1979.)

ally intubated patients to ensure a safe airway when
anesthesia is discontinued.

Postoperative care

Usually these children do well, so that severe postoperative respiratory dysfunction should suggest a retained foreign body. Upper airway obstruction due to
laryngeal or epiglottic edema usually responds to a few
treatments with racemic epinephrine using a saline
mist unit.[1] Mild to moderate tracheobronchitis may
persist for a few days. Foreign bodies containing oils
such as peanuts may produce lipid pneumonia with
persistent infiltrates.

We have generally treated these children with ultrasonic mist by face mask or tent and have added postural
drainage and chest physiotherapy when the foreign
body has been present for more than a few hours or
when there is residual atelectasis.

Prevention

The medical profession, especially those members
in primary care activities, could do much to prevent
these life-threatening accidents by cautioning parents
not to let infants put small objects in their mouths.

FOLLOW-UP OF NEONATAL
SURGICAL CONDITIONS

One of the joys of neonatal surgery is that so
many of the entities, once treated, are cured for
life. Nevertheless, certain late problems do present
themselves, and awareness will lead to early correction.

Respiratory distress

The lesions presenting in the newborn period
with respiratory distress are often life threatening to the child; however, once these lesions are
cured and the child recovers, the long-term complications are few. *Diaphragmatic hernia,* once
repaired, rarely breaks down. However, the child
with severe difficulties from diaphragmatic hernia
in the newborn period may, if he survives, go
on to develop persistent pulmonary hypertension. This entity is often the cause of death in
the immediate postoperative period; and if the
child survives, it may cause the child to have
long-term problems in increased pulmonary hypertension leading to cor pulmonale. Such infants have chronic lung disease and chronic
congestive heart failure. The treatment of these
conditions is complex and requires the consultation of an able pediatric cardiologist and neonatologist, since the long-term follow-up requires
considerable attention to detail.

Tumors

Children with *malignant tumors* in infancy will usually be followed jointly by the primary care physician and the pediatric oncologist. However, an exception is usually made in the care of sacrococcygeal teratoma, since it is unlikely to result in malignant consequences if it is excised in the newborn period. Since it is poorly responsive to drugs and radiation therapy, the multimodal therapy clinics are usually not involved in the follow-up of these patients. The pediatric surgeon should follow the patient on a long-term basis, seeking evidence of recurrence, but the primary care physician may have to fill this gap. Recurrence is a possibility, although a less likely one, when the tumor is excised in the newborn period. The highest recurrence rates occur when the tumor is inadequately resected, particularly when the coccyx is not excised with the tumor. Recognition of such failure should lead to reexcision by a more experienced surgeon. Otherwise, careful follow-up with rectal examinations seeking the presence of masses in the retrorectal presacral space is most important. Although functional disability is unusual after proper excision of a sacrococcygeal teratoma, these children must be followed for evaluation of their continence mechanism. Constipation is a frequent problem but responds to the usual treatment routines. The common retroperitoneal and intra-abdominal malignancies, such as *neuroblastomas* and *Wilms' tumors,* are best followed by a multidisciplinary pediatric oncology service. Even if the initial surgery was not accomplished under the auspices of such a program, referral for follow-up care is important.

Esophageal atresia and gastroesophageal reflux

Esophageal atresia with distal tracheoesophageal fistula, the most common variety, may be complicated by postoperative esophageal stenosis and occasionally by recurrent fistula. *Gastroesophageal reflux* is also common.[5,53] The child who has recurrent aspiration pneumonia or "dying spells" in the months following surgery should be investigated for either gastroesophageal reflux or recurrent tracheoesophageal fistula. A carefully performed cine-esophagogram is essential to differentiate the two. If the injection of the dye into the esophagus is not carefully controlled, it may be regurgitated and aspirated; and the presence of dye in the residual diverticulum of the previous tracheoesophageal fistula may give the appearance of a recurrent fistula when none exists. A balloon catheter occluding the upper esophagus may help to avoid this confusion. The most successful approach has been cannulation of the fistula under fluoroscopy so that the passage of both the catheter and the dye into the trachea is clearly demonstrated.[37] This maneuver requires the skill of an experienced pediatric radiologist. Endoscopy with the pediatric telescopic bronchoscopes, although highly successful in identifying the original tracheoesophageal fistula,[25] has not been successful in evaluating recurrent fistulas, because a small diverticulum is expected to be present at the site of the original fistula (Fig. 15-26). Often a catheter cannot be passed from the tracheal to the esophageal side, and a false-negative impression may be gained. Even injecting methylene blue into the trachea and ventilating the infant forcefully while he is under anesthesia has failed to demonstrate fistulas that were subsequently found to be present by fluoroscopic catheterization techniques.

If no fistula is found and gastroesophageal reflux is either demonstrated or suspected, the child should be treated for it medically by the use of

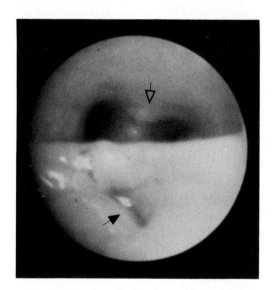

Fig. 15-26. Telescopic bronchoscopic view of a child previously having undergone repair of eosphageal atresia with a tracheoesophageal fistula between the trachea and the distal esophagus. The persistent "pit" (closed black arrow) is seen in the trachea just above the carina (open black arrow). (From Filston, H. C.: The surgical neonate: evaluation and care, New York, 1978, Appleton-Century-Crofts.)

an antireflux board elevated 45 degrees; the child is placed prone on the board and maintained in this position. When the child reaches infancy, 6-inch blocks can be placed at the head of the crib for elevation. Small, frequent feedings and the avoidance of large feedings before sleeping are also helpful. If the gastroesophageal reflux cannot be corrected by these means, an antireflux procedure such as the Nissen fundoplication may be necessary.

Stenosis after esophageal repair, although frequently discussed in the pediatric surgical literature, should occur infrequently if the anastomosis is accomplished with meticulous attention to detail. Leaks from the anastomosis should be infrequent in experienced hands, and it is generally only the anastomosis that leaks that results in stricture. Although some pediatric surgeons have recommended routine dilatations of the esophageal anastomosis after surgery, we have not found it to be necessary and have had a very low incidence of stenosis after eosphageal repair. Severe stricturing of a properly accomplished anastomosis may indicate gastroesophageal reflux with reflux esoph-

agitis of the suture line. That complication, too, has been infrequent in our experience despite the fact that we have had patients who clearly had severe gastroesophageal reflux. The more likely reason for stenosis at the anastomotic site is failure to include the mucosa, particularly that of the upper pouch, in the anastomotic suture line. The result is a raw area that is filled in by granulation tissue, leading to webbing across the anastomosis and thus severe stricture formation.

One complication that most of these children do have is the inability to pass a foreign body that may be ingested through the anastomosis. Even though the anastomosis may appear open and pliable on barium swallow, it generally will not tolerate the passage of coins, pins, and other objects that a child may ingest (Fig. 15-27). Thus, endoscopic extraction will usually be necessary. At the time, the anastomosis should be evaluated for stricture and dilatation accomplished if needed.

Neonatal lesions requiring abdominal exploration

Any lesion, whether it be atresia, malrotation, pyloric stenosis, intussusception, or whatever, that requires entry into the peritoneal cavity may result in adhesions that may, at any time, result in mechanical obstruction of the bowel. Thus, any child in whom the peritoneal cavity has been entered should be evaluated thoroughly for any signs of distention or vomiting. Such evaluation may become a burden during periods when gastrointestinal viruses are causing similar symptoms in the rest of the population, but the risk of bowel loss from strangulation obstruction is so great that these children should be screened early for mechanical obstruction whenever they have symptoms of vomiting and distention. If these symptoms are accompanied by cessation of stooling, a simple screening abdominal radiograph is indicated. The presence of persistent diarrhea helps to confirm an enterovirus etiology and to rule out mechanical obstruction, but the passage of a few stools after mechanical obstruction is not unusual. Ingestion of a small amount of barium is often a helpful maneuver in ruling out intestinal obstruction when the plain films do not clearly show a completely obstructive pattern. There should be no problem with putting barium into the gastrointestinal tract from above, since this concern applies primarily to the adult patient with an obstructing colon carcinoma.

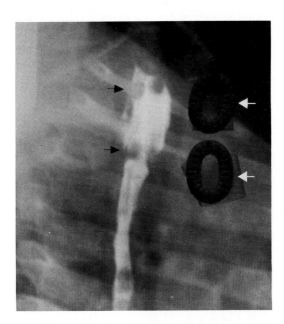

Fig. 15-27. This child had a successful repair of esophageal atresia and tracheoesophageal fistula and had no difficulties with swallowing until the age of 3 years, at which time he had acute obstruction of the esophagus. The radiograph of the barium swallow shows filling defects in the proximal esophagus (black arrows), representing large plastic beads from a baby bracelet that were ingested (white arrows).

Congenital intestinal atresias that require the anastomosis of disparately sized bowel may result in complications of this disparity in subsequent years. It is generally the practice to resect the most dilated proximal bowel to achieve a more uniform anastomosis. However, when the atresia is high in the jejunum and the bowel is dilated well back into the duodenum, it is often impossible to accomplish this maneuver. Even though modern techniques involve placing the anastomosis at the most distal end of the proximal dilated segment, the disparity may lead to overriding of the proximal segment beyond the anastomosis and result in the same type of blind loop syndrome that was common when side-to-side anastomoses were routinely performed.[50] The stasis of bowel content with overgrowth of bacteria that occurs in the blind loop may lead to an imbalance of acid base and bacterial flora in the gut, thus changing the ratio of bile salts to bile acids and lead to poor absorption and a cathartic effect. This chronic diarrhea and flora change may thus result in a chronic state of malabsorption and lead to a failure to thrive, which may be of an insidious degree and be prolonged for years.

Another common sequel to neonatal bowel problems is some form of short gut or *malabsorption syndrome*.[18] Where either congenital atresia has led to extensive loss or a missed volvulus due to malrotation has resulted in gangrene and massive bowel resection, there may be inadequate bowel left for proper digestion and absorption (Fig. 15-28). This complication may lead to an intolerance of certain foods and require a special diet. Although these problems will usually have been solved before the child is released from the care of the neonatologist and pediatric surgeon, the primary care physician should be aware that minor gastrointestinal disturbances in these children may lead to a resumption of the malabsorption problem or to massive diarrhea. Thus, these children should be treated more vigorously for the routine gastrointestinal upsets of childhood. Bowel rest is generally required, and hospitalization with intravenous fluid support may be necessary to prevent severe dehydration. Erring on the side of excess caution in these children will be rewarded.

Most of the *abdominal wall defects* will have been completely corrected; the major long-term problems are those of ventral hernias and adhesions leading to mechanical obstruction of the bowel.

The discussion on *imperforate anus* in Chapter 10 in the section on the newborn should be referred to for follow-up of this condition, since the long-term follow-up is such an essential part of success in this entity.

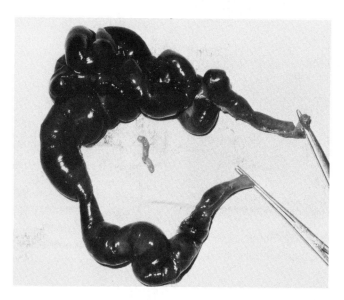

Fig. 15-28. Extensive resection of distal ileum required in an infant with strangulating obstruction of the mesentery secondary to malrotation and volvulus. (From Filston, H. C.: The surgical neonate: evaluation and care, New York, 1978, Appleton-Century-Crofts.)

REFERENCES

1. Adair, J. C., and others: A ten-year experience with IPPB in the treatment of acute laryngotracheobronchitis, Anesth. Analg. **50:**649, 1971.
2. Adelman, S.: Prognosis of uncorrected biliary atresia: an update, J. Pediatr. Surg. **13:**389, 1978.
3. Altman, R. P.: The portoenterostomy procedure for biliary atresia—a five year experience, Ann. Surg. **188:**351, 1978.
4. Amanullah, A.: Neonatal jaundice, Am. J. Dis. Child. **130:**1274, 1976.
5. Ashcraft, K. W., and others: Early recognition and aggressive treatment of gastroesophageal reflux following repair of esophageal atresia, J. Pediatr. Surg. **12:**317, 1977.
6. Barton, L. L., and Feigin, R. D.: Childhood cervical lymphadenitis: a reappraisal, J. Pediatr. **84:**846, 1974.
7. Benson, C. D.: Surgical implications of Meckel's diverticulum. In Ravitch, M. M., and others, editors: Pediatric surgery, ed. 3, Chicago, 1979, Year Book Medical Publishers, Inc., p. 955.
8. Bill, A. H.: Malrotation of the intestine. In Ravitch, M. M., and others, editors: Pediatric surgery, ed. 3, Chicago, 1979, Year Book Medical Publishers, Inc., p. 912.
9. Bill, A. H., Haas, J. E., and Foster, G. L.: Biliary atresia: histopathologic observations and reflections upon its natural history, J. Pediatr. Surg. **12:**977, 1977.
10. Blei, C. L., Gooding, G. A., and Rector, W.: Ultrasonic and fluorescent scanning: a combined noninvasive diagnostic approach to extrathyroidal neck lesions, Am. J. Surg. **134:**369, 1977.
11. Boix-Ochoa, J.: GI pressure studies in GER/hiatal hernia *and* pH monitoring in GER/hiatal hernia. In Gellis, S. S., editor: Gastroesophageal reflux: report of the Seventy-sixty Ross Conference on Pediatric Research, Columbus, Ohio, 1979, Ross Laboratories, pp. 65-76.
12. Boley, S.: New modification of the surgical treatment of Hirschsprung's disease, Surgery **56:**1015, 1964.
13. Bray, P. F., and others: Childhood gastroesophageal reflux: neurologic and psychiatric syndromes mimicked, J.A.M.A. **237:**1342, 1977.
14. Byrne, W. J., and Ament, M. E.: Gastroesophageal reflux (GER): the management of infants, children, and adolescents. In Gellis, S. S., editor: Gastroesophageal reflux: report of the Seventy-sixth Ross Conference on Pediatric Research, Columbus, Ohio, 1979, Ross Laboratories, p. 81.
15. Carré, I. J.: A historical review of the clinical consequences of hiatal hernia (partial thoracic stomach) and gastroesophageal reflux. In Gellis, S. S., editor: Gastroesophageal reflux: report of the Seventy-sixth Ross Conference on Pediatric Research, Columbus, Ohio, 1979, Ross Laboratories, pp. 1-12.
16. Carré, I. J.: Postural treatment of infants and young children with a hiatal hernia (partial thoracic stomach). In Gellis, S. S., editor: Gastroesophageal reflux, report of the Seventy-sixth Ross Conference on Pediatric Research, Columbus, Ohio, 1979, Ross Laboratories, p. 86.
17. Chow, C. W., Chan, W. C., and Yue, P. C.: Histochemical criteria for the diagnosis of Hirschsprung's disease in rectal suction biopsies by acetylcholinesterase activity, J. Pediatr. Surg. **12:**675, 1977.
18. Cywes, S.: The surgical management of massive bowel resection, J. Pediatr. Surg. **3:**740, 1968.
19. Duhamel, B.: A new operation for the treatment of Hirschsprung's disease, Arch. Dis. Child **35:**38, 1960.
20. Ein, S. H.: Leading points in childhood intussusception, J. Pediatr. Surg. **11:**209, 1976.
21. Follette, D., and others: Gastroesophageal fundoplication for reflux in infants and children, J. Pediatr. Surg. **11:**757, 1976.
22. Friedland, G. W., and others: The apparent disparity in incidence of hiatal herniae in infants and children in Britain and the United States, A.J.R. **120:**305, 1974.
23. Gaisford, J. C., and Anderson, V. S.: First branchial cleft cysts and sinuses, Plast. Reconstr. Surg. **55:**299, 1975.
24. Gans, S. L., and Berci, G.: Advances in endoscopy in infants and children, J. Pediatr. Surg. **6:**199, 1971.
25. Gans, S. L., and Berci, G.: Inside tracheoesophageal fistula: new endoscopic approaches, J. Pediatr. Surg. **8:**205, 1973.
26. Gellis, S. S., editor: Gastroesophageal reflux: report of the Seventy-sixth Ross Conference on Pediatric Research, Columbus, Ohio, 1979, Ross Laboratories.
27. Golladay, E. S., and others: Intestinal obstruction from appendiceal abscess in a newborn infant, J. Pediatr. Surg. **13:**175, 1978.
28. Herbst, J. J., Johnson, D. G., and Oliveros, M. A.: Gastroesophageal reflux with protein-losing enteropathy and finger clubbing, Am. J. Dis. Child. **130:**1256, 1976.
29. Hirsig, J., Kara, O., and Rickham, P. P.: Experimental investigations into the etiology of cholangitis following operation for biliary atresia, J. Pediatr. Surg. **13:**55, 1978.
30. Hitch, D. C., and Lilly, J. R.: Identification, quantification, and significance of bacterial growth within the biliary tract after Kasai's operation, J. Pediatr. Surg. **13:**563, 1978.
31. Hitch, D. C., Shikes, R. H., and Lilly, J. R.: Determinants of survival after Kasai's operation for biliary atresia using actuarial analysis, J. Pediatr. Surg. **14:**310, 1979.
32. Horwitz, S. J., and Amiel-Tison, C.: Neurologic problems. In Klaus, M. H., and Fanaroff, A. A., editors: Care of the high-risk neonate, Philadelphia, 1979, W. B. Saunders Co., p. 362.
33. Johnson, D. G., and Jones, R.: Surgical aspects of airway management in infants and children, Surg. Clin North Am. **56:**263, 1976.
34. Johnson, D. G., and others: Evaluation of gastroesophageal reflux surgery in children, Pediatrics **59:**62, 1977.
35. Johnson, D. G., and Stewart, D. R.: Management of acquired tracheal obstructions in infancy, J. Pediatr. Surg. **10:**709, 1975.
36. Kasai, M.: Treatment of biliary atresia with special reference to hepatic portoenterostomy and its modifications, Prog. Pediatr. Surg. **6:**5, 1974.
37. Kirks, D. R., Briley, C. A., Jr., and Currarino, G.: Selective catheterization of tracheoesophageal fistula, A.J.R. **133:**763, 1979.
38. Kleinhaus, S., and others: Hirschsprung's disease: a survey of the members of the Surgical Section of the American Academy of Pediatrics, J. Pediatr. Surg. **14:**588, 1979.

39. Koop, C. E.: Visible and palpable lesions in children, New York, 1976, Grune & Stratton, Inc., p. 2.

40. Landing, B. H.: Considerations of the pathogenesis of neonatal hepatitis, biliary atresia and choledochal cyst—the concept of infantile obstructive cholangiopathy, Prog. Pediatr. Surg. 6:113, 1974.

41. Leape, L. L.: Gastroesophageal reflux as a cause of sudden infant death syndrome. In Gellis, S. S., editor: Gastroesophageal reflux: report of the Seventy-sixth Ross Conference on Pediatric Research, Columbus, Ohio, 1979, Ross Laboratories, p. 30.

42. Lilly, J. R.: Hepatic portocholecystostomy for biliary atresia, J. Pediatr. Surg. 14:301, 1979.

43. Lilly, J. R., and Altman, R. P.: Hepatic portoenterostomy (the Kasai operation) for biliary atresia, Surgery 78:76, 1975.

44. Lilly, J. R., and Randolph, J. G.: Hiatal hernia and gastroesophageal reflux in infants and children, J. Thorac. Cardiovasc. Surg. 55:42, 1968.

45. Lindholm, C.: Prolonged endotracheal intubation, Acta Anesthesiology (Scand.) [Suppl.] 33:1, 1969.

46. Martin, L. W., and Caudill, D. R.: A method for elimination of the blind rectal pouch in the Duhamel operation for Hirschsprung's disease, Surgery 62:951, 1967.

47. McCauley, R. G.: Radiological demonstration of gastroesophageal reflux and hiatal hernia in infants and children. In Gellis, S. S., editor: Gastroesophageal reflux: report of the Seventy-sixth Ross Conference on Pediatric Research, Columbus, Ohio, 1979, Ross Laboratories, pp. 48-54.

48. Miller, R. C., and others: The incidental discovery of occult abdominal tumors in children following blunt abdominal trauma, J. Trauma 6:99, 1966.

49. Moore, K. L.: The developing human: clinically oriented embryology, Philadelphia, 1973, W. B. Saunders Co., pp. 181-188, 192.

50. Nixon, H. H.: Surgical conditions in paediatrics, London, 1978, Butterworth & Co. (Publishers), Ltd., pp. 260-263.

51. Othersen, H. B., Jr.: Steroid therapy for tracheal stenosis in children, Ann. Thorac. Surg. 17:254, 1974.

52. Othersen, H. B., Jr.: The technique of intraluminal stenting and steroid administration in the treatment of tracheal stenosis in children, J. Pediatr. Surg. 9:683, 1974.

53. Parker, A. F., Christie, D. L., and Cahill, J. L.: Incidence and significance of gastroesophageal reflux following repair of esophageal atresia and tracheoesophageal fistula

54. Persky, L., and Forsythe, W. E.: Renal trauma in childhood, J.A.M.A. 182:709, 1962.

55. Puri, P., and O'Donnell, B.: Appendicitis in infancy, J. Pediatr. Surg. 13:173, 1978.

56. Quick, C. A., and Lowell, S. H.: Ranula and the sublingual salivary glands, Arch. Otolaryngol. 103:397, 1977.

57. Randolph, J. G., Lilly, J. R., and Anderson, K. D.: Surgical treatment of gastroesophageal reflux in infants, Ann. Surg. 180:479, 1974.

58. Ravitch, M. M.: Intussusception. In Ravitch, M. M., and others, editors: Pediatric surgery, ed. 3, Chicago, 1979, Year Book Medical Publishers, Inc., p. 1000.

59. Roediger, W. E., and Kay, S.: Pathogenesis and treatment of plunging ranulas, Surg. Gynecol. Obstet. 144:862, 1977.

60. Rosenkrantz, J. G., and others: Intussusception in the 1970s: indications for operation, J. Pediatr. Surg. 12:367, 1977.

61. Seashore, J. H.: Breast enlargements in infants and children, Pediatr. Ann. 4:542, 1975.

62. Shandling, B., and Auldist, A. W.: Punch biopsy of the rectum for diagnosis of Hirschsprung's disease, J. Pediatr. Surg. 7:546, 1972.

63. Singer, R.: A new technic for extirpation of preauricular cysts, Am. J. Surg. 111:291, 1966.

64. Strickland, A. L., and others: Ectopic thyroid glands simulating thyroglossal duct cysts, J.A.M.A. 208:307, 1969.

65. Swenson, O., and Bill, A. H., Jr.: Resection of rectum and rectosigmoid with preservation of the sphincter for benign spastic lesions producing megacolon, Surgery 24:212, 1948.

66. Talwalker, V. C.: Intussusception in the newborn, Arch. Dis. Child. 37:203, 1962.

67. Telander, R. L., and Deane, S. A.: Thyroglossal and branchial cleft cysts and sinuses, Surg. Clin. North Am. 57:779, 1977.

68. Thaler, M. M.: Jaundice in early infancy, Pediatr. Ann. 6:286, 1977.

69. Ward, C. F., and Benumof, J. L.: Anesthesia for airway foreign body extraction in children, Anesthesiol. Rev. 4(12):13, 1977.

70. Yoo, R. P., and Touloukian, R. J.: Intussusception in the newborn: a unique clinical entity, J. Pediatr. Surg. 9:495, 1974.

and the need for antireflux procedures, J. Pediatr. Surg. 14:5, 1979.

CHAPTER 16

Urologic considerations

JOHN W. DUCKETT and HOWARD C. FILSTON

GENERAL CONSIDERATIONS

If any indications of urogenital abnormality have been identified in the newborn period, investigation of the entire urologic system will probably have already been undertaken. However, when they are unassociated with obvious abnormalities in other systems and when the genitalia are normal, marked abnormalities of the urinary tract can exist without symptoms for a considerable period of time. In the infant-toddler age group, the likely manifestations of urinary tract disease are the palpation of a flank mass; the palpation of abdominal or suprapubic masses; and such symptoms as failure to thrive, fevers of unknown origin, and frank urinary tract infections. Hematuria rarely presents as a symptom of urinary tract disease in this age group.

Any child with failure to thrive or fevers of unknown origin should be examined for urinary tract abnormalities as part of the general workup for these conditions. A carefully obtained urine culture and urinalysis are the first steps. In the male infant, a voided specimen obtained after preparing the perineal skin is usually adequate; in the female infant, however, a suprapubic bladder tap or carefully performed catheterization is required. The dividing line of 100,000 organisms per milliliter of urine is usually taken as an indication of significant infection, although some believe that in children this number should be as low as 10,000.[17] Most would consider one urinary tract infection in a male infant an indication for a thorough urologic workup, whereas they would allow two or more infections in the more susceptible female infant before undertaking a complete workup. Others believe that one urinary tract infection in either sex that is confirmed by culture should lead to a urologic evaluation.

Evaluation. Evaluation should consist of a voiding cystourethrogram (VCUG) followed by an intravenous pyelogram (IVP). The decision to proceed with further urologic investigation is based on the results of these two studies. The most likely entities to be found are obstructive uropathy and vesicoureteral reflux (VUR).

OBSTRUCTIVE UROPATHY

Obstruction may occur at any level in the urinary drainage tract but is commonly found at the ureteropelvic junction, the ureterovesical junction, or at the bladder outlet or proximal urethra. These entities are described in detail in Chapter 11 in the section on the newborn. The goal of treatment is to preserve renal function and to correct the obstruction. Almost all of these obstructions can be satisfactorily corrected and should be if the residual renal tissue is functionally adequate. Diversion of the proximal urinary tract may be indicated before major surgical correction of the obstruction is done if the child is severely maldeveloped or if marked infection is present. This may allow improvement in renal function and clearing of infection. On the other hand, such entities as posterior urethral valves that can be excised by transurethral resection can usually be treated without prior diversion. In choosing the method of diversion, the surgeon must pay heed to the need for subsequent reconstruction or "undiversion."

VESICOURETERAL REFLUX

VUR is a common problem in children with urinary tract infections and is abnormal. A VCUG (Fig. 16-1) and IVP should be obtained in every child with a documented, culture-proved urinary tract infection with greater than 100,000 colonies. The infection should be cleared 3 to 4 weeks befor the x-ray studies are begun.

VUR is associated with renal scarring in 20% to 30% of cases. Chronic pyelonephritis in children and young adults almost always is associated with VUR. With repeated urinary infections in the face of VUR, the kidney is at considerable risk for cortical scarring or growth failure. Renal scars rarely develop in the face of sterile reflux in children receiving prophylactic doses of antibacterial agents.

Medical treatment. Once VUR has been demonstrated, the object of therapy is to protect the kidney from pyelonephritis by avoiding further bouts of cystitis. The primary care physician must institute a conscientious program of prophylactic medication and continual surveillance. Nitro-

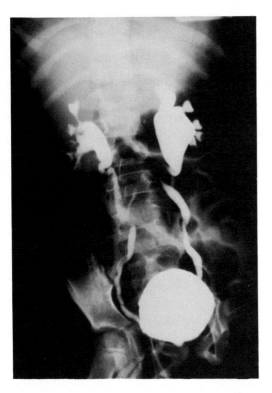

Fig. 16-1. Cystourethrogram showing marked bilateral reflux to the level of the calyces.

furantoin, sulfisoxazole, and trimethoprim with sulfamethoxazole (Bactrim, Septra) are the most commonly used prophylactic antibacterials. The urine should be cultured every 3 to 4 months, or whenever symptoms or fever appear. Uricult dip slides may be used in the office to screen the urine for infections. A VCUG or a nuclear cystogram, if available, and an IVP are repeated annually to determine the status of the VUR and to measure renal growth. When VUR ceases, medication may be discontinued. However, surveillance of urine cultures must continue for the next 2 years and a repeat cystogram (conventional or nuclear) the year after that is preferable. Excretory urography is used in follow-up if there have been intervening infections or if scarring was present on a previous study.

Cystoscopy, urethral dilatation, and urethrotomy. Cystoscopy is useful in assessing the anatomy of the ureterovesical junction. It is done with the idea that surgery will be needed and not as a baseline for later comparison. The fixation of the ureter into good trigonal muscle and its close proximity to the bladder neck with a good submucosal segment of ureter is the normal arrangement. If the ureter is laterally placed with poor trigonal attachment and little muscular backing, the reflux is very likely to persist. Paraureteral weaknesses causing a diverticulum with voiding and chronic cystitis cystica may also be assessed cystoscopically.

Urethral dilatation may be beneficial in a few cases by breaking the cycle of urethral irritation and sphincter spasm. It is our contention, however, that urethrotomy has very little place in the treatment of the child with urinary tract infections and reflux, although this position is controversial.

Surgical options. VUR has been graded on the basis of the amount of contrast that reaches the kidney and the degree of dilatation of the calyces and ureter: grade I is a wispy reflux into the lower ureter; grade IIa is reflux to the pelvis with no effect on any of the structures, that is, no hydroureter or hydronephrosis; grade IIb involves a wide ureter with pyelectasia and upper pole caliectasis; grade III involves a dilated tortuous ureter with or without secondary ureteropelvic obstruction and more advanced hydronephrosis with total caliectasis; and grade IV is associated with massive hydroureter and hydronephrosis and loss of renal parenchyma. In grades I and II, the likelihood of the reflux ceasing spontaneously is high and reimplantation surgery is rarely needed. In grades III and IV, the likelihood for cessation is much less; however, other factors should be taken into consideration before surgery is elected. Difficulty in maintaining a sterile urine in the face of prophylactic antibacterials should be considered; however, one breakthrough infection does not dictate surgery. The presence of significant renal scarring is not an indication for surgery in itself; when it is combined with other factors, however, it tends to tip the scale toward surgery. Intrarenal reflux has become a subject of recent concern and is very likely an indication of papillary deficiencies and susceptibility to scarring. Some children have pain from the distention of the ureter and collecting system on the side of the reflux, and this is taken into consideration.

Prognosis. Antireflux surgery has been quite successful and therefore should not be withheld because of the consideration of surgical risk.[1] The chances of persistent reflux or obstruction postoperatively should be less than 10%. Always remember that surgical statistics are obtained from centers where large volumes of this type of surgery are handled; results may be less than optimal in the hands of the occasional surgeon.

After successful surgical repair of the reflux, 15% to 25% of patients will still have recurrent bladder infections. These are more easily controlled and the chances of pyelonephritis diminished if the surgery was successful.

VUR is also present with a number of congenital abnormalities, such as urethral valves, prune-belly syndrome, and neurogenic bladder dysfunction. Optimal management of VUR involves close cooperation and communication between the primary care physician, the radiologist, and the pediatric urologist. It is true that in the majority of instances, VUR will cease spontaneously; however, there is certainly a place for appropriately selected surgical repair in the treatment of this condition.

CALCULUS DISEASE

Fortunately, stones in children are quite rare. Many are due to metabolic disorders such as cystinuria. Renal tubular acidosis is a common cause for stones and nephrocalcinosis in children. A metabolic workup should be done in all children with calculus disease. The most common etiology is infection associated with urologic anomalies such as VUR, hydronephrosis, and hydrocalyx.

Aggressive metabolic control and control of infection are as important as aggressive surgical correction.

FLANK MASSES

Palpation of a flank mass in the infant-toddler age group should lead to the suspicion of a tumor. Fortunately, most of these children will prove to have obstructive uropathy and the mass will be that of a hydronephrotic kidney. Multicystic or dysplastic kidneys missed on the newborn evaluation may also present in this fashion. An IVP will either fail to demonstrate function on that side, typical of the dysplastic kidney, or will show the marked hydronephrosis. Occasionally, such severe ureterovesical obstruction exists that the ureters will be hugely dilated and hypertrophied and will be palpable as masses.

WILMS' TUMOR AND NEUROBLASTOMA

Tumors, either of renal origin or of neural crest origin, will usually be demonstrated by an IVP. With the nephroblastoma or Wilms' tumor, there is marked distortion of the caliceal pattern caused by an intrarenal mass, usually at one pole of the kidney (Fig. 16-2). Usually, the caliceal system at one pole is maintained. Nonvisualization is unusual on the IVP and usually indicates invasion of the collecting system with obstruction or renal vein invasion. Bilateral Wilms' tumors occur in 5% to 10% of cases.[2]

Neural crest tumors arising from either the suprarenal gland or the paravertebral ganglia will usually displace the kidney with minimal distortion of the caliceal pattern (Fig. 16-3). Although crossing of the midline, the presence of calcifications, and the presence of hypertension have classically been associated with the neuroblastoma, each of these may be found with Wilms' tumor as well. Any tumor, including giant hydronephrosis, that enlarges enough may cross the midline. Hypertension may be associated with a renal artery stenosis and "Goldblatt kidney" effect on the renal glomerular blood flow. Fine, stippled calcifications are more commonly found in neuroblastoma, but occasionally gross calcification is noted in Wilms' tumors. Hematuria is present in only 10% of cases.

Evaluation. Further evaluation, once the presence of a tumor is confirmed, should consist of a spot urine specimen and 24-hour urine collec-

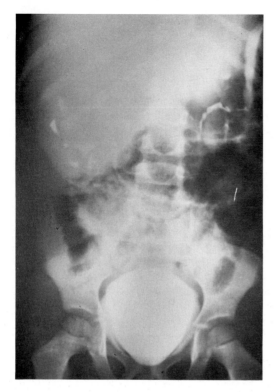

Fig. 16-2. IVP of an infant showing a mass effect on the right side with distortion of the calyces of the right kidney, indicating the probability of Wilms' tumor. This is a polar tumor with the lower pole calyceal appearance being maintained while the tumor exists primarily at the upper pole.

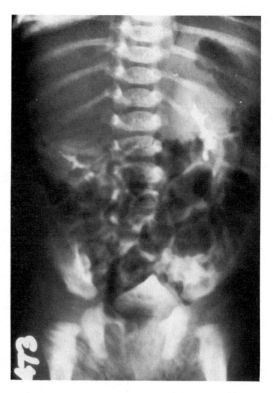

Fig. 16-3. IVP in a patient with a suprarenal neuroblastoma showing rotation and depression of the right kidney beneath a right upper quadrant mass. Displacement rather than distortion distinguishes neuroblastoma from Wilms' tumor. (From Filston, H. C., and Izant, R.: The surgical neonate: evaluation and care, New York, 1978, Appleton-Century-Crofts.)

tion for vanillylmandelic acid excretion and a search for the presence of metastases. Since Wilms' tumors classically metastasize to the lung, a good anteroposterior (AP) and lateral chest radiograph should be the first screening test obtained. When neuroblastoma is suspected, a bone marrow aspiration used to search for metastases to the bone marrow and a bone scan will complete the metastatic survey. A liver scan may be useful, but the liver can usually be evaluated at the time of exploratory laparotomy. An inferior venacavogram will demonstrate tumor invasion if it is present and provides an important "road map" during excision of the tumor (Fig. 16-4).

Medical versus surgical treatment. Since both of these tumors are most successfully treated when they are completely excised, surgical therapy should be the primary mode of treatment. However, great success in the cure of Wilms' tumors

has been achieved by multimodal therapy that combines surgical excision with radiation and chemotherapy. Such success has not yet been demonstrated for neuroblastoma, and surgical excision of the entire tumor is still associated with the highest cures.[5,7] However, since both of these tumors have a high rate of cure in an infant under the age of 1 year—Wilms' tumor because it is usually at an early stage in that age group and the neuroblastoma because of the interaction between the tumor and the child's immune mechanisms—early referral for surgical excision should be the goal. Best results are obtained when a team approach (taking into account the knowledge obtained by the national study groups) allows the surgeon, the radiotherapist, and the oncologist to interact both before surgery in planning the best overall approach to the child's therapy and during and after surgery in completing the multi-

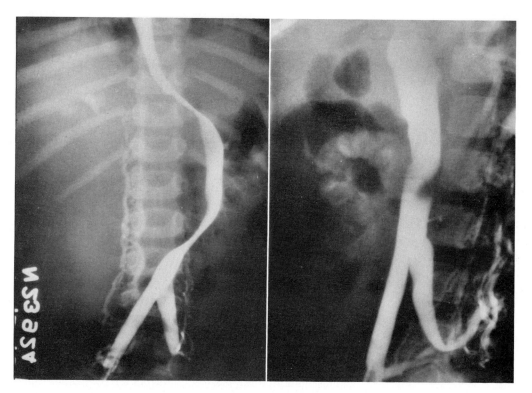

Fig. 16-4. Anteroposterior (AP) and lateral views of the inferior venacavogram in a patient with right-sided Wilms' tumor showing the marked displacement of the cava as the enlarging tumor crosses the midline. There is no evidence of tumor extension into the cava.

modal therapeutic course. Many protocol decisions depend on accurate observation on the part of the surgeon, and newer approaches in Wilms' tumor that enable radiotherapy and chemotherapy to be reduced depend on expert surgical excision combined with evaluation of any possible extension of the tumor. Thus, the practice of having the tumor excised by an inexperienced local surgeon with the intent of then referring the child to a major center should be condemned. Such an approach leads to inadequate therapy, incomplete excisions, the need for repeated surgery, the need for excessive radiotherapy and chemotherapy to make up for the lack of total surgical evaluation and excision, and reduced survival.

Prognosis. The cure rate for Wilms' tumor is now about 90%. Neuroblastoma, the most common solid tumor in childhood, unfortunately has a poor prognosis except in the infant under 1 year of age. In most cases, multiorgan spread occurs before the tumor is discovered. Therapy has not significantly improved the survival rate, which is about 30%, in the last 20 years. Immunotherapy may offer new hope.

OTHER TUMORS
Rhabdomyosarcoma

Tumors of the bladder, prostate, or vagina in infants and children are most likely rhabdomyosarcomas. They may present with symptoms of urinary urgency, frequency, and obstruction. Hematuria is rarely present. The solid embryonal type may arise from the pelvic floor without more precise origin or may start in the prostate. The polypoid type (sarcoma botryoides) grows into the lumen of the bladder or vagina and may present a "cluster of grapes" at the introitus. Radical surgery in the past was the only hope for survival. Much of the ablative surgery has now been replaced by aggressive chemotherapy, which in most cases will offer regression of the tumor so that surgical removal can be more precise and less extensive.[13] A survival rate of 80% can be expected in those of urogenital tract origin.

Renal cell carcinoma

Although Wilms' tumor is the most common tumor of the kidney in childhood, adult-type renal cell carcinoma, or hypernephroma, does occur; over 88 cases have been reported in the literature.[6] Hypernephroma in childhood has been reported in a range of from 2.3% to 3.8% of all childhood renal malignancies. Classically presenting with a triad of pain, hematuria, and a palpable abdominal mass in adults, hypernephroma in children, like the more common Wilms' tumor, most frequently presents as an asymptomatic abdominal mass. Case reports of hypernephroma found underlying blunt abdominal trauma and of spontaneous rupture with presentation as an acute abdominal crisis can be found in the literature.

Survival statistics generally indicate that this tumor has a less favorable prognosis than Wilms' tumor, although long-term tumor-free survival and apparent cures have been reported. The rarity of the tumor obviously has precluded studies of sizable numbers of cases using adjuvant radiotherapy and chemotherapy. A general impression exists that the tumor can persist or recur many years after apparent cure, so that careful long-term follow-up is essential. The tumor has been reported in the infant-toddler age group, but the majority of cases in children have been reported in the childhood and teenage years.

Testicular tumors

In the infant, testicular tumors are characteristically yolk sac carcinomas of the endodermal sinus type and not the typical embryonal tumors of the adult testis.[8,9,11] Radical orchiectomy and periaortic lymph node dissections are of questionable need in the younger age group. In the child under 1 year of age, alphafetoprotein is a reliable tumor marker.[15] Rhabdomyosarcoma of the paratesticular tissues is treated similarly to the other rhabdomyosarcomas.

Multilocular cysts

Also known as cystic adenoma or cystic partially differentiated nephroblastoma, a multilocular cyst is currently thought to be related to Wilms' tumor; consequently, nephrectomy is usually performed. Diagnostic studies fail to differentiate such a lesion from Wilms' tumor. Cystectomy with the upper and lower poles of the kidneys left intact is a feasible procedure if the diagnosis can be made at exploration.

Solitary renal cyst

Although the solitary renal cyst is the most common renal mass in adults and is considered an acquired lesion, simple cysts can occur in children and are usually an incidental finding with no clinical symptoms. They are treated as adult cysts with the same radiologic criteria, including ultrasonography and cyst puncture. Renal exploration is not necessary. Frequently, after cyst puncture, the mass disappears and no further cysts are seen on subsequent x-ray films.

Childhood polycystic disease

Blyth and Ockenden[3] have presented a classification of a spectrum of polycystic kidney disease that includes juvenile and childhood subheadings. Children with this disease present signs of portal hypertension from bleeding varices and succumb from the liver disease rather than the renal disease. The kidneys are, however, enlarged and may have splayed-out collecting systems similar to those of adult polycystic kidneys. The diagnosis is suspected when enlarged kidneys are palpated and from the dysmorphic appearance on the IVP.

Adult polycystic disease

Adult polycystic disease is an autosomal dominant condition with a strong family history. Presentation is at about age 40 and includes renal failure, infection, hypertension, or hematuria. It is rare that adult polycystic disease is diagnosed in the infant or child, since the cysts are formed as the child grows, compressing the renal parenchyma. Beware of the diagnosis of adult polycystic disease in children and suspect, instead, bilateral Wilms' tumor.

URINARY TRACT INFECTIONS

Although urinary tract infections in little girls may occur without underlying abnormalities of the urogenital system, urinary tract infections in little boys are unusual. The occurrence of a urinary tract infection in a male infant should lead to a urinary tract workup that should include, as a minimum, an IVP. Careful physical examination of the child's abdomen and genitalia, including a careful inspection of the urethral meatus, should precede the radiologic examination.

The female child developing a urinary tract infection in this age group should be carefully examined as well, both abdominally and perineally. Attention should be directed to the anus to be certain that it is, in fact, an anus and not an anteriorly placed fistula and that the perineal structures appear normal. Recurrent urinary tract infection in a little girl should lead to further urologic evaluation including intravenous urography and a cystogram with a VCUG.

If any doubt as to the normalcy of the urinary tract exists in either sex, urologic referral for cystoscopy and possibly retrograde pyelography should be considered early. Most urologic conditions that would be discovered are correctable, but failure to diagnose an abnormality that may be a source of chronic infection or reflux pressure may lead to permanent damage to the urinary tract and kidney.

MALE GENITAL TRACT LESIONS
The foreskin

There are very few medical indications for circumcision. Routine infant circumcision is a questionable ritual in this country. Certainly, every parent should have the option of informed consent before signing for a routine circumcision. The care of the uncircumcised penis is important, however, and many that are unaccustomed to dealing with the uncircumcised condition feel that the freeing of the fusion by stripping the foreskin back is important for daily cleansing. This maneuver causes harm and is painful. Therefore, no stripping of this fusion need be done until after puberty. Most of the natural fusions will separate with time and without the aid of the physician. It is only after puberty that regular cleansing is required.

Paraphimosis will occur when the foreskin is retracted and not returned to its normal position. Swelling and irritation occur, and reduction is sometimes difficult. A circumcision is then required.

Meatal ulcers and meatal stenosis

In the circumcised penis, ammonia formed from the breakdown of urinary urea leads to "diaper rashes" on the glans and meatal ulcers, which may result in scarring and meatal stenosis. Meatal stenosis in itself is not a significant obstruction, even with a pinpoint opening. There is no need for a urographic workup with meatal stenosis and certainly no need for cystoscopy or urethral dilatation. The primary indications for meatotomy are upward deflection of the stream and a pro-

longed voiding time. In cooperative children it may be possible to do the meatotomy as an office procedure using local anesthesia.

Testicular and scrotal abnormalities
Hydroceles and hernias

The most common entities found in the infant-toddler age group are hydroceles and hernias. A hydrocele in the child is essentially a hernia with a narrow entry tract from the peritoneum. Generally, only fluid from the peritoneum can pass down the tract into the distal enlarged sac. Occasionally, however, the tract has an hourglass shape and the upper processus vaginalis is wide open and will admit a loop of bowel. Thus, the possibility of incarceration exists with hydroceles as well as with hernias, and a not unusual story is that of a child in whom the physician has observed an obvious hydrocele who then develops incarceration of a loop of bowel in the internal ring.

Hydroceles can also occur along the course of the cord, with a narrow proximal tract and a narrow distal processus. The only part of the processus that fills with fluid and enlarges is that along the central length of the cord.

This lesion can occur in infant girls as well, and is known as a hydrocele of the canal of Nuck.

These lesions are discussed in detail in Chapter 15.

Tender, swollen scrotum

When one side of the scrotum becomes acutely swollen and tender, it is a surgical emergency. These boys should be seen immediately and evaluated to determine if torsion of the testicle is present. Manual or surgical reduction of the twisted testicle is vital to its being saved. Detorsion can be monitored effectively with a Doppler stethoscope so that orchiopexy may be done on a more elective basis if manual reduction is accomplished. Manual reduction also relieves the acute pain that the patient is suffering.

Neonatal torsion occurs during the perinatal time or during labor and usually presents as a nontender mass in the scrotum. Salvage of the testicle in neonatal torsion is extremely rare, so that emergency surgery is usually not warranted.

Another possibility with a tender, swollen scrotum is a twisted appendix testis, which is usually a pinpoint discrete area on the upper inner portion of the testicle. This organ has no function, and its removal is only for symptomatic improvement or when the diagnosis of torsion of the testicle remains a possibility.

A more detailed discussion of these entities can be found in Chapter 21 in the section on the child from 2 to 12.

Epididymitis

Epididymitis is a rare finding in children and constitutes less than 10% of acute scrotal conditions. Urinalysis should be done on all children to determine the presence of an infection.

Orchitis

Orchitis may occur in connection with such viral illnesses as mumps, but unless a clear etiological factor of this type is present, testicular tenderness should be thought of as torsion until proved otherwise.

FEMALE GENITAL TRACT LESIONS
Labial fusion

In labial fusion, the labia minora are fused together, so that the urethral opening is up near the base of the clitoris. Separation can be achieved by applying a local anesthetic topically and separating the labia minora with an applicator or probe, starting from the superior portion and applying pressure in a vertical fashion. Application of an estrogen cream for a few days causes hyperplasia of the area and will usually prevent recurrence of the fusion. Separation can often be achieved in thick fusions by applying the estrogen cream for several days. Urinary tract infections commonly result from this condition if it is untreated.

Urethral stenosis

Not many years ago, urethral stenosis was the most common diagnosis in female children in pediatric urology and urethral dilatations and urethrotomies were commonly being performed. It is becoming more apparent that this type of stenosis, though present occasionally, is unusual. It is not considered the cause for reflux or recurring infections but may be related to some voiding symptoms in little girls, especially symptoms associated with uninhibited contractions.

Urethral prolapse

The lining of the urethra may prolapse through the meatus in black female children and cause irritation and pain (Fig. 16-5). Reduction of the

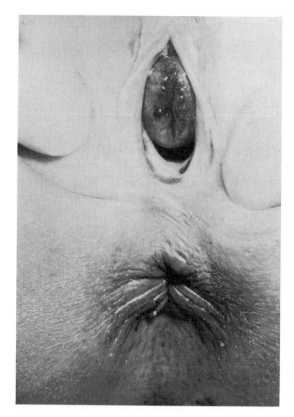

Fig. 16-5. Circumferential prolapse of the urethra, which appears as a mass filling almost the entire vulva.

prolapse is not a permanent cure. Excision of the prolapsing tissue is the best management.

Congenital absence of the vagina

The Mayer-Rokitansky-Kuster-Hauser symdrome is a complex of conditions associated with agenesis of one kidney and lack of formation of the müllerian structures on the ipsilateral side.[16] There is, therefore, a dysmorphic development of the female genital tract with atresia of the vagina and an abnormal uterus. Both of the ovaries are normal. This condition should be considered whenever a solitary kidney is identified in a female infant. Hydrocolpos may occur secondary to stenosis of the vagina or may be due to an imperforate hymen. Incision of the imperforate hymen allows drainage of this minor condition. Vaginal stenosis may be difficult to manage and requires more extensive surgical intervention. This lesion may remain asymptomatic and undiscovered until puberty leads to cyclic pain and primary amenorrhea (see Fig. 25-3).

NEUROPATHIC BLADDER DYSFUNCTION

Myelomeningocele (spina bifida cystica) and congenital sacral deformities are the most common anomalies associated with neurogenic vesical dysfunction in children. If the bladder fails to empty properly, the ureters and kidney rapidly suffer obstruction and renal failure may be the unwanted outcome. Continual surveillance of bladder function, conscientious attention to infection control, and periodic radiographic evaluation are required for all children with myelomeningoceles.

It is not possible to correlate bladder behavior with the level of the spinal lesion or the degree of paralysis of the limbs. Likewise, it is difficult to use the usual neurologic classification for neuropathic bladder in order to determine the management program for these children. We prefer to use the functional classifications of (1) failure of bladder emptying and (2) failure of urine storage.

Children with myelomeningoceles who have increased bladder outlet resistance due to the inability of the outlet to relax during detrusor contraction are the ones most likely to develop upper tract deterioration. Because the bladder is chronically distended, the ureterovesicular junction is lengthened and resistance to inflow into the bladder is increased. The ureters then become dilated, and caliectasis and hydronephrosis develop. Stasis leads to urinary tract infection, which is most difficult to manage unless adequate bladder emptying is achieved. VUR is ultimately present in 75% of these children.[4] If a bladder infection is present, the kidneys are at great risk in the face of VUR.

Management. Management is therefore directed toward ensuring that the bladder empties adequately, whether on its own or with assistance. Credé has classically been used as the assistance maneuver. This maneuver is potentially dangerous, however, especially in the face of VUR. The bladder pressure achieved with Credé is enormous; and if backflow into the kidneys is present, this pressure is exerted directly on the renal parenchyma. Credé should be used very cautiously.

Clean intermittent catheterization (CIC) has proved to be a safe and effective treatment modality for bladders that fail to empty.[10] In female infants we use a No. 10 or 12 French hollow metal sound that is soaked in an antiseptic solution and rinsed with tap water. The metal catheter may be

wrapped in foil and sterilized in a hot oven for 20 minutes. With clean hands and without sterile gloves, it is then inserted in the female urethral meatus with ease to empty the bladder on a regular basis. This technique is especially effective in the older child, who eventually can learn to manage it herself. In the male child, a more flexible polyethylene feeding tube or rubber catheter is inserted through the penis in a clean manner.

Vesicostomy. At the Children's Hospital of Philadelphia, children who have emptying problems at an early age are managed with temporary cutaneous vesicostomy. This procedure is quite simple and effectively brings the dome of the bladder to the lower abdominal skin as a fistula. It can be achieved in a child because the bladder is an abdominal organ, not a pelvic organ, as in the adult. The procedure allows for a pop-off valve for the system and eliminates the need for regular CIC. The child is managed in diapers until he reaches an age where continence is desirable. At that time, the vesicostomy can be closed and a program of CIC instituted. If VUR is present, reimplantation of the ureters can be done at the time of closure of the vesicostomy. We do not consider vesicostomy an adequate form of permanent diversion.

Antibacterials. All of these children should be given suppressive doses of medications: either nitrofurantoin, sulfisoxazole, or trimethoprim with sulfamethoxazole. Cultures should be obtained on a regular basis (every 3 months) by using suprapubic aspiration in younger boys, catheterized specimens in girls, or clean-voided specimens, if possible. It is not necessary to discontinue the prophylactic medication before culturing.

X-ray surveillance. During the child's initial admission to the hospital to have the myelomeningocele repaired, an IVP should be obtained for baseline studies. If there is dilatation of the urinary tract at that time, a voiding cystogram is necessary to determine the presence of reflux. The child begins receiving suppressive medication at that time. The parents are taught a gentle bladder expression technique by bladder massage or by gentle Credé. If resistance is encountered, a program for better emptying should be established, either with cutaneous vesicostomy or CIC. As infections become a problem, it is most likely that stasis and obstruction are present; and these must be eliminated before eradication of the infection will be successful. Chronic bacilluria is not acceptable in the patient with myelomeningocele.

Continence. About one third of these children have bladders classified as "failure to store," meaning that the outlet resistance is so low that urine will not remain in the bladder in sufficient quantity to achieve social continence. These children are the most difficult to manage; however, they are usually the ones whose upper tracts are preserved and who have little trouble with infections. When the child reaches an age when social dryness is desirable, imipramine (25 mg 3 times a day) can be used to increase bladder capacity and outlet resistance and propantheline bromide added (7.5 to 15 mg 3 times a day) to diminish the uninhibited bladder contractions that lead to bladder instability. These parameters are monitored by cystometrograms. The success of this program is about 50% to 60%.

Unfortunately, some of these children cannot be made acceptably continent, and other, more radical procedures are necessary. The newly developed artificial sphincters (Scott prosthesis) have been partially successful in carefully selected children with myelomeningoceles, but the device is still in its developmental stage.[14]

Permanent urinary diversion. In the past, the ileal conduit or, more recently, the colon conduit with an antireflux ureterocolonic anastomosis was advocated as a solution to the long-term management of these children. However, it seems appropriate today to utilize this form of diversion only as a last resort.

Bladder stimulators. Recent experience with these electrical devices indicate that they offer very little benefit over CIC.

Sacral dysgenesis

Neuropathic bladder dysfunction is also associated with congenital dysplasia of the sacral nerve roots, and the management of these children is similar to that described above. Early diagnosis of the condition is most important in proper management. Careful assessment of all spinal films in children with bladder dysfunction is important.

Idiopathic neurogenic bladder

An unusual group of children seem to develop neurogenic bladders because of dysfunctional voiding patterns. Ultimately they have urinary tract infections, VUR, and upper tract deterioration, requiring management as children with "neuropathic bladders." Specific neurologic disorders are not found, and the etiology of the bladder dysfunction is not clear. Relearning normal voiding patterns has been effective therapy.

• • •

Close surveillance of vesical function is mandatory for maintenance of a sound urinary tract in children with myelomeningoceles. This includes the use of prophylactic antibacterials, regular radiographic studies, and extremely conscientious follow-up. Permanent urinary diversion should be discouraged until all other modalities have been attempted.

REFERENCES

1. Bauer, S. B., and others: Long-term results of antireflux surgery in children. In Hodson, J., and Kincaid-Smith, P., editors: Reflux nephropathy, New York, 1979, Masson Publishing U.S.A., Inc., p. 287.
2. Bishop, H. C., and others: Survival in bilateral Wilms' tumor—review of 30 National Wilms' Tumor Study cases, J. Pediatr. Surg. **12:**631, 1977.
3. Blyth, H., and Ockenden, B. G.: Polycystic disease of kidneys and liver presenting in childhood, J. Med. Genet. **8:**257, 1971.
4. Duckett, J. W., and Raezer, D. M.: Neuromuscular dysfunction of the lower urinary tract. In Kelalis, P. P., King, L. R., and Belman, A. B., editors: Clinical pediatric urology, Philadelphia, 1976, W. B. Saunders Co., p. 401.
5. Evans, A. E., D'Angio, G. J., and Koop, C. E.: Diagnosis and treatment of neuroblastoma, Pediatr. Clin. North Am. **23:**161, 1976.
6. Futrell, J. W., Filston, H. C., and Reid, J. D.: Rupture of a renal cell carcinoma in a child: five-year tumor-free survival and literature review, Cancer **41:**1565, 1978.
7. Grosfeld, J. L., and others: Metastatic neuroblastoma: factors influencing survival, J. Pediatr. Surg. **13:**59, 1978.
8. Houser, R., Izant, R. J., Jr., and Persky, L.: Testicular tumors in children, Am. J. Surg. **110:**876, 1965.
9. Juckes, A. W., Fraser, M. M., and Dexter, D.: Endodermal sinus (yolk sac) tumors in infants and children, J. Pediatr. Surg. **14:**520, 1979.
10. Lapides, J., and others: Follow-up on unsterile, intermittent self-catheterization, J. Urol. **111:**184, 1974.
11. MacKinnon, A. E., and Cohen, S. J.: Archenteronoma (yolk sac tumors), J. Pediatr. Surg. **13:**21, 1978.
12. Normand, I.C., and Smellie, J. M.: Vesicoureteric reflux: the case for conservative management. In Hodson, J., and Kincaid-Smith, P., editors: Reflux nephropathy, New York, 1979, Masson Publishing U.S.A., Inc., p. 281.
13. Pratt, C. B., Huster, H. O., and Fleming, I. D.: Coordinated treatment of childhood rhabdomyosarcoma with surgery, radiotherapy, and combination chemotherapy, Cancer Res. **32:**606, 1972.
14. Scott, F. B., Bradley, W. E., and Timm, G. W.: Treatment of urinary incontinence by an implantable prosthetic urinary sphincter, J. Urol. **112:**75, 1974.

15. Tsuchida, Y., and others: Alpha-fetoprotein, prealbumin, albumin, alpha-1-antitrypsin and transferrin as diagnostic and therapeutic markers for endodermal sinus tumors, J. Pediatr. Surg. **13:**25, 1978.

16. Welch, K. J.: Abnormalities and neoplasms of the vagina and uterus. In Ravitch, M. M., and others, editors: Pe-

diatric surgery, ed. 3, Chicago, 1979, Year Book Medical Publishers, Inc., p. 1457.

17. Welch, K.J.: Diagnosis of urologic conditions. In Ravitch, M. M., and others, editors: Pediatric surgery, ed. 3, Chicago, 1979, Year Book Medical Publishers, Inc., p. 1133.

CHAPTER 17

Neurosurgical considerations

W. JERRY OAKES and ROBERT H. WILKINS

MACROCRANIA

Macrocrania is enlargement of the head so that the maximum frontal occipital head circumference is equal to or greater than the ninety-eighth percentile. The condition is a relatively common one with diverse etiological factors, including hydrocephalus, subdural effusions and hematomas, physiologic and familial macrocephaly, intracranial cysts and tumors, achondroplasia, nutritional macrocephaly, encephalopathies (lead intoxication and Vitamin A deficiency), and cerebral storage diseases (Tay-Sachs disease, metachromatic leukodystrophy, and Hurler's syndrome), among others. The vast majority of patients with macrocrania have benign disease that can usually be effectively treated.

Routine examination for age. Every infant being followed by a primary care physician should have sequential head circumference measurements made and recorded. With this simple assessment, a physician can accurately screen patients for an early sign of increased intracranial pressure. A measuring tape is placed around the head, and the maximum frontal occipital circumference is measured. Three readings are routinely taken and should vary no more than 2 mm. The circumference is then plotted on an appropriate growth chart according to the infant's age. Premature infants require a special chart that takes into consideration their shortened gestation (Fig. 17-1). To complement the head circumference measurement, the infant's intracranial tension is assessed by holding the infant vertically and determining the anterior fontanelle tension and position. For this, it is necessary that the infant be calm and not crying or agitated. In the vertical

position the anterior fontanelle is normally flat or concave. The tension is appreciated subjectively by palpating the anterior fontanelle. The pulse and respiratory rate can frequently be seen to be reflected in an anterior fontanelle pulsation. Skull percussion should also be performed to help assess the intracranial tension and is done by stabilizing the head with one hand held flat against the fronto-parietal area and percussing the skull over the opposite hemisphere (Fig. 17-2). The percussion note can be both felt and heard. With these methods an estimate of the current intracranial pressure can be obtained.

Additional information can be gained by transilluminating the skull in a dark room with a strong light. It should be remembered, however, that there are many causes of a false-positive transillumination; the most frequent of which include subgaleal hematomas and infiltration of the scalp with fluid from an intravenous infusion. Every skull examination should also include auscultation of the head and palpation of the cranial sutures.

Possible findings. Patients who would eventually develop macrocrania can be diagnosed prior to the development of gross enlargement of the skull by early determination of an accelerated *rate* of head growth. If they are serially plotted, the head circumference measurements will show that the patient is crossing percentile lines of growth and yet may not have reached the point of macrocrania (Fig. 17-1). This sign of abnormality is usually the earliest and only one that can be detected clinically. The significance of the finding increases when the child's length and weight are similarly plotted and found to be growing parallel to expected growth curves. An accel-

Boys' head circumference vs. age (10th, 50th, and 90th percentiles)

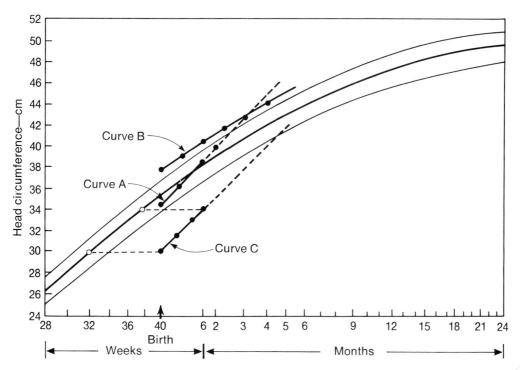

Fig. 17-1. Chart of head circumference versus age. *Curve A:* Infant with accelerated head growth. Although the absolute size of the head is still normal, the patient is demonstrating an accelerated *rate* of growth and needs elective evaluation. *Curve B:* Infant with absolute macrocrania but a normal rate of head growth. Although the patient may very well have familial or physiologic macrocephaly, elective evaluation is still required, as well as careful follow-up. *Curve C:* If the head circumference of premature neonates is plotted on standard growth curves without consideration for the degree of prematurity, the rate of head growth may appear accelerated. When the head circumference is plotted at the appropriate point on the curve, however, the rate of head growth is seen to be normal.

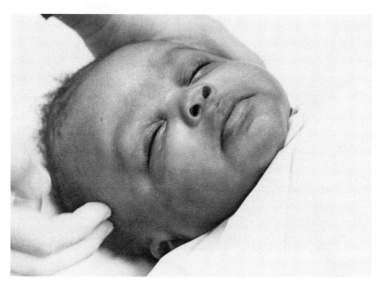

Fig. 17-2. MacEwen's sign. The head is stabilized with one hand and percussed with the other. The percussion note can be both felt and heard.

erated rate of growth is more indicative of an active pathologic process than is a single measurement of head circumference. This finding is particularly helpful in diagnosing physiologic or familial macrocephaly, where the rate of head growth is normal and parallels the expected growth curves but the head circumference measurements are in the range of macrocrania (Fig. 17-1). When a premature infant's head circumference is plotted on a routine growth chart and no allowance is made for the infant's shortened gestation, the rate of growth may seem excessive (Fig. 17-1). ''Catch-up'' growth of the head in prematurity as well as following nutritional deprivation may be difficult to differentiate from pathologic growth. Careful follow-up as well as radiographic investigation will help to determine the true nature of the accelerated head growth.

A variety of abnormalities can be detected to support a diagnosis of accelerated head growth secondary to increased intracranial pressure. The percussion note may become dull and the superficial scalp veins prominent. Palpation of the sutures may show them to be separated, and the tension of the anterior fontanelle will be excessive. The fontanelle may bulge externally and lose its spontaneous pulsations. The skull configu-

ration may change in the presence of a subdural effusion or chronic subdural hematoma (becoming square or boxy when viewed from the vertex). Transillumination will usually be positive over the lesion (Fig. 17-3). Acute and subacute subdural hematomas and subdural empyema may not demonstrate abnormal transillumination because of the high density of the fluid. In hydranencephaly and severe hydrocephalus, where the cortex is thinned to less than 1 cm, there may be diffuse and symmetric transillumination of the entire supratentorial compartment. Focal transillumination is also seen in superficially placed arachnoid cysts or porencephalia. Abnormal transillumination present over the posterior fossa may indicate the presence of a Dandy-Walker cyst or posterior fossa extracranial cyst.

As the intracranial contents expand and the pressure increases, the cranial sutures separate. By compensating in this way, the infant may not develop alarming symptoms requiring medical attention until late in the course of the disease. The fact that the neurologic examination will characteristically remain normal except for increased irritability and mild developmental delay again emphasizes the importance of early detection by assessing the rate of head growth. When the neu-

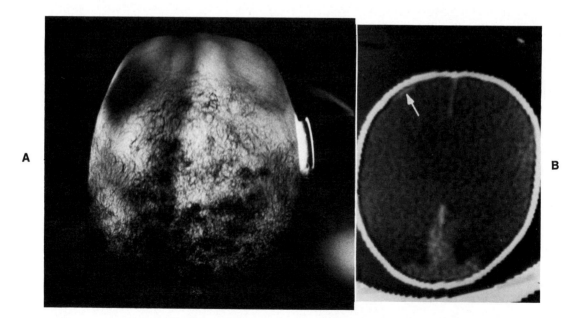

Fig. 17-3. A, Diffuse transillumination of an infant with hydranencephaly. **B,** Computerized tomographic (CT) brain scan of the same patient demonstrating that the only residual cortex present is in the left frontal area (arrow). This finding corresponds with the area of diminished transillumination.

rologic examination does begin to show focal abnormalities, eye signs are frequently the first to occur and include abducens nerve palsy with inability to fully abduct the involved eye on lateral gaze. This condition may be seen unilaterally or bilaterally and has no localizing neurologic value. The "setting sun" sign can also be seen, with the sclera prominently visible above the superior portion of the iris (Fig. 17-4). Papilledema is rare in infancy because of the ability of the immature skull to expand and relieve increased intracranial pressure. A late sign of severe increased intracranial pressure is the development of respiratory irregularity and stridor, which is thought to be secondary to medullary compression or ischemia. If it develops, it is a sign of severe neurologic compromise and potential respiratory distress. Infants with increased intracranial pressure are generally irritable, feed poorly, and may have a high-pitched "cerebral cry." Vomiting is common and occurs after feeding and on awakening. Vomiting secondary to increased intracranial pressure differs from simple regurgitation, which is commonly seen in normal infants, in that it usually involves the entire meal or feeding whereas simple regurgitation involves only a small portion of the feeding. Following an episode of vomiting, the infant frequently rests more comfortably than before. This composure and decreased irritability,

however, are short-lived. The projectile nature of vomiting secondary to increased intracranial pressure has been overemphasized in the past and is seen in many other conditions. Late in the course of the condition, the infant may show periods of decerebrate rigidity with marked arching of the back and extension of the neck and extremities. The untreated infant will become progressively more lethargic, eventually losing the decerebrate rigidity, and finally becoming flaccid immediately before death.

Common occurrences. Hydrocephalus is the most common cause of macrocrania.[41] It may be present at birth or occur during infancy as a consequence of trauma or meningitis. It may occur spontaneously with limitation of cerebral spinal fluid (CSF) flow at the aqueduct of Sylvius without known precipitating factors. As discussed earlier, patients with myelodysplasia have a 60% to 90% chance of developing hydrocephalus, depending on the level and extent of their spinal lesion—lumbodorsal lesions have a much greater association with hydrocephalus than do sacral lesions. Occasionally, hydrocephalus may be the presenting sign of an intracranial cyst (Fig. 17-5) or tumor (Fig. 17-6), or the consequence of a strategically located arteriovenous malformation. Hydrocephalus that has its onset in later childhood, when skull expansion is more limited, will

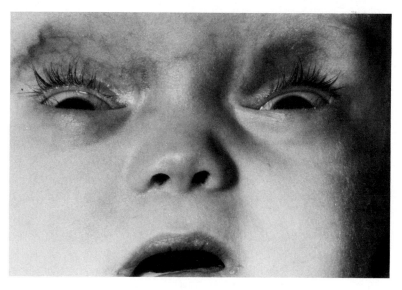

Fig. 17-4. Infant with "setting sun" sign. The sclera is visible above the iris bilaterally when the eye is in the primary position. Venous engorgement is easily appreciated in the upper eyelids.

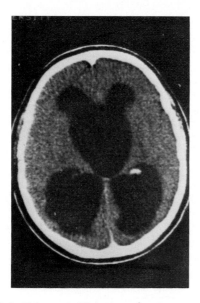

Fig. 17-5. Enhanced CT brain scan of a patient with an anterior third ventricular cyst. Symmetric internal hydrocephalus occurred secondary to obstruction of the foramina of Monro. The patient is a teenage boy with a bobbing motion of the head as though it were suspended from a coiled spring (bobble-head doll syndrome). (Courtesy S. Rothman, M.D., Durham, N.C.)

not present with macrocrania but with the classic triad of headache, vomiting, and papilledema, implying increased intracranial pressure.

In the vast majority of patients, hydrocephalus results from the obstruction to CSF flow.[40] CSF produced by the choroid plexus is not allowed to flow freely out of the ventricular system to be reabsorbed in the arachnoid granulations in the subarachnoid space. Common points of obstruction to flow within the ventricular system include the aqueduct of Sylvius, outlets of the fourth ventricle (foramina of Magendie and Luschka), and the two foramina of Monro. The hydrocephalus that results is termed internal or noncommunicating. Ventricular enlargement in these cases occurs proximal to the point of obstruction (Fig. 17-7). Commonly, in cases of myelodysplasia the occipital horns of the lateral ventricles will dilate first and most extensively (Fig. 17-8). This enlargement will be followed by dilatation of the bodies and temporal horns of the lateral ventricles, followed by enlargement of the frontal horns and third ventricle. Following decompression of the ventricular system by the insertion of a ventriculoperitoneal shunt, the sequence is reversed, so that the occipital horns are the last portion of the enlarged ventricular system to diminish in size.

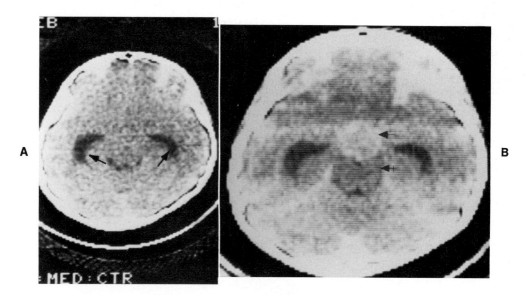

Fig. 17-6. A, Unenhanced CT brain scan through the suprasellar area. No tumor can be seen; but the cerebrospinal fluid (CSF) cisterns, which can usually be seen in this area, are absent. The temporal horns are easily seen (arrows) and are pathologically dilated. **B,** Enhanced study at the level of **A** demonstrating the enhancing tumor (→) compressing the brain stem (↠).

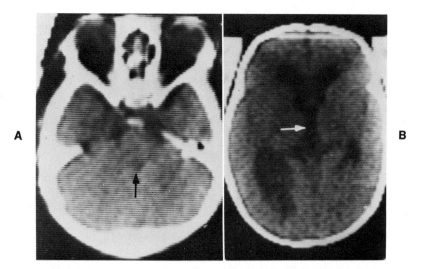

Fig. 17-7. Unenhanced CT brain scan of an infant with hydrocephalus secondary to congenital aqueductal stenosis. **A,** The fourth ventricle is normal in size and position (arrow). **B,** The third ventricle is easily visualized and pathologically dilated (arrow).

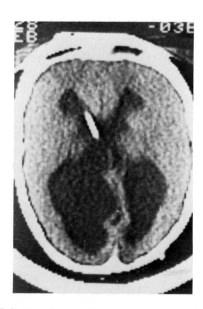

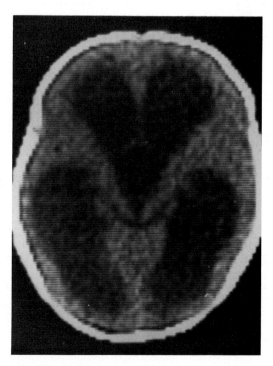

Fig. 17-8. Unenhanced CT brain scan of a child with myelodysplasia and shunted hydrocephalus. Occipital horns are dilated out of proportion to the rest of the ventricular system.

Fig. 17-9. Unenhanced CT brain scan of an infant with external or communicating hydrocephalus. The entire ventricular system is symmetrically dilated. The section is through the third and lateral ventricles, all of which are moderately to severely dilated.

Characteristic points of CSF obstruction outside the ventricular system include the basal cisterns and the arachnoid granulations themselves. With obstruction to CSF flow at these points, the entire ventricular system will enlarge (Fig. 17-9). In addition, there can be some degree of exaggeration of the subarachnoid space when the obstruction to flow is at the level of the arachnoid granulations. This form of hydrocephalus is termed external or communicating.

A rare but interesting cause of hydrocephalus is the excessive production of CSF, so that the physiologic limits of the normally functioning resorptive pathway are exceeded. This situation has been shown to occur only with tumors of the choroid plexus (choroid plexus papillomas).[42] The tumors that present in this fashion characteristically occur in infancy in the posterior portion of the lateral ventricle. The successful removal of these neoplasms will actually return the CSF production to the normal range and restore normal CSF dynamics in some patients without the need for a shunting procedure. If hydrocephalus persists following removal of the tumor, it is thought to be secondary to diminished CSF resorption in association with previous subarachnoid hemorrhage from the tumor.[50]

In the past several years, patients have been identified with pathologic enlargement of the ventricular system but with normal CSF pressure as recorded from a lumbar puncture. This entity of "normal-pressure hydrocephalus" was first described in adults[1] and is associated with the clinical triad of mental deterioration, gait disturbance, and urinary incontinence. When these patients are treated by the insertion of a ventriculoperitoneal or ventriculoatrial shunt, there frequently is clinical improvement. Recently it has been discovered that if the intracranial pressure is constantly monitored over a 24- to 48-hour period, the normal CSF pressure of these patients is interrupted by frequent and prolonged bouts of intracranial hypertension, which are resolved spontaneously.[36,57] These periods of elevated pressure characteristically occur during the rapid eye movement phase of sleep. Therefore, the condition is not truly normal-pressure hydrocephalus; rather, it involves intermittent elevation of the intracranial pressure. Similar findings have subsequently been reported in children.[41]

An additional category of hydrocephalus encompasses patients who are thought to have "com-pensated" or "arrested" hydrocephalus. These patients do not have any of the classic triad of symptoms associated with increased intracranial pressure (headache, vomiting, and papilledema). Characteristically, they are clinically and neurologically "stable," although frequently they are subnormal mentally. Their general neurologic examination will be unchanged from previous examinations except during periods of stress. These patients may become symptomatic with the development of headache, vomiting, and papilledema following relatively minor insults, including minor head trauma or systemic infection. With the resolution of the superimposed stress, the patient will spontaneously resume his previous status. CSF circulation in these patients is finely balanced, with little to no reserve of CSF absorption to compensate for periods of stress. Intracranial pressure monitoring in this group of patients has also revealed a large subgroup of patients with periodic elevations of intracranial pressure, predominantly during sleep.[31] In this group, ventriculoperitoneal or ventriculoatrial shunting has been shown to cause the ventricular system to diminish in size, eliminating the periods of pathologic elevation of intracranial pressure associated with stress. In addition, there is some evidence that intellectual function benefits significantly from the return of the ventricular system toward normal size and normalization of the intracranial pressure.[31]

Extracerebral fluid collections may imitate hydrocephalus in their presentation and clinical findings. Chronic subdural hematomas in infancy are the second most frequent cause of macrocrania.[41] Subdural hematomas that present acutely and are associated with cerebral contusion and laceration are included in the discussion on trauma (see Chapter 27 in the section on the teenager) and are not considered here. Chronic subdural hematomas frequently result from previously unrecognized trauma, with the fall or blow having occurred several weeks or months before the infant is brought in for evaluation. The trauma in some cases is associated with a difficult delivery and is unknown to the parents. However the trauma occurred, cutaneous signs of head injury are generally lacking; there are no subcutaneous hematomas or skin abrasions. As previously mentioned, the head may transilluminate in the area of the fluid collection and the skull shape may change, taking on a boxy or square appearance. If the examination shows retinal hemorrhages or healing fractures, parental abuse should be strongly considered.[21] Appropriate measures to investigate this possibility should then be taken.

Following meningitis, a collection of sterile fluid will occasionally accumulate in the subdural space (subdural effusion) (Fig. 17-10). This occurrence is particularly common following meningitis caused by *Hemophilus influenzae*.[5] Small collections will generally disappear without specific therapy. When the collection is large, it may be the cause of macrocrania and may be associated with increased intracranial pressure. The clinical presentation may be separated from the bout of meningitis by several weeks. If the fluid becomes infected (subdural empyema), it may be a source of continued bacterial contamination of the subarachnoid space and result in recurrent or persistent meningitis. Patients with bacterial meningitis and a poor clinical response to appropriate therapy need to have subdural effusion or empyema excluded during their evaluation.

Physiologic or familial macrocephaly is also commonly encountered in the evaluation of macrocrania. These infants are neurologically normal and reach appropriate developmental milestones. Although the head is large, serial measurements of the infant's head circumference will show that the head growth parallels rather than crosses the percentile lines (Fig. 17-1). Macrocrania is frequently present in other family members as

well. In addition, there are no supportive signs of increased intracranial pressure, such as bulging of the anterior fontanelle or prominence of the scalp veins. It is our view, however, that patients

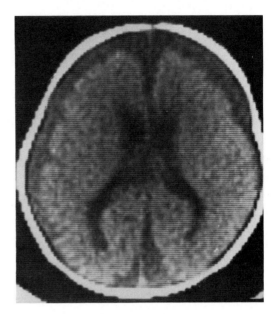

Fig. 17-10. CT brain scan of an infant 2 weeks after the onset of symptoms from *Hemophilus influenzae* meningitis. Low-attenuation fluid collections (subdural effusions) are symmetrically distributed over both cerebral hemispheres. The subdural effusion fluid is also seen in the longitudinal fissure separating the cerebral hemispheres.

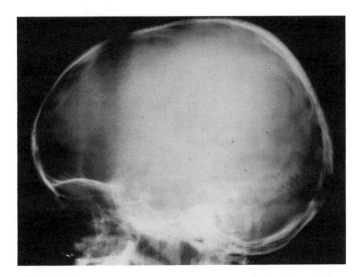

Fig. 17-11. Lateral radiograph of the skull. Coronal sutures are widely separated, and the interdigitations in the lambdoid sutures are exaggerated.

with macrocrania and growth of the head parallel to the normal growth curve should all be evaluated further with x-rays films of the skull and a computerized tomographic (CT) scan of the brain. It is also best to include these patients in follow-up clinics so that their subsequent developmental and neurologic examinations can be monitored carefully for early signs of deterioration if the presumed diagnosis of physiologic macrocephaly proves to be incorrect.

Evaluation. Evaluation of the infant with macrocrania begins with x-ray films of the skull and a CT brain scan. The skull films are obtained to document suture separation or secondary evidence of increased intracranial pressure, such as erosion of the dorsum sellae or a beaten silver appearance of the cranial vault (Fig. 17-11). Intracranial calcification may also be seen and assessed. The single best test with the highest diagnostic accuracy in the presence of macrocrania is the CT brain scan. By this one noninvasive technique, the size, position, and configuration of the entire ventricular system can be outlined (Fig. 17-12). Infants and neonates may need sedation to maintain the head in a single position, which is required for the examination. The newer CT brain scanners require less than 10 seconds of scan time for each section of the study, and the vast majority of infants can be adequately sedated for the study without the use of general anesthesia. Contrast enhancement by the intravenous infusion of an iodine-containing contrast agent is advised during the initial evaluation of all patients with macrocrania. Contrast enhancement helps to visualize areas of alteration in the blood brain barrier (neoplasm, vascular malformation, recent infarction, trauma, etc.). The presence of bilateral symmetric subdural hematomas, which appear to have the same attenuation as brain, may be difficult to diagnose with the CT brain scan.[18] If clinical suspicion is high even in the face of a "negative" CT brain scan, diagnostic subdural taps or cerebral angiography may be necessary to exclude this possibility. In addition to computerized scanning, ventricular size can be estimated by ultrasonography, a convenient way of *following* ventricular size without using ionizing radiation. During the initial evaluation, however, CT brain scanning remains the most reliable method of diagnosis currently available.

The need for angiography, ventriculography, and pneumoencephalography has decreased drastically since the introduction of CT brain scanning. These tests are now reserved for difficult diagnostic problems that cannot be solved with the CT brain scan or for outlining the vascular system in the presence of suspected vascular disease or in anticipation of surgery. Air studies continue to be used occasionally to evaluate suprasellar masses or to resolve fine anatomy that is not clearly visualized by other means.

Fig. 17-12. Normal enhanced CT brain scan. **A:** *A,* streak artifact across the brain stem; *B,* inferior portion of the cerebellum; *C,* basilar artery seen end-on; *D,* petrous ridge; *E,* mastoid air cells; *F,* temporal lobe within the middle fossa; *G,* sphenoid ridge; *H,* inferior portion of the frontal lobes; *I,* sella turcica. **B,** Section through the suprasellar cistern (circle of Willis) and fourth ventricle: *A,* fourth ventricle; *B,* cerebellar vermis; *C,* cerebellar hemisphere; *D,* brain stem; *E,* posterior cerebral arteries; *F,* basilar artery seen end-on; *G,* suprasellar cistern; *H,* middle cerebral artery; *I,* anterior cerebral arteries. **C,** Section through the upper brain stem: *A,* fourth ventricle; *B,* tentorium cerebri—dural separation of the superior aspect of the cerebellum and the inferior aspects of the occipital lobe (cut on edge); *C,* brain stem; *D,* middle cerebral artery complex seen end-on; *E,* anterior cerebral artery complex; *F,* falx cerebri—dural separation of the cerebral hemispheres— note that the temporal horns are not normally visualized with this degree of scan resolution. **D,** Section through the area of the third ventricle: *A,* occipital lobes; *B,* straight sinus; *C,* vein of Galen; *D,* occipital horns of the lateral ventricle; *E,* internal cerebral veins lying in the roof of the third ventricle; *F,* frontal horns of the lateral ventricles; *G,* frontal lobes. **E,** Section through the body of the lateral ventricles: *A,* body of the lateral ventricles; *B,* falx cerebri—differentiation of peripheral gray matter from slightly lower attenuation white matter can be appreciated. **F,** Section near the vertex: *(A)* differentiation between white (centrum semiovale) *(A)* and surrounding gray matter *(B)* can be appreciated.

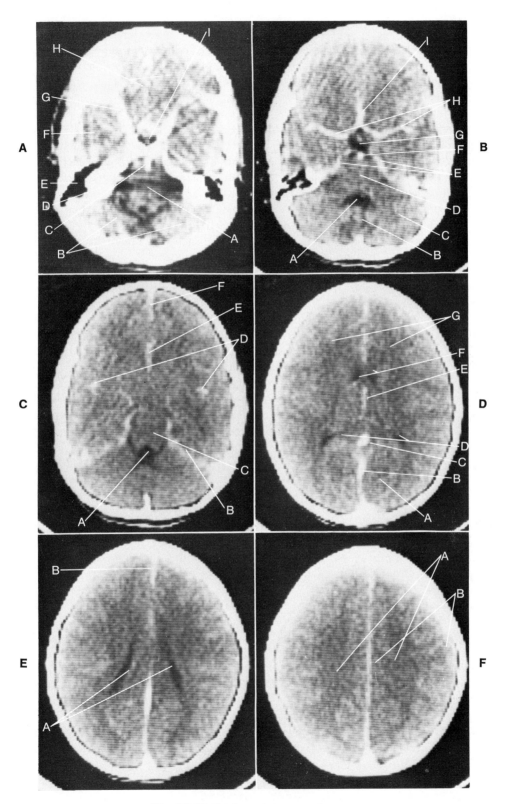

Fig. 17-12. For legend see opposite page.

The electroencephalogram (EEG) is a useful test in the presence of episodic disorders of cerebral dysfunction, but its role in the evaluation of increased intracranial pressure and hydrocephalus is limited. The EEG should not be relied on to screen patients for the presence of structural disease of the brain.

Referral. All children with macrocrania and evidence of increased intracranial pressure need neurologic evaluation. Those with respiratory stridor, decerebrate rigidity, or an altered mental status need urgent evaluation. Patients with a slowly enlarging head or chronic symptomatology can be evaluated on a nonurgent basis. As emphasized earlier, in addition to the infant with obvious macrocrania, the infant whose head circumference measurements are crossing percentile lines of growth should be evaluated. These infants can usually be referred on an elective basis for outpatient assessment and evaluation. However, there is no indication for a "wait and see" policy once macrocrania or accelerated head growth has been documented. The patient will obviously benefit by early diagnosis and prompt treatment of his condition. In cases of child abuse, the primary care physician will frequently be asked to take an active role in helping the family and local supporting services arrive at a plan of action that will ensure the infant's health and well-being once he is returned to the community.

Medical versus surgical treatment. The therapeutic alternatives in macrocrania are a function of the etiology of the condition. When hydrocephalus is diagnosed, the therapeutic alternatives are limited. Although numerous medications are known to decrease CSF production transiently (e.g., acetazolamide) or lower intracranial tension (e.g., isosorbide, mannitol, glycerin), none is a long-term answer to hydrocephalus. Currently the only effective means of treating hydrocephalus is by shunting of the CSF into a body cavity able to reabsorb the fluid. Ventriculoperitoneal or ventriculoatrial shunts are now commonly employed to relieve increased intracranial pressure and treat hydrocephalus.

Another approach to accelerated head growth secondary to hydrocephalus has recently been popularized. This involves intermittently wrapping the infant's head with an elastic bandage in an effort to avoid shunting by physically limiting the growth of the head. It is hoped that in this way alternative CSF resorptive pathways will be opened. The number of infants treated by this method is small and the follow-up short,[13] and this procedure has yet to be proved effective or safe. Of primary concern is the prolonged exposure of the developing nervous system to elevated intracranial pressure. Although ventricular shunting procedures have many complications and disadvantages, they remain the best proved long-term method of controlling increased intracranial pressure due to hydrocephalus.

The treatment of chronic subdural hematomas and effusions has changed significantly in the past several years. Treatment has generally become more conservative; when surgery is performed, it is usually less extensive than the craniotomy and membrane stripping previously advised.[38] Subdural fluid collections other than pus are initially managed with repeated subdural taps. This procedure is performed on the fully shaved and meticulously cleaned anterior fontanelle. A short beveled needle is placed through the dura at least two finger breadths lateral to the midline into the subdural space. The needle is advanced through the skin, periosteum, and dura in an oblique path (to enhance the creation of a watertight seal once the needle is removed). With each millimeter of advancement, the stylet is removed and the presence of fluid in the hub of the needle checked. If fluid is present in the subdural space, it will flow freely out of the needle when the needle is properly positioned. The needle is never aspirated during a diagnostic subdural tap for fear of damaging nearby cortical veins and causing further hemorrhage in the extracerebral space.[37] Fluid is allowed to flow out until either fresh blood appears (indicative of bleeding as a consequence of the tap) or the flow of fluid becomes negligible. The same procedure is then repeated on the opposite side. Although the actual quantity of fluid removed may appear relatively insignificant, repeated taps can lead to serious anemia, electrolyte imbalance, and negative protein balance. All these factors must be corrected as the situation dictates. If more than 30 ml of fluid are removed at a single setting, care should be taken to monitor the infant closely. Deterioration of the vital signs or clinical condition is an indication to terminate the procedure immediately. Provisions for immediate transfusion should also be available when large quantities of fluid are being removed.

Subdural taps are repeated whenever the anterior fontanelle becomes full or the head circumference increases. The frequency of tapping is dictated by the rate of formation of the subdural fluid. Initially, taps may be required once or twice a day. Eventually, the interval between taps gradually increases until they finally become unproductive. Objective factors to follow and record include the quantity of fluid removed from each tap and the protein content of the fluid. Both of these factors should gradually decrease if this form of therapy is effective. Samples should also periodically be taken for culture to ensure continued sterility of the fluid.

Subdural tapping is continued until the subdural space no longer yields a significant amount of fluid, or for 10 to 14 days. At the end of that period, the situation is reassessed; and if significant improvement has occurred, with a decrease in the volume of fluid obtained or an increasing interval between taps, the procedure may be continued for an additional 7 to 10 days. If, on the other hand, the frequency of tapping and the volume of fluid have remained constant, a change in tactics is indicated. The child is then anesthetized, and burr holes are placed over the lesion to allow for complete drainage of the contents of the subdural space via an indwelling subdural catheter. The external drain is left in place for 24 to 48 hours and then removed. This procedure will prove effective in the vast majority of subdural collections that are resistant to tapping. It should also be noted that a simple burr hole is associated with minimal risk and no manipulation of cerebral tissue. If this procedure also fails because of recurrence of the fluid collection, a subdural-pleural or subdural-peritoneal shunt can be placed and left for 2 to 3 months. The pleural space is ideally suited for the acceptance of this fluid because of its negative pressure and ability to absorb highly proteinaceous fluid. Small infants, however, may not tolerate this procedure because of respiratory embarrassment. By necessity the peritoneal cavity must then be used.

Surgical options. Following the revelation of Dandy and Blackfan[10] that CSF is produced by the choroid plexus, removal or cauterization of that tissue within the lateral ventricles was proposed to control communicating or external hydrocephalus.[8] Bilateral choroid plexectomies were performed through the 1950s despite their limited rate of success. It has subsequently been shown that following postoperative recovery, choroid

plexus removal does not alter CSF production.[43] To control internal or noncommunicating hydrocephalus, Dandy suggested an alternative procedure[9] that involved creating a perforation or window in the lamina terminalis to communicate the expanded and obstructed ventricular system with the subarachnoid space. This procedure was further refined by Stookey and Scarff[55] in 1936. As late as 1976 this approach still had its supporters, although the method had been modified to allow the communication to be created stereotactically.[26]

In 1939 Torkildsen published an innovative article describing a surgical procedure to bypass the intraventricular obstruction to CSF flow by placing a tube between a dilated lateral ventricle and the cisterna magna.[60] Since this system was completely within the normal CSF pathway, no valve was required to regulate the CSF pressure or flow. Once the CSF had bypassed the obstruction, normal resorption could take place over the cerebral hemispheres in the arachnoid granulations. This procedure proved very effective in some settings but not in others. If congenital aqueductal stenosis was present, the procedure was ineffective; but patients with acquired occlusion of the aqueduct from a tumor or vascular malformation could be improved significantly. It was postulated that the arachnoid granulations were also defective in congenital aqueductal stenosis and did not possess the capacity of adequate CSF resorption.

It was not until 1951 that Nulsen and Spitz[45] introduced the valve-regulated ventriculoatrial shunt. Many modifications of this scheme have subsequently occurred, mainly in the placement of the distal catheter. All of the following positions for the distal catheter have been tried and advocated at some time: the sagittal sinus, the mastoid air cells, the eustachian tube, Stensen's duct, the thoracic duct, the heart (by direct cardiac implantation), the gallbladder, the ureter (with sacrifice of the kidney), and the fallopian tube. By and large, these have all been abandoned, with only the occasional zealot advocating their continued use. Currently the three sites of placement that are favored are the peritoneal cavity, the right atrium (via the jugular vein), and the pleural space.

Placement of the distal catheter in the peritoneum has the advantages of the ready accessibility of the peritoneal cavity and the lack of a need for critical positioning of the catheter tip (Fig. 17-13).

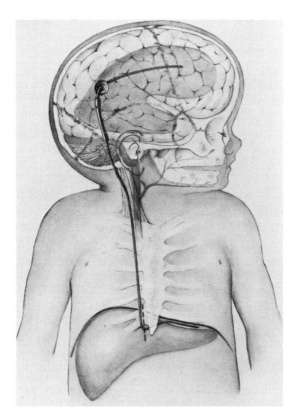

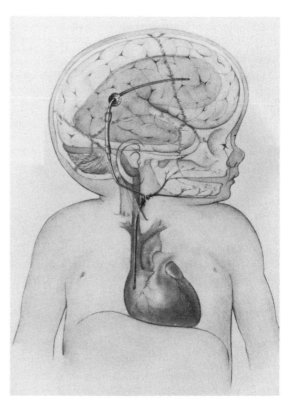

Fig. 17-13. Ventriculoperitoneal shunt. (From Matson, D. D.: Neurosurgery of infancy and childhood, 1969, Courtesy Charles C Thomas, Publisher, Springfield, Ill.)

Fig. 17-14. Ventriculoatrial shunt. (From Matson, D. D.: Neurosurgery of infancy and childhood, 1969. Courtesy Charles C Thomas, Publisher, Springfield, Ill.)

Peritoneal placement is particularly advantageous in the neonate and infant because sufficient excess tubing can be placed in the abdomen to allow for future rapid body growth. The function of ventriculoatrial shunts is significantly influenced by the position of the distal catheter tip; therefore, these shunts are more difficult to maintain during the years of rapid growth (Fig. 17-14). Distal catheter tips located below the T-6 vertebra are associated with increasing infection rates the more caudal they are in location.[4] As the catheter tip rises above the T-5 vertebra, the tendency for the catheter to be encased in fibrous tissue or occluded by thrombus and excluded from the circulation also increases. In addition, distal-end revision or replacement is technically simpler with peritoneal shunts than with atrial shunts. The pleural space is used infrequently because of its limited resorptive capability, particularly in children younger than 5 years old. It is, however, ideally suited to accept small amounts of proteinaceous fluids, as is occasionally necessary in the treatment of chronic subdural hematomas. In addition, the pleural space has a small negative pressure, which enhances flow.

There are currently available many varieties of shunt equipment, each with its own advantages. Ventricular catheters may be simple or flanged. The regulating valve may be located under the scalp (Hakim, Holter, and Pudenz) or be located in the distal catheter as a slit valve (Accuflow, Ramondi) (Fig. 17-15). Additional accessories that can be placed in the shunt system include reservoirs or tapping chambers to allow sampling of CSF, flushing devices, and antisiphon devices (Fig. 17-16). Flushing devices or chambers work under the principle that the CSF within the chamber can be forced out of the chamber only if the distal catheter is patent and will then refill only if the proximal catheter is patent. Although theoretically correct, the devices are plagued with inaccuracy. The high incidence of false-positive and false-negative information generated by the devices make their use questionable.[47] Antisiphon

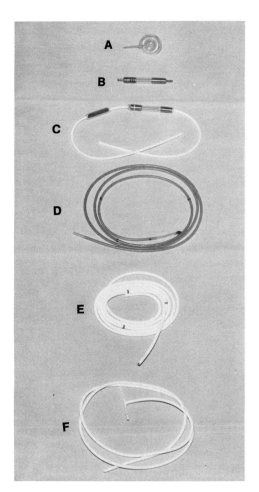

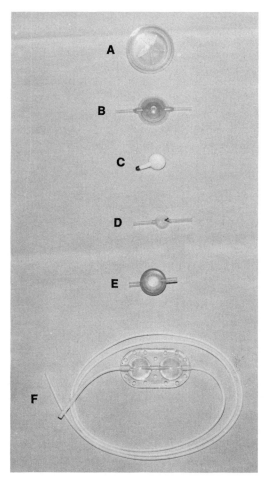

Fig. 17-15. Regulating valves used for ventriculoatrial and ventriculoperitoneal shunting (*A* to *E*) and for lumboperitoneal shunting (*F*).

Fig. 17-16. Shunt accessories. **A,** Reservoir used to inject intraventricular medication and repeatedly sample CSF. **B,** Double-lumen reservoir. **C,** Metal-based reservoir used as part of the shunt assembly. **D,** Antisiphon device. **E,** In-line shunt filter for the exclusion of malignant cells. **F,** Double-chamber flushing device.

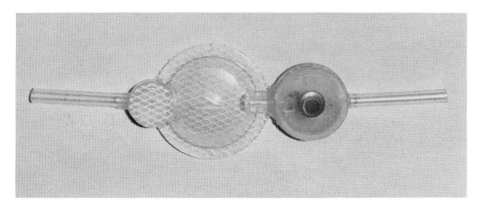

Fig. 17-17. On-off flushing device.

devices were designed to eliminate the position-dependent siphoning effect through the shunt system. One additional attachment is the millipore filter, designed to filter out malignant cells and prevent seeding through the vascular system or into the peritoneal cavity.[27] The multipurpose valve, composed of a flushing device, on-off switch, and antisiphon device, is of some concern to the primary care physician because of the on-off switch built into the system (Fig. 17-17). With percutaneous pressure on the switch, the system can be permanently occluded. Because of this feature, these devices are somewhat dangerous and should be inserted only under very special circumstances.

An additional shunting system sometimes encountered is the lumboperitoneal shunt. This system was designed to treat pseudotumor cerebri or communicating hydrocephalus where difficulty in canulating the lateral ventricle is anticipated. With this system, a T tube is placed in the lumbar subarachnoid space and tunnelled subcutaneously in the abdominal wall to be inserted into the peritoneal cavity.[28] The shunt is usually equipped with a slit valve to regulate flow, but initially these patients almost always suffer orthostatic headaches on assuming the erect position. An additional problem with the placement of this device is the development of kyphosis, scoliosis, or limited back mobility. Their use is therefore restricted to patients who cannot be shunted adequately by some other means.[34]

As mentioned previously, the treatment of extracerebral effusions or chronic subdural hematomas is initially conservative. Therapeutic subdural taps are continued for at least 10 days before some other form of therapy is resorted to. If the character and quantity of the fluid is improving, the period of tapping may be continued. If no improvement has taken place, burr holes are made over the fluid collection to wash out the remaining blood products adequately and to permit complete drainage of the space for 48 hours. Rarely, this too will fail; in such cases a subdural-pleural shunt is recommended.[59]

Postoperative course. Following the routine placement of a ventriculoatrial or ventriculoperitoneal shunt, the infant may gradually be brought to the sitting position the day after surgery. If the preoperative evaluation has shown massive ventricular enlargement, the advancement to the erect position is slower and may take place over

several days. This is done in an attempt to minimize the sudden decompression of the ventricular system and the creation of subdural hematomas as the bridging cortical veins tear from the sagittal sinus. Additional findings that can be seen with rapid decompression of the ventricular system on assuming the upright position include tachycardia, blanching of the face and scalp, lethargy, and an increase in the concavity of the anterior fontanelle. If signs of intracranial hypotension develop, the infant or child should be allowed to lie flat and be brought to the vertical position gradually over a period of days. Usually by the seventh postoperative day the sutures are ready for removal and the infant is discharged. With peritoneal shunts, oral feeding is delayed until bowel sounds return. Postoperative ileus may occur, but it is unusual for this to last more than 24 hours. Patients with pleural shunts must be followed carefully for the appearance and extent of pleural effusion. This in itself is not a reason for alarm; but if the infant becomes dyspneic or if signs of respiratory embarrassment occur, the distal end of the shunt must be replaced into another body cavity. Subdural-pleural shunts, which are occasionally placed for the management of chronic subdural hematomas, may be removed electively after 2 to 3 months.[58] Rarely, following the placement of a ventriculoatrial shunt for massive hydrocephalus, cardiac failure may occur because of the large volume of CSF presented to the circulation.

Following the placement of burr holes for drainage of subdural effusion or chronic subdural hematomas, care should be taken that fluid is not reaccumulating in the subdural space. This can easily be checked by repeating the subdural taps and CT brain scan. Following successful therapy, the patient is discharged from the hospital to be followed closely as an outpatient for the possible recurrence of the extracerebral fluid collection.

Prognosis. The eventual outcome of patients with shunted hydrocephalus is a function of multiple factors: the underlying cause of the hydrocephalus, the effectiveness of the therapy, and the presence of neural damage that occurred before shunting. Although the cause of the condition is "benign" in the majority of patients, follow-up of one large group of shunted hydrocephalics has shown a survival of only 70% after 5 years.[41] This same series showed that only two thirds of those surviving 5 years had an IQ greater than 75. The longer any particular series is followed, the more it becomes apparent that there is a gradual decrease in the number of survivors and in the quality of life of those who do survive. Determination of the thickness of the cerebral mantle before shunt insertion is of only limited value in predicting eventual intellectual function.[56] A discouraging finding is the presence of significant areas of cerebral destruction following meningitis or intracerebral hemorrhage. Effective shunting in these patients will do nothing to restore function in the damaged cortical areas. Secondary signs of hydrocephalus and increased intracranial pressure (such as sixth nerve palsy, the ''setting sun'' sign, and noninfectious respiratory stridor) may or may not be reversible with adequate therapy, depending on the presence of irreparable damage before the reduction of the intracranial pressure.

Chronic subdural hematomas of infancy or subdural effusions are associated with an excellent chance of survival. Significant sequelae, however, commonly occur and include mental retardation, seizure activity, and spastic weakness.

Important aspects of follow-up. Following the placement of ventriculoperitoneal and ventriculoatrial shunts, the most sensitive indicators of shunt function are those factors that originally aroused clincial suspicion of increased intracranial pressure. When shunt dysfunction occurs, the patient's parents will frequently comment that ''This is just how he became ill originally.'' In the majority of infants the anterior fontanelle will bulge, the rate of growth of the head circumference will increase, and the infant will become irritable and vomit frequently. However, if the child's initial symptom was respiratory stridor, the ''setting sun'' sign, decreased visual acuity, or focal weakness, this symptom may be the presenting sign of recurrent elevation of intracranial pressure secondary to shunt malfunction. If a question arises, the CT brain scan should be repeated. Of great help in this situation is a postoperative CT brain scan done several weeks following successful shunting at a time when the patient is clinically well. This scan will act as a baseline for subsequent evaluations of the patient's ventricular system and will help rule out the presence of clinically silent complications of the shunting procedure such as subdural hematomas.

A controversial subject is elective shunt revision. Numerous authors would advise allowing some elevation of the intracranial pressure and waiting until shunt malfunction is clinically obvious before committing the patient to a shunt revision.[24,59] Hopefully, the patient would develop additional CSF resorptive pathways or areas of constriction of flow would become dilated, allowing natural resorption and bulk flow to occur. Then, hopefully, fewer patients would be shunt dependent. An alternative approach would be for patients to be electively scheduled for shunt revision at specific points of time along their growth curve.[41] With elective revision of the shunting system, emergency revision may, hopefully, be avoided. The ideal shunt length is maintained by periodically lengthening the distal catheter rather than waiting for the shunt to malfunction and allowing increased intracranial pressure to become clinically evident. Ordinarily the procedure involves lengthening the distal catheter while simply testing the ventricular catheter for patency. Weighing against this approach is the fact that since the child is normal before this elective procedure, any complication would be difficult to justify. Yet, it would be clearly beneficial to be able to avoid periods of increased intracranial pressure. The conversion of patients to shunt independence by not electively revising their shunts occurs infrequently, if at all. However, data strongly supporting either view are not available.

Complications. With all ventriculoperitoneal and ventriculoatrial shunting operations, the two most prevalent serious complications are shunt obstruction and infection. If shunt obstruction is thought to be present clinically because of recurrent evidence of increased intracranial pressure, radiographs of the entire shunt system may be helpful. These may show disconnection or poor positioning of the shunt and may give a good clue as to the nonfunctioning portion. The CT brain scan is then repeated and the ventricular size compared with that seen in the initial postshunt period when the child was clinically well. If there is evidence of increased intracranial pressure or ventricular enlargement, shunt revision is undertaken. Anything short of surgical revision, including shunt pumping routines and medical regimens aimed at altering CSF production, are generally ineffective on a long-term basis and are not advised. Proximal and distal end obstructions are about equally responsible for shunt failures. Proximal end failures are frequently due to choroid

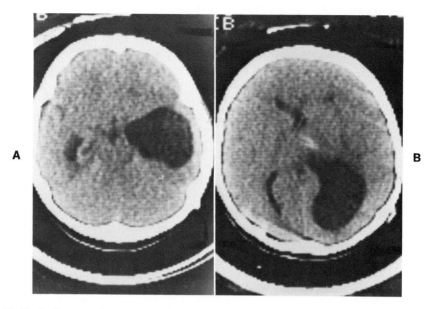

Fig. 17-18. Brain scan of a child with hydrocephalus following meningitis and compartmentalization of the right temporal (**A**) and occipital (**B**) horns following shunting. An intraventricular septum prevented free communication within the ventricular system.

plexus or ventricular debris blocking the ventricular catheter. Occasionally, the catheter will become embedded in the cerebral substance and will be associated with gliosis around the catheter tip. Distal-end failure may be due to debris in the valve or to omentum or other soft tissue enveloping the catheter tip. Occasionally, a cyst will form around the catheter tip within the abdomen, interfering with CSF absorption. In this case, lysing the cyst wall or moving the catheter to an alternate abdominal location may prove effective.[48]

Infection occurs in approximately 10% of shunt insertions and revisions.[53] The infection may take the acute form, becoming clinically manifested by a painful, indurated, and draining surgical wound, frequently with a visible area of erythema extending down along the shunt tract. Or, the condition may be chronic and present as meningitis, abdominal pain, or superficial wound infection months or years following the shunt insertion. Not infrequently, the patient with an infected shunt system will simply have shunt obstruction and debris occluding the valve mechanism. Synechia may develop within the ventricular system as a result of infection or bleeding, causing loculation or compartmentalization (Fig. 17-18). These patients will have a presentation clinically similar to that of patients with shunt obstruction. *Staphylococcus aureus* and *Escherichia coli* are commonly associated with acute shunt infection, whereas *S. epidermidis* is by far the most common organism causing chronic infection. It is important to realize that organisms that are frequently considered contaminants in other situations may be the infectious agent in the presence of a shunting system.[15,16] The presence of acute infection in a shunt system usually necessitates its removal. The infection is then treated with systemic antibiotics (in addition to intraventricular antibiotics if ventriculitis is present). While no shunt is present, external ventricular drainage or occasional ventricular puncture may be necessary to control increased intracranial pressure and to administer intraventricular antibiotics. An exception to this management is chronic infection caused by *S. epidermidis* or other, less virulent organisms. In an attempt to salvage the shunt system without its removal, systemic and intraventricular antibiotics may be given.[39] If this conservative therapy fails to eradicate the infection after 14 days of therapy, removal of the shunt and immediate replacement with a new shunt at an alternate site are per-

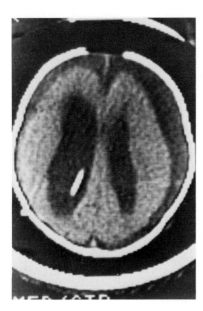

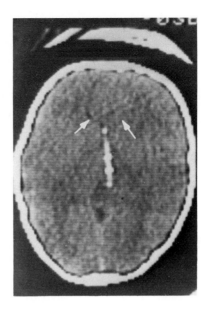

Fig. 17-19. Bilateral subdural hematoma following shunting of moderate to severe hydrocephalus.

Fig. 17-20. Unenhanced CT brain scan of a child with the small ventricle syndrome. The ventricular catheter is in a good position in the body of the right lateral ventricle. The ventricular system is collapsed and only faintly visible (arrows.)

formed.[49] Infected ventriculoatrial shunts have been associated with bacterial endocarditis, septic pulmonary emboli, and shunt nephritis.[54,62] Multiple pulmonary emboli of a noninfectious nature may also be seen.[44] All of these life-threatening conditions require the immediate removal of the shunt and subsequent replacement of the distal catheter at an alternate site, usually the peritoneum.

Infrequent complications from peritoneal catheters include perforation of the abdominal wall or an intra-abdominal or pelvic structure (vagina, bladder, gastrointestinal tract). Although it is not thought that inguinal hernias are caused by ventriculoperitoneal shunts, clinical presentation of the hernia may be hastened by a functioning peritoneal shunt.[41] Following rapid decompression of a grossly dilated ventricular system, a subdural hematoma may occur with any shunting system as the cortical veins inserting in the sagittal sinus tear as the cerebral cortex falls away (Fig. 17-19). Such a hematoma may remain clinically silent for weeks to months, or it may present acutely in the immediate postoperative period. If the patient is symptomatic from the lesion, it must be treated. This usually requires occlusion of the shunt and drainage of the subdural fluid. Small

asymptomatic subdural hematomas are usually followed conservatively with repeated CT brain scans and allowed to reabsorb spontaneously. If repeat CT scans show enlargement of the extracerebral fluid collection, conservative therapy is abandoned, the shunt is occluded, and the lesion is drained.

An uncommon complication of shunting is the development of the small ventricle syndrome.[14] In this situation the ventriculoperitoneal or ventriculoatrial shunt functions with little resistance to CSF flow down the shunt and the child becomes totally shunt dependent. Because of the low resistance in the shunt system, the ventricles maintain an excessively small size (Fig. 17-20). An element of shunt obstruction then occurs; and before the ventricular system can dilate, the patient becomes desperately ill, showing evidence of increased intracranial pressure. The presentation usually includes an altered mental status of short duration. A CT brain scan done at this time will show small ventricles that may be slightly larger than when the patient was scanned during an asymptomatic period. Treatment of this condition on an emergency basis may be quite difficult. If the shunt obstruction is found to be in the ventricular catheter and the ventricles are small,

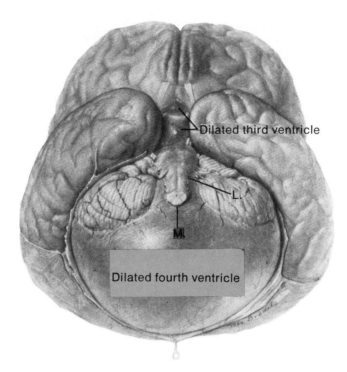

Dilated third ventricle

L.

M

Dilated fourth ventricle

Fig. 17-21. Gross specimen of brain with a Dandy-Walker cyst. The cerebellum appears hypoplastic and displaced laterally. (From Dandy, W. E.: The brain. In Mark, V. H., editor: Neurosurgery, vol. 11. Lewis' practice of surgery, Hagerstown, Md., 1947, W. F. Prior Co., Inc.)

removal of the malfunctioning catheter and recannulation of the small ventricle may prove technically challenging. A better approach would be to try to decrease intracranial pressure with emergency medical measures and allow time for the ventricular system to dilate and then revise the shunt on an elective basis, substituting a higher resistance valve system for the one in place. Subtemporal decompression in selected cases may be beneficial.[14]

Other, less common lesions. The Dandy-Walker cyst is a form of hydrocephalus worth special mention. Ventricular enlargement in this condition is associated with hypoplasia of the cerebellar vermis (Fig. 17-21). Fourth ventricular enlargement is greater than either third or lateral ventricular enlargement. It was originally thought that the hydrocephalus was secondary to obstruction to the outflow of the fourth ventricle via the foramina of Magendie and Luschka. However, both surgical observation and pathologic study have shown this not to be true in all cases.[22] The exact origin of the condition is still not fully understood. Therapy consists of shunting of the loculated CSF compartments. If the lateral and third ventricles are in free communication with

the greatly enlarged fourth ventricle, a single ventricular catheter is sufficient for adequate decompression of the dilated ventricular system. If, however, the compartments are not in free communication, two ventricular catheters are necessary for adequate therapy. One is located in the enlarged lateral ventricle, and a second is placed in the loculated fourth ventricle. These proximal catheters are then connected by a Y connection and attached to a distal outflow system.

OCCULT SPINAL DYSRAPHISM

Congenital malformations of the spinal cord resulting in improper fusion of the neuroectoderm, as well as surrounding mesoderm, that are not obvious at birth are conveniently grouped together under the heading *occult spinal dysraphism*. These lesions are thought to be etiologically related to each other and to myelomeningoceles. They commonly occur together and have similar clinical presentations and physical findings. As with myelomeningoceles, these lesions are almost universally associated with the nonunion of the posterior elements of one or more vertebral arches (spina bifida occulta). This finding in itself is common and occurs in at least 4% of the adult popula-

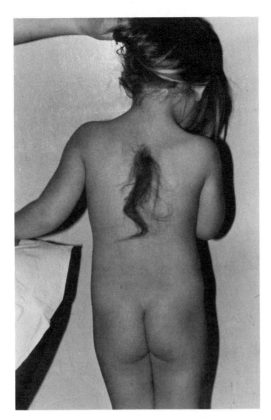

Fig. 17-22. Midthoracic "hairy patch" overlying diastematomyelia with a bony median septum and a large cervical syrinx. The child was neurologically normal.

tion. These bifid laminae occur predominantly in the S-1 and S-2 vertebral arches and less commonly in the L-5 arch. They are also seen to occur in the upper cervical spine, particularly at the level of C-1.

The vast majority of patients with spina bifida occulta are neurologicaly normal and will remain so throughout their lives. A small group will show evidence of neurologic deterioration. In this group the spinal cord, conus medullaris, or cauda equina may be involved in the developmental malformation. Such patients may have diastematomyelia, a tethered spinal cord, a lipomeningocele, a neurenteric cyst, or a dermal sinus tract with an intraspinal dermoid tumor. These lesions commonly become evident clinically when the child is beginning to walk and gain voluntary control of bowel and bladder function. In the screening of children for neurologic compromise, simple delay in walking or bladder control is less indicative of a structural spinal abnormality than is actual regression and loss of function. The normal de-

velopmental history should be one of a progressive increase in skills.

Physical examination. Although no nervous tissue may be present on the skin surface with these conditions, there are frequently cutaneous signs of occult spinal dysrhaphism. The skin of the back is abnormal in 75% of patients with clinical signs of occult spinal dysraphism.[30] These signs include focal hirsutism over the spine, capillary hemangiomas, dermal sinus tracts or skin dimples, and abnormal accumulation of subcutaneous fat.

The base of the hairy tuft occurs in the midline and tapers laterally, frequently taking on a diamond configuration (Fig. 17-22). The texture of the hair varies from fine and silky to short and curly. The texture of the hair over the spine usually matches the hair texture on other parts of the body. It may obtain a length of several inches to several feet and is sometimes referred to as a faun's tail. This particular cutaneous abnormality may be the patient's or parent's only complaint and should never be dismissed without further investigation. Focal hirsutism over the spine seems to have a particularly high association with diastematomyelia.[19] The spinal cord abnormality need not be directly under the hairy patch; not infrequently, it will be at some distance from the patch. For this reason, it is important not to limit the clinical or radiographic investigation to the area immediately under the cutaneous abnormality.

Capillary hemangiomas are common in neonates and infants. They are frequently seen over the occiput and in this location have no specific clinical significance. However, when they are located over the spine, especially in conjunction with other cutaneous abnormalities, they take on increased importance and demand further investigation. The accumulation of fat in the subcutaneous tissues is normal. This accumulation, however, should not be discrete and identifiable as a focal mass. Congenital subcutaneous lipomas over the spine occur almost exclusively in the area of the lumbosacral junction (Fig. 17-23). They are always present at birth but may be small and not arouse clinical suspicion. The lesions may, however, be quite large, covering most of the lower back. In this case, the family will frequently seek medical attention for cosmetic removal of the subcutaneous aspect of the lesion. The presence and significance of the possible un-

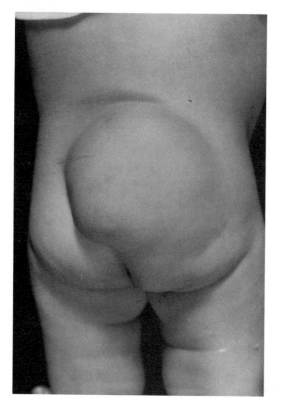

Fig. 17-23. Lipomeningocele. The lesion is fully covered by skin with multiple faint capillary hemangiomas over its surface. The infant was nuerologically intact. (Courtesy G. L. Odom, M.D., Durham, N.C.)

derlying spinal cord abnormality may not be appreciated. The surface of the lipoma is characteristically covered by full-thickness skin, which may be smooth, or dimpled and irregular.

Dermal sinus tracts may occur at any point along the craniospinal axis (Fig. 17-24). The most frequent location is over the lumbosacral spine. The cutaneous opening is easily missed when it is small. The course of the tract is dictated by its embryologic development. Spinal dermal sinus tracts course cephalad toward their eventual termination. Cranial dermal sinus tracts characteristically occur over the occiput with extension of the tract caudally. The tract may terminate anywhere along its course, from the subcutaneous tissues to the substance of the spinal cord or the floor of the fourth ventricle. Along the tract are periodic expansions, which represent accumulation of sebaceous material, hair, and keratin (dermoid cyst) or simply keratin (epidermoid cyst). More than one tumor may be found along a tract, giving the appearance of beads along a string.

It is important to be able to assess the clinical significance of openings in the skin over the lumbar sacral spine. Neurologically significant spinal dermal sinus tracts course cephalad. The specific course of a lesion can be determined by the direction in which the lesion is tethered. With movement of the skin adjacent to the lesion, the defect

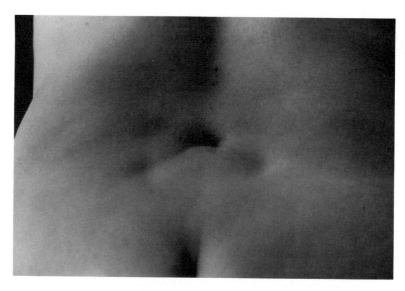

Fig. 17-24. Lumbosacral dimple and dermal sinus tract leading to an intraspinal dermoid tumor. (Courtesy G. L. Odom, M.D., Durham, N.C.)

will either be made more pronounced and limit movement or become less pronounced (Fig. 17-25). Tracts that run in a cephalic direction are of neurosurgical interest and concern. Tracts that are tethered caudally and occur between the buttocks are pilonidal sinuses and of little neurologic significance.

Kyphosis or scoliosis may be present in as many as one third of the infants and children with occult spinal dysraphism.[6] It may, in fact, be the presenting and only complaint. With all congenital spinal deformities, care should be taken to survey the patient for any sign of neurologic involvement that might indicate the coexistence of some form of occult spinal dysraphism. Other common or-

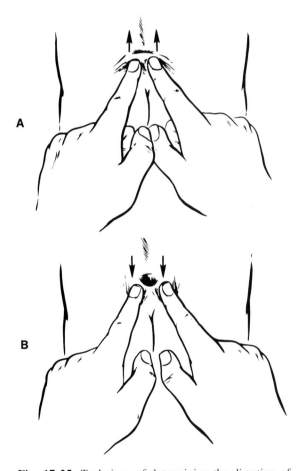

Fig. 17-25. Technique of determining the direction of tethering of a sinus tract. If the defect becomes less obvious with cephalic movement of the adjacent skin (**A**) and deepens with caudal traction (**B**), the lesion is tethered superiorly. Lesions tethered superiorly carry a much higher risk of having intraspinal and intradural extension. Caudal tethering is indicative of a pilonidal sinus tract and has the opposite characteristics.

thopedic presentations of intraspinal anomalies include a variety of foot deformities, such as talipes cavus, talipes equinovarus, and talipes valgus. There may be discrepancies in the bony length of the feet or legs, which may first be manifested clinically by an abnormal gait or stance. With chronic lesions involving the lower motor neuron, the muscles of the foot and calf may be atrophic; deep tendon reflexes are absent, and contractures of the gastrocnemius and hamstring muscles are common. Toe walking is frequently the only disturbing factor during the first few months the infant is learning to walk.

Sensory changes are difficult to document in infants, but the presence of seemingly painless ulceration of the foot in ambulatory patients implies an element of sensory loss and should be taken as a strong sign of sensory neurologic compromise. The skin in the involved distal lower extremities may appear cold and somewhat cyanotic. If the spinal cord and upper motor neurons are primarily affected, the leg may have increased tone, exaggerated deep tendon reflexes, and extensor plantar responses. Incontinence of the bladder and bowel are commonly seen and sometimes are not associated with other neurologic abnormalities. Bladder involvement is manifested clinically by frequent urinary tract infections and involuntary control of urination with frequent and small voidings and excessive postvoiding residual urine volumes. Frequently, urine can be expressed from the bladder by abdominal pressure. The rectal tone may be flaccid with loss of the anal wink reflex. The development of a neurogenic bladder secondary to an intraspinal anomaly is almost always accompanied by a change in the rectal sphincter tone.

Older children may be able to localize pain to the back or leg, whereas children younger than 5 years of age will simply be irritable. Spinal mobility may also be limited, with restrictions in forward bending, straight-leg raising, and neck flexion. Percussion over the involved area of the spine may demonstrate local tenderness with or without a radicular component.

Common occurrences. Diastematomyelia is a condition in which the spinal cord is separated into two parts by a sagittal cleft. Between the divided segments of spinal cord, a dural-covered septum usually exists. The septum is frequently osseous, but it may be cartilaginous or fibrous. The cleft in the cord may be complete or partial, with penetration only to the central canal. The cleft may divide the cord in the midline, but more frequently the division is paramedian. Normal nerve roots exit laterally from the divided spinal cord. Adhesions or abortive nerve roots may extend from the medial aspect of each cord segment and course toward the dural sleeve covering the septum. These roots as well as other fibers may pass through the dura and be attached to the surrounding bone and muscle. They may then act as additional tethering forces on the spinal cord. The conus medullaris is usually displaced caudally. With the septum in a fixed position, the spinal cord cannot move freely in the spinal canal, and repeated trauma occurs to the cord surrounding the septum.[19]

Diastematomyelia with a median septum is seen primarily in female patients, with a 4-to-1 predominance.[19] Occasionally, the lesion may be discovered during the evaluation of an asymptomatic hairy patch or other cutaneous anomaly associated with occult spinal dysraphism. At least 75% of the patients found to have diastematomyelia will have a cutaneous anomaly. Not uncommonly, the patient has congenital scoliosis or a gait abnormality. The predominant location of the septum is in the lumbar or low dorsal spine. The lesions located in the thoracic region appear to have a higher incidence of scoliosis.[19] It is not unusual to find diastematomyelia associated with other forms of spinal dysraphism, including myelomeningocele and intraspinal dermoid tumor. Neonates with diastematomyelia and a median septum are characteristically found to be normal on the neurologic examination at birth. The lesions usually come to clinical attention in infancy and childhood; occasionally, however, a teenager or adult will seek medical attention for symptoms referable to this lesion. Clinical deterioration with a gradual onset of paraparesis has been seen to develop in adults in the fifth or sixth decades of life.[12,17] Rarely, ''asymptomatic'' diastematomyelia with a median septum will be an incidental finding on autopsy.

An abnormal focal accumulation of fat over the lumbosacral spine may be associated with spina bifida occulta. The lesion may be found to terminate above the lumbodorsal fascia, but it frequently extends through the dura and is attached to a caudally displaced conus medullaris (Fig. 17-26). The subcutaneous lipoma is always present and recognizable at birth.[11] These neonates

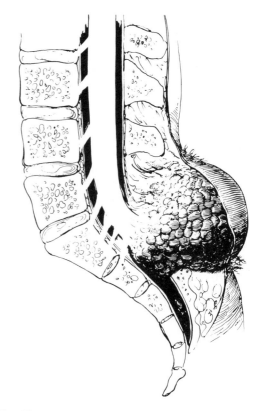

Fig. 17-26. Sagittal section of a lipomeningocele. Note how the subcutaneous fat merges with the caudally displaced conus medullaris. Nerve roots are commonly encountered within the deeper portions of the lipoma. (From Milhorat, T.H.: Pediatric neurosurgery, Philadelphia, 1978, F.A. Davis Co.)

are also characteristically found to be normal on the orthopedic and neurologic examination at birth. This lesion, like other forms of occult spinal dysraphism, is commonly seen in association with the other manifestations of developmental abnormality, including meningocele and myelomeningocele. The lipoma that is somewhat laterally positioned is more likely to be associated with an unrecognized meningocele. The elements of the cauda equina are intermingled among the fat and fibrous tissue making up the lipoma. The tumor frequently has a complex association with the conus medullaris. Although its natural history is not as well known as that of diastematomyelia, a lipomeningocele will frequently be associated with progressive neurologic deterioration.[41,61]

The tethered spinal cord has been recognized clinically and studied in the past 25 years.[23,29,32] This lesion is pathologically characterized by elongation of the conus medullaris below the L1-2

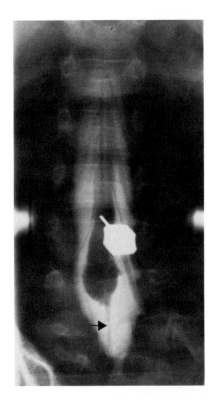

Fig. 17-27. Myelogram of a 4-year-old child with marked lower extremity weakness. The spinal cord is displaced caudally, and the most caudal portion is enlarged. A thick tethering band can be seen leaving the mass inferiorly (arrow). Although the enlargement was composed largely of fat, elements of striated muscle, dorsal root ganglion, and nerve were also present.

disc space, in association with a thickening of the filum terminale (usually more than 2 mm) and a more transverse course of the lumbar and sacral nerve roots in the subarachnoid space (Fig. 17-27). The clinical presentation of these patients is similar to the presentation of those with other forms of occult spinal dysraphism (orthopedic deformity of the spine, legs, and feet; neurologic compromise with weakness and wasting of the lower extremities; urologic abnormalities with development of a neurogenic bladder; and pain). Cutaneous signs of occult spinal dysraphism are present in only 45% of patients,[29] which is less frequent than with other lesions in this group. Older children commonly will demonstrate limited spinal mobility and limitation of forward bending and straight-leg raising.

Recurrent bouts of bacterial or aseptic (chemical) meningitis should alert the clinician to an abnormal communication between the subarach-noid space and the environment. One of these abnormal communications occurs over the lumbo-sacral spine and is termed a dermal sinus tract (Fig. 17-28). As mentioned previously, these sinus tracts may be particularly difficult to find on clinical examination, and manipulation of the skin is of help. If necessary, the skin over the back should be examined with the use of magnification. Palpation will occasionally cause pus or sebaceous material to be expressed from the sinus opening. Along the sinus tract, there may be enlargements containing keratin, hair, and sebaceous material (dermoid tumor), or simply keratin (epidermoid or pearly tumor). The tract may terminate at any level from the subcutaneous tissue to the central canal of the spinal cord. If meningitis has occurred, subarachnoid if not intramedullary extension is assured. Even a primary bout of meningitis associated with foot deformity, leg weakness or atrophy, or a neurogenic bladder should make the clinician highly suspicious of an intradural dermoid tumor and dermal sinus tract. Ideally, all dermal sinus tracts should be diagnosed and prophylactically excised before the onset of meningitis.[38,64]

Neurenteric cysts are included here because of their congenital origin. They too may occur in conjunction with other forms of spinal dysraphism, including myelomeningocele and diastematomyelia.[46,63] These lesions are relatively rare and are thought to result from an abnormal or persistent communication between embryonic endoderm and neuroectoderm. Such cysts are lined by gut or respiratory epithelium but may have other histologic elements in their walls. The lesions are typically located within or anterior to the spinal cord in the cervical region. Associated with the cyst may be a bony defect through the vertebral body. A tract may then connect the intraspinal cyst with the respiratory or gastrointestinal system. The clinical presentation varies with location but is usually characterized by spinal cord compression, which occurs over a period of years.

Evaluation. When any of the above lesions is suspected on clinical grounds, radiographic evaluation begins with anteroposterior (AP) and lateral x-ray films of the spine. The occurrence of multiple levels of bony abnormality is so common that total spine films are indicated. Tomography may be of additional help in complex spinal anomalies. With diastematomyelia and a median

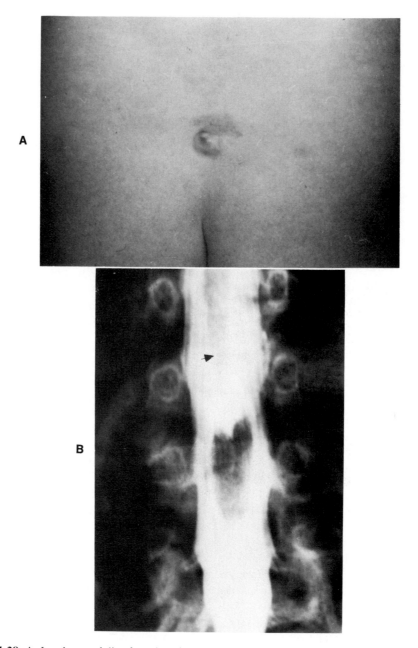

Fig. 17-28. A, Lumbosacral dimple and angioma. **B,** Myelogram of the same patient demonstrating a filling defect at the level of L-4, indicating a dermoid tumor. The conus medullaris is caudally displaced to lie over the body of L-3 (arrow). (Courtesy N. Grant, Hospital for Sick Children, London, Eng.)

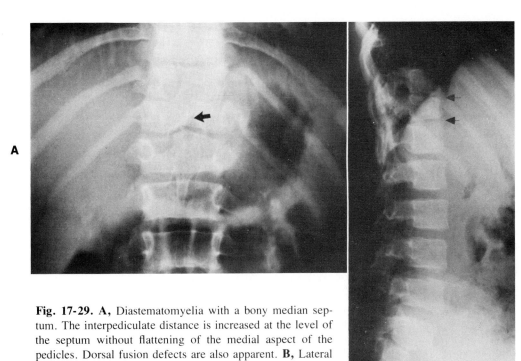

Fig. 17-29. A, Diastematomyelia with a bony median septum. The interpediculate distance is increased at the level of the septum without flattening of the medial aspect of the pedicles. Dorsal fusion defects are also apparent. **B,** Lateral radiograph of the same patient showing narrowing of the disc space at T10-11 (arrow).

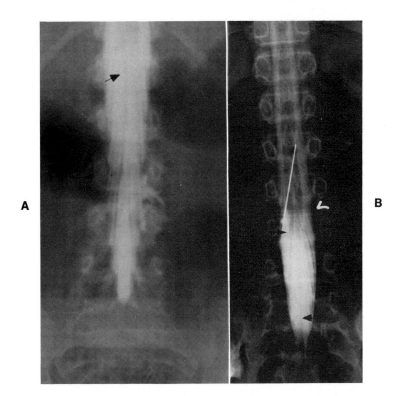

Fig. 17-30. A, Normal myelogram showing the typical position of the conus medullaris over the body of L-1 (arrow). **B,** Myelogram of a patient with a tethered spinal cord (extending to the body of L-3) (→). The filum terminale is thickened (→).

septum, plain films usually show widening of the interpediculate distance, fusion abnormalities of the laminae, spina bifida (usually at multiple levels), and shortening of the sagittal diameter of the vertebral body under the septum[26] (Fig. 17-29). In only 50% of patients can the septum actually be recognized prior to tomography or myelography. With a lipomeningocele or dermal sinus tract that enters the dura or with a tethered spinal cord, x-ray films of the lower spine almost always show spinal bifida over multiple segments. In addition, the interpediculate distance may be increased if there is a significant intraspinal tumor (lipoma or dermoid).

When surgery is contemplated, myelography is advised to demonstrate the extent of the lesion and to survey those areas that will not be exposed at the time of the surgery to rule out any associated anomalies. The myelogram is performed with the patient under general anesthesia, usually with a water-soluble myelographic contrast medium (metrizamide). Both prone and supine views are frequently needed. No myelogram can be called normal that does not visualize the dorsal surface of the cord and accurately determine the caudal extent of the conus medullaris (Fig. 17-30).

A CT scan of the spine has proved helpful in a limited number of patients. With further experience this diagnostic modality may prove to be a valuable adjunct to myelography.[51]

Injection of contrast medium into a dermal sinus to demonstrate the depth of its penetration is unwise. It carries the significant risk of meningitis if the sinus tract does communicate with the subarachnoid space and adds little diagnostic information.

Referral. Referral of patients with occult spinal dysraphism for neurosurgical evaluation is by and large elective. Sudden deterioration of neurologic function and meningitis may occur, in which case urgent referral is indicated. The vast majority of patients, however, come to the primary care physician because of cutaneous abnormalities, progressive scoliosis or kyphosis, a neurogenic bladder, gait abnormality, a foot deformity, or weakness in one or both legs. Ideally, all lipomeningoceles and spinal dermal sinus tracts should be diagnosed at birth, before a neurologic deficit develops and should receive evaluation and therapy from early infancy. Diastematomyelia should also be evaluated within the first few weeks of life, before a neurologic deficit develops. Once

neurologic function has been lost, it may not return completely with treatment. The longer the deficit has been present, the less likely function is to return, even with prompt action. The existence of a fixed foot deformity or simple spina bifida of L-5 or S-1 is unlikely to be indicative of an underlying neurologic abnormality.

Medical versus surgical treatment. Opinion differs over the management of many of these lesions. Little doubt exists that a dermal sinus tract needs surgical attention. Many of these simply end outside of the subarachnoid space and are of little neurologic interest. However, to wait for the development of meningitis to prove that the sinus does, in fact, penetrate the dura and arachnoid is unwarranted and unwise. If meningitis has developed, spinal exploration is postponed until the infection is controlled. The only exception to this rule is the patient with neurologic deterioration during the medical treatment of the meningitis. Such deterioration can come about with abscess formation in an intraspinal dermoid tumor. In this case, the abscess requires immediate drainage and the likelihood of complete and successful surgical excision of the dermoid is lessened.[38]

We, like others, believe that the presence of diastematomyelia with a median septum in childhood is an indication for excision because of the low risk of increasing the neurologic deficit by surgery and the high probability that neurologic deterioration will follow conservative therapy.[19,52] Neurenteric cysts are quite unusual; when such cysts are diagnosed, however, they should also be excised. The operative risk with section of the tethered filum terminale in the tethered spinal cord syndrome is so low that almost all authorities advise prompt surgery once the diagnosis has been established.

Treatment of lipomeningoceles with attachment to the conus medullaris is more controversial. Some surgeons advocate elective surgical exploration during the first few months of life,[41,61] others recommend waiting until serial examinations have clearly proved clinical deterioration.[38] The more aggressive surgeons argue that, as with diastematomyelia, the operative risk is low and once a neurologic deficit has developed, even prompt surgery frequently will not reverse the existing neurologic deficit. Other, more conservative surgeons argue that intradural exploration of a lipomeningocele is not without significant risk and that the risk of progression is less than that of diastematomyelia with a median septum. It is our view that an aggressive approach is justified. Microsurgical techniques decrease the risk of neurologic damage during the procedure and make exploration justified.

Surgical options. All patients undergo surgery under general anesthesia. Pelvic and chest supports are used to allow the abdomen free excursion, which decreases venous pressure in the epidural space and thereby decreases intraoperative bleeding. A tethered spinal cord is approached through a limited laminectomy at a single level over the thickened filum terminale. The dura mater is opened, and the filum terminale is located and sectioned. Spinal exploration for diastematomyelia requires laminectomy at multiple levels and initial extradural removal of as much of the bony spicule as possible. The dura mater is then opened in an elliptical fashion around the septum, and intradural adhesions from the surrounding spinal cord to the dural sleeve are lysed. The dural sleeve and ventral portion of the septum are then removed. Ventrally located neurenteric cysts are removed through a wide laminectomy so that the surgeon may work anterior to the cord with as little manipulation of the spinal cord as possible. The cyst is excised along with any anterior communication through the vertebral body. Any intrathoracic or intra-abdominal component of the cyst is removed during a second procedure once the spinal cord has been decompressed. Intraspinal dermoid lesions that have not been associated with meningitis are usually distinct and easily separated from the surrounding cauda equina and conus medullaris. Once meningitis has occurred, however, the plane of dissection between tumor and neural tissue becomes difficult to define and impossible to dissect without damage to the surrounding neural structures. Subtotal excision is then accepted and recurrence assured.

The removal of a lipomeningocele with extensive attachment to the conus medullaris and cauda equina is technically challenging. The surgical goal is to release any tethering effect from the lipoma's attachment to surrounding structures and to debulk the intradural and subcutaneous aspects of the tumor without damaging the surrounding neural tissue. Functioning spinal roots are found coursing through the lipoma; in addition, fat will be found embedded in the substance of the spinal cord. Removal of the portion of the lipoma intimately associated with neural tissue carries great risk and is not justified. Recurrent growth of tumor following subtotal removal is unusual. However, cosmetic procedures to remove the subcutaneous component of the tumor, leaving the deeper portions, are ill advised. When these patients do develop neurologic symptoms because of the continued tethering effect and the intradural component of the tumor must be explored, this procedure is significantly more difficult because of the one preceding it. During surgery the conus medullaris will be found lying at the level of the lumbosacral junction. At the cephalic point of emergence of the lipoma through the dura mater, a dense transverse band will frequently be present.[2] Angulation and traction on the spinal cord at this point is often significant and may be the cause of neurologic deterioration.

Postoperative course. If the dura mater in the lower portion of the spine has been opened, the child is nursed prone and horizontal for 5 to 7 days to allow time for the dural opening to seal properly. Following this time, the skin sutures are removed and the patient is slowly allowed up. The total time for postoperative recovery in the hospital is 7 to 10 days. The neurologic examination following recovery from the anesthetic is of particular importance to establish the existence of any damage resulting from the surgical exploration. In addition, the examination is used as a baseline for subsequent examinations to determine neurologic progress. Bladder function is frequently retarded immediately following surgical exploration; and if no urine has appeared spontaneously after 8 to 10 hours, intermittent bladder catheterization is necessary and is continued until the patient begins to void spontaneously. Voiding is enhanced once the patient is allowed to be upright.

Hematoma formation in the operative site occurs rarely. If neurologic function regresses significantly from that noted on the immediate postoperative examination, this possibility must be entertained. Infection, either superficial (causing a wound abscess) or deep (causing meningitis), can occur. This is particularly true since many of the incisions are placed near the anus and the adjacent contaminated skin. Proper surgical technique minimizes this possibility.

A more common problem is maintaining a watertight closure of the dura mater. Postoperative iatrogenic meningoceles form because the dural closure is inadequate. They are more common the more caudal the dural incision. The hydrostatic force of the CSF column makes adequate dural closure more difficult in the sacral and low lumbar areas. A repeat procedure for closure of a dural leak may be necessary if conservative measures fail to eradicate the problem.

Prognosis. After successful surgery, patients with a tethered spinal cord, diastematomyelia with a median septum, a dermal sinus tract and intradural dermoid tumor, or a neurenteric cyst can expect no further loss of neurologic function. In addition, they may achieve some return. This, however, is not an excuse to wait until major deficits have developed before a surgical opinion is requested. Areas in which improvement is more likely to take place include strength, sensation, and limited bladder control. Of these, bladder control is the function most easily lost and the least likely to improve. Orthopedic bony deformities involving the feet and legs, as well as scoliosis and kyphosis, do not usually improve after successful removal of the offending intraspinal lesion. Scoliosis and kyphosis not infrequently continue to progress despite successful intraspinal surgery.[19,30] Partially excised dermoid lesions and lipomeningoceles may continue to grow at a relatively slow rate, causing continued loss of neurologic function. Secondary explorations of these lesions are sometimes necessary.

Important aspects of follow-up. Depending on their degree of disability, these children can best be managed as myelodysplastic patients in a multispeciality clinic. Of particular importance is orthopedic attention to the lower extremities and spinal deformity. The presence of a neurogenic bladder continues to be life threatening because of acute urinary tract infection and septicemia and progressive renal failure. The urologist directs this aspect of the child's care. As with other forms of spinal dysraphism, genetic counseling is of major importance. Subsequent siblings of the patient are at a higher risk ($>4\%$)[7] of being born with one of the more obvious and disabling forms of dysraphism (myelomeningocele or anencephaly). These mothers should receive screening of the maternal serum concentration of alphafetoprotein and ultrasonography of the fetus during the second trimester of pregnancy, as outlined in the discussion on myelodysplasia and encephalocele.

Complications. From a neurologic standpoint,

the subsequent complications following surgery for occult spinal dysraphism may result in progressive worsening of neurologic function. This remains a possibility with all forms of occult spinal dysraphism where there is involvement of the nervous system. Thus, continued observation is advised at 6-month intervals throughout childhood and adolescence. Partially resected dermoid tumors and lipomeningoceles are necessarily followed more closely. Occasionally, neurologic deterioration will occur but be unrelated to the known spinal abnormality; associated abnormalities commonly occur and may be found distant to the involved neural segment.

Chiari malformations and hydrocephalus are not associated with these lesions. Syringomyelia does appear to be associated occasionally with diastematomyelia, dermal sinus tracts, and intradural dermoid tumors.

Other, less common lesions. Teratomas occur in the sacrococcygeal area and are of major surgical importance. These lesions should not be confused with lipomeningoceles or meningoceles. Sacrococcygeal teratomas require early surgical removal to prevent malignant transformation.

Syringomyelia and hydromyelia are cystic dilatations of the spinal cord.[3] Hydromyelia is a cystic enlargement of the central canal of the spinal cord that communicates with the caudal portion of the fourth ventricle (obex). Patients with hydromyelia come to clinical attention with complaints of spastic weakness of the extremities, loss of pain and temperature appreciation, orthopedic deformity (scoliosis, kyphosis), or a neurogenic bladder. Hydromyelia may be seen in association with Chiari malformations, communicating hydrocephalus, myelomeningocele, and basal arachnoiditis. Syringomyelia is a paramedian cystic dilatation within the spinal cord that can be seen in association with spinal cord tumors and following spinal cord trauma. The diagnosis of communicating cavitation of the spinal cord is confirmed by myelography with collapse of the dilated spinal cord as a result of a change in position of the patient. Therapy depends on the etiology of the condition. Those associated with hydrocephalus are most effectively treated by ventriculoperitoneal shunt insertion. Patients with communication of the cavity with the fourth ventricle may be helped by placing a muscle plug in the opening of the cavity near the obex.[20] Noncommunicating cavities may be treated by communicating the cavity with the subarachnoid space. The prognosis is dependent in large part on the etiology of the condition.

REFERENCES

1. Adams, R. D., and others: Symptomatic occult hydrocephalus with ''normal'' cerebrospinal-fluid pressure: treatable syndrome, N. Engl. J. Med. **273:**117, 1965.
2. Anderson, F. M.: Occult spinal dysraphism, J. Pediatr. **73:**163, 1968.
3. Barnett, H. J. M., Foster, J. B., and Hudgson, P.: Syringomyelia, London, 1973, W. B. Saunders Co., Ltd.
4. Becker, D. P., and Nulsen, F. E.: Control of hydrocephalus by valve regulated venous shunt: avoidance of complications in prolonged shunt maintenance, J. Neurosurg. **28:**215, 1968.
5. Bell, W. E., and others: Infections of the brain and spinal cord. In Swaiman, K. F., and Wright, F. S., editors: The practice of pediatric neurology, St. Louis, 1975, The C. V. Mosby Co.
6. Burrows, F. G. O.: Some aspects of occult spinal dysraphism: a study of 90 cases, Br. J. Radiol. **41:**496, 1968.
7. Carter, C. O., Evans, K. A., and Till, K.: Spinal dysraphism: genetic relation to neural tube malformations, J. Med. Genet. **13:**343, 1976.
8. Dandy, W. E.: Extirpation of the choroid plexus of the lateral ventricles in communicating hydrocephalus, Ann. Surg. **68:**569, 1919.
9. Dandy, W. E.: An operative procedure for hydrocephalus, Bull. Johns Hopkins Hosp. **33:**189, 1922.
10. Dandy, W. E., and Blackfan, K. D.: Internal hydrocephalus: an experimental clinical and pathological study, Am. J. Dis. Child. **8:**406, 1914.
11. Dubowitz, V., Lorber, J., and Zachary, R. B.: Lipoma of the cauda equina, Arch. Dis. Child. **40:**207, 1965.
12. English, W. J., and Maltby, G. L.: Diastematomyelia in adults, J. Neurosurg. **27:**260, 1967.
13. Epstein, F. J., Hochwald, G. M., and Ransohoff, J.: Neonatal hydrocephalus treated by compressive head wrapping, Lancet **1:**634, 1973.
14. Epstein, F. J., and others: Subtemporal craniectomy for recurrent shunt obstruction secondary to small ventricles, J. Neurosurg. **41:**29, 1974.
15. Everett, E. D., Eickhoff, T. C., and Simon, R. H.: Cerebrospinal fluid shunt infections with anaerobic diphtheroids (Propionibacterium species), J. Neurosurg. **44:**580, 1976.
16. Fokes, E. C.: Occult infections of ventriculoatrial shunt, J. Neurosurg. **33:**517, 1970.
17. Freeman, L. W.: Late symptoms from diastematomyelia, J. Neurosurg. **18:**538, 1961.
18. Grumme, T., and others: Intracerebral space-occupying lesions with brain density (isodense lesions). In Wullenweber, R., and others, editors: Treatment of hydrocephalus: computerized tomography, Berlin, 1978, Springer-Verlag.
19. Guthkelch, A. N.: Diastematomyelia with median septum, Brain **97:**729, 1974.
20. Hankinson, N. J.: The surgical treatment of syringomyelia, Adv. Tech. Stud. Neurosurg. **5:**129, 1978.
21. Harcourt, B., and Hopkins, D.: Ophthalmic manifestations of the battered-baby syndrome, Br. Med. J. **3:**398, 1971.
22. Hart, M. N., Malamud, N., and Ellis, W. G.: The Dandy-Walker syndrome, Neurology **22:**771, 1972.
23. Heinz, E. R., and others: Tethered spinal cord following meningomyelocele repair, Radiology **131:**153, 1979.
24. Hendrick, E. B.: The treatment of hydrocephalus—a philosophy. In Morley, T. P., editor: Current controversies in neurosurgery, Philadelphia, 1976, W. B. Saunders Co.
25. Hilal, S. K., Marton, D., and Pollack, E.: Diastematomyelia in children, Radiology **112:**609, 1974.
26. Hoffman, H. J.: The advantages of percutaneous third ventriculostomy over other forms of surgical treatment for infantile obstructive hydrocephalus. In Morley, T. R., editor: Current controversies in neurosurgery, Philadelphia, 1976, W. B. Saunders Co.
27. Hoffman, H. J., Hendrick, E. B., and Humphreys, R. P.: Metastasis via ventriculoperitoneal shunt in patients with medulloblastoma, J. Neurosurg. **44:**562, 1976.
28. Hoffman, H. J., Hendrick, E. B., and Humphreys, R. P.: New lumboperitoneal shunt for communicating hydrocephalus, J. Neurosurg. **44:**258, 1976.
29. Hoffman, H. J., Hendrick, E. B., and Humphreys, R. P.: The tethered spinal cord: its protean manifestations, diagnosis, and surgical correction, Child's Brain **2:**145, 1976.
30. James, C. C. M., and Lassman, L. P.: Spinal dysraphism: spina bifida occulta, London, 1972, Butterworth & Co. (Publishers), Ltd.
31. Johnson, I., and Wright, J.: Intracranial pressure changes in ''arrested'' hydrocephalus; presented at the Fourth International Symposium on Intracranial Pressure, Williamsburg, Va., June 1979.
32. Jones, P. H., and Love, J. G.: Tight filum terminale, Arch. Surg. **73:**556, 1956.
33. Keucher, T. R., and Mealey, J.: Long-term results after ventriculoatrial and ventriculoperitoneal shunting for infantile hydrocephalus, J. Neurosurg. **50:**179, 1979.
34. Kushner, J., and others: Kyphoscoliosis following lumbar subarachnoid shunts, J. Neurosurg. **34:**783, 1971.
35. Lorber, J.: Systematic ventriculographic studies in infants born with meningomyelocele and encephalocele, Arch. Dis. Child. **36:**381, 1961.
36. Maria, G., Rossi, G. F., and Vignati, A.: Intracranial pressure and pathogenesis of ''normotensive'' hydrocephalus. In Lundberg, N., Ponten, U., and Brock, M., editors: Intracranial pressure II, New York, 1975, Springer-Verlag New York, Inc.
37. Martin, G., Wallace, J. C., and Ross, I.: A dangerous way to treat subdural hematoma, Dev. Med. Child Neurol. **17:**517, 1975.
38. Matson, D. D.: Neurosurgery of infancy and childhood, Springfield, Ill., 1969, Charles C Thomas, Publisher.
39. McLaurin, R. L.: Treatment of infected ventricular shunts, Child's Brain **1:**306, 1975.
40. Milhorat, T. H.: Hydrocephalus and the cerebrospinal fluid, Baltimore, 1972, The Williams & Wilkins Co.
41. Milhorat, T. H.: Pediatric neurosurgery, Philadelphia, 1978, F. A. Davis Co.
42. Milhorat, T. H., and others: Choroid plexus papilloma:

proof of cerebrospinal fluid overproduction, Child's Brain **2:**273, 1976.

43. Milhorat, T. H., and others: Normal rate of cerebrospinal fluid formation five years after bilateral choroid plexectomy, J. Neurosurg. **44:**735, 1976.

44. Noble, T. C., and others: Thrombotic and embolic complications of ventriculo-atrial shunts, Dev. Med. Child Neurol. [Suppl.] **22:**114, 1970.

45. Nulsen, F. E., and Spitz, E. B.: Treatment of hydrocephalus by direct shunt from ventricle to jugular vein, Surg. Forum **2:**399, 1952.

46. Odake, G., Yamaki, T., and Naruse, S.: Neurenteric cyst with meningomyelocele, J. Neurosurg. **45:**352, 1976.

47. Osaka, K., and others: Correlation of the response of the flushing device to compression with the clinical picture in the evaluation of the functional status of the shunting system, Child's Brain **3:**25, 1977.

48. Parry, S. W., Schuhmacher, J. F., and Llewellyn, R. C.: Abdominal pseudocysts and ascites formation after ventriculoperitoneal shunt procedures, J. Neurosurg. **43:**476, 1975.

49. Perrin, J. C. S., and McLaurin, R. L.: Infected ventriculoatrial shunts, J. Neurosurg. **27:**21, 1967.

50. Raimondi, A. J., and Gutierrez, F. A.: Diagnosis and surgical treatment of choroid plexus papillomas, Child's Brain **1:**81, 1975.

51. Resjo, I. M., and others: Computed tomographic metrizomide myelography in spinal dysraphism in infants and children, J. Comput. Assist. Tomogr. **2:**549, 1978.

52. Shaw, J. F.: Diastematomyelia, Dev. Med. Child Neurol. **17:**361, 1975.

53. Shurtleff, D. B., Christie, D., and Foltz, E. L.: Ventriculo-auriculostomy-associated infection, J. Neurosurg. **35:**686, 1971.

54. Stauffer, U. G.: "Shunt nephritis": diffuse glomerulonephritis complicating ventriculo-atrial shunts, Dev. Med. Child Neurol. [Suppl.] **22:** 161, 1970.

55. Stookey, B., and Scarff, J. E.: Occlusion of the aqueduct of sylvius by neoplastic and nonneoplastic processes with a rational surgical treatment for relief of the resultant obstructive hydrocephalus, Bull. Neurol. Inst. N.Y. **5:** 348, 1936.

56. Sutton, L. N., Bruce, D. A., and Schut, L.: Hydranencephaly versus maximal hydrocephalus: an important clinical distinction, Neurosurgery **6:**35, 1980.

57. Symon, L., Dorsch, N. W. C., and Stephens, R. J.: Pressure waves in so-called low-pressure hydrocephalus, Lancet **2:**1291, 1972.

58. Till, K.: Subdural haematoma and effusion in infancy, Br. Med. J. **3:**804, 1968.

59. Till, K.: Paediatric neurosurgery, Oxford, 1975, Blackwell Scientific Publications, Ltd.

60. Torkildsen, A.: A new palliative operation in cases of inoperable occlusion of the sylvian aqueduct, Acta Chir. Scand. **82:**117, 1939.

61. Villargjo, F. J., Blazquez, M. G., and Gutierrez-Dias, J. A.: Intraspinal lipomas in children, Child's Brain **2:** 361, 1976.

62. Wald, S. L., and McLaurin, R. L.: Shunt-associated glomerulonephritis, Neurosurgery **3:**146, 1978.

63. Wilkins, R. H., and Odom, G. L.: Spinal intradural cysts, In Vinken, P. J., and Bruyn, G. W., editors: Handbook of clinical neurology. Vol. 20. Tumors of the spine and spinal cord, Amsterdam, 1976, North Holland Publishing Co.

64. Wright, R. L.: Congenital dermal sinuses, Prog. Neurol. Surg. **4:**175, 1971.

CHAPTER 18

Orthopedic considerations

ROBERT J. RUDERMAN and PETER W. WHITFIELD

EXAMINATION: GENERAL CONSIDERATIONS

The initial orthopedic assessment takes place in the newborn nursery, but it must not end there. At each return visit during the ensuing weeks and months, a musculoskeletal review should be part of the routine evaluation. A number of conditions that are, in fact, "congenital" become apparent only with abnormal growth or failure to develop. Trigger thumb, fibromuscular torticollis and dislocation of the hip are three well-known examples of important congenital conditions that may be diagnosed only after the child leaves the newborn nursery.

After the first 6 to 12 weeks of life, the range of motion of the joints should approach that of the older child or adult. If it does not, the examiner should be alert to possible underlying problems. For example, congenital dislocation of the radial head probably is present at birth or occurs shortly thereafter. If the proximal radius is dislocated posteriorly or laterally, the abnormal prominence and alteration in contour of the elbow are easily recognized. However, if the dislocation is anterior, there may be no gross external deformity; the infant's failure to flex the elbow fully may be recognized only during the next few months.

It is during this period that the child begins to walk. Since the gait matures fully in later years, it is dealt with in more detail in Chapter 23 in the section on the child from 2 to 12. There is enormous variability in the gait of infants and toddlers, and there are few well-documented guidelines for its assessment. Therefore, the examiner will probably have to rely on personal experience and judgment in evaluating a child in

the toddler age group. One important point does need to be repeated: even the child with severe bilateral clubfeet will be up and about at approximately the appropriate age. Failure of the child to do so implies a failure of motor development rather than structural deformity, and the appropriate causes should be sought. Similarly, children who have already reached a milestone generally do not regress for structural reasons. Thus, a child may refuse to walk because of hip pain but not because his feet turn in, his toes curl, or he "trips a lot."

Because the orthopedic-musculoskeletal assessment is inseparable from the neurologic evaluation, the reader is referred to the chapters on neurosurgical considerations throughout the text; but it is well to remember here that the period of most rapid growth of the brain continues during the first 6 months of life and that it is not until almost 2 years of age that the central nervous system is fully differentiated. Abnormalities of strength and tone and the persistence or absence of primitive or developmental reflexes are often perceived in structural terms by the parents but should not fool the alert examiner.

LOWER EXTREMITY ALIGNMENT

Some variation of static or dynamic alignment of the lower extremity (toe-in, toe-out, bowleg, knock-knee, flatfeet) is by far the most common reason for referral to a pediatric orthopedist. An understanding of normal anatomy and skeletal development will make these problems of lower extremity alignment much easier to understand, but the greatest difficulty is in imparting this understanding to parents and grandparents. Young parents, in particular, are often anxious and un-

285

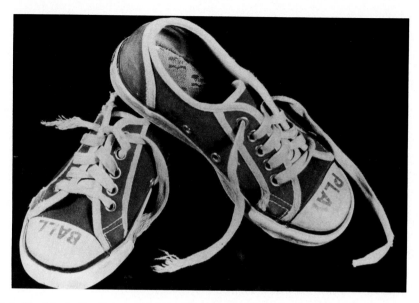

Fig. 18-1. The North Carolina Orthopedic Shoe. This multipurpose orthosis was designed by rehabilitation engineers at Duke University Medical Center. It has proved to be effective for all forms of physiologic torsional variations and angular deformities.

der great pressures from family and friends. They may want their child's legs to be "straight" and may not be above shopping around until they find a physician who is willing to "treat" the infant. It is no more appropriate to prescribe corrective shoes, bars, or splints for an otherwise normal child than it is to prescribe high-dose vitamins for an infant who eats an adequate diet (Fig. 18-1). Patience and understanding are most important. The goal is to keep a consultation from becoming a confrontation. Even when the primary care physician has confidence in the diagnosis of physiologic variation, a referral to a pediatric orthopedist may be appropriate for confirmation and reassurance of the parents. On the other hand, there are many conditions that are not self-limiting and that will demand orthotic and even surgical management. These conditions may be difficult to distinguish at first. Physiologic variation, when carried to its extreme, can interfere with cosmesis or function. When reasonable, correction should be done, but it is required less frequently than one might think. Every referral to an orthopedist should not be interpreted as a request for corrective therapy.

Normal development

There is a normal inward inclination of the femur and an outward inclination of the tibia. This configuration is achieved only after a period of development that occurs during the first 6 to 8 years of life.[47] Development occurs along the longitudinal axis of the leg as well.[11] In the first stages of embryologic development, the lower limb buds project at right angles to the body and the preaxial, or tibial, border of the leg (great toe) points cephalad. At about the third intrauterine month, the leg undergoes a 90-degree medial rotation about its long axis, which positions the great toe medially and directs the kneecap cranially. At this point the entire lower extremity is in a flexed and abducted position. Subsequent adduction and extension, through an additional 90 degrees, bring the limb beneath the trunk with the preaxial border (great toe) now pointing medially and the extensor border (kneecap) pointing anteriorly. Development continues in postnatal life and accounts for the changing angular and torsional alignment of the extremity during infancy and early childhood. The angular extremes are recognized as bowlegs (genu varum) or knock-knees (genu valgum). Torsional changes are most prominent in the femur but may be seen, as well, in the tibia or foot. These torsional variations are recognized as out-toeing or in-toeing and can be measured as the deviation of the long axis of the foot from the line of progression in gait[22] (Fig. 18-2).

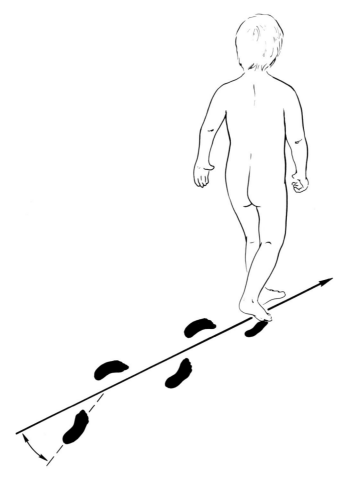

Fig. 18-2. The degree of in-toeing or out-toeing can be documented by recording the angle of gait. This angle is measured as the deviation of the long axis of the foot from the line of progression in gait.

Torsion

Femoral anteversion

As the femur rotates medially, the axis of the femoral neck does not come to lie in the frontal plane. Rather, it points forward in the infant approximately 40 degrees. Anatomically this angle is measured as the difference between the anterior inclination of the femoral neck and the transcondylar axis of the distal femur (Fig. 18-3). During the ensuing 6 to 8 years, remodeling of the femur gradually decreases this angle to the normal adult level of approximately 20 degrees[49] (Fig. 18-3). When femoral anteversion is exaggerated or persists to the degree normally seen in fetal life, one is dealing with femoral torsion. With increasing femoral anteversion, the hip will have a greater range of internal rotation than of external rotation. Internal rotation may be as great as 90 degrees, and external rotation may be only 10 to 20 degrees.

This may be clinically assessed with the child in the supine position with the hips and knees extended. The legs are simultaneously rotated, and the patellas are utilized as markers for the degree of rotation available. A simpler technique is to place the child prone with the buttocks level and the pelvis stabilized parallel to the table top (Fig. 18-4).

Clinical presentation. Anteversion is a very common cause of in-toeing ("pigeon toes"). The child has in-turning of the entire lower extremity, the patellas point medially, and there is an inward deviation of the angle of gait. In the younger child, the feet may actually overlap in gait. The child steps on his own toes or catches the toe as it is brought forward in the swing phase of gait. These children appear clumsy and fall frequently.

There may be a bowed appearance to the lower extremities because of the internal rotation. This

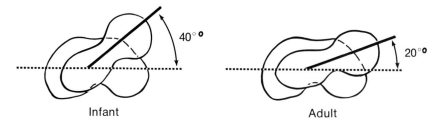

Fig. 18-3. Femoral anteversion is the angle formed by the transcondylar axis of the distal femur and the axis of the femoral neck. Anteversion gradually decreases over the first 8 years of life to the adult level of 20 degrees.

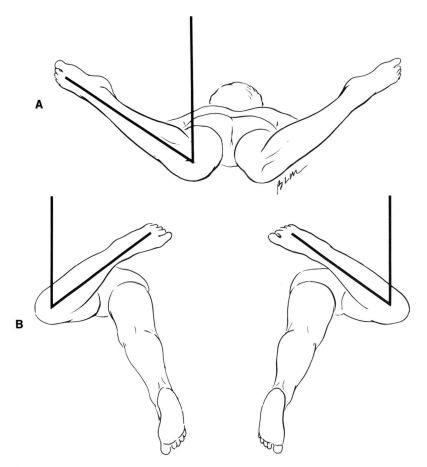

Fig. 18-4. Hip rotation is easy to estimate with the child prone. **A,** Internal rotation. **B,** External rotation.

posture will be exaggerated if there is true genu varum or internal torsion of the tibia. More commonly, an adaptive posture of external rotation of the knee and ankle and valgus of the hindfoot occurs as time goes by. Because of the increased range of internal rotation at the hip, these children sit in the "reverse tailor" position. This sitting position is also referred to as the "TV squat" or "W sitting" (Fig. 18-5). It is important to note that this is the result, not the cause, of the structural alignment of the extremity.

Evaluation. The degree of anteversion is usually estimated indirectly from the clinical range of motion. When surgery is being considered, radiographic measurements are often obtained as well. There are a variety of indirect radiographic techniques.[41] Recently, computerized transaxial tomography has been utilized for direct observation of the inclination of the femoral neck. All radiographic techniques are highly specialized and are likely to be inaccurate unless performed under rigid control in an experienced radiology department. The studies are unnecessary for most clinical purposes and need be performed only if surgery is being considered.

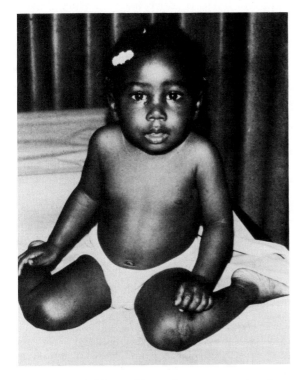

Fig. 18-5. Children with persistent anteversion have an increased range of internal rotation. This variation allows them to "W sit" (reverse tailor position).

Treatment. The most important consideration in treating femoral anteversion is maintaining a perspective on whom we are treating—the parent or the child. Few of us would consider it reasonable to hang a child by his thumbs in an attempt to produce a taller child in order to satisy the parents. Why then should we twist children by the feet in an attempt to alter the intrinsic bony structure of their hips so that the legs will be "straight"? There is no question that bone will respond to externally applied mechanical forces. Indeed, this is the basis of Wolf's law,[53] which is one of the underlying principles of dynamic skeletal biology, and which accounts for the so-called biologic plasticity of bone. However, this alteration occurs only when the forces are applied directly and continuously over a long period of time, as in orthodontia. Thus, most devices are unlikely to have a significant effect. The apparent alteration in the limb position and gait is the result of changes in alignment or range of motion at distal segments and joints. There is *no* place for the use of corrective shoes, wedges, or Denis Browne splints in the management of in-toeing that results from femoral anteversion. Nor is forced alteration in the sleeping or sitting posture likely to be effective. All of the above measures are usually accompanied by parental nagging, which has also proved to be ineffective.

One must remember that we are dealing with variations in normal structure and development. Longitudinal studies of children have shown that the angle of anteversion does change significantly during the first 7 to 8 years of life.[19] It is not until the child has reached the age of 8 that one can make any final estimate of adult alignment.

The only appropriate treatment during the early years of life is continued observation and reassurance. There will occasionally be children in whom anteversion persists beyond the age of 8 years and in whom the deformity is extremely unsightly or functionally disabling. These children are surgical candidates for derotational osteotomy of the femur—the only effective surgical approach. The osteotomy is usually performed at the subtrochanteric level of the proximal femur.

Since anteversion is often symmetric, the surgical procedure is frequently done bilaterally. Both extremities can be corrected simultaneously or at least during the same hospitalization. The osteotomy will be stabilized with one of a variety of plates, pins, or screws. The decision to employ the additional support of a body cast depends on the size of the child and the security of the fixation. It is unusual for the internal fixation to be strong enough to allow immediate unguarded ambulation. Usually a wheelchair or, at least, crutches will be necessary for the first 4 to 6 weeks following surgery. The hospitalization period may not extend beyond a week.

Postoperative course. Postoperative considerations include the usual problems of wound and cast care. A sudden increase in pain or a change in position of the extremity may indicate failure of the fixation device and loss of position of the osteotomy. Healing of the osteotomy can be anticipated in 6 to 12 weeks with gradual return to normal activity at that time. Complete healing and remodeling of the bone occur only after several months. A secondary surgical procedure is often required to remove the fixation device.

Femoral retroversion

A decrease in the normal anterior inclination of the femoral neck can be referred to as retroversion. It is probably quite unusual for absolute retroversion to exist, but relative degrees are seen. In these instances, increased external rotation and out-toeing are the presenting complaints. The same general principles regarding anteversion apply to this condition, but this condition is much less common.

Tibial torsion

As indicated in Chapter 13 in the section on the newborn, the degree of tibial torsion is the angular difference between the transcondylar axis of the distal femur and the transmalleolar axis of the ankle. The intrinsic rotation at the knee and ankle make these axes difficult to estimate, particularly that of the femur. The measurement of the ''thigh-foot angle'' (p. 170) is probably as good a measure of tibial torsion as any and has the virtue of expediency. A variety of radiographic measurements have been described, but none are clinically useful. As with femoral anteversion, the degree of tibial torsion changes in early life. While the average newborn may have only a very few degrees of external torsion of the tibia, by the time the child is 5 years of age this angle averages 10 degrees and by adulthood 15 to 20 degrees.[34]

INTERNAL TIBIAL TORSION

Clinical presentation. Some degree of internal tibial torsion is not unusual. It is probably over-emphasized as a cause of in-toeing. More commonly, it is one part of a pattern and is associated with a degree of metatarsus adductus and tibial bowing (Fig. 18-6). Femoral anteversion may also be present. This rather typical pattern has something to do with intrauterine constraint, although familial patterns are also recognized. The presenting clinical complaint is either pigeon toe, bowleg, or in-toeing, depending on the age of the child and whether the child has begun to walk. In this setting, it is important to define which elements of hip, knee, or foot variations are primarily responsible for the apparent torsional deformity. As noted, the etiology is usually a combined one, with multiple levels of involvement.

Treatment. The guidelines are the same as those for femoral anteversion. Spontaneous correction almost invariably occurs with time and growth. The incidence of internal tibial torsion severe enough to cause functional disability in the adult is exceedingly small. Treatment with shoes or splints is rarely necessary. The only definitive method of correction is derotation osteotomy, but surgery is rarely necessary.

EXTERNAL TIBIAL TORSION

External tibial torsion is much less common than significant internal tibial torsion. It may develop as a secondary adaptive posture as a result of femoral torsion or genu valgum. Actually, the out-toeing in these instances may occur with ankle rotation and valgus alignment of the hindfoot as opposed to true torsion of the tibia. External tibial torsion occurs in certain neuromuscular problems such as polio or myelodysplasia as a result of contracture of the iliotibial band or muscle imbalance. These are special circumstances and are not likely to be confused with the more common anatomic variant.

Angular deformities: bowleg and knock-knee

Angular deformities of the lower extremity, like torsional abnormalities, are quite common and frequently cause great parental concern. Fortunately, they represent, for the most part, physiologic variations that rarely require treatment. Fig. 18-7 demonstrates, in accordance with a num-

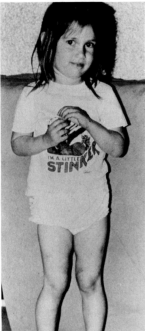

Fig. 18-6. In-toeing in often the result of several torsional variations: femoral anteversion, internal tibial torsion, bowing, and metatarsus adductus. In this child increased internal rotation, resulting from femoral anteversion was believed to be the predominant feature.

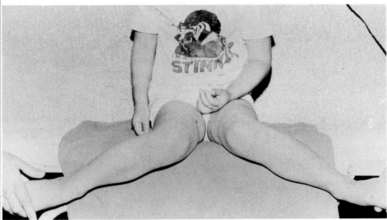

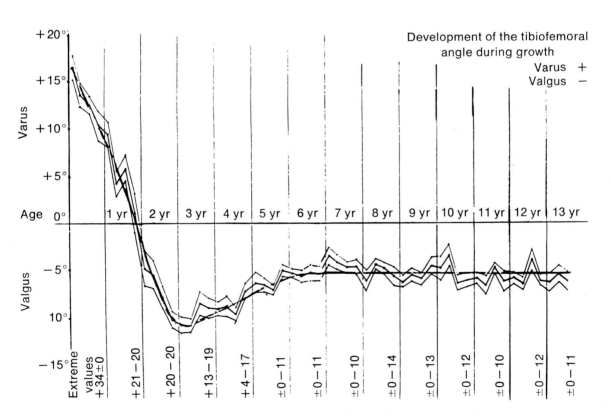

Fig. 18-7. Bowlegs and knock-knees in infants and toddlers are less worrisome when one appreciates the natural history of these deformities. (From Salenius, P., and Vankka, E.: Bone Joint Surg. **57A:**259, 1975.)

ber of other studies, the normal bowleg posture of children under the age of 2 years. This posture is frequently accentuated by an element of internal rotation of the femur and tibia. Most commonly, bowing is bilateral. The child will walk with a marked in-toeing deformity or else an adaptive pronation and pes planus. Radiographs are usually unnecessary but, if obtained, will reveal lateral bowing of the femur in a gentle curve at the junction of the middle and distal thirds and similar changes in the tibia at the junction of the proximal and middle thirds. The physeal plate and metaphysis are normal, but some flaring and wedging may be present. Mild thickening and sclerosis of the medial cortex may also be seen.

Between the ages of 18 months and 2 years the pendulum begins to swing toward knock-knee, which peaks at about age 3. Then there is a gradual return and leveling off at about the age of 7 or 8. By the age of 10 the adult alignment is achieved. Most adults have a mild degree of genu valgum (slightly more in women than in men but rarely above 5 to 7 degrees). If the genu valgum is moderate to marked in the younger child, the gait may be awkward; the knees tend to rub together, and external rotation of the tibia and pronated feet develop as compensatory mechanisms. In the average case, radiographs are not necessary; if they are obtained, they show only the variations similar to genu varum, with no obvious abnormality of growth or development.

Evaluation. The deformity can usually be documented by simple clinical means. To measure bowlegs, one aligns the legs with the patellas or feet pointing forward and the medial malleoli touching; one then measures the distance between the medial femoral condyles. In knock-knee, the legs are similarly aligned and the distances between the medial malleoli are recorded.

Treatment. Once the natural history is recognized, one can be more comfortable with the only appropriate treatment: reassurance of the parents and regular follow-up of the child. Both bowleg and knock-knee are self limiting, and there is no role for shoe corrections, splints, or exercises.

There is a point when physiologic variation becomes so severe and persistent that it borders on the pathologic. Although there are no firm guidelines to define the pathologic state, after the age of 24 months varus of greater than 20 to 30 degrees may require intervention. Similarly,

knock-knees that persist well beyond the age of 7 or are greater than 15 to 20 degrees should be treated. Bracing at a young age may be useful; more often, however, surgical correction is required in the form of either epiphyseal stapling or an osteotomy.

The choice of these two surgical procedures depends on individual judgment and the etiology of the abnormality. Stapling is effective only when the cause of the abnormality is such that significant growth remains at the physeal plate (on the medial side in bowleg and on the lateral side in knock-knee). One or two metallic staples are placed across the growth plate on the long side. This procedure allows continued growth on the opposite side and subsequent straightening of the deformity (Fig. 18-8). In theory, when the staple is removed, growth will resume on the retarded side and this reversibility will allow for variations in epiphyseal growth.[14] The procedure is not always as predictable as one would hope but is, in general, satisfactory and does provide flexibility. The placement of the staples is a limited surgical procedure, and removal is not complicated. Hospitalization for stapling lasts only a few days, and postoperative care should be routine.

When the deformity is corrected at an advanced age, or where an injury or disease process has directly affected the growth potential of the physeal plate, stapling will not suffice. In these instances, angular deformity is corrected with an osteotomy. The level of the osteotomy will depend on the site of the abnormality. If the deformity in genu valgus is in the femur, the femur becomes the site of the osteotomy; genu varum is usually corrected in the tibia. If correction and internal fixation are satisfactory, weight bearing can be allowed immediately. Usually weight bearing is delayed for several weeks.

Complications. A major postoperative complication is vascular or neurologic embarrassment, which is most common with proximal tibial osteotomies. Great care must be taken in any procedure that effectively lengthens the tibia and places longitudinal stress on the peroneal nerve. Anterior compartment syndrome can occur in any procedure on the proximal tibia; thus, prophylactic anterior compartment fasciotomy is usually included in any osteotomy procedure. Neurovascular complications are less of a concern once the patient is past the initial postoperative period.

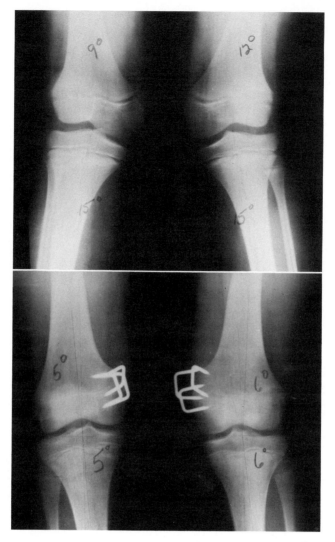

Fig. 18-8. There are several ways to correct pathologic angular deformities. Unilateral stapling of the epiphysis has limited indications but is an effective technique when utilized in the appropriate patient. These preoperative and postoperative x-ray films were taken approximately 1 year apart.

Pathologic angular deformity

When the angular deformity fails to follow the normal developmental curve, one becomes concerned that one is dealing with more than physiologic variation. This concern is particularly great if there is a strong familiy history of short stature. An epiphyseal or metaphyseal dysplasia or an endocrinopathy may be present. The distal femur and proximal tibia are the most rapidly growing and metabolically active physeal centers in the body. Tumor or infection should always be kept in mind, especially if the angular deformity is unilateral, very asymmetric, or particularly sharp.

RICKETS

In recent years our understanding of calcium, phosphorus, and vitamin D physiology has increased.[21] Along with this understanding, the list of causes of osteomalacia of childhood has grown. Vitamin D—resistant rickets of the sex-linked dominant form remains the most common cause of rickets (in addition to being the only common sex-linked dominant disease), but many genetic patterns have been identified, as well as a host of varying metabolic abnormalities (Fig. 18-9). It is rare that one sees the full-blown picture of rickets, and one almost never sees nutritional

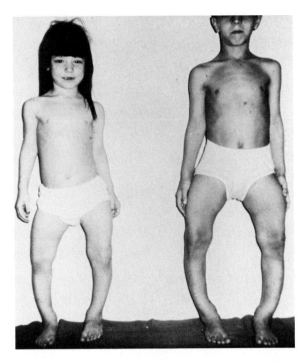

Fig. 18-9. Several features distinguish this bowing from physiologic variation. The children are older than one would expect with physiologic variation, the bowing is more severe, the femurs are involved, there is widening of the metaphyseal region of the bone (particularly at the wrist), and the condition is familial. In fact, these children were found to have the sex-linked dominant form of Vitamin D–resistant rickets.

rickets. However, the other entities are not as rare as one might imagine, and any child with significant angular deformity should at least have screening calcium and phosphorus studies done and probably should also have an assay done of vitamin D metabolites. We are seeing children with severe genu varum or valgus who do not have x-ray evidence of rickets but in whom more sophisticated techniques clearly document a metabolic abnormality. The ability to measure vitamin D metabolites gives one a direct and powerful tool for monitoring treatment. Many rachitic children have their obvious radiographic abnormalities corrected but fail to grow normally on more traditional treatment regimens. The recognition that phosphate must be replaced adequately to achieve normal growth has helped, and specific replacement therapy is most promising.[45]

One additional entity needs mentioning: "Dilantin-induced rickets." Liver microsomal hydroxylation of cholecalciferol at the 25 position is retarded by phenobarbitol as well. In children with severe neuromuscular disorders who have associated seizure problems, a combination of dietary and feeding difficulties and seizure medication may lead to significant osteomalacia. We have seen children in whom the resultant hypercalcemia has aggravated the seizure problem. The vicious circle of increased medication leading to increased calcium imbalance has been interrupted only when the metabolic defect was identified and corrected, resulting in improvement in the seizure management.

Treatment. There are two important principles in the surgical management of angular deformities in rickets. First, appropriate medical management must be instituted and the bone disease stabilized if one is to hope for satisfactory correction of the deformity and bone healing. Second, vitamin D and calcium replacement should be stopped or at least carefully monitored in the perioperative period. Immobilization hypercalcemia coupled with replacement therapy may lead to severe systemic effects or to renal calculi. This complication should be avoidable, however, with proper recognition and cooperation between the medical and surgical teams.

BLOUNT'S DISEASE (TIBIA VARA)

Blount's disease is usually described as an osteochondrosis, which actually says little about the true etiology. Blount's disease is often classified with the vascular disturbances of bone, but there is really no evidence that avascular necrosis is the underlying problem. There is a suggestion that obesity and relatively lax ligaments contribute to the development of Blount's disease. There is a hereditary component, and blacks are thought to be more severely affected. Whatever the etiology, all observers agree that there is a disturbance of growth of the proximal medial tibial physeal plate and metaphysis.[13,27] There are two major clinical forms of Blount's disease. In the juvenile form, the onset is between the ages of 6 and 14, the disease is usually unilateral, and the deformity is relatively mild. The infantile form is usually bilateral and more severe.

In the infantile form, the bowing becomes evident between the ages of 1 and 2. Mild cases seen at an early age are difficult to distinguish from physiologic bowing. Unilateral cases are easier to distinguish, particularly if there is a sharp angular bow, proximal medial tibial metaphyseal beak, and no femoral bowing (Fig. 18-10).

Radiographs are not diagnostic before the child is 18 months of age. There are several degrees of radiographic involvement,[38] ranging from mild irregularity of the physis and hypoplasia of the medial epiphysis with mild beaking to complete disruption of growth, severe deformity, wedging of the epiphysis, and medial closure of the physis. This continuum of changes probably represents degrees of involvement as well as stages of progression. If metaphyseal disruption does not progress beyond the mild form, complete restoration is possible. In the more advanced stages, some degree of permanent deformity is expected and surgical correction is necessary.

Tibia vara progresses because of the permanent disruption of the growth complex. The greatest progression occurs during the first 3 or 4 years of life, but the condition continues throughout growth. Simple observation may be all that is required in a young patient with mild deformity. Bracing is often recommended for the early case;

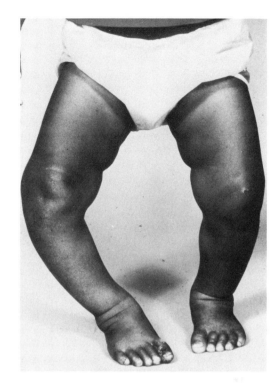

Fig. 18-10. Tibia vara in a 3-year-old child. The unilateral, sharp, angular deformity distinguishes this condition from physiologic bowing.

but it is difficult to assess the results of brace programs objectively, since complete, spontaneous restoration has been described. When the varus deformity exceeds 15 degrees and has not improved by the time the child is 2 years of age, and where an advanced stage of Blount's disease is evident radiographically, surgery in the form of an osteotomy must be considered. The correction achieved from an osteotomy may be permanent if the operation is done early. When surgery is delayed beyond the time the child is 6 to 8 years of age, multiple procedures are often required.

Trauma

Any injury or fracture that adversely affects the physeal plate of the tibia or femur may result in angular deformity, particularly when a partial bridge is formed across one portion of the physis but the rest remains open. One specific fracture should be mentioned: the innocent-appearing, undisplaced fracture that occurs in the proximal, medial tibia. For reasons not entirely understood, this apparently innocuous injury often results in a severe growth disturbance and progressive valgus deformity.[48] It is important to recognize this fracture and not undertreat it. However, even aggressive management may not prevent late deformity. The parents should be warned of the possibility of angulation and the need for surgical correction in the future.

Angulation in the sagittal plane
The femur

The femur has a normal anterolateral bow. If the bowing is accentuated bilaterally, it may be a physiologic variation or it may be the result of a systemic metabolic disorder or bone dysplasia. These pathologic conditions are quite rare, however. More commonly, pathologic bowing is unilateral and the cause more mundane. Intrauterine or birth fracture should be considered and x-ray films obtained. Congenital pseudarthrosis of the femur has been described but is also quite rare. Proximal bowing may be associated with coxa vara as part of the short femur, coxa vara, proximal femoral focal deficiency (PFFD) group of disorders. Limb length inequality should be carefully followed.

The tibia
POSTEROMEDIAL BOWING

Posteromedial bowing of the tibia is a distinct congenital anomaly for which no etiology has been determined. The deformity is in the middle third or at the junction of the middle and distal thirds of the tibia, and the bowing is directed posteriorly or posteromedially (Fig. 18-11). There may be associated foot deformities, usually calcaneus, with contracture of the anterior tendinous structures. These foot deformities are not fixed and will stretch out with time and range of motion exercises. Since the bowing itself is not associated with underlying bony disease and is generally resolved within the first 2 to 4 years of life, no braces or surgical procedures are needed.[31]

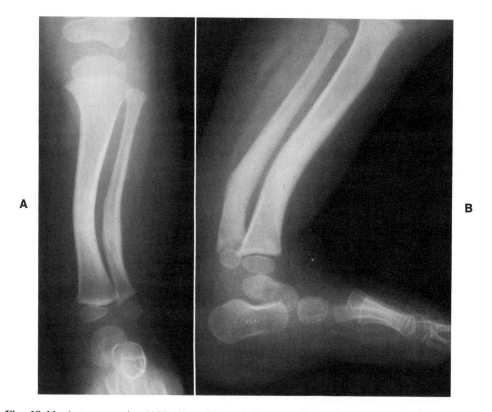

Fig. 18-11. Anteroposterior (AP) **(A)** and lateral **(B)** x-ray films of an infant with posteromedial bowing of the tibia and fibula. This condition is not associated with underlying bony disease; in addition, no braces or surgical procedures are necessary, since the bowing invariably resolves spontaneously.

ANTERIOR BOWING

Anterior bowing of the tibia is always an indication of severe underlying disease. The presence of anterior bowing alone should warrant referral to a pediatric orthopedic center. There are two groups of patients with anterior bowing. In one group the deformity is a result of congenital absence of the fibula or another significant developmental anomaly. In the other group the entity involved is known as *congenital pseudarthrosis of the tibia* (Fig. 18-12) and is a rare disorder in which there is anterior angulation of the tibia and often of the fibula with dysplastic changes in the bone.[1]

In congenital pseudarthrosis of the tibia, the apex of the bow generally occurs in the middle to distal portion of the tibia, which is usually sclerotic and narrowed; less frequently, there are cystic changes of the cortex. The lesion is usually unilateral. The tibia is bowed anteriorly or anterolaterally at birth; and fracture may occur with birth, or it may not occur until later in life. It should be remembered that *traumatic* fracture below the level of the knee is extremely rare in the newborn.

There is a strong association with neurofibromatosis.[10] Indeed, many authors feel that with long-term follow-up and careful investigation, evidence of neurofibromatosis will be found in all patients or their families. Despite this relationship with neurofibromatosis, biopsies of the bony defects reveal hamartomatous and vascular changes of the soft tissue but not classical neurofibromas.

Treatment. The initial treatment for patients with congenital pseudarthrosis of the tibia when no fracture has occurred is to protect the bone with a cast or orthosis. Once the fracture occurs, it is extremely resistant to all forms of treatment. The fracture never heals with conservative measures, and progressive atrophy and tapering of the bone ends occur with the development of true pseudarthrosis. At least 20 or 30 different surgical procedures have been described for obtaining union of these fractures, but the overall results of surgical treatment are not good.[15] Multiple procedures are often required; and even if union is obtained, bracing until skeletal maturity is always required. Repeat fracture is not infrequent and can be disastrous. Significant limb length inequality is common. A significant percentage of children with congenital pseudarthrosis ultimately require amputation despite a childhood devoted to multiple surgical procedures. Recently there have been promising reports of the use of free vascularized composite tissue grafts.[52] Equally promising are the results of electrical enhancement of fracture healing with the use of pulsed electromagnetic fields.[12]

Regardless of the form of treatment elected, it should be apparent that the techniques are highly specialized and that only major children's orthopedic centers will have adequate cumulative experience in the management of congenital pseudarthrosis to achieve even modest success. Early referral is mandatory.

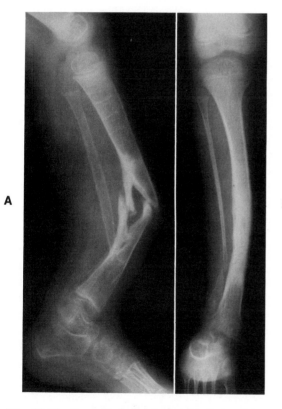

Fig. 18-12. Congenital pseudarthrosis of the tibia associated with neurofibromatosis. The apex of the bowing is directed anteriorly and laterally. **A,** X-ray film taken following an unsuccessful attempt at bypass bone grafting. **B,** Union was finally achieved after two further surgical procedures. A persistent nonunion of the fibula is evident.

COXA VARA

Coxa vara is a congenital abnormality of the proximal femur in which the angle formed by the long axis of the femoral neck and the femoral shaft is reduced from its normal 125 to 135 degrees to 90 degrees or less. There is commonly a defect in the ossification of the neck of the femur, as well as alteration in the growth afforded by the proximal femoral physeal plate. The shortening associated with this condition results not only from the alteration in the neck-shaft angle but from the limitation of growth. Since the proximal femur contributes only some 30% of the growth of the femur, the total limb length discrepancy should not be unmanageable. The condition may be bilateral, has no sex preference, and only a slight familial incidence. The etiology is unknown. Similar alterations in the femoral neck–shaft angle are seen in a variety of systemic bone dysplasias, such as Morquio's disease; in coxa vara, however, the problem is limited to the proximal femur.[9]

Clinical presentation. In the newborn period the findings may mimic those of congenital dislocation of the hip (CDH). The extremity will be shortened, and the trochanter can be palpated proximal to its normal level. The perineum may be widened, and there may be restriction of abduction. The signs of instability usually noted with CDH will not be present. However, since instability may be variable, the two conditions are difficult to distinguish. The older child has a short stature (if the condition is bilateral), limb length inequality, and a waddling gait. This gait defect is the result of proximal migration of the insertion of the hip abductors. Trendelenburg's sign will be positive. There will be excessive lumbar lordosis if the child has developed a hip flexion contracture. Pain does not become a problem until late childhood or adolescence.

Evaluation. Radiographs will demonstrate the change in the neck-shaft angle as well as the irregularity of the femoral neck. There is a characteristic triangular defect of the medial border of the neck of the femur, and the physeal plate may be almost vertical. The defect in the femoral neck will range from mild radiolucency to gross pseudarthrosis.

Treatment. In mild forms of coxa vara, the femoral neck will ossify eventually; if a limp is the only symptom and it is not severe, no treatment is necessary. In more severe cases, fragmentation of the femoral neck may occur with progressive displacement of the shaft in relationship to the proximal femur. The greater trochanter

impinges on the acetabulum, and secondary degenerative changes develop. When the neck-shaft angle is less than 100 to 110 degrees, or if the deformity is progressive, surgical correction by proximal femoral abduction osteotomy is indicated to avoid secondary changes and the development of pain.[40]

CONGENITAL DISLOCATION OF THE HIP

In the typical instance, the hip is not dislocated at birth but is dislocatable; the displacement may occur several days after birth. While this hip laxity should be identifiable in the newborn nursery with the maneuvers outlined in Chapter 13 (see that chapter for a more complete discussion of the entity and treatment), it may be missed. Careful reexamination of the hip during early well-baby follow-up is necessary. The classical findings on examination result from hip instability. After several weeks of dislocation, it may be impossible to reduce the hip and the important diagnostic feeling of reduction will be lost. In that instance one has to rely on asymmetry of thigh folds, apparent shortening of the extremity, limitation of abduction, and proximal positioning of the trochanter in making the diagnosis.

Radiographs are often not useful in the first few weeks of life. After the child is 6 to 8 weeks of age, however, one begins to see the first shadows of the capital femoral epiphysis and x-ray films become extremely important. If any doubt exists, an arthrogram should be diagnostic. As dislocation persists, secondary changes begin to develop and the various radiographic signs of dislocation become apparent. Fig. 18-13 outlines some of these changes and the more frequently used radiographic indices. Unfortunately, x-ray films are not always completely diagnostic and must always be correlated with the clinical examination. By the time an x-ray study has been ordered and the radiographic abnormalities become apparent, the child should have been referred for orthopedic evaluation. The essence of successful treatment of CDH, early therapeutic intervention, requires early recognition.

ABNORMALITIES OF THE CERVICAL SPINE AND SHOULDER GIRDLE
Congenital fibromuscular torticollis

The sternocleidomastoid muscle has both a sternal and a clavicular origin, and the two heads

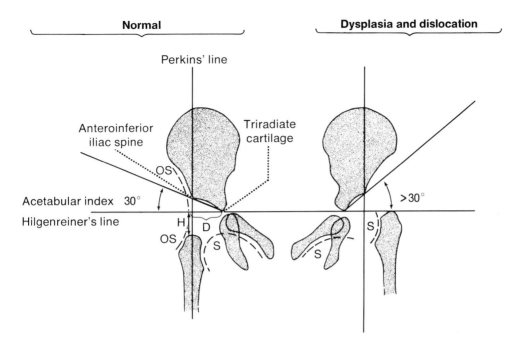

Fig. 18-13. Radiographic criteria for CDH. Most "views," "lines," and other "criteria" are based on secondary adaptive changes in the pelvis. The position of the child is critical. Perfect symmetry of the pelvis is mandatory, and minor rotation may distort normal relationships and alter the diagnostic value of the "lines." Hilgenreiner's horizontal line (through triradiate cartilage) intersects Perkin's vertical line (perpendicular to the lateral rim of the acetabulum) to create quadrants. The ossific nucleus or the medial beak of the metaphysis in a normal hip falls in the inner lower quadrant. A dislocated hip will fall in the upper or outer quadrants. *H,* The vertical distance from the femoral neck to Hilgenreiner's line decreases with proximal migration. *D,* The horizontal distance from the triradiate cartilage to the center of the ossific nucleus or the metaphyseal beak increases with lateral migration. *S,* Shenton's curved line (medial metaphysis to the superior border of the obturator foramen) should be smooth and unbroken. *OS,* The line along the ilium and lateral femoral neck should also be smooth and unbroken. The intersection of the line connecting the medial and lateral acetabulum with Hilgenreiner's line creates an angle that is known as the acetabular index and reflects the slope of the bony roof. The upper limits of normal in the newborn period is 30 degrees. Other common findings include delayed ossification of the capital femoral epiphysis on the dislocated side and the presence of a false acetabulum on the lateral iliac wing.

coalesce into a longitudinal muscle that inserts on the mastoid bone. When contracted, in congenital fibromuscular torticollis, the muscle tilts the head to the ipsilateral side and rotates it to the contralateral side. This posture is the typical "wry neck" appearance in the infant with torticollis (Fig. 18-14). The condition may not be apparent at birth but is usually discovered within the first 6 to 8 weeks of life. A nontender olive-shaped mass in the central portion of the muscle is typical but transient and in some series has been recognized in only 20% of patients with otherwise characteristic disease. The right side will be affected in approximately 75% of cases. Sec-

ondary facial asymmetry resulting from abnormal muscle pull and sleeping posture may not be evident in the neonatal period but will become progressively more prominent if the condition remains untreated. The diagnosis is not difficult, particularly when the fusiform mass can be detected; but congenital anomalies of the vertebrae and occipital cervical junction must be excluded, and every patient should have radiographs made of the cervical spine.[26]

Treatment. Once the diagnosis is made, therapy is instituted immediately and consists initially of manipulation and stretching exercises performed by the parents. These exercises should

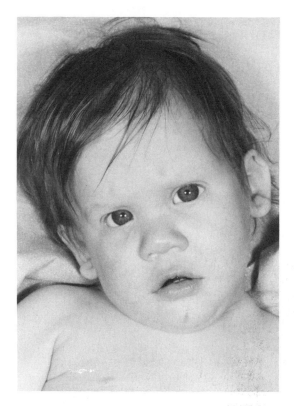

Fig. 18-14. Typical posture in fibromuscular torticollis. The head tilts to the ipsilateral side and rotates toward the contralateral side.

include rotation toward the side of the lesion and lateral flexion of the neck with the ear positioned opposite the contracted muscle adjacent to the shoulder. Maximal stretch will be accomplished when these maneuvers are performed with the neck in extension. Several repetitions of the exercise are performed with each diaper change. The child's toys, his position during feeding, the position of the crib and radio—indeed the child's entire environment—are modified so that his attention is always drawn to the affected side and he is encouraged to rotate in that direction. A photographic record of progress is extremely useful in documenting improvement, and the parents should be encouraged to keep a snapshot record of the child for comparison of facial asymmetry and resting posture.

When such a regimen is instituted early, nearly complete resolution can be expected in better than two thirds of all affected children.[18] If contracture persists beyond the age of 4 to 6 months, referral is indicated for surgical release and/or excision of the sternocleidomastoid muscle. Often

release of the distal insertions will suffice but may leave an unsightly scar. Some surgeons combine this procedure with a proximal release through a separate incision. Our preference is for resection of the midportion of the muscle through a single transverse incision. The more severe the contracture and the older the child at the time of surgery, the more extensive must be the resection of the fibrotic muscle and its surrounding fascial investments. In the young child, a soft dressing or a foam collar will be all that is required postoperatively, perhaps in combination with a period of resumption of stretching exercises. The results of such surgery have been highly satisfactory; there has been only mild residual deformity and alteration in the contour of the sternocleidomastoid muscle. The degree of resolution of facial asymmetry depends on the age of the child when the procedure is performed and may be complete in the infant.

In the older child, where the case has gone undiscovered or has been neglected for some period of time, a more extensive procedure is required. Moreover, postoperative bracing or casting in the overcorrected position may be necessary for several weeks, and complete resolution of facial asymmetry should not be expected.

Complications. Complications from this surgical procedure, though few, might include damage to the adjacent major vessels and nerves, in particular the spinal accessory nerve as it innervates and passes through the sternocleidomastoid muscle before reaching the trapezius muscle. The resultant trapezius paralysis will be detected as an alteration in the contour of the neck, inability to shrug the shoulders against resistance, and inability to stabilize the scapula and elevate it laterally. There is also weakness of shoulder motion and inability to abduct the arm fully. The trapezius muscle is not readily substituted for by other, adjacent muscles. Therefore, if this weakness is detected, reexploration with anastomosis or nerve grafting is indicated. While this is not a neoplastic condition and in that sense does not recur, scarring about the operative site or inadequate excision during the initial procedure can result in residual deformity or limitation of motion, indicating the need for additional surgery.[25]

Klippel-Feil syndrome

The Klippel-Feil syndrome (brevicollis) is characterized by the clinical triad of a short, thickened

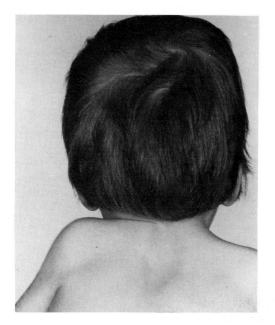

Fig. 18-15. The triad of a short, thickened neck, limitation of motion of the cervical spine, and a low posterior hairline defines the Klippel-Feil syndrome.

neck; limitation of motion of the cervical spine; and a low posterior hairline[28] (Fig. 18-15). Webbing of the neck may be associated. There are all degrees of severity. The abnormality is apparent at birth in the severely involved patient but may be diagnosed only on radiographs later in life in the child with mild involvement. Torticollis and facial asymmetry may be present. The fixed nature of the asymmetry and the associated congenital abnormalities should distinguish Klippel-Feil syndrome from congenital fibromuscular torticollis.

The etiology of the condition is unknown, but familial cases have been reported. The central abnormality is failure of segmentation of two or more of the cervical vertebrae. Associated anomalies are quite common and often are of greater clinical significance than the vertebral lesion. A third of the patients have congenital elevation of the scapula, and more than half have scoliosis or kyphosis of a significant degree. A third have an abnormality of the urinary tract that may be detectable only on an intravenous pyelogram (IVP), which is always indicated in these children. Anomalies of the ear are common and may be associated with hearing loss. Cardiac abnormalities are not rare, and anomalies have been described in almost every organ system.

Twenty percent of children with Klippel-Feil syndrome will exhibit synkinesia, or "mirror motion."[30] This is probably due to an intrinsic abnormality of the cervical spinal cord rather than mechanical impingement by the vertebral abnormalities. Synkinesia may interfere with two-handed activities requiring dexterity. Occupational therapy for adaptation may be of benefit.

Treatment. The cervical anomalies are fixed and are not usually amenable to modification. Stretching or bracing has no value, although if the cervical fusion is limited and there is a significant degree of cervicothoracic scoliosis, use of a Milwaukee brace may be beneficial. If webbing of the neck is severe, plastic surgery may be of value. For the most part, the abnormalities of the cervical spine are relatively asymptomatic during childhood. Treatment is usually directed at the associated abnormalities, which are so frequent.

Sprengel's deformity (congenital elevation of the scapula)

The upper limb bud makes its appearance opposite the cervical segments during the third week of embryonic development. About 2 weeks later, the scapula appears. Normally, by the third month of intrauterine life the scapula has migrated caudally to its adult position on the upper thorax from the second through eighth vertebral segments.

In congenital elevation of the scapula,[32] the caudal migration does not occur. In addition to being abnormally high, the congenitally elevated scapula is adducted, rotated, hypoplastic, and deformed. There is an increase in scapular width and a reduction in height. The supraspinous portion may be angulated as it contours to the upper thorax and shoulder. The "omovertebral" bone is a trapezoidal band extending from the superomedial border of the scapula to the lower cervical vertebra. This abnormal structure may be osseous, chondroid, fibrous, or a mixture of these. A well-developed omovertebral bone is seen in approximately one third of cases of congenital elevation of the scapula. Deformation of the clavicle and first rib and hypoplasia of one or more of the shoulder girdle muscles are common. Greater than 90% of children with Sprengel's deformity also have some abnormality in development of the cervical spine, thoracic spine, or rib cage.[29] An increased incidence in families has been reported, and there is a definite association with the Klippel-

Feil syndrome. Sprengel's deformity may be bilateral, or unilateral; when it is unilateral, it occurs more frequently on the left. There is no sex preference.

Evaluation. Congenital elevation of the scapula may be evident at birth or shortly thereafter. There is progression with subsequent growth. In addition to the scapular elevation, there is an alteration in contour of the affected side of the neck (Fig. 18-16). This neck asymmetry may give the appearance of torticollis, or true torticollis may exist from congenital anomalies of the cervical vertebrae or from shortening of the sternocleidomastoid musculature. Limitation of motion of the shoulder is common. Radiographs will confirm the clinical impression. Radiographic examination should include the spine so that the commonly associated abnormalities can be identified.

Treatment. The treatment considerations are twofold: cosmesis and function. Range of motion exercises may be useful in the young infant and child to maximize function but have little major effect on the long-term results. There is no conservative therapy of any value; surgery is the only treatment option. In the mildest cases, where the deformity is minimal and function is almost complete, correction is probably unnecessary. In the most severe cases, usually with associated anomalies, the deformity may be so great that the benefits of correction are marginal. In the intermediate grades, significant cosmetic improvement can be achieved but functional improvement is less assured.

Complications. The ideal age for surgical correction is 3 years. The procedure is formidable in the smaller child, and in the older child there is a significant increase of complications resulting

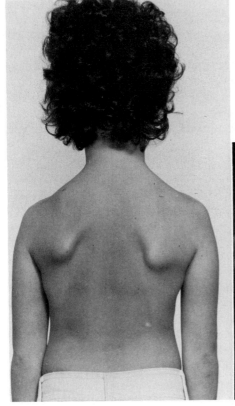

A

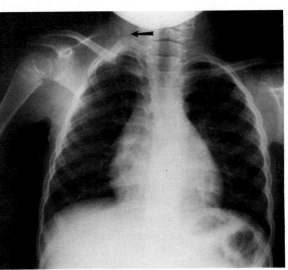

B

Fig. 18-16. A, Scapular elevation was detected in this child as an incidental finding during a routine examination. The degree of deformity is mild, but the elevation and alteration in coutour of the affected side of the neck is readily apparent. **B,** The arrows point to the level of the scapular spine in this chest radiograph of a child with a moderately severe degree of Sprengel's deformity.

from stretching or compression of the brachial plexus. Brachial plexus injury is the most common major complication and is the result of overcorrection or compression by the abnormal clavicle. This injury usually heals over the first several postoperative months, but recovery may not be complete. Additional complications include recurrence of the deformity, regeneration of the omovertebral bone, and the development of heterotopic bone at the medial border of the scapula with subsequent loss of functional improvement. Scarring may be severe, and this possibility should be taken into consideration when one is planning correction, particularly in the mild case.

Neurologic disorders

Spinal cord tumors, cerebellar lesions, syringomyelia, ocular dysfunction, and bulbar palsies have all been reported as being associated with torticollis and should, of course, be included in the differential diagnosis of neck pain or deformity.

Trauma

Because major trauma is so common in our society, cervical spine injuries in the child are not rare. Unlike in the adult, injuries to the lower cervical spine are uncommon; the child most frequently experiences injury in the upper cervical

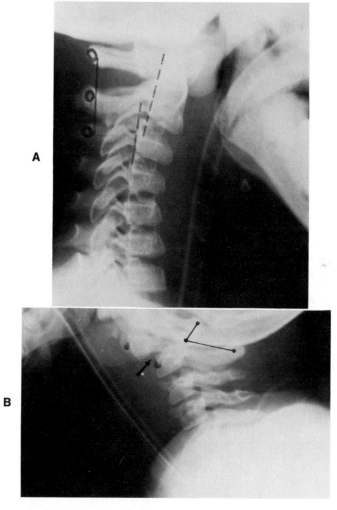

Fig. 18-17. A, Pseudosubluxation of C-2 on C-3. As much as 3 to 4 mm of displacement may be normal. This must be distinguished from fracture dislocation as seen in **B,** where there is a fracture through the base of the odontoid (arrow).

spine. Fractures of the odontoid have been documented and may be mistaken for congenital abnormalities.

Pseudosubluxation of C-2 on C-3

In the child below the age of 8 years, it is not unusual in hyperflexion for C-2 to ride forward on C-3 as much as 2 to 3 mm (Fig. 18-17). This displacement is often mistaken for a major cervical injury, and many children have spent weeks in skull tongs for treatment of what is a normal anatomic variant. In the absence of pain, fracture, or associated soft tissue injury (as demonstrated by prevertebral swelling, displacement of the prevertebral fat pad, or retropharyngeal hematoma), the anterior displacement of C-2 on C-3 is probably a normal variant.[17]

Other, less common abnormalities
Assimilation of the atlas

Failure of segmentation of the atlas from the occiput is not uncommon and may result from fibrous adhesions joining the two structures or from a complete bony synostosis.[43] In and of itself, assimilation is probably an asymptomatic anatomic variation. It is important, however, to realize its frequent association with other abnormalities of the occipital cervical region as well as with the Klippel-Feil syndrome and basilar impression. The latter is a congenital malformation of the base of the skull that allows proximal migration of the odontoid, which may then impinge on the space available in the foramen magnum for the brain stem and upper cervical spine.

In addition, compensatory hypermobility of adjacent segments may be present. Hypermobility may increase the propensity for neural injury, particularly if there are vertebral anomalies or fusion of adjacent segments.

Atlanto-occipital instability

The odontoid and the anterior rings of C-1 and C-2 normally move together in flexion and extension. The ring of C-1 encircles the spinal cord, the spinal epidural space, and the odontoid process, each of which accounts for one third of the available diameter. Where trauma or rheumatoid arthritis weakens the strong retaining ligaments of the odontoid, it may be displaced posteriorly in flexion. There it impinges on the space available for the spinal cord and may result in neurologic injury. In flexion and extension, a space greater than 4 mm between the posterior arch of C-1 and the anterior body of the odontoid is abnormal and represents atlantoaxial instability. Assimilation of the atlas and the occiput is commonly seen in association with this instability. It is assumed that the additional stress placed on the C1-2 articulation by occipital assimilation is the underlying cause of the atlanto-occipital instability. Intrinsic laxity of this articulation is seen commonly in Down's syndrome and has been reported as causing unexpected sudden death in these children.[20]

Atlantoaxial rotary subluxation

Wry neck from such paracervical inflammatory diseases as an upper respiratory tract infection, adenitis, or retropharyngeal abscess is common and is usually easily managed with attention to the underlying infectious process. Occasionally, the associated torticollis will be more severe and more resistant to treatment. Radiographs may demonstrate asymmetry of the proximal cervical spine; and if appropriate views (including tomography and cineradiography) are obtained, rotational subluxation of the first and second cervical vertebrae will be evident. The subluxation is presumed to be a result of hyperemia and capsular swelling of the facet joints of C-1 and C-2.[25] The torticollis is fixed and is painful when forced reduction is attempted. Neurologic deficit is unusual. Rotary subluxation usually responds to rest and the use of a cervical collar and/or head-halter traction. Less commonly, the condition is resistant even to skeletal traction and upper cervical fusion is required.

Odontoid anomalies

The odontoid process of the second cervical vertebra actually represents the embryologic remnant of the centrum of the first cervical vertebra.[24] Developmental abnormalities of the odontoid are congenital, but it is rare to make the diagnosis in childhood. Symptoms are all referable to relative instability of the atlantoaxial joint: upper cervical myelopathy, vertebral artery compression, or local neck symptoms of pain and headache. Once odontoid dysplasia is identified, careful follow-up is indicated. Surgical stabilization may be necessary, even in childhood, to prevent the major neurologic sequelae, including sudden death. Hypoplasia of the odontoid is a common feature of several of the dwarfing syndromes, particularly the spondyloepiphyseal dysplasias and the mucopolysaccharidoses. The symptoms in childhood may be quite subtle, and the generalized weakness that accompanies upper cervical compression is often incorrectly attributed to metabolic or skeletal disease.

SCOLIOSIS

Congenital spinal anomalies are the most common cause of scoliosis in the infant-toddler age group. In their text on scoliosis, Moe and co-workers[42] list at least 20 different forms of congenital spinal deformity, each with many subheadings. For purposes of cohesion, management of these defects is included in the discussion on scoliosis in Chapter 23 in the section on the child from 2 to 12. However, since the curvature may become apparent during the first 2 years of life, one cannot overemphasize the need for early recognition, accurate diagnosis, and referral to an experienced scoliosis center. There is no room in this condition for observation by anyone not equipped to provide comprehensive management. Watchful waiting can be disastrous. Fusion to prevent spinal deformity may be necessary as early as 6 months to 1 year of age. The worst tragedies occur when inappropriate delay allows curves to progress to grotesque proportions or where neurologic complications develop.

LIMB DEFICIENCIES

Individuals working regularly with limb-deficient children need a comprehensive taxonomy and nomenclature for communication and categorization. These individuals may move comfortably in a world of *intercalary, terminal, meromelias, hemimelias,* and *amelias,* but the average practitioner is rapidly lost. For the most part, the nonspecialist can satisfactorily describe any deficiency identified by simply grouping it into the complete amputations (terminal transverse deficiencies) and partial absences (longitudinal deficiency) and accurately describing the anatomic level of the deficiency or missing part. An understanding of the natural history and the approach to treatment far outweighs any semantic considerations.

The pediatric amputee poses special physiologic and emotional problems that are not well managed in the standard amputee clinic, crippled children's clinic, or limb and brace facility. The juvenile amputee is best managed in a multidisciplinary clinic at a referral center with broad experience in amputations and limb deficiencies in children.[6] Even some university medical centers do not have such specialized facilities. The effort and inconvenience involved with identifying and attending such a clinic will be rewarded with better adaptation to the disability and improved function.

The emotional impact of a congenital or acquired amputation falls on the family as well as on the patient. The task of dealing with parental anger, rejection, and guilt begins in the newborn nursery, and the educational process must begin there as well. If the parents are unable to come to terms with their child's deficiency, it will be extremely difficult to integrate a prosthetic program into the child's life.[5] When a limb-deficient child does not use his prosthesis, the problem is as often with the parents as it is with the patient. On the other hand, often in our attempts to get the child to accept a limb replacement as part of "self" rather than an external device and in our concern with such noble goals as "cosmetic restoration" and "integration into the community," we forget that function is the ultimate touchstone against which any prosthesis should be measured. The missing element in any terminal prosthetic device is sensation, and partial or distal amputees or those with residual appendages may elect not to use a prosthesis. In those instances it might be a rational choice.

Transverse deficiencies

Most childhood amputee centers report that 60% of the deficiencies of their patients are congenital and 40% are acquired.[51] This statistic is probably inaccurate, since many conventional, acquired amputations are managed in less specialized settings and the more complex, congenital problems are referred to the specialty center.

Acquired amputations

Trauma is the leading cause of acquired amputations in childhood. Usually only one limb is involved, and the lower extremity is affected in about 60% of cases. Males outnumber females (3:2) in large series. During the infant-toddler years, accidents involving power equipment and machinery, such as lawn mowers, are the most frequent causes of amputations. In the older age groups, vehicular accidents, gunshot wounds, household injuries, and burns become important. About one third of the total group will have an amputation performed for a disease process. Malignant tumors account for the majority of disease-related amputations, particularly in the older child. Vascular malformations or neurogenic disorders account for most of the other amputations and are frequent in children up to the age of 4 years.[37]

Modifications of general surgical principles. The recurrent theme throughout the orthopedic chapters of this text is consideration of growth and development. Here again, although most of the general surgical principles that are applicable to the adult are also applicable to the child, the first rule in managing an acquired amputation in the child is to preserve limb length whenever possible. In the child, stump scarring, closure under tension, and skin grafting are all acceptable in the name of preserving length.[7] Because longitudinal growth occurs at the physeal plate, transarticular amputation is performed, if possible, rather than the diaphyseal amputation that one might perform in an adult. For example, an above-knee amputation would sacrifice the distal femoral physeal plate, which accounts for 70% of the longitudinal growth of the femur. What might seem like a disproportionately long above-knee stump in a 2-year-old will be extremely short and probably not functional when the child grows to adult size.

Complications. Terminal overgrowth, the most common complication of acquired amputation, occurs when a bone is transected through its shaft.[2] The overgrowth results from appositional new bone growth from both the remaining segment of bone and the overlying soft tissues. Overgrowth does not occur with disarticulation and is another major reason for selecting that form of amputation in a child. If terminal overgrowth is allowed to continue it will not only interfere with the wearing of a prosthesis but the expanding bone can actually penetrate the skin, requiring repeated stump revisions until skeletal maturity is reached.[36] Bony spurs not infrequently develop at the corners and margins of amputations and are the result of periosteal irritation. Bursas overlying the end of a stump or adjacent bony spurs may be the result of a poorly fitting prosthesis. Maintaining a perfect total contact prosthesis may be difficult in the growing child, and the intermittent development of painful bursas is not unusual. Socket modification, rest, or even injection and aspiration may relieve the painful bursa; surgical resection of the underlying bony prominence, however, may be necessary.

The development of a neuroma at the end of a transected nerve is a natural biologic process; but if the neuroma is bound in scar tissue or is in a superficial position where it will be exposed to pressure from the prosthesis, pain may result, requiring socket modifications or even surgical resection and placement of the transected nerve in a more protected position.

Phantom sensation does not occur in congenital amputations,[51] but the sensation of a persisting part (or *phantom limb sensation*) always occurs in any acquired amputation whether the patient is a child or an adult. Often the patient is reluctant to discuss these feelings because he thinks he is somehow "crazy." Recognizing that they exist and discussing them may help the patient deal with them. Children under the age of 10 rapidly lose phantom sensation, and it usually recedes from consciousness in the older child and adult. In contrast to this normal sensation, *phantom limb pain* is a complex psychologic as well as physiologic process. Phantom limb pain may occur in the teenage amputee but never occurs in children.

Congenital amputations

For the most part, congenital amputations can be thought of in the same terms as an acquired loss with some important differences. With multilimb involvement or very proximal amputations, powered prostheses and special bucket orthoses become necessary. These are very special circumstances, and the prostheses can be managed only in highly specialized centers. However, all congenital deficiencies may have abnormalities of the remaining segments, such as proximal joint instability, malrotation of remaining skeletal elements, or deficient musculature, which may significantly alter prosthetic management.[5] The dictum that one always attempts to maintain length still holds true; small, unstable, or apparently useless remaining segments may well prove to be functional in an appropriately designed prosthesis, particularly in the upper extremity. One should not casually attempt to modify a congenital amputee to conform to standard expectations for adult or acquired amputees without careful forethought.

Considerations for prosthetic replacement

The goal of prosthetic replacement in a limb-deficient child is to maximize adult function and allow the child to progress through the normal developmental sequence during early infancy and

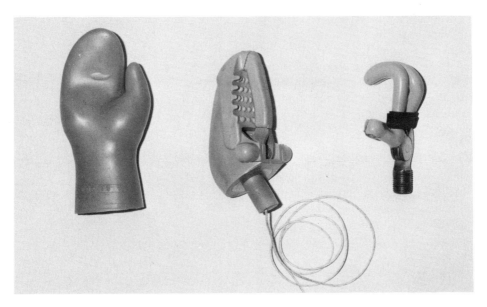

Fig. 18-18. Three commonly used terminal devices. On the left is a passive mitten, on the right a standard hook. The device in the center is known as a Child Amputee Prosthetics Project (CAPP). This device was developed at the University of California–Los Angeles.

childhood. Thus, in the upper extremity it is important to encourage two-handed prehensile activities and to develop a concept of placing the hand in space. Once the child begins to develop sitting balance and would normally begin utilizing a two-handed grasp, prosthesis fitting should be initiated. The first terminal device may be a passive mitten or a small passive hook that will allow the child to pull to a standing position (Fig. 18-18). Sometime after the child has reached the age of 1 year, cable activation of the terminal device will be introduced. Activation of the terminal device is timed to coincide with the time that children begin to pick up objects with one hand. If the deficiency is above the elbow, some form of elbow lock activation can be incorporated at this time; however, the usual remote-control shoulder mechanism will not be introduced until the third or fourth year.

The same general adherence to the developmental schedule is important in the lower extremity. Before the age of 8 to 12 months, the child will be crawling, and having two symmetric lower extremities is not absolutely necessary. However, the general symmetry and sense of body function in space may be important, and prosthesis fitting can begin as early as 6 months of age. Certainly, the lower extremity amputee should be fitted by 8 to 12 months of age, when the child is beginning to pull to stand and develop standing balance (Fig.

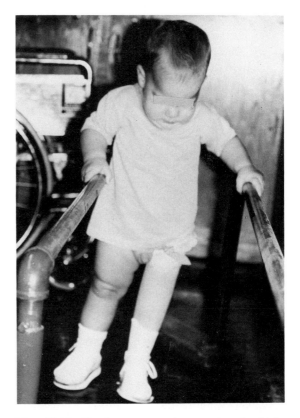

Fig. 18-19. The lower extremity amputee should be fitted with a prosthesis no later than age 8 to 12 months.

18-19). If the amputation is above the knee, knee stability will be provided by a lock. It is only after several months of walking that a free knee will be provided. One should not expect development of a heel-toe pattern of gait until the child is 4 or 5 years of age, any more than one would expect to see an adult pattern of gait in a normal child of that age.

Longitudinal (intercalary) deficiencies

Longitudinal deficiencies cause the greatest confusion because a wide variety and combination of defects occur in this group. Since the thalidomide tragedy in the 1950s, special emphasis has been placed on limb deficiencies that are the result of teratogens.

The major upper extremity longitudinal deficiencies are discussed in Chapter 13. This separation of material has been chosen because of the high incidence of associated congenital defects of other organ systems in the upper extremity. Such associated defects do occur with lower extremity deficiencies but not with the same frequency. The incidence of other organ involvement appears to be higher in children with bilateral or multilimb involvement.

Fibular hemimelia (congenital absence of the fibula)

Fibular hemimelia is the most common long bone deficiency.[44] It may be partial or complete and is usually unilateral, although bilateral cases are described (Fig. 18-20). Males are affected much more often than females (2:1). Involvement of other segments of the limb is frequent. Commonly, portions of the lateral rays of the foot are absent, and there may be tarsal coalition. The tibia itself is often bowed anteriorly, and there are abnormalities of the distal tibial growth center. PFFD occurs in approximately 50% of cases.[23] This combination of abnormalities presents a typical clinical picture of a short extremity with anterior bowing and an unstable valgus and equinus foot in which the lateral rays are often hypoplastic or absent (Fig. 18-21, *A*). A dimple may overlie the bowed tibia. The major prosthetic and clinical problems relate to the foot deformity, ankle instability, and limb length inequality.

If the foot is satisfactory and the shortening will not be severe, attempts at maintaining limb length and stabilization of the ankle and knee may be made to preserve a functional limb. The re-

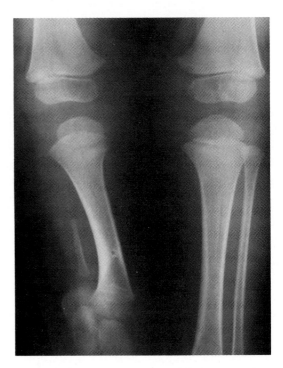

Fig. 18-20. Fibular hemimelia. In addition to the almost completely absent fibula, the lateral rays of the foot are missing as well.

sultant extremity may be functional, but it is certainly not going to be normal. Shoe lifts and/or braces may be necessary. In marked deficiencies, prostheses modified to accommodate the hypoplastic foot can be utilized; these are often awkard, however, and are not particularly cosmetic. Because of the difficulties of attempting reconstruction, early amputation through the ankle joint (Syme's amputation) is often recommended with subsequent management as a long, below-knee amputation.[54] Most candidates for ablative surgery can be identified before the age of 1 year, and early ablation seems to offer the best opportunity for a good functional and psychologic result.

Paraxial tibial hemimelia (congenital absence of the tibia)

Paraxial tibial hemimelia is the next most common limb deficiency. Unlike most of the other isolated congenital limb deficiencies, tibial hemimelia has a familial incidence. Other skeletal anomalies are frequent, especially CDH.[4] The leg is always severely shortened and the knee unstable, frequently with severe knee flexion contracture and popliteal webbing. The hindfoot is usually in marked varus, and the sole of the foot may

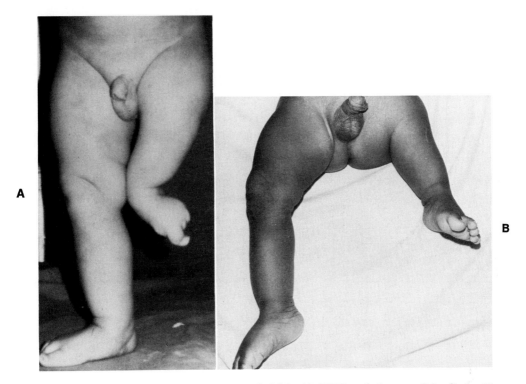

Fig. 18-21. A, Clinical appearance of a typical child with PFFD and absence of the fibula. Note the abnormal foot and valgus deformity. **B,** In the typical case of PFFD the thigh is rotated, shortened, abducted, flexed, and bulky in appearance. The soft tissues are telescoped over the short skeletal segment.

face the perineum. Deficiencies of one or more of the medial rays are common.

In the milder forms of the deficiency, where segments of the proximal tibia remain, surgical procedures to create a one-boned leg are possible; if the deficiency of the tibia is complete or the foot and ankle are unstable, however, amputation may be required.

Proximal femoral focal deficiency

PFFD is a congenital abnormality of both the proximal femur and its pelvic articulation.[3] It is the next most common abnormality after tibial deficiency. Unilateral involvement is most common, but bilateral cases are frequent (2:1). There is an even distribution of the sexes in the unilateral cases, but males are more frequently involved than females in the bilateral cases (2:1). More than half of these patients will have other congenital malformations, the most frequent of which is absence of the fibula (50% of cases). The varying degrees of absence and/or deformity of the osseous structures that make up the proximal fe-

mur and hip joint may combine to give severe hip instability and marked shortening of the thigh. The typical clinical picture is that of a shortened, flexed, abducted, and rotated thigh with a bulky appearance of the musculature about the hip as the soft tissues are telescoped over the short skeletal segment (Fig. 18-21, B). If there is concomitant fibular deficiency, there will be deformity of the leg and foot as well and the overall shortening may be such that the foot is at or above the level of the contralateral knee. The final clinical result depends on the other associated anomalies, the extent of the shortening of the limb, and the stability of the foot and hip.[35] In 75% of cases limb shortening is so great that even heroic surgical measures cannot create a functional extremity and conversion to an amputation is necessary. In the remaining cases limb length equalization and joint stabilization are possible but the surgical course will be complex, requiring multiple surgical procedures. The surgical approach is more conservative in bilateral cases, since these children can use their dwarfed extremities for mobility.

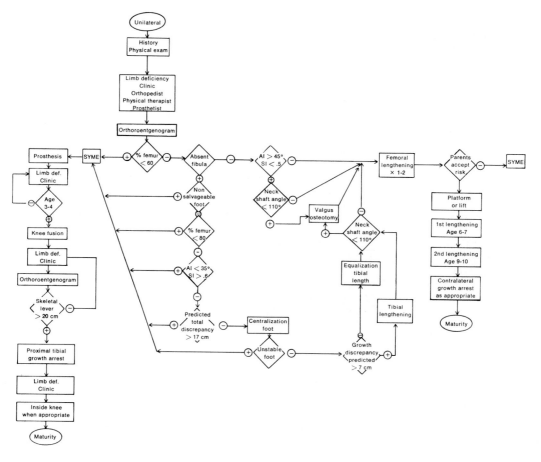

Fig. 18-22. Algorithm for the management of the unilaterally involved child with PFFD. The complexity of the decision-making process in this type of congenital abnormality is evident. (From Koman, L. A., Meyer, L. C., and Warren, F. H.: Clin Orthop., in press.)

Fig. 18-22 represents an algorithm for management of the unilaterally involved child that was developed after extensive review of a large series of patients at the Greenville Shriners Hospital.[35] This treatment plan is an excellent example of the complexity of the decision-making process in this type of congenital abnormality and demonstrates why children with PFFD and similar problems should be referred early to specialized centers.

Children are remarkably adaptive. Regardless of the extent of their individual skeletal problem, and independent of the type of treatment chosen, most of these children will ambulate before the age of 2 and, barring major anomalies in other organ systems, will lead functional and active lives.

CONSTRICTION WITH A FOREIGN BODY

The child can constrict a digit or acral part with any form of circular foreign body, and this constriction may lead to severe vascular obstruction and distal edema. In the infant, the offending material is commonly the mother's hair, which may become entwined about the digit in question. If this entwinement is unnoticed, severe constriction, distal edema, swelling, secondary infection, and even impending autoamputation may ensue (Fig. 18-23). Treatment consists of accurately diagnosing the condition, releasing the foreign material, and adequately draining any infection. With subsequent elevation, soaks, and antibiotics, one can anticipate complete resolution of the problem. Involvement of the fingers,

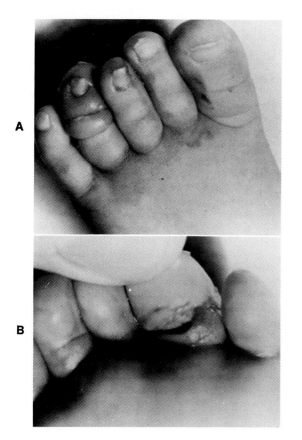

A

B

Fig. 18-23. Dorsal **(A)** and plantar **(B)** views of a child with foreign body (thread) circular constriction of the fourth toe. Amputation almost occurred.

toes, and even the penis has been described. Child abuse should be considered in unusual cases.

REFERENCES

1. Aegerter, E. E.: The possible relationship of neurofibromatosis, congenital pseudarthrosis and fibrous dysplasia, J. Bone Joint Surg. **32A:**618, 1950.
2. Aitken, G. T.: Surgical amputation in children, J. Bone Joint Surg. **45A:**1735, 1963.
3. Aitken, G. T.: Proximal femoral focal deficiency—classification and management. In a symposium on Proximal Femoral Focal Deficiency: A Congenital Anomaly, Washington, D.C., 1969, National Academy of Sciences.
4. Aitken, G. T.: Tibial hemimelia. In a symposium on Selected Lower Limb Anomalies: Surgical and Prosthetic Management, Washington, D.C., 1971, National Academy of Sciences.
5. Aitken, G. T.: The child amputee—an overview; Orthop. Clin. North Am. **3**(2):447, 1972.
6. Aitken, G. T., and Frantz, C. H.: The juvenile amputee, J. Bone Joint Surg. **35A:**659, 1953.
7. Aitken, G. T., and Frantz, C. H.: Management of the child amputee. In American Academy of Orthopaedic Surgeons: Instructional course lectures, vol. 17, St. Louis, 1960, The C. V. Mosby Co., pp. 246-298.
8. Amstutz, H. C.: Natural history and treatment of congenital absence of the fibula, J. Bone Joint Surg. **59A:**1349, 1972.
9. Amstutz, H. C., and Wilson, P. D., Jr.: Dysgenesis of the proximal femur (coxa vara) and its surgical management, J. Bone Joint Surg. **44A:**1, 1962.
10. Anderson, R. S.: Congenital pseudarthrosis of tibia and neurofibromatosis, Acta Orthop. Scand. **47:**108, 1976.
11. Bardeen, C. R., and Lewis, W. H.: Development of the limbs, body-wall, and back in x-ray, Am. J. Anat. **J:**1, 1901.
12. Bassett, C. A. L., Pilla, A. A., and Pawluk, R. J.: A nonoperative salvage of surgically resistant pseudarthrosis and non-unions by pulsing electromagnetic fields, Clin. Orthop. **124:**128, 1977.
13. Blount, W. P.: Tibia vara-osteochondrosis deformans tibial, J. Bone Joint Surg. **19**(1), 1937.
14. Blount, W. P., and Clark, G. R.: Control of bone growth by epiphyseal stapling, J. Bone Joint Surg. **31A:**464, 1949.
15. Boyd, H. B., and Sage, F. P.: Congenital pseudarthrosis of the tibia, J. Bone Joint Surg. **40A:**1245, 1958.
16. Cattell, H. S., and Filtzer, D. L.: Pseudo subluxation and other normal variations in the cervical spine in children, J. Bone Joint Surg. **47A:**1295, 1965.
17. Cavendish, M. E.: Congenital elevation of the scapula, J. Bone Joint Surg. **54B:**395, 1972.
18. Coventry, M. B., and Harris, L.: Congenital muscular torticollis in infancy—some observations regarding treatment, J. Bone Joint Surg. **41A:**815, 1959.
19. Crave, L.: Femoral torsion and its relation to toeing-in and toeing-out, J. Bone Joint Surg. **41A:**421, 1959.
20. Curtis, B. H., Blank, S., and Fisher, R. L.: Atlanto-axial dislocation in Down's Syndrome, J.A.M.A. **205:**464, 1968.
21. Drezner, M. K., and Harrelson, J. M.: Newer knowledge of vitamin D and of metabolites in health and disease, Clin. Orthop. **139:**206, 1979.
22. Engel, G. M., and Staheli, L. T.: Natural history of torsion and other factors influencing gait in childhood, Clin. Orthop. **99:**12, 1974.
23. Farmer, A. W., and Laurin, C. A.: Congenital absence of the fibula, J. Bone Joint Surg. **42A:**1, 1960.
24. Fielding, J. W.: The cervical spine in the child, Curr. Pract. Orthop. Surg. **5:**31, 1973.
25. Fielding, J. W., and Hawkins, R. J.: Atlanto-axial rotary fixation, J. Bone Joint Surg. **59A:**37, 1977.
26. Fielding, J. W., Hawkins, R. J., and Hensinger, R. N.: Atlantoaxial rotary deformities, Orthop. Clin. North Am. **9**(4):955, 1978.
27. Golding, J. S. R., and McNeil-Smith, J. D.: Observations on the etiology of tibia vara, J. Bone Joint Surg. **45B:**320, 1963.
28. Gray, S. W., Romaine, C. B., and Skandalokis, J. E.: Congenital fusion of the cervical vertebrae, Surg. Gynecol. Obstet. **118:**373, 1964.
29. Green, W. T.: The surgical correction of congenital elevation of the scapula (Sprengel's deformity): proceedings of the American Orthopedic Association, J. Bone Joint Surg. **39A:**149, 1957.
30. Hensinger, R. N., Lang, J. R., and MacEwen, G. D.:

The Klippel-Feil syndrome: a constellation of related anomalies, J. Bone Joint Surg. **56A:**1046, 1974.

31. Heyman, C. H., Herndon, C. H., and Heiple, K. G.: Congenital posterior angulation of the tibia with talipes calcaneus: a long-term report of elevan patients, J. Bone Joint Surg. **41A:**476, 1959.

32. Horwitz, A. E.: Congenital elevation of the scapula—Sprengel's deformity, Am. J. Orthop. Surg. **6:**260, 1908.

33. Kempe, C. H.: Approaches to preventive child abuse, Am. J. Dis. Child. **130:**941, 1976.

34. Kheumosh, O., Lior, G., and Weissman, S. L.: Tibial torsion in children, Clin. Orthop. **79:**2, 1971.

35. Koman, L. A., Meyer, L. C., and Warren, F. H.: Proximal femoral focal deficiency, Clin. Orthop., in press.

36. Lambert, C. N.: Amputation surgery in the child, Surg. Clin. North Am. **3**(2):473, 1972.

37. Lambert, C. N.: Etiology in the child with an acquired amputation, Washington, D.C., 1972, National Academy of Sciences.

38. Langenskjiold, A., and Riska, E. B.: Tibia vara (osteochondrosis deformans tibiae), J. Bone Joint Surg. **46A:**1405, 1964.

39. Lloyd-Roberts, C. G., and Pilcher, M. F.: Structural idiopathic scoliosis in infancy: a study of the natural history of 100 patients, J. Bone Joint Surg. **47B:**520, 1965.

40. MacEwen, G. D., and Ramsey, P. L.: The hip. In Lovell, W. W., and Winter, R. B., editors: Pediatric orthopaedics, Philadelphia, 1978, J. B. Lippincott Co.

41. Magilligan, D. J.: Calculation of the angle of anteversion by means of horizontal lateral roentgenography, J. Bone Joint Surg. **38A:**1231, 1956.

42. Moe, J. H., and others: Scoliosis and other spinal deformities, Philadelphia, 1978, W. B. Saunders Co.

43. Nicholson, J. S., and Sheik, H. H.: Anomalies of the occipito-cervical articulation, J. Bone Joint Surg. **50A:**295, 1968.

44. O'Rahilly, R.: Morphologic patterns in limb deficiencies and duplications, Am. J. Anat. **89:**135, 1951.

45. Peacock, M., Heyburn, P., and Aaron, J.: Vitamin D resistant hypophosphataemic osteomalacia: treatment with 1 alpha-hydroxyvitamin D_3, Clin. Endocrinol. (Oxf.) **7**(Suppl.):231, 1977.

46. Robinson, R. A.: The surgical importance of the clavicular component of Sprengel's deformity, J. Bone Joint Surg. **49A:**1481, 1967.

47. Salenius, P., and Vankka, E.: Development of the tibiofemoral angle in children, J. Bone Joint Surg. **57A:**259, 1975.

48. Salter, R. B., and Best, T.: The pathogenesis and prevention of valgus deformity following fractures of the proximal metaphyseal region of the tibia in children, J. Bone Joint Surg. **55A:**1324, 1973.

49. Shands, A. R., Jr., and Steele, M. K.: Torsion of the femur, J. Bone Joint Surg. **40A:**803, 1958.

50. Solomons, G.: Child abuse and developmental disabilities, Dev. Med. Child Neurol. **21:**101, 1979.

51. Tooms, R. E.: The amputee. In Lovell, W. W., and Winter, R. B., editors: Pediatric orthopaedics, Philadelphia, 1978, J. B. Lippincott Co.

52. Urbaniak, J. R.: Personal communication, 1978.

53. Wolff, J.: Uber die innere architecture der Rnochen and ihre Beckutung fur die Frage Von Knochen Wachstum, Virchows Arch. [Pathol. Anat.] **50:**389, 1870.

54. Wood, W. L., Zlotsky, N., and Westing, W.: Congenital absence of the fibula: treatment by Syme amputation—indications and technique, J. Bone Joint Surg. **47A:**1159, 1965.

55. Woodward, J. W.: Congenital elevation of the scapula—correction by release and transplantation of muscle origins, J. Bone Joint Surg. **43A:**219, 1961.

SECTION FOUR

The child from 2 to 12

CHAPTER 19

General considerations

HOWARD C. FILSTON

The most common childhood problems first become evident during the years from 2 to 12. In addition, many lesions discussed under the infant-toddler age group, such as malrotation, intussusception, and hernias, first become evident during the early years of this older age group.

Adding to the primary care physician's difficulty in making proper evaluations of some of these lesions is the tendency of parents to stop bringing their children for regular well-child care after the infancy period has passed. Most children are healthy during these years, and the parents do not seek medical attention except for acute care. The primary care physician, thus, is often confronted with a child with an acute illness whom he has not seen for years.

CHAPTER 20

Specific problems

HOWARD C. FILSTON

ABDOMINAL EMERGENCIES

The most frequent and difficult acute problem that the primary care physician is faced with in children in the age group of 2 to 12 years is the acute abdomen. It probably causes the primary care physician the greatest concern and is the area in which he feels least secure. Those of us with years of experience at children's surgery continue to look on the acute abdomen as a mystery, the unraveling of which presents us with our greatest challenges and threatens us with our greatest failures. The ability to perform a thorough, thoughtful examination of the abdomen and an attitude of willingness to respond to symptoms and signs without demanding a secure diagnosis will go far toward providing proper management for these diseases.

Examination of the abdomen. The examination of the abdomen is the most important part of data gathering in dealing with the acute abdomen. Laboratory values and radiographic findings rarely give information that is diagnostic outside the context of the abdominal findings. Although occasional children are so out of control that adequate abdominal examination is impossible, the physician who approaches the child in a concerned, thoughtful, and organized fashion can usually obtain a wealth of information from this examination.

To begin with, certain principles of dealing with all patients, and particularly with pediatric patients, must be adhered to in approaching a sick child with an acute abdomen. Some socialization with the child and his family should take place before the physical examination is begun. Although adults will tolerate, though not appreciate,

being "attacked" by an eager physician wanting to get to the "meat" of the problem, all patients appreciate a chance to get to know and feel secure with the examining physician. A few minutes of conversation with the child and his family will help to relax the child.

Probably the worst advice I received as a medical student was never to sit on the patient's bed. The physician examining a child's abdomen should make himself comfortable, and if that requires sitting on the bed or examining table, he should not hesitate to do so. He must be in a position to continue the examination for a prolonged period so that it can be done gently and in such a manner that the child's confidence can be gained.

As always, it is important to accomplish a complete physical examination, and I like to do this before proceeding to the abdominal examination itself. Such entities as pharyngitis, otitis media, and lower lobe pneumonia can present with abdominal pain, tenderness, and even guarding, especially in the younger child. These entities must be looked for and eliminated as possible sources of the abdominal complaint. Information about the degree of abdominal tenderness can be gained during this part of the examination by observing the child's behavior and willingness to cooperate with motion. The examination of the abdomen therefore really begins with an overall evaluation of the child, which may include the speed and gait with which the child enters the room and the ease with which he gets onto the examining table. Observation of the child's breathing, particularly for motion of the abdominal wall, is helpful. Distension or the lack thereof should be noted. Sometimes an abdominal mass is clearly

316

visible. The child should be in a supine position with the hips and knees flexed to relax the rectus muscles.

I find a warm stethoscope a useful device for palpating the abdomen before actually using my hands. Often the child will not realize that palpation is being done with the stethoscope. While listening for bowel sounds, one can apply gentle pressure on the stethoscope to allow evaluation of each area of the abdomen for tenderness and guarding while the child is distracted. A few children will be uncooperative and resist all attempts at palpating the abdomen, and information gained from the stethoscope examination may become invaluable. Others will have experienced considerable discomfort during palpation by inconsiderate previous examiners and will be set to resist manual palpation but will allow gentle pressure examination with the stethoscope. In general, the quadrants that are least likely to cause discomfort should be examined first, because demonstration of their benignity will assure that generalized peritonitis is not present.

The general attitude of the examiner should be a considerate and cooperative one. If the child is old enough for discussion, an explanation of what is being done should be offered and the child assured that any maneuver that causes pain will be stopped. Once this promise is made, it must be adhered to. Nothing is to be gained by continued pressure that causes pain to the child. It will only cause the child to resist, whereas backing off from the examination will win most children's cooperation because it makes them realize that the examiner is considerate and will not persist in a painful examination. Once the examiner has backed off from a painful spot, gentle reexamination with assurance to the child that the examination will again cease if tenderness is elicited will frequently lead to the child allowing a more thorough examination.

As with the "auscultatory palpation," palpation with the hand should progress from the areas least likely to cause discomfort to those more likely to be tender. Conversation with the older child at this point may be highly productive. Often lesions that are not representative of acute surgical emergencies, such as gastroenteritis and chronic constipation, will produce moderate tenderness at initial palpation of the abdomen; but with release of the pressure and more gentle recompression of the spot, the tenderness will abate and deeper

examination will be possible. The reason for this is that the major pain stimulus to bowel is stretch. If a loop of bowel is distended and then pressed on, this further stretch will result in pain. Release of the pressure and then more gentle reinstitution of the pressure may allow the gas to escape from the intestinal lumen and eliminate the pain caused by distention. The examiner's hand may then progress to deep palpation of the area of the abdomen without eliciting further tenderness.

It is important to be certain that complete examination of the posterior peritoneal area is possible after initially eliciting such tenderness and having it ebb. The same type of finding as described above may be noted with a retrocecal inflamed appendix in that the initial impulse is transmitted through the distended bowel to the inflamed appendix, causing tenderness. Then, with more gentle palpation and the escape of gas from the intestinal lumen, fairly deep palpation can be accomplished without further tenderness. However, examination of the posterior peritoneal area will result in actual pressure on the appendix itself and once again elicit tenderness. This finding, consistently reproducible, is a direct indication for surgery.

It is important to differentiate rigidity, involuntary guarding, and spasm from voluntary guarding. This usually can be done by careful, prolonged evaluation of the abdomen while seeking the child's cooperation. Involuntary guarding or spasm represents peritonitis, whereas voluntary guarding merely represents tenderness without reflex spasm of the abdominal muscles.

Percussion of the entire abdomen should be accomplished, and the most important finding is the presence or absence of liver dullness. The normal liver produces a dull percussion note that disappears when intestinal perforation leads to the presence of free air under the abdominal wall between the abdominal wall and the liver. Failure to seek this sign has led to missing free perforation.

Rebound tenderness has long been a mainstay of the evaluation of the acute abdomen. It is mentioned here only to be deprecated. The examining maneuvers required for the demonstration of rebound tenderness go against all the principles of dealing with children. The mainstays of dealing with the sick child are truthfulness and careful preparation for the events that are to take place. The most hurtful procedures can be accomplished in children if careful preparation, explanation, and an attitude of concern and understanding are maintained. A major part of this involves explaining carefully what is being done, why it is being done, and what the child can do to cooperate and facilitate the procedure. In this regard, thoughtful use of analgesic agents should be part of the program to relieve both the child's pain and the child's anxiety. With careful explanation and truthful preparation for hurtful procedures, the child will tolerate much and will cooperate with further evaluations appropriately.

Rebound tenderness, however, is elicited by getting the cooperative child to relax his abdominal wall and allow the examiner to palpate deeply in one or more quadrants of the abdomen. At that point, without informing the child of the next step, the examiner quickly releases the pressure on the abdominal wall, allowing it to snap back from the depressed position. Pain caused by this maneuver is considered a positive sign of peritonitis. The child, however, has been hurt without having been told that pain will occur or the reason for it. At this point, any intelligent child would object and fail to cooperate with this examiner and probably with all subsequent examiners. After all, it was the relaxation of his guard that led to his being hurt in such a manner.

What, on the other hand, has the examiner learned from duping the child in this manner? Although the textbooks have long championed positive rebound tenderness as being a sure sign of peritonitis,[6,47] the same pain would be elicited by compressing the gas out of a loop of bowel and then suddenly releasing it, allowing the gas to return to the bowel and distend it.[100] When the bowel is inflamed by gastroenteritis, such a stretch will evoke severe pain, which may erroneously lead the examiner to conclude that peritonitis is present. Thus, the demonstration of rebound tenderness is almost guaranteed to lose the child's cooperation and may confuse the examiner. Seeking rebound tenderness when abdominal spasm or involuntary guarding has already suggested the presence of peritonitis is sadistic, and the finding of "positive" rebound tenderness when previous examination failed to demonstrate signs of peritonitis is contradictory. The same information can be better elicited by asking the child to elevate his buttocks off the bed and allow his body to drop back onto the bed or table. This jolt may demonstrate the same kind of tenderness that rebound

elicits, but it is now under the child's control and he can refuse to do it again if it caused undue pain. At the same time, it is not involved with palpation of the abdomen, so that he has no reason to object to subsequent evaluations.

Finally, rectal examination is an important part of the examination of the abdomen, but not for the reasons that most physicians might think. Most children are tender on rectal examination, and in the smaller child palpation to the right will almost always cause more tenderness than palpation to the left because the sigmoid curves to the left. Pushing the examining finger to the right distends the wall of the sigmoid, again eliciting pain from the stretch reflex. The important parts of the rectal examination are, therefore, palpation for the presence of masses, fullness, or fluctuant swelling and a careful bimanual examination performed with one hand on the abdomen and the examining finger in the rectum. Thus, I find it most useful to examine the rectum with the child remaining in the supine position with the knees and hips flexed as in the routine abdominal examination. The knees are allowed to fall laterally, and the well-lubricated finger is carefully and gently passed into the rectum. After the pelvis is examined with this finger, the physician's other hand is placed on the abdomen and gentle pressure again maintained until the child relaxes. An attempt is then made to bring the two hands together.

Again, release of pressure when the child objects will often gain further cooperation and allow a more thorough subsequent examination. In the female child, these maneuvers will allow careful evaluation for abnormalities of the ovary and tube. Torsion of the ovary, a ruptured cyst, salpingitis, and ovarian tumors may all present with signs of an acute abdomen.

There are literally hundreds of maneuvers that have been described to confirm the presence of an inflamed appendix, none of which are consistently useful. By far, the gentle, thorough evaluation of the abdomen with a palpating hand, with careful attention given to the signs that are elicited, is the most important factor in the diagnosis. No child should be released from the physician's care until a complete examination of all areas of the abdomen with deep palpation of the posterior peritoneal structures convinces the physician that there are no consistently tender areas. Until this can be accomplished, the child should be reevaluated at frequent intervals. Depending on the family's situation, the location of the home, and the physician's degree of concern after his initial evaluation, this reevaluation may involve return trips to the office, admission to an observation unit, or actual admission to a hospital. Failure to diagnose appendicitis resulting in rupture and generalized peritonitis, is not caused as often by failure to make the diagnosis at the initial evaluation as by failure of the primary care physician to provide continued follow-up until all signs of abdominal illness have abated. Too often, the physician settles on a diagnosis such as gastroenteritis and releases the child from follow-up. It is this release and the assurance given to the parents that lead to delay in reevaluation and allow a period of progression of the acute abdominal process to a more serious state.

Evaluation, referral, and recommendations for treatment. We must now discuss the range of findings in the acute abdomen and try to give some indication of when referral and surgery should be accomplished. The two extremes present little difficulty. In the child with a rigid abdomen with diffuse tenderness usually accompanied by fever, collapse, and an elevated leukocyte count, the diagnosis is easy to make. At the other extreme, the case of the child who complains of abdominal pain that is often crampy in nature, who is otherwise active and healthy, and whose abdominal examination reveals no areas of persistent tenderness in a soft, easily examined abdomen likewise causes little confusion. Between these two extremes, however, a wide range of presentations is possible. The most important concept for the primary care physician to grasp is that it is not his duty to make the diagnosis of a specific acute abdominal emergency, such as appendicitis. His only concern is to confirm the presence of some degree of intra-abdominal disease. Once this is done, referral to a surgeon who will give careful evaluation and consideration to the problem should be accomplished. The sign that the primary care physician should seek is involuntary guarding representing actual peritonitis in any of the abdominal quadrants. In addition, the consistent demonstration of tenderness in a discrete area that is not relieved by easing the pressure and approaching it more gently should also lead to surgical consultation.

Certain entities may lead to confusion. Although some authorities have said that constipation does not present with abdominal symptoms, there are certainly children who present with severe abdominal pain, fever, and elevated white blood cell counts whose total symptom complex is relieved by enema evacuation of a constipated stool. Whether these children, in addition to their chronic constipation, have some low-grade enterocolitis on either an infectious or allergic basis is not known. Perhaps these children are suffering from a minor allergic enteritis or short-term viral or bacterial gastroenteritis that without the constipation would lead to a few loose stools and some abdominal cramps. In the presence of the constipation, they develop a distended inflamed tender bowel that may mimic all the signs of peritonitis. Thus, I find it helpful to evaluate the child for the presence of constipation and to provide enema relief of this entity. If the abdominal findings are improved after the enema, further observation is warranted but referral may not be needed. Once again, however, the consistent demonstration of point tenderness should lead to referral even though frank peritoneal signs such as involuntary guarding are not present.

The idea of an enema in the face of an acute abdomen may cause concern among many physicians. Laxatives and enemas have often been blamed in the past for causing rupture of the inflamed appendix. Realization, however, that appendicitis is an obstructive disease, usually caused by inspissation of a fecalith or hypertrophy of lymphoid tissue in the appendix, should suggest that simple enema evacuation of the constipated stool will not result in explosive rupture of the appendix. The fact that in the past many children had a ruptured appendix after having received enemas and laxatives is related to the time lost in proper evaluation and treatment because the physician, often over the telephone, suggested to the parent that the cause of the child's abdominal symptoms was constipation. The parent would then give a laxative or enema, and hours or days of delay would elapse before medical attention was again sought. The resultant rupture of the appendix was the result not of the laxative or enema but of the delay that allowed the inflammatory process to progress.

Once the child is referred to the surgeon, this physician's goals should again be to evaluate the child's abdomen for signs of peritonitis or the consistent demonstration of localized tenderness. Once again, the surgeon should avoid attempts to pin down a secure diagnosis but need only be convinced that the required signs are present. Once these are demonstrated, surgery should be accomplished expeditiously with delay only for proper hydration and institution of antibiotic therapy when indicated.

Some thought as to the time course of the disease is also helpful in making decisions. The child brought in for treatment shortly after the onset of symptoms who has persistent point tenderness without peritoneal signs is a candidate for surgery to resect an early stage of appendicitis before the complications of gangrene and rupture ensue. On the other hand, the child whose similar symptoms are of several day's duration can well be watched with such limited findings for a period of time to assure that the findings are persistent. The child with an acute onset of what appears to be generalized peritonitis should be operated on urgently, because some intra-abdominal catastrophe has probably occurred. On the other hand, the child brought in for treatment after several days of illness who is in a state of collapse with generalized peritonitis would probably benefit from a period of rehydration, antibiotic therapy, improvement of his cardiovascular status, and reevaluation of the process. Prolonged delay is not warranted, but the child will do better if his hypovolemia and septic state are under control before he undergoes anesthesia and surgery. This delay also allows a short period of time for further evaluation and confirmation of the presence of the peritoneal signs and the elimination of any possible confusion from coincident diseases such as pneumonia or otitis media.

Finally, some mention should be made of laboratory and x-ray evaluations. The absolute value of the white blood cell count is of little help in decision making. Lymphocytosis in a child whose abdominal evaluation is equivocal and who is known to be capable of generating a neutrophil response would cause me to pause in considering surgery. A high white blood cell count with a marked shift to the left is possible in a child after a few episodes of vomiting; and if the abdominal findings are not consistent with a peritoneal process, reevaluation of the white blood cell count after adequate hydration may show a normalization of the total count as well as of the shift. Persistence of a high white blood cell count after such rehydration where the abdominal findings remained suggestive but equivocal would push me toward exploration.

Radiographic evaluation is important for what it rules out. A chest x-ray examination is important when the abdominal findings are not clear-cut to rule out lower lobe pneumonia presenting with abdominal pain and tenderness. Identification of a fecalith on plain radiographs is infrequent enough in my experience that it is generally not helpful (Fig. 20-1). When one is found, however, appendicitis is highly likely to be present.[23] When surgery is not clearly indicated by the abdominal findings, radiographic evaluation of the abdomen should be accomplished to look for signs of mechanical obstruction of the bowel as well as the presence of free air. Fluid levels are common in gastroenteritis in children, so that these are not necessarily indicative of an obstructive process if bowel gas through the large intestine can be demonstrated. Recent enthusiasm for the routine use of barium enema examination in the diagnosis of appendicitis is probably excessive.[69] In the equivocal or confusing case, particularly if other reasons for abdominal symptoms are present, such as the coincidental presence of pneumonia or otitis media, barium examination may be helpful. Careful evaluation of the cecum for evidence of intrinsic compression or inflammation is the crux of the examination—not just the filling or failure of filling of the appendix itself.

Appendicitis

Since Duke University Medical Center is a major regional referral center for children's problems, we see a great many complicated problems there following appendicitis and appendectomy. Many of these could be prevented by intelligent management of the child with appendicitis. Although the primary care physician cannot direct the surgical management intraoperatively, he is often deeply involved in postoperative management considerations; and it is in this capacity that he can make considerable contributions to a successful outcome for the child.

The child with early acute or even early ruptured appendicitis usually has little in the way of complications. The surgical procedure is straightforward, the soilage of the peritoneal cavity is minimal, and appendectomy is usually curative. Although drainage is often cited as being an essential part of management for the child with a gangrenous or early ruptured appendix, when there is no necrotic tissue or frankly purulent material left behind, drainage of the peritoneal cavity is not essential. On the other hand, drainage is es-

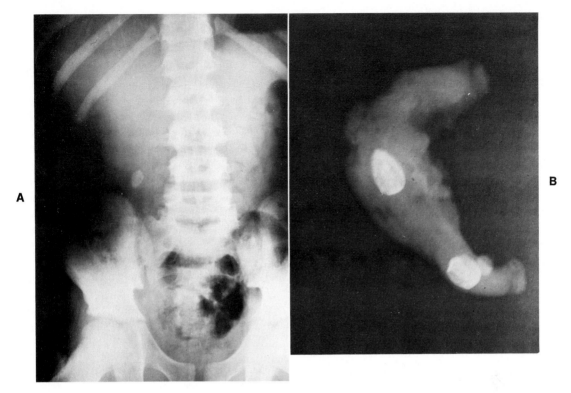

Fig. 20-1. A, A fecalith is clearly identifiable on this abdominal radiograph just above the medial aspect of the right iliac crest. **B,** A second fecalith is seen in the radiograph of the specimen.

sential when abscess formation has occurred, when there is necrotic or edematous material left behind or severely damaged periappendiceal tissue remains, or when the perforated appendix has resulted in extensive generalized peritonitis with purulent collections in other areas, such as the pelvis or the suprahepatic, infrahepatic, or infradiaphragmatic areas. Drainage will not help in generalized peritonitis; when extensive purulent exudate is present in the general peritoneal cavity, however, the surgeon would be wise to explore the subdiaphragmatic and subhepatic spaces and drain these appropriately if purulent collections have already formed. When such drainage is indicated, we prefer a sump-type drain with suction and institute short periods of postoperative irrigation to ensure that the drains are functioning adequately.

Antibiotic coverage for the patient with a suspected or confirmed ruptured appendix is essential, and we generally prescribe a preoperative broad-spectrum coverage that includes ampicillin, gentamycin, and often clindamycin. Although anaerobic flora is common in the gastrointestinal tract, anaerobic infections are unlikely unless necrotic tissue or abscess formation is present. The choice of preoperative antibiotics should depend on the surgeon's estimate of the extent of the disease and the length of time it has been present. The one clearly demonstrated fact about antibiotic coverage is that it is most successful when the antibiotics are begun preoperatively and a definite level of antibiotics is present in the tissues before surgical manipulation is attempted.[126] We are therefore liberal in beginning antibiotics with our patients but are just as quick to discontinue them if we see no indication for their use postoperatively. If the appendix is neither gangrenous nor ruptured, a simple appendectomy suffices; and if antibiotics were begun preoperatively, additional doses are withheld.

One of the biggest failings in postoperative management for gangrenous or perforated appendicitis, particularly for the child with established peritonitis, either local or generalized, is the failure to continue antibiotics for a long-enough time. They should be given for at least 10 days to 2 weeks. Too often, if the child remains febrile with an elevation of the white blood cell count after 48 to 72 hours of receiving antibiotics, the antibiotics are changed. Changes in the antibiotic regimen should be dictated by culture results that show a need to change the regimen on the basis of antibiotic sensitivity. Cultures obtained should be planted anaerobically so that anerobic organisms can be identified. It is not unusual for the fever and elevated white blood cell count to persist for several days after rupture of the appendix and peritonitis, and the antibiotic program should be maintained.

The other failure after surgery for ruptured appendicitis is too early removal of drains. This, combined with failure of the simple Penrose drain to clear collections of necrotic debris or abscess cavities adequately, leads to reaccumulation of purulent material and persistence of abscesses. It is for this reason that we prefer to irrigate our drains and use a suction type of sump catheter that will enable us to clear the necrotic debris better.

Finally, late complications after appendicitis are the formation of abscesses in the subhepatic and subphrenic spaces and the development of adhesive bowel obstruction. The latter may present within a few days following surgery for appendicitis. The perforated appendix with its marked inflammation, especially when generalized peritonitis is present, may lead to extensive adhesive bowel obstruction. Such a development should be thought of and watched for in the postoperative period, for missing it may lead to strangulation obstruction and the loss of considerable segments of bowel, resulting in the complications of postoperative anastomotic breakdown and fistula formation.

When fever and leukocytosis continue unabated after several days of antibiotic therapy following surgery for perforated appendicitis, subphrenic and subhepatic abscesses should be looked for. When the appendicitis has been missed for several days before surgery, these lesions may present sooner after the surgical procedure than is usually anticipated. Ultrasonography may be helpful in defining these lesions and computerized tomography has also been useful.

Although recently some surgeons have preferred to treat subphrenic and subhepatic collections in adults for several days with the expectation of allowing the abscess wall to "firm up" and make extraperitoneal drainage possible, such expectant treatment is contraindicated in children because the abscess may be poorly contained and may re-

rupture into an adjacent cavity.[31,90] We have seen two cases of children in whom the subphrenic abscess eroded through the diaphragm. One presented as an empyema; the other eroded into a bronchus and flooded the lung with purulent drainage from the abscess cavity, resulting in overwhelming purulent pneumonia and death. Thus, a fairly aggressive approach to the problem of abscess formation following ruptured appendicitis in the child is warranted and reexploration of any suspected areas should be undertaken early. Pelvic abscesses may spontaneously drain transrectally or may be drained by the surgeon transrectally, and pelvic abscesses in the female child may be drainable through the vaginal vault. Regardless of the route, thorough evacuation of purulent material followed by sump drainage is mandatory.

With proper use of antibiotics (particularly when they are begun before surgery), with the intelligent use of drains and their maintenance for adequate periods following surgery, and with an aggressive approach to possible secondary purulent collections, severe morbidity and mortality following rupture of the appendix can be reduced. Ultimately, the goals should be better education of parents so that children are brought to the primary care physician for treatment earlier in the course of an abdominal illness and more astute diagnosis on the part of the primary care physician so that more cases of appendicitis can be diagnosed and treated early, before gangrene and rupture supervene.

Pancreatitis

Although it is not a common lesion in childhood, pancreatitis does occur, and its diagnosis is highly dependent on the physician considering it and obtaining the necessary laboratory investigation that will confirm its presence.

Etiology. Pancreatitis may be caused by one of several etiological factors and includes a familial relapsing form as well as a similar but nonfamilial chronic relapsing form.[16,26,30,143] These entities are not clearly understood. Pancreatitis may also be due to metabolic abnormalities, including lipoidosis. It may accompany or follow such viral illnesses as mumps or coxsackie viral infections, and it may be due to congenital abnormalities of the biliary tree or pancreatic duct system. Duplications of the duodenum buried in the head of the pancreas may obstruct the pancreatic duct.[46,144] Trauma is perhaps the most common cause of pancreatitis in the child and is certainly the most common etiological factor for the complications of pancreatitis, which include the formation of a pancreatic pseudocyst and pancreatic ascites.*

Clinical presentation. Pancreatitis usually presents with severe abdominal pain, which may or may not radiate through to the back. It is usually associated with some fever and elevation of the white blood cell count. Nausea and vomiting may be present. The pain is usually epigastric; in severe pancreatitis, however, the abdominal findings may be most striking. It is probably only in severe pancreatitis that a true rigid or boardlike abdomen exists. Severe pancreatitis may result in marked blood loss, hypocalcemia, and marked internal fluid shifts with vascular volume depletion and collapse. Such extreme presentations are, fortunately, unusual in children.

Evaluation. The demonstration of an elevated amylase level, either in the serum or in the urine, is essential to the diagnosis of pancreatitis. Both investigations should be undertaken early. A urinary collection is especially important; if the pancreatitis resolves, the serum amylase may fall back toward normal levels very quickly and the diagnosis may be confirmable only by the persistent elevation of urinary amylase.

Pancreatic ascites and pseudocysts. Pancreatic ascites or the formation of a pancreatic pseudocyst may follow known trauma to the pancreas or may develop insidiously after seemingly mild epigastric trauma in which initial pancreatitis was not apparent.[22] Such a pseudocyst may present as a painless, enlarging epigastric mass, and pancreatic ascites may present silently with the formation of ascites. The serum amylase may be elevated in the patient with pancreatic ascites not because of persistent pancreatitis but because of resorption of amylase from the ascitic fluid. The serum amylase may not be very elevated and may, in fact, be within normal limits. The ability of the kidneys to clear amylase from the serum may hide the elevation in serum aymlase, but the urinary amylase will usually be elevated. Paracentesis usually reveals bloody ascites, although hemorrhage into the ascitic fluid is not always present. The diagnosis of pancreatic ascites is based on the finding of an elevated amylase level in the ascitic fluid combined with an elevation of the

ascitic fluid albumin that approaches the serum level.[33]

A pancreatic pseudocyst may be identified by noting the anterior displacement of the stomach on a lateral view of an upper GI series or may be clearly delineated by ultrasonography.

Medical versus surgical treatment. Most pancreatitis will be resolved with medical therapy, which usually involves supportive therapy with intravenous fluids, bowel rest with or without nasogastric tube decompression, and perhaps the use of antibiotics. There seems to be no convincing evidence that antibiotics aid in the treatment of pancreatitis,[78] but many authors recommend their use.[16,49] Peritoneal lavage has also been advocated.[16,107] When the amylase level fails to return to normal under these circumstances, a complication such as an evolving pseudocyst or pancreatic ascites should be suspected and looked for. There is little role for surgery in the treatment of acute pancreatitis. In fact, if a surgeon inadvertently explores an abdomen for peritonitis and finds acute pancreatitis, he should probably back out gracefully with as little trauma to the pancreas as possible.

Surgical options. For the child with recurrent pancreatitis, further investigation of the integrity of the pancreatic duct system is warranted and may be accomplished either by operative pancreatography during a quiescent phase of the disease or by endoscopic retrograde cholangiopancreatography.[58] We have been able to accomplish visualization of the pancreatic duct in a child as young as 5 years of age, and this study should be obtained when recurrent or relapsing pancreatitis is diagnosed.[46,138] If duct obstruction is identified, some diverting procedure is probably warranted.

For the child with pancreatic ascites, the endoscopic investigation should be carried out as soon as the child is stabilized; and if an obstructive lesion of the duct or a traumatic leakage from the duct is identified, some pancreatic duct-intestinal diversion should be performed. A pancreatic pseudocyst can be drained into the stomach by performing a transgastric pseudocyst-gastrostomy; or if that is not feasible, a Roux-en-Y intestinal drainage limb can be constructed.[22] Another option is external drainage, but many authors believe that it leads to persistence or recurrence of the pseudocyst and fails to cure the problem in a significant number of cases.[138]

Prognosis. For the child with pancreatic ascites

---

*See references 17, 22, 25, 97, and 115.

or a pseudocyst following trauma or duct obstruction, successful surgical drainage should lead to cure. Long-term problems of adhesive bowel obstruction are at least as common in these children as in other children undergoing abdominal exploration. For the child with chronic recurrent pancreatitis, the disease may ultimately produce the ravages of the pancreas that are common to the alcoholic pancreatitis of the adult.

Other abdominal emergencies

Many of the lesions discussed in Chapter 15 in the section on the infant and toddler may not present until the child is beyond the age of 2 years. These include such lesions as malrotation with volvulus and strangulation of the mesentery, intussusception, and the various complications of Meckel's diverticulum. In addition, such congenital lesions as stenoses, duplications, and mesenteric cysts may remain silent until later childhood. These lesions are discussed in detail in Chapter 10 in the section on the newborn and in Chapter 15, and the reader is referred to these chapters for in-depth discussion. A few comments about the variations and presentation of these lesions in the older child are warranted.

Malrotation may present in the older child as an acute abdominal emergency with duodenal obstruction, bilious vomiting, abdominal pain, rapid collapse, and strangulation of the mesentery with or without bloody stools. This presentation is more likely in the early childhood years and becomes less likely as the child ages. In fact, as the child reaches late childhood and the early teenage years, malrotation is more likely to present as recurrent abdominal pain, especially postprandial pain. Often the older child with malrotation will have chronic recurrent symptoms that lead to psychologic or psychiatric evaluation. Any child presenting with recurrent abdominal pain of a crampy nature, particularly if it is postprandial, merits an upper GI series looking for malrotation as the cause before the child is forced to undergo an extensive psychologic evaluation for psychosomatic illness.

Until recently it was thought that *intussusception* presenting in the later years of childhood was more likely to be caused by a defined anatomic leading point other than a Peyer's patch. Some authorities considered this difference to be so prevalent that they did not think hydrostatic barium reduction was indicated in the older child. A re-

cent study by Toronto's Hospital for Sick Children indicates that although leading points are more common in the older child, it is unlikely that an anatomic leading point can be reduced by hydrostatic enema, at least not permanently[37,38]; thus, it is reasonable to utilize this diagnostic and therapeutic modality in all children with intussusception uncomplicated by peritonitis or free perforation.[114] Nevertheless, it may be expected that few of these children will be completely relieved of their intussusception, and more explorations will be needed to discover the anatomic leading points in the older child. Leading points should be suspected particularly when the intussusception is higher in the small bowel rather than in the usual ileocolic location. In fact, exploration is warranted for any intussusception presenting in the proximal small intestine.

The presentation of *Meckel's diverticulum* and its complications in the older child is similar to that in the younger age groups, and the discussions of this entity in Chapters 10 and 15 should be reviewed in dealing with this lesion in the older child.

CONSTIPATION

Although many children have occasional problems with constipation, when this symptom becomes persistent or recurrent, a thorough evaluation is warranted. Without such an examination, many children will go on to have complex problems stemming from the constipation, including difficulties in toilet training, intermittent or constant soiling or actual encopresis, perianal and rectal inflammatory lesions, recurrent bouts of abdominal pain, and eventually severe problems in emotional and social adjustment. Constipation is not diagnosed solely by the failure to have a bowel movement daily. In fact, many children who have daily bowel movements are severely constipated. The frequency of bowel movements, the amount of waste passed, the amount retained in the rectum and distal colon, the dryness and hardness of the bowel movement, and the amount of stool normally carried in the rectal ampulla must all be evaluated.

To understand constipation, one must understand the normal physiology of gastrointestinal tract functioning. Although much water is removed from the intestinal content in the distal ileum, a great deal of additional water is removed in the colon, as noted by the difference in liquidity of ileostomy drainage and distal colostomy or anal output. To a considerable extent, the longer a stool remains in the colon, the drier it becomes. The newborn infant and the undomesticated animal respond to the ingestion of food and the presence of food in the stomach by an urge to evacuate; this gastrocolic reflex can be seen in the infant, who most often has a stool following each nursing period. Although there may be some natural adaptation in that the presence of a small amount of food fails to elicit a major evacuation in the later infancy years, the major change in functioning comes with the advent of toileting. The use of the gastrocolic reflex as an aid to toilet training has not been a widespread practice in American pediatric care. Consequently, the toilet training program is generally an unscientific and highly individualized one, usually left to the parents, with minimal guidance from the pediatrician or family practitioner. The usual approach is to take advantage of the child's willingness to please the parent. Under a system of reward and punishment, the child is urged to perform his evacuations in the appropriate receptacle.

However, this period in the child's development is also one during which the child is becoming more independent and wandering farther afield. He therefore is often presented with the choice of giving up an enjoyable activity or soiling. Since the child cannot conceptualize time and space relationships at this age, he cannot conceive that he can leave an enjoyable play activity for a few minutes to evacuate his bowels and then find the activity available to him when he returns. He is therefore faced with a marked conflict and must choose between soiling his pants, with its attendant parental disapproval, and giving up the enjoyable activity. Soon a solution to the conflict appears: the child learns to constrict his anal sphincter voluntarily and suppress the gastrocolic reflex. As he does this, his rectal ampulla, which should be a temporary storage area and conduit for the stool, becomes stretched and accommodates to increased amounts of stool, so that it acts more like a bladder. With this stretching comes a lessening of the urge to defecate and suppression of the gastrocolic reflex. Once this adaptation is accomplished, the child's gastrocolic reflex may become almost nonexistent. Most children tolerate this situation reasonably well and succeed in evacuating an adequate amount of stool each day at some convenient time, such as at bedtime.

At that time, with the child relaxed and no longer distracted by the multiple daily activities, his sense of fullness leads him to evacuate his distal bowel. Although, as mentioned above, most individuals can tolerate this situation and have no complications from it, it occasionally is the start of numerous and varied problems related to the retention of stool. It is when the problem becomes symptomatic that attention must be paid to it, and the solution often involves changing the stooling pattern.

History. The history of the constipation problem may vary from that of the child who occasionally has crampy abdominal pain and difficulty in passing stool to the child who has had a lifelong problem with irregular bowel movement schedules, hard stools, chronic soilage, and even failure to thrive. When soiling is a major component of the problem, marked emotional problems may either have existed previously in the family or are certainly likely to develop with persistence of the soiling problem. Such problems may include conflicts between the parents as to their views on child rearing and discipline and severe emotional problems between the child and his parents and the child and his peers.

The most important aspect of the history in evaluating a constipation problem is to ascertain the age at which the problem first developed. As noted in Chapter 15, constipation problems developing in the early weeks or months of life are highly likely to represent aganglionic megacolon (Hirschsprung's disease). On the other hand, children who do not develop problems until after the first year of life are equally likely to have a basic constipation problem unrelated to anatomic or physiologic malfunction of the gastrointestinal tract. The confidence factor for such a historical factor is well over 90%, but it must be remembered that approximately 1 in 20 children with an unusual history will turn out to have Hirschsprung's disease even though they apparently had no problems with constipation in the early months of life. Generally, children with constipation problems developing after the first year of life can initially be considered as having primary constipation rather than Hirschsprung's disease, with the more thorough workup for Hirschsprung's disease reserved for the child who fails to respond to the constipation program.

Other factors in the history include soiling, which is unusual in Hirschsprung's disease except for the liquid overflow soiling that may occur during periods of enterocolitis. The ability to pass a large, bulky stool is most unusual in Hirschsprung's disease. It is not uncommon, on the other hand, for many children with chronic constipation to go several days without a movement and then pass a stool so large that it stops up the plumbing. Such histories are almost unheard of in Hirschsprung's disease.

Evaluation. Physical examination of a constipated child will frequently reveal palpable stool in the sigmoid colon, which may range from a bowel of relatively normal caliber containing firm though still liquid contents to a massive enlargement of the rectosigmoid arising out of the pelvis and filled with rock-hard stool. The bowel may be slightly tender to firm palpation. The older child with longstanding chronic constipation may be of short stature and, except for his protuberant abdomen, be very thin. If a low grade of colitis has existed, the child may also exhibit chronic anemia.

Staining of or frank stool in the underwear is the first notable finding on the anorectal examination. The most frequent finding is that of a smear of moderately firm stool in the underwear, caused by the presence of stool in the overdistended rectal ampulla, which protrudes from the patulous anus when the child is engaged in normal activities. The child does not actually pass a bowel movement into his underpants but simply soils his pants as they rub against his anus. The hallmark of chronic constipation is the presence of stool in the anal canal and rectal ampulla. The absence of stools from these areas in a constipated child whose anorectum has not been recently cleaned out is highly suggestive of Hirschsprung's disease. Further examination may reveal that the child has a large impacted mass of stool in an extremely overdistended rectum and rectosigmoid.

As noted above, if the history suggests that the constipation problem developed after the first year of life, and if the physical examination confirms stool in the rectum, with or without soiling, a further evaluation for Hirschsprung's disease generally need not be pursued at this time. If the possibility of anemia exists, it should be evaluated with a complete blood count, of course, and further workup to identify the source of the anemia. Guaiac testing should confirm any suspected blood in the stool. Plain films of the abdomen may be helpful in confirming the level to which the stool is backed up in the colon.

If the history and physical evidence point to constipation rather than Hirschsprung's disease, a barium enema is not needed and the child should be given a program to overcome his constipation. The most important part of this program is strong support to the parents, providing enough information that they understand the various aspects of the problem and will have the patience to deal with it as a long-term one with a long-term solution. Many parents seek a one-shot solution to a problem that may have been chronic for many years. Careful discussion of all aspects of the problem is the first step in appropriate therapy. Furthermore, the parents need to feel supported by the physician and to know that he recognizes the problem as a serious one. Too often, the primary care physician, in seeing a myriad of youngsters with constipation problems, fails to identify the child whose constipation problem is a serious one. Once it becomes chronic and openly symptomatic, he may tend to refer the child to a surgeon for evaluation for Hirschsprung's disease. Unless the surgeon has a particular interest in constipation problems, which is unusual, after an extensive radiographic evaluation is accomplished, eliminating Hirschsprung's disease as the diagnosis, the constipation is ignored and the parents are left once again unsatisfied and unsupported.

Treatment. Any program designed to deal with the chronically constipated child must begin by thoroughly cleaning out and decompressing his overstretched lower intestine. No program will be successful as long as the child's lower intestine is impacted or his rectal ampulla is continuously overdistended. Occasionally, the child must actually be admitted to the hospital, anesthetized, and his lower intestine disimpacted manually in the operating room. If this procedure is necessary, it should be done. Some children can undergo manual disimpaction while they are awake. Disimpaction is followed by repeated oil retention enemas and saline enemas. Subsequently laxatives are used until the stool is finally cleared from the rectum, rectosigmoid, and even descending and transverse colons if required.

Once clearing of the stool is accomplished, it is essential to keep the bowel decompressed for a period of time to allow it to regain tone and a more normal caliber. Daily enemas and laxatives may be required for days or weeks at a time. The physician should follow the child during this period and judiciously utilize plain abdominal x-ray films to evaluate the progress.

There are several aspects to the attack on a constipation problem after disimpaction and resolution of the overdistention have been achieved. We try to use a multimodal attack that involves necessary changes in the diet, the use of stool softeners, a primary reliance on retraining toward postprandial defecation, and the judicious use of laxatives and enemas as an aid in the early management of the problem. This program has been highly successful over a period of about 9 years. It requires a commitment on the part of the physician to long-term follow-up with the family and the realization that habit patterns and physiologic dysfunctions that have developed over years in the child's life will not be cured in the short time span that both the physician and the parents would prefer.

Our program, outlined below, is discussed in detail with the parents at the first visit. Frequent reinforcement of the fact that the problem developed over a long time and will take a definite time to resolve itself is essential. We usually ask the parents to bring the child back frequently to assure that the bowel is decompressed and kept empty if overstretching has been a major problem. Once the bowel is empty and regaining tone, we ask the parents to follow the program religiously for a month or two and then report back to us on a definite date concerning the results of the efforts. It will often take more than one visit and discussion with the family to get them started on the program. However, once parents are committed to it, the vast majority find definite success in retraining the child and improving bowel habits. Few require use of the laxative and enema routine beyond the first time or two. The continued use of stool softeners over a considerable period of time is required, however, until the child develops improved bowel habits on his own.

Although our intention is to do a workup for Hirschsprung's disease on any child who fails to respond to this program after a month or two of

---

PROGRAM OF BOWEL RETRAINING FOR _____

Discipline

After each meal child is to sit on commode for 15 minutes. No toys, books, or other diversions. Do not comment on failure to stool, but praise success. Discipline as needed to enforce cooperation with sitting, but no discipline for failure to stool.

Diet

Decrease milk to 16 ounces a day. Increase all other liquids, especially juices. Add roughage—salad, green vegetables.

Mineral oil

Start with 1 tablespoon of mineral oil daily. Increase or decrease a teaspoon at a time to achieve soft, greasy stool without free oil running out. Do not give within 2 hours of nap or bedtime.

Laxative/enema routine

1. Allow _____ free days (1 to 3 days)
2. _____ day _____ ounces milk of magnesia (1/3 to 1 ounce)
3. _____ day _____ ounces milk of magnesia (1½ to 2 ounces)
4. _____ day _____ ounces milk of magnesia (same as step 3) plus ½ to 1 teaspoon cascara liquid
5. _____ day adult Fleet's enema (fifth to seventh day)

Then begin again. Any day child moves bowels go back to beginning. Even if he has a good movement in his pants this counts.

Remember that the most important factor is to remove the emotional upset surrounding the problem and retrain the child's habit pattern. Most children have achieved some negative gain from the turmoil.

This retraining program may take several months to achieve success. Be patient. It has taken years to develop the problem.

Please report monthly on progress.

dedicated effort, we have found that very few children require barium enemas and none required a rectal biopsy when the decision that the child has chronic constipation is based on the combination of historical and physical findings described on pp. 325-326. Unfortunately, we temporarily missed a case of Hirschsprung's disease when the initial barium enema failed to confirm a highly suggestive history and physical examination. If little progress has been made after 4 or 5 months of effort, a workup for Hirschsprung's disease is indicated.

Important aspects of follow-up. In following these children, frequent discussion of the entire problem with the parents may be necessary. The parents are often looking for easy solutions, and a pattern of physician shopping is not unusual among them. An acceptance on the part of the physician of the chronicity and difficulty of the problem will often be supportive to the parents and help in gaining their cooperation to follow through with the program. It is essential that the stool be kept soft, even if that requires the chronic use of mineral oil for a protracted period. Many primary care physicians object to the use of mineral oil, in infants particularly, because of the risks of aspiration and lipoid pneumonia. These risks can generally be avoided by giving the mineral oil just after the child arises, so that considerable hours pass before the child's next sleep time. The unpalatability of mineral oil has usually not been a major problem. For the child who objects strenuously, it can be flavored with chocolate or hidden in an appropriate juice.

Occasionally, constipation problems lead to such severe emotional problems in the older child that psychologic or psychiatric consultation will be mandatory. Some children become so unacceptable to themselves and their peers that years of psychotherapy may be needed. The primary care physician who deals thoroughly with the constipation problems in his infant population will do a great service in preventing the serious maladjustments that may later arise in a child whose chronic constipation has led to soiling and encopresis in older childhood.

Constipation related to perianal lesions

Occasionally but very infrequently, constipation will be found to be related to an anatomic lesion at the anus. This may involve a stenotic anus that will not distend elastically in a normal fashion or a form of imperforate anus with a perineal fistula that may not have been recognized previously as being an anatomic anomaly. Among the vast number of patients with constipation problems, however, these findings will be most unusual. Particularly in the infant, however, local trauma to the anus may be a significant factor in the development of constipation. Either a hard, constipated stool or an episode of diarrhea may produce an anal canal irritation or actual fissure, which may cause sphincter spasm and painful movements and lead the infant to withhold bowel movements. Often, the chronic constipation dates back to such an episode. The anal lesion may persist and years later still be the source of constipation problems for the child, or it may resolve but leave the child with an established habit of constipation.

When the local problem persists, effective stool softening should be the prime component of treatment. Local care to the lesion with sitz baths and topical ointments may also be effective. A deep fissure may require surgical excision, but it must be remembered that following such a procedure the local care, sitz baths, and stool softening will still be required. Often with stool softening, the repeated trauma is eliminated and the lesion will heal. The bowel retraining program described on p. 327 should then be used to deal with the secondary constipation problem.

RECTAL PROLAPSE

Rectal prolapse is an unusual occurrence in childhood despite the significant incidence of constipation problems in this age group. I have seen rectal prolapse occur in a normal anus in only two situations: in the child with myelodysplasia who has deficient or absent innervation to the anorectum and in the child with cystic fibrosis. Obviously, the child with an imperforate anus, particularly the child who has required a major pull-through procedure for reconstruction, may commonly have rectal prolapse as a complication of anal surgery.

When an otherwise healthy child presents with rectal prolapse, cystic fibrosis should be the major consideration. Careful history taking will often elicit the fact that the child has bulky, foul-smelling, greasy, and sometimes strange-colored stools, often a brick red. The parents may complain more of the foul-smelling stool than of the prolapse itself.

Prolapse must be differentiated from a prolapsing or intussuscepting polyp, but such differentiation is usually readily done by careful inspection and palpation.

Evaluation. Since the diagnosis can usually be made by inspection and palpation, no extensive radiologic evaluation is necessary. However, the diagnosis of cystic fibrosis should be pursued with appropriate sweat tests, chest x-rays films, and stool evaluation for trypsin. On the other hand, if the child lacks normal anal sphincter tone and voluntary control, appropriate radiographs seeking spinal dysraphia should be obtained. If evidence of myelodysplasia is confirmed, further evaluation of the urogenital system is warranted.

Medical versus surgical treatment. When the prolapse is due to cystic fibrosis, the institution of a regimen for supplementing pancreatic enzymes will often relieve the prolapse. Surgery is rarely necessary. However, if the prolapse persists, a decision between a local mucosal excision and a more extensive rectal suspension procedure must be made. Certainly, conservative medical therapy is indicated initially. Rarely is stool softening necessary in these patients. The child with myelodysplasia is more likely to require extensive surgical correction of the prolapse, and long-term success may be difficult to achieve.

For the child with cystic fibrosis, the other manifestations and complications of the disease far outweigh the rectal prolapse in their impact on the child's life and survival. The importance of prolapse in this disease is its frequent initial indication of the presence of the underlying systemic illness.

MASSES

Since almost every major tumor that arises in the childhood age group presents as a painless mass, the physical examination, particularly of the abdomen, takes on considerable importance. Cancer is the second leading cause of death in childhood after trauma.[128] The primary care physician must not disregard mass lesions. The high curability rates for many childhood tumors found in early stages makes such early diagnosis mandatory. Some tumors are easily palpable; others are noted merely because of the child's protuberant abdomen or a feeling of fullness (Fig. 20-2). Such signs should not be ignored but thoroughly investigated. If the physician, on one or two examinations in a short period of time, cannot assure himself that no mass lesion is present, a more extensive evaluation including radiologic investigation should be initiated. Examination with the child under sedation or anesthesia may be warranted in an equivocal case.

The major tumors are those that arise in the abdomen, the brain, and the extremities. Tumors

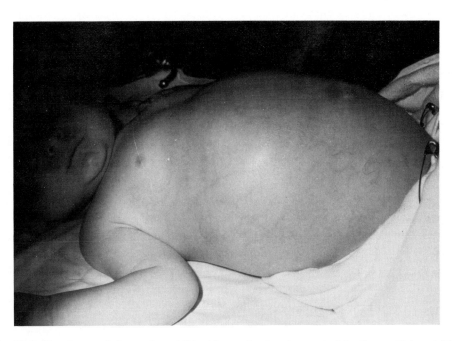

Fig. 20-2. Protuberant abdomen in a child with massive involvement of the liver with hepatoblastoma.

of the lymphoma group usually present first with nodal involvement, often of the cervical lymph glands. However, they may present first as intra-abdominal masses.

Neck masses

Lesions in the neck that first present in childhood are generally benign except for those associated with the cervical lymph nodes. Routine examination should always include careful palpation of the neck, including the area behind the sternocleidomastoid muscles and the paratracheal area.

When a mass is found, attention to the presence of tenderness, heat, and erythema in the area is important. Inflammatory lesions present with these characteristics, whereas neoplastic lesions, except when secondarily infected or inflamed, do so less frequently.[99] Nevertheless, persistent adenopathy should lead to early biopsy.

In evaluating cervical lesions, attention should be paid to identifying the common benign entities, which are usually identifiable by their location. They are discussed in detail in Chapter 15 and include such entities as the midline thyroglossal duct cyst, the second branchial cleft cysts or sinuses occurring along the course of the sterno-cleidomastoid muscle, and the first branchial cleft remnants, extremely rare lesions, which occur at the angle of the jaw[52] (Fig. 20-3). Dermoid cysts often occur at the lateral aspect of the eyebrow, and epidermoid lesions present in the midline of the neck. These lesions are all discrete, rounded, cystic ones that are usually identifiable as such. Secondary inflammation and infection may lead to surrounding erythema, tenderness, and actual abscess formation.

Inflammatory lesions of the cervical lymph nodes are characterized by their rapid onset, tenderness, and progression to fluctuant swelling. Often, systemic symptoms of fever and malaise accompany them. These characteristics are true for the acute suppurative inflammatory conditions of the cervical nodes; in the more chronic infections, however, such as those due to tuberculosis, atypical mycobacteria, cat scratch disease, and chronic viral or bacterial infections, these acute inflammatory signs may be absent.* Differentiating these nodes from those of the malignant lym-

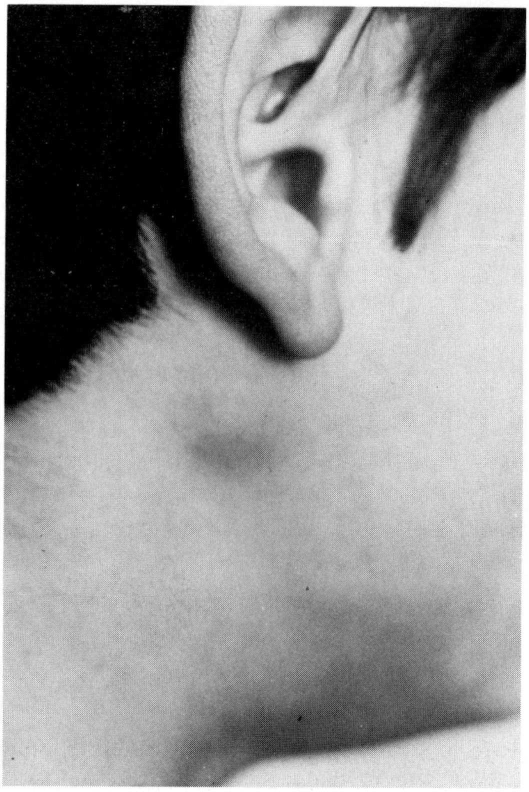

Fig. 20-3. This mass at the angle of the jaw proved to be a first branchial cleft cyst. (Courtesy Donald Serafin, M.D., Durham, N.C.)

phomas may be very difficult. Early biopsy or excision is essential.[3,116]

Evaluation. In dealing with neck masses in children, the amount of prereferral or preoperative workup necessary is usually limited. The common cystic lesions due to thyroglossal duct remnants, branchial cleft remnants, dermoid cysts, and so on, can usually be diagnosed by their characteristic location and their cystic nature. When a thyroglossal duct cyst is suspected, having the child protrude the tongue may indicate the attachment of the thyroglossal cyst to the foramen cecum by the motion of the cyst with such protrusion.

Many authorities have advised that all thyroglossal duct cysts be evaluated by radioisotope scanning to be certain that the child has other, normal thyroid tissue.[127] It is unusual, however, for ectopic thyroid tissue in a thyroglossal duct cyst to be the patient's only thyroid tissue.[103,132] When this is the case, this thyroid tissue is usually dysplastic, and the child is already sympto-

---

*See references 3, 9, 18, 19, 89, and 116.

matically hypothyroid. Thus, it is unusual to remove a thyroglossal duct cyst from a child, find it to be a dysplastic ectopic thyroid, and find that postoperatively a previously euthyroid child is hypothyroid. For this reason, in the asymptomatic child, thyroid scanning preoperatively is unnecessary exposure to radiation and an unnecessary expense for the vast majority of children whose thyroglossal duct cyst has no influence on their thyroid functioning. My general approach to the problem is to take a thorough history for thyroid dysfunction, and if any is suggested by symptoms, to obtain a preoperative thyroid function analysis. If histopathologic examination of the specimen reveals thyroid tissue in the wall of the thyroglossal duct cyst, a postoperative thyroid function analysis should be obtained.

Branchial cleft cysts require no further evaluation, although as noted previously, injection studies of a branchial cleft sinus or fistula may be helpful to the surgeon. A tangential skull film of the area of a dermoid cyst of the eyebrow will show the erosion of the outer table with the inner table intact—a common occurrence with dermoid cysts.

Acute suppurative cervical lymphadenitis is usually immediately apparent, and the child can be started on a regimen of antibiotic therapy. Needle aspiration of the lesion may help to resolve it and also provide material for culture and sensitivity analysis. Evaluation of nonsuppurative cervical lymphadenopathy requires screening for mycobacterial infection, as well as skin tests and a chest film. If these prove negative, a careful history should be obtained for cat-scratch exposure and an inoculum site should be sought.[19]

Referral and treatment. Surgery for cervical lesions requires experience with such lesions in children and a knowledge of the correct surgical procedures. Too many thyroglossal duct cysts in children are excised locally without the extensive surgical procedure that is required. This almost universally results in recurrence, requiring repeated procedures in the child's neck. Each additional surgical procedure increases greatly the risks of damage to the normal anatomy. A great many vascular and neural structures course through the areas in the neck that these cysts and sinuses occupy, and such lesions should never be approached by a surgeon lacking extensive experience in the surgery of the neck, particularly in that of the child.

Excision of a thyroglossal duct cyst requires

removal of the cyst and its tract (Sistrunk procedure).[123] This dissection is carried through the central portion of the hyoid bone, which is removed with it.[132] The dissection is then carried en bloc to the base of the tongue, where excision of the tract is completed and suture of the final connection to the foramen cecum accomplished. Although this procedure is a delicate and extensive one, when it is properly performed, the upset to the child is minimal and he is often ready to be discharged the following day.

The more common second branchial cleft remnants are easier to remove than those of the first branchial cleft because of the latter's involvement with the facial nerve. Perhaps more than any other lesion of the neck, first branchial cleft cysts require the experience of a surgeon who frequently works in this area and is familiar with the ramifications of the facial nerve. Second branchial cleft remnants generally course upward through the bifurcation of the carotid artery and extend on to the tonsillar fossa. Radiographic evaluation of the tract following injection with contrast medium is helpful in demonstrating the course and extent of the lesion (see Fig. 15-19). Branchial cleft *cysts,* however, are generally unassociated with such tracts. Dermoid and epidermoid cysts are easily removed by any surgeon familiar with the nature of these lesions. Cosmetic considerations are the primary focus.

Surgical considerations with regard to inflammatory lesions of the cervical nodes include judgment as to the proper timing of surgical intervention and the proper use of prophylactic as well as therapeutic antibiotics. The chronic inflammatory lesions due to tuberculosis and atypical mycobacterial infection require knowledge of these two entities. Nodal involvement with tuberculosis represents spread from the pulmonary focus and involves the lower cervical or supraclavicular nodes.[62] The diagnosis can be made by skin testing or by noting an obvious tuberculous lesion on the chest radiograph. Surgery is not usually required for these lesions, since antituberculous medication will often achieve resolution of them over the course of several months. Only when this therapy fails should surgical excision be entertained. For atypical mycobacterial lymphadenopathy, however, surgical excision is the only treatment. These organisms respond poorly to antituberculosis medication, and complete excision provides the greatest chance for cure.[3,89]

When cervical lymphadenopathy persists and a clear-cut diagnosis of an inflammatory condition cannot be made, early biopsy is essential. The primary surgical consideration in such a biopsy is to remove the largest node in the area. This node may not be the easiest or most accessible one to remove, but it is the one that is most likely to carry the diagnosis. Occasionally, repeated nodal biopsies are necessary before a diagnosis can be made. On the other hand, complete surgical excision of cervical nodes for lymphoma is not indicated, since the primary therapeutic modalities are chemotherapy and radiation therapy.

Prognosis. For the child with a benign lesion, the prognosis is obviously excellent. Malignant lymphomatous lesions are generally part of a generalized disease, and it is the extent of the spread of that disease that will determine the outcome rather than the localized involvement of the cervical nodes. A high rate of cure is expected in the atypical mycobacterial infections and in those due to cat-scratch disease. Tuberculosis infection should respond to medical therapy in the usual way. Acute suppurative lesions of the cervical nodes may persist despite incision and drainage, and occasionally excision of the entire node is necessary. Chronic infections of the cervical nodes secondary to viral infections of the pharynx and tonsils may cause hyperplastic enlargement of the nodes that is tenaciously persistent. Excision of these nodes may be required to rule out tumor and to achieve resolution of the problem.

Important aspects of follow-up. The major consideration in the follow-up of children with these lesions is recurrence. As noted above, the thyroglossal duct cyst has a high rate of recurrence if improper surgery is provided at the first attempt. Branchial cleft lesions that are incompletely excised or that have been previously infected also have a significant rate of recurrence. Localized inflammatory lesions are the usual presenting signs of recurrence.

Other, less common masses

Thyroid carcinoma in the childhood age group is uncommon but does occur.[130] Careful examination of the thyroid gland on physical examination should be an important part of the physical examination, particularly in the older childhood age group. Any nodule occurring in these children should be thoroughly investigated for thyroid carcinoma. Nodules appearing in the preteenage child are likely to be malignancies; hyperthyroidism and nontoxic nodular goiter are unusual findings in this age group. Evaluation of these lesions should include a complete thyroid function panel, thyroid scan, and early excisional biopsy. These lesions are best treated by either a pediatric surgeon or a general surgeon who is an expert in diseases of the thyroid gland, since the decisions that must be made must take into account the prognosis of the particular lesion as well as the age of the child and life expectancy considerations.

Abdominal masses

An abdominal tumor presenting in the 2- to 12-year age group is most likely to be Wilms' tumor or a neuroblastoma.[120] Later in this age group, lymphoma becomes a more common entity than either of these but remains relatively rare. Hepatoblastoma occurs primarily in the child under the age of 2; hepatocellular carcinoma, as previously noted, occurs in the child under the age of 2 and in the teenager.[42] Thus, the age group under present consideration is relatively free of hepatic tumors.

For the child who has been followed throughout infancy with repeated well-baby visits and examinations, it is more than likely that congenital anomalies of the kidney and renal collecting systems will have been previously identified. Therefore, a mass first recognized in a child beyond the age of 2 is more likely to be a neoplasm. A flank mass fixed in the retroperitoneum presents the differential diagnosis of a suprarenal or paraspinous neuroblastoma or a nephroblastoma (Wilms' tumor). A mass in the liver in this age group is more likely to be a metastatic neuroblastoma than a primary hepatocellular lesion. Neuroblastomas, of course, may arise from any ganglion tissue in the body. Although the common intra-abdominal locations for these tumors are the suprarenal and paraspinous areas, the tumors have been known to arise in neural tissue in the hilum of the kidney and within the bladder as well as within the pelvis.[32,100]

Rhabdomyosarcomas may present in the retroperitoneum or arise from the pelvic structures. Lymphomas are included in the discussion on less common masses.

Evaluation. Although modern radiologic imaging might suggest ultrasonography as the initial modality for evaluating intra-abdominal masses, the intravenous pyelogram (IVP) remains the mainstay of the workup for retroperitoneal tumors in childhood. This modality may be entirely diagnostic for Wilms' tumor, so that no further evaluation, other than an inferior venacavogram for locating the position of the cava and any tumor extension into the cava, is required. Arteriography is of little help in evaluating Wilm's tumor, and a liver scan is indicated only with a palpable hepatic mass. Of more importance is an excellent chest radiograph, since the lungs are the most frequent site of metastases from Wilms' tumor.

Plain films of the abdomen may confirm a flank mass or other intra-abdominal mass as being a neuroblastoma by the presence of speckled calcifications throughout the mass. An IVP may not be diagnostic but would suggest neuroblastoma by the displacement rather than distortion of the kidney. For a large mass, particularly one crossing the midline, inferior venacavography is essential for the "road map" it provides in locating the vena cava at surgery. Arteriography is more likely to be helpful in neuroblastoma, both in identifying the extent of the lesion and in confirming the tumor nature of the mass. It is not essential, however.

Since neuroblastoma has a high propensity for liver metastasis, a liver scan is extremely helpful. Ultrasonography and computerized tomography have their place in the evaluation of these masses when the expertise of those interpreting the studies allows for proper evaluation.

Referral. The success of multimodal therapy in the treatment of Wilms' tumor under the auspices of the National Wilms' Tumor Study[28] makes it imperative that children with malignant neoplasms be referred to centers where multimodal therapy is available and proper guidance through all phases of the workup and treatment of the disease can be directed by the best pediatric oncologists, surgeons, and radiotherapists. The familiarity of these professionals with the requirements of the national protocols will provide patients with Wilms' tumor the opportunity to benefit from the high curability achievable with properly applied multimodal therapy. In addition, it allows patients to benefit from the reduced therapeutic programs that have evolved with further study of this lesion.[28] Surgical excision by surgeons unfamiliar with this lesion and the protocol requirements may lead to either improper surgical technique or to inaccurate staging of the lesion. The former errors may lead to failure of the overall

therapeutic program, resulting in unnecessary mortality, whereas the latter errors may lead to unnecessarily extensive adjuvant chemotherapy and radiation therapy with their attendant complications.

For patients with neuroblastoma or rhabdomyosarcoma, the prognosis is not as promising as it is for most children with Wilms' tumor. Nevertheless, national protocols again offer the greatest hope for improvement. Carefully applied multimodal therapy, including appropriate dosage reductions for chemotherapy and radiation therapy, offer the child the best balance between attempts at cure and avoidance of excessive therapeutic complications. These carefully thought-out national protocols offer the most hopeful arena for advancing knowledge about these heretofore highly lethal malignancies, and the cooperative team approach to multimodal therapy facilitates application of the protocol requirements.

Medical versus surgical treatment. With the initial success of multimodal therapy, there was a flurry of interest in the possible avoidance of surgery in the treatment of Wilms' tumor. Such avoidance soon led to unacceptable increases in recurrence and mortality, and it is clear today that surgical excision remains an essential part of therapy for these tumors.[11,83,141,142] Nevertheless, surgical considerations can now be modified by the successful adjuvant therapy provided by chemotherapy and radiation therapy. Children in whom Wilms' tumor is extensive may benefit from preoperative radiation therapy and chemotherapy that will enable a second-look procedure or delayed primary excision to be successful.

Similarly, neuroblastomas may respond to radiation therapy and/or chemotherapy and allow a previously unresectable tumor to be removed. Adjuvant therapy has led to the decision that surgical excision of rhabdomyosarcomas need not be as extensive and therefore as mutilating as what previous surgical programs called for.[54,61,93] Results and therefore therapeutic requirements vary with the site of these tumors, so that thorough knowledge of the results of controlled studies is imperative for proper management.

Surgical options. The goal of all surgical approaches to these malignant tumors should be total excision. Nevertheless, there are options based on the degree of involvement of important structures. With the success of adjuvant therapy, radical excision including major organs and vascular structures sometimes can be avoided. Major amputations for extremity rhabdomyosarcoma can be avoided in many instances in favor of wide local excision including the origin and insertion of the major muscle groups. The infiltrating retroperitoneal neuroblastoma that cannot be excised without endangering the major vascular structures of the retroperitoneum can be biopsied and treated subsequently with radiation and chemo-

Table 20-1. Clinical staging: The National Wilms' Tumor Study*

Stage I: Tumor limited to kidney and completely excised—capsule intact.

Stage II: Tumor extends beyond kidney but is completely excised. May have been biopsied or spilled locally.

Stage III: Residual nonhematogenous tumor confined to abdomen. Includes:

  A. Lymph nodes involved in hilum, abdominal periaortic chain, or beyond.
  B. Diffuse peritoneal contamination by tumor, or tumor penetrates peritoneal surface.
  C. Implants on peritoneal surfaces.
  D. Tumor beyond surgical margins microscopically or grossly.
  E. Tumor not completely resectable because of local infiltration into vital structures.

Stage IV: Hematogenous metastases, e.g., to lung, liver, bone, brain.

Stage V: Bilateral renal involvement.

*Adapted from D'Angio, G. J., and others: Cancer **38:**633, 1976, and from D'Angio, G. J.: personal communication, 1980.

therapy. A second-look procedure may then possibly succeed in removing a greater bulk of the tumor. These options are carefully spelled out in the national protocols for these tumors and are familiar to the surgeons working in these conjoined efforts.

Postoperative course and complications. The usual postoperative course after these tumors are excised is a benign one, and the hospital stay expected for the surgical procedure alone is usually about 1 week. Often, however, radiation therapy and chemotherapy are begun during that hospitalization and extend the stay. Extensive excisional therapy, however, still carries with it the threat of bleeding, injury to other tissues, and infection. Disseminated intravascular coagulopathy has been known to occur after excision of major malignant tumors in childhood in the absence of identifiable sepsis.

Prognosis. The prognosis for the child with Wilms' tumor is affected by the age of the child, the stage of the tumor, and the favorable or unfavorable nature of the histology (Table 20-1). Children under 1 year of age do much better with Wilms' tumor, partly because most of them have early-stage tumors. Nevertheless, the overall survival for patients with Wilms' tumor approaches 90%, with stage IV metastatic disease and unfavorable histology being the primary factors that lessen this optimal survival.[7] Table 20-2 lists the recent results of the National Wilms' Tumor Study by groups.

Important aspects of follow-up. For the child

Table 20-2. Results of National Wilms' Tumor Study*

Patient group	Therapy regimen	Survival, disease free (%)	Survival (%)
Group I			
Under 2 years	Radiotherapy + S + D†	90	97
	No radiotherapy	88	94
2 years and above	Radiotherapy + S + D	77	97
	No radiotherapy	58	91
All ages	Radiotherapy + S + D	83	97
	No radiotherapy	71	92
Groups II and III	AMD + S + R	57	67
	VCR + S + R	55	72
	AMD + VCR + S + R	81	86
Group IV	Immediate surgery + R + D		83
	Preop VCR + S + R + D		29

*Adapted from D'Angio, and others: Cancer **38:**633, 1976.
†*S,* Surgery; *R,* radiotherapy; *AMD,* actinomycin D; *VCR,* vincristine; *D,* drugs.

who has been cared for in a children's tumor center, the follow-up will be provided, again, in a multimodal fashion with input from the pediatric oncologist, radiation therapist, and surgeon, either a pediatric surgeon or pediatric urologist. These physicians usually meet together at regular intervals, keep abreast of the protocol requirements, and attend the national meetings frequently. The important aspects of follow-up for children with these tumors relate to identification of recurrence at the primary site and screening for metastases. The common site for metastases for Wilms' tumor is the lung; the common sites for metastases for neuroblastoma are the liver and the bone marrow. Rhabdomyosarcoma may metastasize to all of these locations. For neuroblastoma, reelevation of the vanillylmandelic acid (VMA) in the urine of a patient known to have a secreting tumor may be a helpful sign of recurrence but absence of such elevation does not rule out recurrence.

When the patient with Wilms' tumor or neuroblastoma has received extensive radiation to the retroperitoneum, long-term follow-up of the spine for scoliosis and shortening of stature is important. There is also a definite incidence of new malignancy formation in the radiated bed.[131] The short-term problems with chemotherapy will be carefully monitored by the knowledgeable pediatric oncologist. The long-term problems of chemotherapy have yet to be assessed. These probably will prove to be related primarily to reproductive capacity, genetic malformations, and neo-oncogenesis.

Other, less common masses

Less common abdominal masses include retroperitoneal teratomas and sarcomas and tumors arising in the ovaries. These lesions are generally highly malignant, and the best chance for cure remains that of total excision.

Later in this childhood age group, lymphoma may present initially as an abdominal mass. Non-Hodgkin's lymphoma may present in early childhood and occasionally may present as the leading point of an intussusception if it arises in the bowel. Extensive growth of lymphoma in the mesentery and intestinal wall may take place without symptoms or signs until a low-grade bowel obstruction ensues. Intra-abdominal lymphoma has protean symptoms and must always be included in the differential diagnosis of any abdominal mass, obstructive phenomenon, or nonspecific urinary tract symptoms.[12]

Evaluation. How extensive the preoperative evaluation undertaken should be will be determined by the acuteness of the presenting symptoms. Often when the lesion presents as an acute or subacute abdomen, surgical exploration is the first study undertaken and the lymphoma is discovered at that time. When mass lesions inconsistent with the more common retroperitoneal lesions are found preoperatively, a more extensive search for other sites of involvement should be made. If cervical lymphadenopathy is present, a biopsy of this region may indicate the nature of the intra-abdominal disease without exploratory laparotomy. Usually, however, exploratory laparotomy for diagnosis is essential.

Referral. Again, as in the more common solid tumors, the multimodal team approach to the care of these lesions is most likely to result in successful outcome. The pediatric oncologist and radiation therapist must be able to rely on the surgical findings in their decision-making processes. Inadequate surgical evaluation may lead to too much or too little therapy with consequences at either extreme.

Medical versus surgical treatment. Although the treatment of lymphoma is primarily radiation and chemotherapy, there are surgical options. Biopsy is generally essential to confirm the nature of the lesion. The staging procedure may be necessary to determine the presence or absence of tumor in certain sites in planning subsequent radiation therapy.[41,56] Splenectomy is usually a part of such staging procedures. Finally, the surgeon provides the radiation therapist with a "road map" by outlining the gross lesions with radioidentifiable metal clips (Fig. 20-4). On the other hand, it is rarely necessary to excise the vast tumor masses that may be present in the mesentery and intestinal wall. These lesions usually are easily eliminated with the radiation and chemotherapy programs. Rarely is it difficult in controlling the intra-abdominal mass lesions that leads to an unfavorable outcome in these patients; rather, it is the propensity of non-Hodgkin's lymphoma to underto so-called leukemic degeneration. On the other hand, good results have followed excision of major intra-abdominal tumor masses.[67]

Benign abdominal masses

For the most part, benign abdominal masses are intra-abdominal rather than retroperitoneal. They are usually freely movable, often from quadrant to quadrant. The common ones are mes-

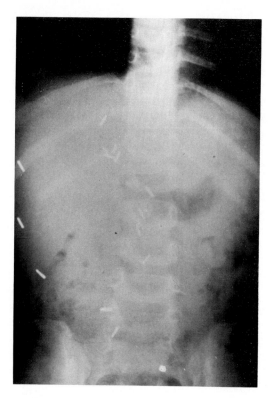

Fig. 20-4. Metal clips placed at the time of surgical excision outline the extent of Wilms' tumor, providing a "roadmap" for the radiation therapist.

enteric cysts and duplications. These masses may be highly mobile, rounded, and cystic in nature (see Fig. 10-44). Ultrasonography is probably the most helpful initial evaluative procedure, since it will identify the cystic nature of the mass. It may also identify an ovarian source for the cyst. Once the cystic nature of such lesions is identified, further evaluation is of little help and one can proceed directly to surgical excision.

Although mesenteric cysts are generally readily removable, some duplications require considerable experience in dealing with other malformations of the intestinal tract and may require the use of techniques that are more common to the armamentarium of the pediatric surgeon than that of the adult surgeon.[147]

On the other hand, any of the lesions may present acutely with either torsion of the lesion itself or with the lesion acting as the leading point for a volvulus of the mesentery (see Fig. 10-45). A duplication can act as the leading point of an intussusception or can become inflamed and present with perforation or peritonitis. Surgical options are few, and the usual procedure is a straight-

forward excision of the lesion. When the duplication is extensive, it may require an endoenteric excision of the mucosa leaving the muscular tube, allowing this to scar, so that the adjacent normal intestinal lumen can be maintained.[147] The postoperative course is generally benign and the hospital stay that of a routine abdominal procedure. The prognosis is excellent, and recurrence is extremely rare. Consequently, follow-up requires little other than the attention to the problems of adhesive bowel obstruction characteristic of any exploratory laparotomy. The possibility of adhesive obstruction of the bowel must always remain in the primary care physician's mind when such a patient at any time after surgery has abdominal distention, crampy pain, or vomiting, particularly if the vomitus is bile stained or feculent.

Other lesions that present as abdominal masses are those of organomegaly, including hepatomegaly and splenomegaly. Splenomegaly may be the first harbinger of portal hypertension secondary to cavernous transformation of the portal vein. Hepatosplenomegaly, on the other hand, may represent chronic liver disease. The presence of a right upper quadrant cystic mass associated with intermittent jaundice and right upper quadrant pain is highly suggestive of a choledochal cyst, an extremely rare lesion.

GASTROINTESTINAL BLEEDING
Upper gastrointestinal bleeding

Gastrointestinal bleeding in this age group is an unusual occurrence but may be of life-threatening proportions when it does occur. The otherwise healthy child with acute upper gastrointestinal bleeding is most likely to be bleeding from *esophageal varices* secondary to either portal hypertension from cavernomatous transformation of the portal vein or from portal hypertension secondary to occult liver disease such as chronic active hepatitis or congenital hepatic fibrosis.[48,137] Upper gastrointestinal bleeding may present with hematemesis, or it may present with either melena or frankly bloody stools. Almost always, the stools are dark red to black rather than bright red when the source of bleeding is from the upper gastrointestinal tract. Other patients with upper gastrointestinal hemorrhage may merely have anemia and be found to have intermittent or continuous guaiac-positive stools.

Other causes of upper gastrointestinal bleeding

in this age group, such as *ulcers* and *gastritis,* are unusual in the otherwise healthy child. They do occur as stress-induced lesions in the hospitalized child with a major neurologic disease or injury or a septic episode related to other medical or surgical illness.[27,110] Burn patients, of course, are also at risk for such stress ulcerations.[110] Rare causes of upper gastrointestinal bleeding in the otherwise healthy child include *arteriovenous malformations, hemangiomas,* and such other rare congenital or acquired abnormalities as *polyps, pancreatic rests,* and *duplications.*

The child who presents with acute life-threatening upper gastrointestinal bleeding should be hospitalized in a center where all necessary evaluations and possible surgical corrections can be achieved. A short-term stay in a less sophisticated hospital may be warranted to stabilize the severely bleeding child.

Physical examination may be helpful in differentiating cavernomatous transformation of the portal vein from intrahepatic causes of portal hypertension. The presence of an enlarged liver favors the latter diagnosis. The liver in cavernomatous transformation is usually normal, whereas the spleen may be quite enlarged. Of course, splenomegaly may be present in relation to portal hypertension from any cause. Other signs of portal hypertension include a prominent venous pattern over the abdomen and occasionally hemorrhoids. The presence of ascites does not favor one entity over the other, since ascites may be due to the portal hypertension alone or to the intrinsic liver disease.

A good-size nasogastric tube should be passed into the stomach and the stomach aspirated and emptied and the nature of the contents noted. The argument that a nasogastric tube should be avoided in a patient with esophageal varices is a specious one, for the continued presence of clot and gastric acid is far more detrimental to the esophageal varix than the trauma from the passage of the tube. Decompression of the stomach and iced saline lavage are the first line of defense against upper gastrointestinal bleeding. A dependable, adequately sized intravenous line should be placed and resuscitation begun with whole blood when it is available. If the patient is already hypovolemic and has signs of shock, initial infusion of Ringer's lactate solution is warranted until blood is available.

Referral. Once the child is stabilized, he should be transferred to a facility where intensive care of children is available, where arteriography and endoscopy can be readily accomplished in the childhood age group, and where surgical consultation is available from surgeons who have experience with managing these problems in children and who have the knowledge and judgment to make the proper choices between medical therapy and emergency surgery.

Medical versus surgical treatment. The vast majority of gastrointestinal bleeding episodes in childhood can be handled by medical means. These should all be exhausted before emergency surgery is resorted to. The latter, far too often, leads to extensive resectional surgery in children with acute problems that have no long-term sequelae if they are handled satisfactorily by nonsurgical therapy. Good medical therapy, however, is aggressive medical therapy. It includes effective nasogastric decompression, lavage, and emptying of the gastric contents. Extensive iced saline lavage may be necessary over a prolonged period of time to control hemorrhage.

Evaluation and initial treatment. Proper diagnosis is essential to proper treatment. Until recently, the first diagnostic maneuver was the ingestion of barium followed by radiographic evaluation of the upper gastrointestinal tract. Modern evaluation begins with endoscopy,[101] which in experienced hands is a highly successful modality in diagnosing esophageal varices and gastritis, particularly if the patient is still bleeding at least moderately. If endoscopy is unsuccessful, or if the bleeding is too extensive to allow satisfactory endoscopy, arteriography is the preferred approach.[68,101] In experienced hands, percutaneous cannulation of the femoral arteries is possible in the youngest infants and is easily accomplished in children. Highly selective arteriography can then be obtained in an organized sequence beginning with aortography and progressing to highly selective cannulation of individual upper abdominal vessels.[44,68,101] Venous-phase angiography can identify the portal venous system and demonstrate obstructions there as well as the presence of esophageal varices (Fig. 20-5).

The diagnosis should be accomplished by endoscopy and/or angiography in well over 90% of patients. When angiography has been utilized and bleeding continues or is likely to continue, a catheter should be left in place for subsequent infusion of vasoconstrictive agents.[5]

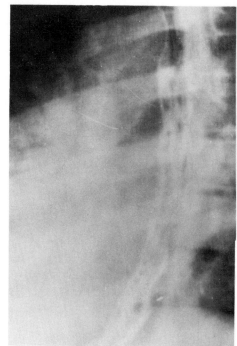

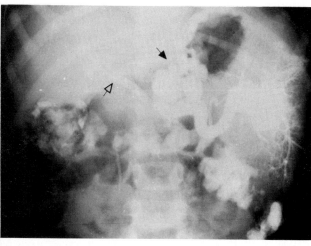

Fig. 20-5. A, Barium swallow examination shows filling defects in the esophagus representing esophageal varices. B, Venous phase arteriography shows the tortuous splenic vein and cavernomatous transformation of the portal vein (open arrow) and clearly shows the esophageal varices (closed arrow).

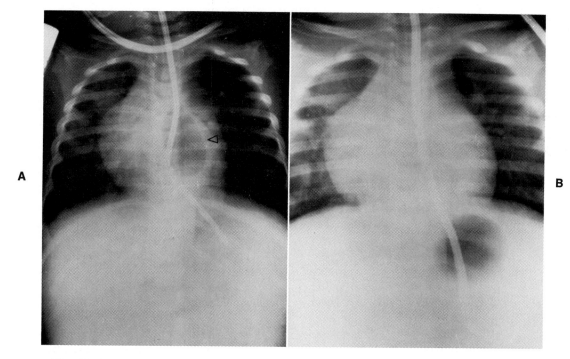

Fig. 20-6. A, Gastric balloon of the Sengstaken-Blakemore tube (arrow) inadvertently inflated in the esophagus. Such an error could lead to rupture of the esophagus. B, Gastric balloon properly positioned in the stomach.

If the patient is not actively bleeding at the time of diagnostic evaluation, angiography may offer little help and endoscopy may also be unsuccessful. Under these circumstances, with a stable patient who is no longer bleeding, standard upper gastrointestinal contrast studies should be obtained. Remember that the ingestion of barium prior to endoscopy and angiography makes both of these modalities more difficult to accomplish.

If esophageal varices are identified as the cause of bleeding and the bleeding continues after iced saline lavage, either angiographic infusion therapy or the Sengstaken-Blakemore tube should be utilized. The latter requires experience, since it is a potentially hazardous instrument. It is best utilized in an intensive care setting, monitored by a nursing staff familiar with the potential problems of the tube. The two major risks of the Sengstaken-Blakemore tube are rupture of the esophagus due to inadvertent pressure expansion of one of the balloons in a malpositioned tube (Fig. 20-6) and the risk of aspiration of oropharyngeal secretions due to complete occlusion of the esophagus by the balloons. The latter problem is avoided by positioning a nasogastric tube in the esophagus above the esophageal balloon of the Sengstaken-Blakemore tube and attaching it to suction. Another potential complication with the tube is necrosis of the nose, which occurs when traction is placed on the tube and the tube is taped to the nose. A sponge rubber block will help to offset this problem, but a more effective and more comfortable method of placing traction on the tube is by putting the child in a football helmet with a face guard and taping the tube to the face guard under traction.

Vasopressin is an effective splanchnic vasoconstrictor and can be utilized for esophageal varices, either by peripheral venous infusion or by direct infusion into the superior mesenteric artery through the angiographic catheter.[29] When selective infusion through the artery is chosen, repeated radiographic checks on the degree of vasoconstriction are essential to avoid necrosis of the bowel. The usual dose for either peripheral venous or direct arterial infusion is 0.1 to 0.4 units of Vasopressin per minute. The least dose that achieves satisfactory hemostasis should be utilized.

Probably the most common complication with the use of Vasopressin is its antidiuretic effect. Vasopressin essentially is an antidiuretic hormone, and as such it causes fluid retention to a degree that may lead to congestive heart failure in the otherwise healthy child. These children are receiving massive intravenous fluid therapy to restore their hypovolemic state from the blood loss; in addition, they may absorb huge quantities of saline from the iced lavage therapy to their stomachs. Central venous pressure monitoring is essential in the management of these patients.

Surgical options. Until recently the general consensus about the lesions causing esophageal varices in children was that those due to portal hypertension secondary to liver disease could be easily treated with a portacaval shunt to prevent esophageal hemorrhage. However, these children usually went on to die of chronic liver disease. It was believed that early shunting was desirable for these children because the repeated episodes of major hemorrhage caused further damage to their already-impaired livers and because the patency of a major portal vessel made accomplishment of a satisfactory shunt relatively easy.

On the other hand, for the more healthy child with cavernomatous transformation of the portal vein and a healthy liver, the repeated bleeding episodes were well tolerated and the liver was rarely permanently damaged by them. The lack of a portal vein made satisfactory shunting less easy to accomplish, since the splenic vein and even the superior mesenteric vein in the child under 10 to 12 years of age was often too small for satisfactory shunting. In these children, therefore, the shunt procedures were often delayed until late childhood or early teenage years. At that time, some form of splenorenal shunt or Marion-Clatworthy caval mesenteric shunt was accomplished.[20]

Recent data suggesting that patients suffer a high incidence of encephalopathy due to ammonia intoxication when the liver is deprived of the mesenteric portal flow has led to a reevaluation of shunting in general.[136,137] Since many children with cavernomatous transformation of the portal vein apparently develop adequate collateral vessels by the teenage years, and since the number of bleeding episodes may lessen as the child reaches adulthood, it is possible that many children can be satisfactorily managed without ever having a shunt. For the child with severe liver disease who is threatened by the repeated hypovolemic episodes secondary to variceal hemorrhage, early shunting may still be warranted.

For all of these children, the shunt suggested by Warren,[139] which is generally known as the distal splenorenal shunt, offers hope for satisfactory control of variceal hemorrhage. At the same time, it eliminates the hepatic encephalopathy risk attendant on depriving the liver of the mesenteric flow. This surgical procedure, which entails dividing the splenic vein just proximal to its entry into the portal vein and anastomosing it to the left renal vein, provides selective decompression of the splenic circuit. The short gastric veins are left intact and provide decompression of the stomach and esophagus. The coronary vein, which is a major tributary from the esophagus and lesser curvature of the stomach to the portal vein, is identified and divided, as are any other collateral vessels extending from the stomach to the portal venous system. This partial devascularization disconnects the esophageal venous plexus from the high-pressure portal system and allows it to drain into the azygos venacaval system superiorly and by way of the short gastric veins into the spleen and thence out the splenic vein into the low-pressure renal vein and vena cava. At the same time, it maintains the mesenteric flow into the liver through the portal system and its various tributaries. Thus, complete bypass of the liver by the portal flow is avoided and the risk of encephalopathy lessened.

• • •

Gastric ulcers are almost unheard of in the childhood age group, and duodenal ulcers are quite rare. Generally, when these occur as chronic peptic ulcer disease, they can be managed satisfactorily by medical means such as diet regulation and antacid therapy. Major hemorrhage from such lesions can usually be controlled by iced saline lavage. Angiography and endoscopy are invaluable in the diagnostic evaluation. Angiographic infusion therapy and occasionally transarterial embolization therapy may control an otherwise difficult hemorrhage.[44,68,101] Individual branches of the celiac vessels can be selectively embolized with autogenous clot or Gelfoam to control a major hemorrhage from an ulcer (Fig. 20-7). When such attempts fail to control the hemorrhage or when the ulcer disease presents with perforation as its primary complication, selective surgical management should err on the side of minimizing the initial surgical procedure. Oversewing the ulcer or the bleeding point without further surgery may be warranted. If some preventive ulcer procedure is desirable based on the chronicity of the

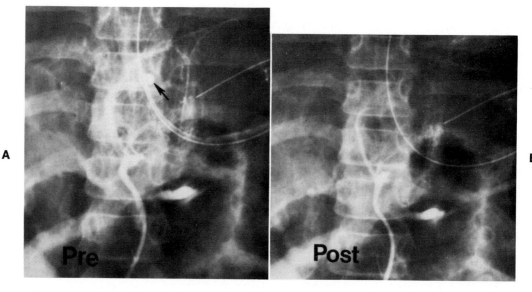

Fig. 20-7. A, Selective arteriogram with a bleeding point in the left gastric circulation (arrow). **B,** Following embolization with Gelfoam, the bleeding point is fading. (From Filston, H. C., Jackson, D. C., and Johnsrude, I. S.: J. Pediatr. Surg. **14:**276, 1979.)

previous ulcer disease, a surgical procedure with the least degree of destruction to normal physiology should be performed.[27,117] In this regard, the highly selective vagotomy is an appealing procedure, and the truncal vagotomy with pyloroplasty or gastroenterostomy would be the next indicated procedure.[71] Extensive resectional surgery is contraindicated. Children will tolerate repeated massive hemorrhages well if they are properly resuscitated; thus, it is not mandatory that a one-shot, guaranteed hemorrhage-preventing procedure be done in these children, such as might be indicated in an older individual with multiple-system diseases.

Postoperative course. The postoperative course after any of these procedures is similar to that of any major abdominal surgical procedure, with the usual hospitalization extending 7 to 10 days. The Warren shunt has been highly successful in controlling variceal hemorrhage in adult patients, but its efficacy in childhood is only beginning to be evaluated.[113,139] The procedures mentioned for control of an ulcer are standard ones with a low risk and morbidity rate and a high degree of success.

Complications. Following shunt procedures, splenic function should be repeatedly evaluated. Improvement in hypersplenism may be a good sign that a shunt is working, although hypersplenism will not always be controlled by a shunt. Ascites is a frequent problem occurring in children with cavernous transformation of the portal vein when their albumin level drops during a major hemorrhage. Usually, adequate intravascular albumin levels help to offset the tendency to ascites. When ascites does present as a complication, mild diuretic therapy such as with spironolactone will often serve to control the ascites until the intravascular oncotic pressure builds back up to a level where physiologic control is maintained. The main complication after a shunt procedure is clotting of the shunt with renewed bleeding. Propagation of a thrombus from a splenic vein into the renal vein could lead to venous thrombosis of the kidney, but that is unlikely because of the collateral vessels to the left renal vein from the genitalia and from the adrenal gland. On a long-term basis, the usual complication of adhesive bowel obstruction must be kept in mind for any patient having had an intra-abdominal procedure.

Other, less common causes of bleeding

Less common lesions causing upper gastrointestinal hemorrhage are those of the arteriovenous malformation or hemangioma group. These can usually be identified by angiography when they are actively bleeding. They may also be identifiable by selective angiography when hemorrhage is not occurring. We had a patient with a large hemangioma of the proximal jejunum that presented with chronic upper gastrointestinal bleeding, anemia, guaiac-positive stools, and chronic low-grade bowel obstruction due to intussusception of the hamartoma. Such entities are rare, but their presence must be sought for in any child with occult bleeding when the source of the bleeding is not found on standard approaches.

Lower gastrointestinal bleeding

Bleeding from the lower gastrointestinal tract rarely presents as a life-threatening hemorrhage in a child. *Meckel's diverticulum* may bleed massively, and large amounts of blood may be passed. Other lesions usually present with intermittent bloody stools or even chronic anemia.

Evaluation. Physical examination is rarely helpful is the diagnosis of lower gastrointestinal bleeding except when a fissure or very low rectal polyp is the source. Rectal examination usually does produce a stool sample that can be tested for blood to confirm that the substance seen is, in fact, blood. Red-colored gelatin and fruit punches can pass through the gastrointestinal tract in a state so unaltered as to leave them with their same color and appearance, simulating bleeding and clots. Massive lower gastrointestinal bleeding in the infant and early childhood age groups is strongly suggestive of Meckel's diverticulum. This entity occurs in 2% of the population and becomes symptomatic in approximately 25%.[10,96] Hemorrhage is not the only symptom of Meckel's diverticulum; other patients may present with intussusception, perforation, or generalized diverticulitis of the diverticulum as the complicating factors.

A properly performed and evaluated technetium scan may be helpful in demonstrating Meckel's diverticulum if the diverticulum has created an ulcer and caused bleeding from the adjacent normal bowel.[73,145] Also, if the gastric mucosa in the diverticulum is extensive enough, it may be noted on the scan (Fig. 20-8). When active bleed-

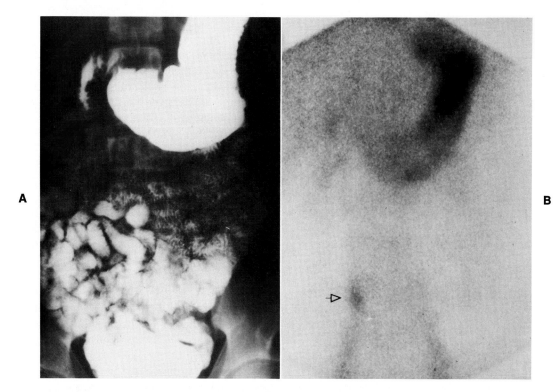

Fig. 20-8. A, Upper GI series with small bowel follow-through rarely will demonstrate Meckel's diverticulum, as illustrated by this normal study. The ^{99}Tc scan in **B** demonstrates Meckel's diverticulum (arrow).

ing is occurring from any lesion, angiography may identify the bleeding point. Often, however, the acute bleeding has ceased and the physician is left with the time-honored proctosigmoidoscopy and barium enema evaluations. Properly performed, these may be very helpful in identifying polyps. Occasionally, colonoscopy may be successful in reaching more proximal lesions in the large intestine. This procedure is usually unsuccessful in reaching lesions proximal to the sigmoid colon in young children because the sigmoid is overly distensible and the colonoscope cannot be easily manipulated into the descending colon.

When evaluation of the lower gastrointestinal tract fails to identify a source of bleeding, it is extremely important to evaluate the upper gastrointestinal tract, for chronic slow bleeding from the upper gastrointestinal tract may present solely as lower gastrointestinal bleeding. It must not be assumed that lower gastrointestinal bleeding is always from the distal ileum and colon.

Referral. Just when a child is referred to a major center for surgical care depends on the primary care physician's ability to evaluate the problem in his own institution and on the availability of knowledgeable and capable surgical consultants. The surgeon who deals exclusively with bleeding problems of the lower gastrointestinal tract in adults is usually too malignancy conscious and therefore too aggressive in the management of bleeding lesions in children. Seldom is malignancy found to be the source of bleeding in this age group. The three most common lesions causing bleeding in this age group are Meckel's diverticulum, polyps, and local anorectal lesions such as fissures.

Medical versus surgical treatment. When Meckel's diverticulum is identified or highly suspected, it should be removed. There is no successful medical therapy for Meckel's diverticulum. It is a congenital anomaly often containing gastric mucosa, which causes ulceration of the normal adjacent ileum by its acid secretions. The possible consequences of persistent Meckel's diverticulum are protracted bleeding, perforation, diverticulitis, and intussusception.[10] The surgical procedure is a simple one of the magnitude of a straightforward appendectomy and should be attended by few and minimal complications.

Polyps, on the other hand, require thoughtful management. If there is no family history for polyposis or Gardner's syndrome, the overwhelming likelihood is that polyps in the colon, even though multiple, will be of the juvenile mucosal variety.[133] These lesions are not premalignant. They do cause hemorrhage but often slough on their own. Polyps easily reached through the anus or through the sigmoidoscope should be removed. Exploratory laparotomy for the removal of a polyp higher in the colon is indicated only if persistent or recurrent massive hemorrhage complicates the polyp or if biopsy of a polyp further distally has shown it to be adenomatous. Colonoscopic removal of juvenile polyps would be a desirable procedure if it were easily accomplished; as previously discussed, however, colonoscopy is extremely difficult in young children because of the redundant sigmoid loop and the thin, highly elastic bowel wall. The fact that the child generally requires general anesthesia for such a procedure makes the risk of perforation greater in such patients, since they cannot advise the operator of pain from distention of the bowel wall by either excess insufflation of gas or direct pressure of the colonoscope.

Most fissures and other irritative phenomena in the perianal region can be managed with stool softeners and sitz baths. A deep, chronic, persistent fissure may require excision or curettage of the tract.

Postoperative course and prognosis. The postoperative course for most of these procedures should be benign and the hospital stay short. The prognosis after excision of Meckel's diverticulum or a juvenile polyp should be excellent, and the complication rate should be negligible. After excision of a polyp, the child should be screened on a long-term basis for anemia or evidence of continued or recurrent lower gastrointestinal bleeding, since additional polyps may be present or develop.

Less common causes of bleeding

Less common lesions in this age group that may present with lower gastrointestinal bleeding are ulcerative colitis and regional enteritis. Usually with the latter, other symptoms of pain and diarrhea are present. Nevertheless, bleeding may be the first presentation of regional enteritis and not uncommonly is the initial presentation for ulcerative colitis. Early in the course of the disease, barium contrast studies may not define these lesions; and when persistent bleeding occurs and no definitive bleeding site can be identified, biopsy of the bowel is indicated. Biopsy can usually be accomplished transanally, but the risk of full-thickness perforation must be kept in mind if the biopsy site chosen is above the pelvic peritoneal reflection.

Again, be reminded that if no lower gastrointestinal source of bleeding is found, the entire proximal gastrointestinal tract must be evaluated, since the site of bleeding may well reside therein.

CHEST WALL DEFORMITIES

Although there are a wide variety of minor deformities in the thoracic cage, the most common lesions that attract attention are the pectus deformities: pectus excavatum and pectus carinatum. The more common of the two is pectus excavatum. This lesion is more likely to cause concern and has been shown to have some degree of physiologic effect on cardiac output. The pectus carinatum, or pigeon breast, deformities are of no physiologic consequence and are usually of less cosmetic importance. This is not always the case, however. For many years, despite frequent attempts to show a degree of pulmonary embarrassment in these children, none was demonstrable by the usual pulmonary function studies. Thus, the lesions were treated primarily for cosmetic and emotional reasons. Recently, however, the patient with pectus excavatum has been shown on stress exercising to have a reduced cardiac output.[8] Although this reduced output is probably not of a degree to affect the child in performing the normal activities of daily living or even in the average exercise situation, in extensive, trained athletic endeavors these children probably have a reduced cardiac reserve due to malposition of the heart by the compression of the pectus deformity.[109] The degree of this reduced reserve will vary with the extent of the reduction in the size of the chest cavity.

Although pectus deformities are relatively common entities and are readily recognized, several tumors present in the chest wall and must be differentiated from these deformities. Certainly, any mass presenting in a more lateral location must be judged a tumor first and a deformity second.

These tumors range from the benign hemangiomas arising in the muscles of the chest wall and diaphragm to frank malignancies such as Ewing's sarcoma and osteosarcoma arising in the ribs.

Treatment. There is no medical therapy for the lesion other than nontreatment, which is a valid decision in many cases. Surgical procedures usually involve dividing the costal cartilages that are the cause of the deformity, elevating the sternum back into its normal anterior position, and supporting it by suturing the muscles and fascia of the chest wall behind it. This procedure is relatively benign and has few complications, the most frequent being inadvertent entry into the pleural cavity, resulting in the creation of a pneumothorax and requiring the short-term use of a chest tube.

Some surgeons utilize prosthetic plates or struts for periods of time, particularly in the older child. Those surgeons who prefer to perform the surgery in the preschool age group have found that the strut is rarely needed.[109] None of the procedures has met with 100% success, and recurrence of some degree of the deformity must be anticipated. However, a second surgical procedure is rarely required.

The decision for surgery is usually made on the basis of the child's cosmetic appearance and his reaction to the problem. Particularly when the child is bothered or embarrassed by the abnormality, surgical correction is warranted. We generally point out the physiologic changes that have been demonstrated but downplay these as reasons for surgery, believing that the cosmetic and emotional factors are more important. Nevertheless, this surgery should not be classified as cosmetic, since it is to correct a definite congenital deformity and does produce physiologic changes.

Referral. Referral of children with pectus deformities should certainly be to surgeons who have considerable experience in treating these lesions. Only in their hands will the success of the procedure be dependable.

TUMORS OF THE CHEST WALL, MEDIASTINUM, AND LUNGS

Tumors of the chest wall, mediastinum, and lungs may present at any age, although they are less frequently found in newborns or in the infant-toddler age group. Tumors of the chest wall are generally asymptomatic and present as painless masses found by the patient, his parents, or the physician on routine examination. Tumors of the

mediastinum may be found on chest x-ray films obtained for other symptoms or as part of an evaluation for the extent of tumor spread from another primary site. This is particularly true of the lymphoma group. Occasionally, tumors of the mediastinum may involve pulmonary structures and present with symptoms of respiratory distress, especially in infants. In childhood, these tumors present with dysphagia due to esophageal compression and occasionally cause chest pain.

Tumors of the chest wall

Tumors may arise from any of the structures in the chest wall, but the most common ones arise from the muscles and the ribs. The tumors may be benign or malignant. In the younger infant, hemangiomas and lymphangiomas may be found on routine physical examination or may be discovered by the parents as asymptomatic masses developing somewhere on the chest. In the childhood age group, Ewing's sarcoma and osteosarcoma may arise from the bony structures of the chest, although both of these lesions more commonly arise from the long bones of the extrem-

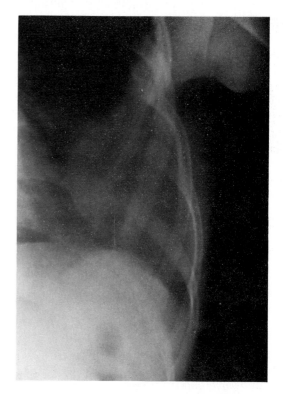

Fig. 20-9. Cone-down view of a chest radiograph of Ewing's sarcoma of the chest wall.

ities.[81] The benign soft tissue lesions are hemangiomas, lymphangiomas, and, very infrequently, lipomas, whereas the malignant lesions are usually embryonal rhabdomyosarcomas. The malignant bony tumors may arise as asymptomatic growths, but occasionally pain calls the patient's attention to the mass.

Evaluation. Chest x-ray films with varying views should be obtained for initial evaluation of the lesion and will confirm involvement of the bony structures in Ewing's sarcoma and osteosarcoma. Some rarifaction of the bone may be present in the extensive soft tissue tumors as well. Differences are fairly characteristic (Fig. 20-9). Further specific evaluation after the routine history, physical examination, and screening laboratory examinations should consist of a computerized tomography (CT) scan to further delineate the extent of the tumor within the chest and to demonstrate any additional lesions, either contiguous or metastatic (Fig. 20-10). When malignant lesions are suspected, a metastatic survey consisting of a bone scan and bone marrow evaluation is indicated.

Medical versus surgical treatment. A diagnostic biopsy is required for all of these lesions before any definitive therapy can be undertaken. Lesions obviously arising from or primarily involving bony structures are most likely to be malignant, and biopsy procedures should be planned with consideration for subsequent excision of the biopsy tract. Biopsies of lesions arising from vascular sources such as hemangiomas and angiomatous malformations should be limited in extent to control the bleeding, since hemorrhage from these lesions can be extensive. Although these angiomatous lesions are usually benign, complete excision may be impossible because of involvement of normal tissues.

Treatment of malignant soft tissue lesions such as rhabdomyosarcoma and those arising from bony sources such as Ewing's sarcoma and osteosarcoma have shown an encouraging response to multimodal therapy in recent reports,[65,81] and the sequence of application of surgery, radiation therapy, and chemotherapy varies in different protocols. Complete discussion of protocol construction is beyond the limits of this text, but the primary care physician should recognize that the most successful therapy for these lesions has been achieved in centers dealing extensively with childhood cancer where the up-to-date applications of the varying treatment modalities are known and can be applied appropriately to the individual child. The primary care physician should be assured that almost all such protocols are designed with the welfare of the patient as the primary consideration. The first goal is for cure of the patient's disease with protection of the patient's normal functioning. To this end, many modern protocols

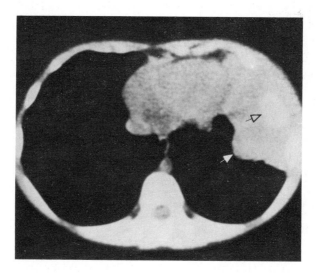

Fig. 20-10. This computerized tomography (CT) scan of the lesion in Fig. 20-9 gives better definition of the extent of impingement of the tumor into the pleural space (white arrow) and also better defines the involvement of the rib (open black arrow).

are demonstrating that less therapy is better. This is most true of tumors that have shown a highly successful response to multimodal therapy. In all instances, the less tested and more experimental drugs are reserved for children who have failed to respond to established therapeutic modalities.

Prognosis. Benign tumors of the chest wall, whether hemangiomas or lymphangiomas, may be surgically removable; and when they are not, they may cause no significant dysfunction. Some, however, may interfere with normal functioning tissue by their presence and mass effect and many times are difficult to excise entirely. Radiation therapy and steroid therapy have occasionally been successful in treating large hemangiomas that are not amenable to excision, but side effects of these modalities must be balanced against the complications of the tumor's presence.

Tumors of the mediastinum

The most common tumor of the mediastinum in childhood is neuroblastoma. This tumor arises from the paravertebral ganglionic chain and may

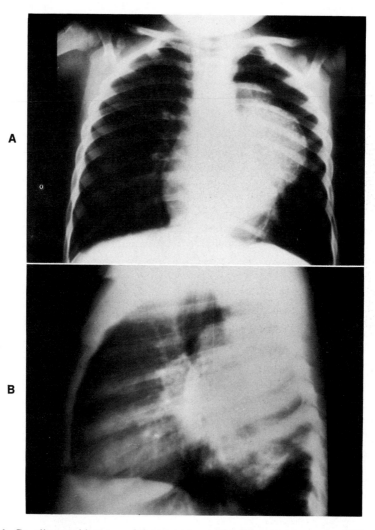

Fig. 20-11. Ganglioneuroblastoma of the chest in a child. The anteroposterior (AP) view **(A)** and lateral chest radiograph **(B)** demonstrate the posterior mediastinal location of the tumor. The tumor is well defined by the CT scan in **C,** and the entire CT scan study showed absence of invasion of the spinal canal. **D** shows the postoperative chest radiograph with metal clips marking the extent of attachment of the tumor in the mediastinum to guide postoperative radiotherapy if indicated.

grow to considerable size before its presence is evident. It may invade a spinal foramen and present initially as acute spinal cord compression with paraplegia or paraparalysis. In the absence of spinal column invasion, the mass may grow to fill a good portion of the hemithorax and present eventually with respiratory symptoms (Fig. 20-11).

Evaluation. Evaluation begins with good chest radiographs, which should demonstrate the posterior mediastinal location of the tumor. When the tumor has already reached considerable size in the thorax, it may appear to be invading the intercostal spaces, resulting in widening of one or more interspaces and compression changes in the adjacent ribs. Further evaluation consists of (1) a metastatic bone survey utilizing either a radioisotope bone scan or radiographs of the skull, long bones, and vertebral column; (2) bone marrow aspiration looking for bone marrow metastases; (3) an IVP looking for the occasional concomitant suprarenal or abdominal paravertebral site of origin; and (4) a collection of urine for VMA excretion, a highly diagnostic sign of neuroblastoma when positive. When no invasion of the spinal column is evident, myelography with a CT scan should be performed to rule out asymptomatic invasion. Failure to do so may result in hemorrhage into the tumor that has invaded the spinal foramen, resulting in compression of the spinal cord during attempted removal of the intrathoracic tumor.[76]

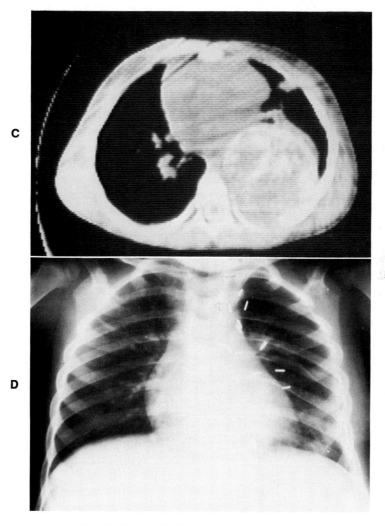

C

D

Fig. 20-11, cont'd. For legend see opposite page.

Medical versus surgical treatment. Although extensive investigations have been carried out in attempts to develop radiation therapy and chemotherapy protocols that will improve the survival of patients with neuroblastoma, there is no conclusive evidence that either of these modalities has influenced the overall survival rate.[80] The best hope of cure still remains surgical excision. Neuroblastoma in the child under 1 year of age still appears to be significantly influenced by the child's immune mechanisms against the tumor; and even when only minimal excision is possible, the child may have a favorable outcome. Beyond the age of 2 years, however, surgical excision of the entire tumor should be the primary therapeutic goal when possible, for in the older child neuroblastoma has an unfavorable prognosis if it cannot be nearly totally excised. When invasion of the spinal column has been demonstrated, laminectomy should be performed initially to remove the tumor and release the compression of the spinal cord. Thoracotomy can then be performed and as much of the residual tumor removed as possible. In most instances, thoracic neuroblastomas can be nearly totally removed. Obviously, microscopic disease is often left behind.

Additional therapy should probably be dictated by national protocols, for these take into account what has previously been learned about unsuccessful therapeutic agents and attempt to amass information regarding newer combinations and modalities.

Prognosis. Despite the fact that no proved increase in survival has been demonstrated by any protocol, the tumor clearly does respond to many chemotherapeutic agents as well as to radiation therapy; thus, combinations of the modalities should be applied on the basis of the extent of the surgical excision. These additional therapeutic efforts are particularly important in the older child, in whom the prognosis for survival from neuroblastoma is much lower than that for the infant.

Other, less common tumors

No other tumors of the mediastinum are common, but bronchogenic cysts, thymic cysts, and lymphomas do occur.[121] The compartmental location of the tumor in the mediastinum may help to suggest the probable diagnosis. Thymomas arise in the anterosuperior compartment but are rare in childhood, and lymphomas arise in the middle mediastinum from the hilar lymph nodes and are second only to neuroblastomas in frequency. When a thymoma is suspected, the child should be evaluated for myasthenia gravis; and when a lymphoma is suspected, the child should be examined carefully for other nodal enlargement. Not infrequently, lymphoma, particularly Hodgkin's disease, can be diagnosed by biopsy of more accessible nodes, such as those in the cervical region or axilla, obviating the need for thoracotomy. Thymic cysts may be difficult to differentiate from cystic hygromas of the mediastinum prior to surgical excision and histopathologic evaluation.

Benign bronchogenic cysts are uncommon lesions and may present any time in childhood from infancy onward. Their usual presentation is that of pressure on the adjacent bronchial structures causing either atelectasis or a ball valve effect with emphysema of a pulmonary segment or segments (Fig. 20-12). There may be a combination of overinflation and atelectasis, depending on the location of the cyst in relation to the bronchial structures. Bronchograms may be required for delineation but should be performed only after bronchoscopy has failed to demonstrate an intrabronchial cause for the obstruction. Bronchograms in young infants are hazardous procedures because of the possibility that the bronchogram dye will be poorly cleared from the bronchial tree, leading to obstruction and interference with pulmonary function. In the young infant, they are best performed with the infant under general anesthesia with a Carlen tube protecting the opposite bronchial tree. Following the procedure, excess contrast agent should be suctioned from the tracheobronchial tree. Postoperative care should consist of extra attention to tracheal toilet to clear the contrast medium from the lung.

Tumors of the lungs

Tumors of the pulmonary parenchyma are extremely unusual occurrences throughout the childhood age group. Benign tumors are rare and consist of occasional hamartomas. Lesions are more likely to be inflammatory or granulomatous lesions than neoplasms. Malignant tumors of the pulmonary parenchyma are almost nonexistent in the childhood age group. Therefore, neoplastic lesions of the pulmonary parenchyma are almost always metastatic from other sources, the most common being Wilms' tumor of the kidney and

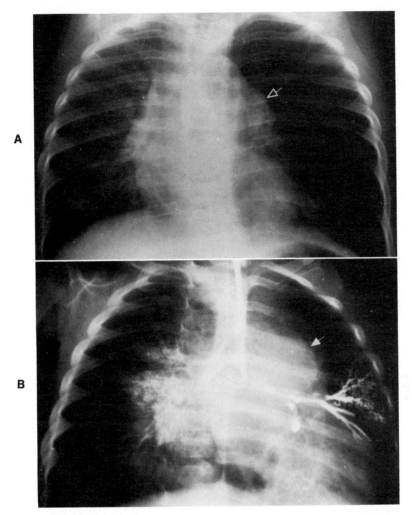

Fig. 20-12. A, Chest radiograph showing a lesion (arrow) near the hilum of the left lung, which is defined in the bronchogram **(B).** This bronchogenic cyst compressing the left main stem bronchus led to atelectasis in the left lower lobe.

bony tumors such as Ewing's sarcoma and osteosarcoma. Pulmonary parenchyma, of course, can be invaded from adjacent tumors of the chest wall.

Evaluation for lesions of the pulmonary parenchyma should consist of skin tests and cultures seeking inflammatory and infectious causes as well as a general body tumor survey seeking primary sources for possible metastatic disease. If no cause can be demonstrated from these evaluations, a biopsy with excision is indicated.

BREAST PROBLEMS: MALE AND FEMALE

Most breast problems develop either in infancy or in the early teenage years. Breast problems are extremely unusual lesions in the childhood years. Occasionally, precocious puberty will develop in late childhood with development of breast tissue as part of the overall picture. Other secondary sex characteristic changes will accompany the breast development under these circumstances, so that the physician must do a complete physical evaluation looking for hair growth in the axillas and pubic area to substantiate the endocrine basis for the breast changes. More commonly, however, breast development occurs as part of an end-organ response to normal adrenal estrogen. This is particularly true when only one breast enlarges. If this occurs in the female child, usually normal puberty will bring about development of the other breast and the overall end result will be a normal one. However, occasionally hypertrophic development of one breast becomes so massive that surgical reduction is indicated. Nevertheless, most parents and children can be assured that such reduction is rarely necessary. Unilateral gynecomastia in the male child, on the other hand, may require surgical excision if the enlargement is enough to be obvious. Attention should be paid by the primary care physician to the technique utilized by the surgeon. Gynecomastia can almost always be treated through an areolar type of incision, which is inapparent after it heals. An incision in the area of the breast that is apparent may lead to as many questions and anxieties as the gynecomastia itself and thereby fail to solve the problem for the child.

ENDOCRINE PROBLEMS

Although endocrine problems are unusual in childhood and rarely require surgical intervention, certain problems with the endocrine glands are best solved by surgical intervention. For instance, *hyperthyroidism,* although usually responsive to medical therapy, may require surgical excision of the gland if the child is uncooperative in taking the daily medications or develops an allergy to them. The alternative of radioactive iodine therapy is believed by some authorities to be contraindicated in the young child[134] because of the possibility of long-term associated risks of hypothyroidism and thyroid carcinoma developing in a radiated gland.[134] An underdeveloped or dysplastic thyroid remnant may be present in a thyroglossal duct cyst and be the only thyroid tissue present in the child. The indicated excision of the thyroglossal duct cyst may remove the little functioning thyroid tissue the child has. Although the dysplastic tissue usually has been hypofunctional preoperatively, the total deprivation of thyroid tissue will increase the child's hypothyroid symptoms. Follow-up on any child who has excision of a thyroglossal duct is therefore important, especially if thyroid tissue is present on histologic evaluation of the specimen. Thyroid function studies obtained several weeks after surgery will indicate the hypothyroidism and alert the physician to the need to provide long-term maintenance therapy.

One of the most insidious endocrine lesions is *islet cell adenoma.* This lesion is an unusual one, and the symptoms may be far from clear-cut. Nevertheless, any child who shows signs of periods of confusion, sleepiness, and certainly of spells of unconsciousness should be investigated

for hypoglycemia. In infancy, these symptoms may be due to islet cell hyperplasia of a diffuse variety and be responsive to medication. In middle to late childhood, however, such symptoms are almost invariably due to an islet adenoma. Whipple's classic triad of spells of unconsciousness that are accompanied by hypoglycemia and responsive to the provision of sugar confirms the diagnosis.[140] Excision of the islet cell adenoma will usually be curative, but multiple adenomas may be present; and if hyperplasia that is unresponsive to medical therapy is the diagnosis, a subtotal or total pancreatectomy may be needed.[140]

Pheochromocytoma is a rare tumor of the adrenal medullary tissue or of any chromaffin tissue throughout the body. This lesion classically produces paroxysms of hypertension, but in children the hypertension is often sustained. It has been reported in children as young as 5 years of age.[13] Bilaterality, extraadrenal locations, and familial occurrences are all more common in children with pheochromocytomas. An association with the multiple endocrine adenopathy syndrome (MEA$_2$) has been reported. A pheochromocytoma should be suspected in any child with symptoms of hypertension, such as headache, sweating episodes, or seizures, in whom hypertension is confirmed. Hypertension in childhood is an unusual lesion and is usually caused either by a neuroblastoma, pheochromocytoma, or renal vascular lesion. The latter can be demonstrated by arteriography, and pheochromocytoma can be diagnosed by increased urinary catecholamines, various incitatory tests, or the response of the patient to phentolamine.[57] Surgical excision is curative, and the incidence of malignancy is low. The surgery is hazardous unless the patient is well prepared by preoperative volume expansion, a short-term course of an alpha blocker such as phenoxybenzamine, and the ready availability of propranolol for any arrhythmias caused during the surgery. Nitroprusside has been useful for hypertensive crises during surgery.[43] The best results are obtained with a team approach wherein careful preoperative planning is done by the team, which should include the surgeon, the anesthesiologist, the primary care physician, and the endocrinologist. General discussion of the possible complications during and after surgery and preoperative preparation for appropriate intraoperative responses usually lead to a problem-free surgical experience.

Precocious puberty is a complex problem with

many causes. Its recognition should lead to early referral to an endocrinologist for a thorough evaluation. The surgeon may become involved when abnormally functioning primary sex organs are contributing to the secondary manifestations of precocious puberty. An indepth discussion of this problem is beyond the scope of this book.

TRAUMA
Major blunt trauma

Major trauma is the most serious entity to afflict the childhood age group. Although most major trauma will require that the primary care physician consult with a surgeon early in the course of the disease and in some cases the child will have been taken directly to an emergency room, where either a surgeon or an emergency care specialist will be attending to the child, in many instances the primary care physician is called first, and his responses may determine the success or failure of subsequent treatment. Despite the multitude of variations in the injury pattern, only four entities are responsible for death: interference with proper ventilation, shock to the point of injurious organ hypoperfusion, permanent injury to the brain, and sepsis. Thus, the resuscitating physician's attention must be directed primarily to correction of blood loss, maintenance of adequate ventilation and oxygenation, careful ongoing assessment of any injury to the brain itself, and prevention of infection.

The principles of resuscitation for major trauma are so basic as to be well-known to anyone who has had a simple first-aid course. However, they are so often forgotten in the confusion of the emergency setting that they must be repeated and emphasized. First, a *clear airway* must be assured and established. This may require aspiration of secretions from the hypopharynx, the placement of an oral airway, or the insertion of a translaryngeal endotracheal tube. Rarely is tracheostomy indicated as an emergency procedure, but it must be instantly available if translaryngeal intubation fails. If the patient is so obtunded as to be incapable of sustaining normal respiratory effort, artificial ventilation must be provided either mouth to mouth, or by bag and mask insufflation or the attachment of a mechanical ventilator by means of an endotracheal tube.

At the same time that respiratory resuscitation is taking place, the *adequacy of the pulse and blood pressure* must be assessed and dependable intravenous cannulas established. This can usu-

ally be achieved by a percutaneous technique[45]; if this technique is difficult, however, a cut-down procedure over any vein that is easily accessible should be rapidly accomplished rather than waste additional valuable time attempting percutaneous puncture. The technique of incisional exposure of the saphenous vein at the ankle should be known to any physician who might ever be involved in an emergency resuscitative effort. Blood should be obtained for cross-match, blood count, and chemistry evaluation. If the pulse and blood pressure are not normal and stable, a rapid infusion of balanced electrolyte solution should be given to stabilize the patient and should be continued as necessary until blood is available. If the patient is in severe shock from blood loss, unmatched O negative blood should be administered until a properly cross-matched supply of blood is available. In giving blood, the bolus technique of providing one fourth of the blood volume of the individual as a push and then observing the patient for stability or instability, rather than a continuous infusion, is most useful. This technique allows evaluation of the stability of the patient and gives information regarding ongoing blood loss.[98]

Three other things should be accomplished almost simultaneously. First, *a record* should be started and someone assigned to keep a continuous account of all the information regarding the patient, including vital signs, drugs administered, and level-of-consciousness evaluations. Determining the patient's *level of consciousness* is the second maneuver that should be accomplished at the earliest possible time in the resuscitation; the patient's level of consciousness should be recorded then and observed frequently over the subsequent resuscitative period. Third, *a nasogastric tube* should be inserted into the stomach, the stomach aspirated of its contents, any abnormalities of the contents noted, and the stomach kept decompressed. The importance of this cannot be overemphasized, since failure to decompress the stomach has led to some of the most serious complications in major trauma and has left many children maimed for life who were not seriously injured in the original accident. The reason for this is the propensity of the child at just about any age to cry, hyperventilate, and swallow air, leading to gastric dilatation, which may produce a severe ileus and which may lead to vomiting with aspiration of recently ingested stomach contents and acid. Pulmonary injury from such aspiration may far outweigh any trauma that ensued from the accident itself, and the severe ileus has led to unwarranted explorations of the peritoneal cavity that resulted in complications and injuries far beyond the direct trauma to the abdomen. If nothing else occurs, the distention that follows may mislead the physician into believing that a serious intra-abdominal injury exists and lead to unnecessary exploration. The following case history illustrates some of the complications of failure to insert a nasogastric tube.

Case history

A 5-year-old boy, having just visited the local hamburger shop with his sister, stepped off a curb while walking home and was struck by an automobile. He was taken to a local hospital, where he vomited and filled his hypopharynx with the recently ingested food material. Because the hypopharynx could not be cleared rapidly enough, an emergency tracheostomy was performed. On further evaluation, the child was found to have a blunt injury to his cranium; this injury was evaluated by arteriography, and no vascular abnormalities were seen. It was believed that he had a severe cerebral contusion, which accounted for his obtunded state. Indeed, with time, the child did recover full mentation.

With observation of the child over the next several days, it was noted that his abdomen had become increasingly distended. No nasogastric tube had been placed. Because of concerns regarding the distension, abdominal films were obtained; these showed a marked dilatation of the bowel gas pattern and a rectal temperature probe that had reached the left upper quadrant. It was believed that the child had a severe intra-abdominal injury and a probable perforation of the distal colon from the temperature probe. Exploratory laparotomy revealed the temperature probe to be intraluminal and showed no intra-abdominal injury whatsoever. When closure of the long midline incision extending from the xiphoid to the pubis was attempted, it was impossible to achieve complete replacement of the intestine because of the marked dilatation of the bowel. Consequently, the transverse colon, which was markedly distended, was left out as an exteriorized loop with the incision being closed above and below it.

Over the next several days, the child failed to regain bowel function and the obstruction persisted. Because the child's symptoms were suggestive of an inflammatory process in his abdomen and because of the marked weight loss that was ensuing, the child was transported to the children's medical center, where on admission he was found to have a clear-cut mechanical bowel obstruction, signs of peritonitis, and a wasted appearance consistent with moderate weight loss. Total parenteral nutrition was established, along with broad-spec-

trum intravenous antibiotic therapy; and after a positive nitrogen balance was reestablished, the child's abdomen was explored. Two loops of small bowel were caught in the incisional closure, and intussusception of the small bowel had occurred secondary to this obstruction. One of the intussuscepted loops was totally necrotic and undergoing autolysis within the intussuscipiens. The bowel was resected, primary anastomosis accomplished, and decompression achieved; abdominal closure concluded the procedure.

The child had a complicated postoperative course but eventually seemed to recover on a regimen of broad-spectrum antibiotics and total parenteral nutrition. He subsequently developed a *Candida* meningitis with a *Candida* abscess of the brain, which left him with a permanent deficiency in mental functioning. This was a secondary insult, the child having totally recovered from his initial cerebral contusion.

The above case is an extreme example of complications that can result from failure to decompress the gastrointestinal tract, but less severe difficulties arise almost daily from failure to observe this important principle.

Once an airway and proper mechanical or autogenous ventilation are achieved, the circulatory status supported and stabilized, a nasogastric tube in place and functioning, and a mental status examination accomplished, other major injuries, such as fractures, dislocations, and major lacerations, should be attended to. Fractures should be splinted on site with traction splinting when available. If the patient must be moved before adequate immobilization of a fracture can be accomplished, he should be moved in such a way that no force is exerted on the fracture line and in such a way that there is traction control of any potential fractures of the extremities. This means dragging the patient by the head, if necessary, to maintain alignment of the cervical vertebrae.

Other considerations in dealing with major trauma include the need for antibiotics and the need for tetanus prophylaxis. Antibiotics are indicated when any major contamination of the peritoneal or pleural cavities occurs or in major lacerations that are severely contaminated. They are also indicated in human bites.

The general principles of tetanus prophylaxis are that for an injury that is not tetanus prone, that is, is not a dirty wound or a wound producing devitalized tissue, the patient does not need a prophylactic tetanus toxoid inoculation booster if he has had the basic series of toxoid and has received a booster within 5 years. Most major trauma leads to tetanus-prone wounds, however. For a tetanus prone wound, the patient should have had a toxoid booster inoculation within 1 year.[118]

Specific injuries

Although a complete discussion of every potential injury that could occur in major trauma is beyond the scope of this text, certain injuries are complicated and require proper attention to avoid life-threatening or crippling complications.

Blunt trauma to the *cranium* is best evaluated by level-of-consciousness evaluations. If the patient is fully conscious and has experienced no period of unconsciousness, a severe injury to the brain is unlikely. If the patient sustained a short period of unconsciousness and then awoke, or if the patient had a lucid interval and then became obtunded, concern for subdural and epidural hemorrhages is indicated. A CT brain scan should be obtained. In most instances of minor trauma to the cranium, skull x-ray films are not indicated; these radiographs have been much overused and abused in the past because of medical-legal considerations. The recent emphasis on decreasing the indications for skull films should be applauded and adhered to.[50] The child who has had no period of unconsciousness, who is fully awake and mentating normally, and who has no palpable fracture in the cranium or other signs of cranial fracture does not need skull films. This is particularly true for the child who sustains minor lacerations about the face and head—injuries common in childhood. However, when major trauma is accompanied by some degree of loss of consciousness, skull films should be obtained. Cervical spine films should probably be obtained in any patient who has had significant blunt trauma such as that sustained in an automobile accident, either as a passenger or as a pedestrian. Missing these injuries can lead to laceration of the cord and death or a lifetime of total paralysis. Thoracolumbar spine films should be obtained in any unconscious patient who has sustained blunt trauma, especially from a fall. They should be selectively obtained in the alert, conscious patient who has any physical signs or symptoms or in whom the type of trauma sustained suggests the possibility of such an injury.

Blunt trauma to the *chest* may produce severe injury to the lung or to the great vessels or heart. These injuries may not be apparent on initial physical examination or on initial radiographs. If evidence of such injury is present or suspected, reevaluation of the chest is mandatory and repeat x-ray films should be obtained with comparison views. Over a period of several hours, severe pulmonary contusion can lead to marked hemorrhage, and failure to provide ongoing evaluation of such injuries may lead to severe pulmonary decompensation just at the time when the patient may be in the operating room undergoing extensive surgery for some other injury, such as femoral fracture or head trauma.

The problem of *cardiac tamponade* must be considered in any blunt trauma to the chest. Although it is not a common complication of such blunt trauma, it is one of the major causes of mortality when it is unsuspected. Reevaluation at frequent intervals is essential for any child who has sustained severe blunt trauma to the chest. The examiner must be assured that the cardiac sounds are strong and that the peripheral pulses remain firmly palpable. A repeat chest x-ray film following the initial evaluative film is a wise maneuver for any child with severe chest trauma, and part of that examination should include a comparison of the size of the heart on the two films. Any evidence of enlargement of the cardiac shadow should lead to suspicion of developing pericardial fluid and tamponade.

Blunt trauma to the *abdomen* can usually be evaluated by a combination of the stability of the patient's vital signs, the abdominal examination—particularly the presence or absence of tenderness—and the evidence on both physical examination and serial radiographs of continued bowel function. In the alert patient, an ongoing evaluation of this type will provide the important information necessary. We therefore do not favor routine paracentesis seeking blood as an indication for the need for exploratory laparotomy. Indications for paracentesis are the presence of neurologic injuries that may interfere with proper evaluation of the abdomen such that the patient does not respond to the tenderness that is present and the presence of multiple major injuries with an equivocal abdominal examination such that early decision regarding severe injury to the abdomen is important. One must accept the fact that paracentesis will be positive in a number of patients who would otherwise stabilize and not require exploratory laparotomy. If one performs this maneuver, one must be willing to act on it. Thus, the finding of free blood on paracentesis or the finding of over 100,000 red blood cells per milliliter of aspirate after a Ringer's lactate lavage of the peritoneal cavity suggests intraperitoneal hemorrhage and warrants exploration.[98] Because significant injuries to the spleen and minor lacerations of the liver can occur and the bleeding stop or be stabilized, the finding of free intraperitoneal blood does not force abdominal exploration in every instance.[34] These decisions, however, must be made by a surgeon who is experienced not only in the care of major trauma but in the care of such trauma in children. It is far better to explore the abdomen of a child unnecessarily, even though no injury is ultimately found, than to miss a serious injury under uncontrolled circumstances and allow the development of complications that may prove more life threatening and crippling than the original injury.

In regard to *splenic injuries,* the realization that splenectomy leads to postsplenectomy sepsis has changed the approach to dealing with the injured spleen over the past several years.[39,40,74] Although it was initially thought that overwhelming postsplenectomy sepsis followed splenectomy only for severe hematologic disorders and this only in the very young infant,[40,74] in recent years it has been found that this entity follows splenectomy for any reason and at any age.[122] Certain factors of both cellular and humoral immunity are found to be lacking in individuals who have been subjected to splenectomy, and this deficit makes them susceptible to overwhelming infec-

tion from such common organisms as the pneumococcus.[21,84,146] For years it was believed that the spleen was of little use to the older individual (that is, beyond early infancy), and at the same time it was thought that repair of the injured spleen was impossible without exceedingly high risks of renewed bleeding. Many recent series have been reported, however, in which even severely injured spleens have been repaired or partial splenectomy achieved, leaving a significant portion of functioning splenic tissue.[14,95,108,119] Thus, just as the liver is amenable to partial resection and repair, the spleen can be salvaged after trauma. Nonetheless, the management of a child with potential intraperitoneal trauma must be in the hands of a competent and experienced surgeon who can weigh the risk factors appropriately and evaluate the overall condition of the child in deciding for observation or exploration, and if exploration is chosen, for resection or salvage of the spleen.

The unstable child suspected of having an intraperitoneal injury should also be explored. Bolus infusions of blood will achieve replenishment of the vascular volume and allow a better estimate of ongoing losses. Continued bleeding is indicated by the child's continued relapse into an unstable vascular state after each bolus infusion.[98]

The spleen is not the only intraperitoneal organ susceptible to injury from blunt trauma; the *liver* is equally susceptible to injury, and the complications of hepatic injury may be considerably more complex. Radiologic investigations may be

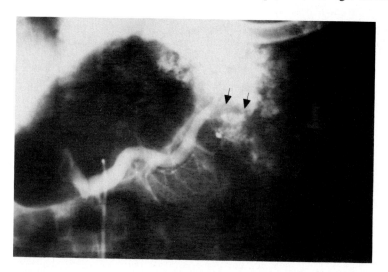

Fig. 20-13. Splenic arteriogram demonstrating a rupture through the central portion of the spleen (arrows). Splenic scans are being used more frequently today to define such injuries. (Courtesy Donald Kirks, M.D., Durham, N.C.)

helpful in demonstrating injury to major intra-peritoneal organs. The least complicated evaluation is probably the radioactive technetium scan, which is a good screening maneuver for the relatively stable patient; arteriography is more accurate in demonstrating the site of bleeding, however, and its use should be considered where a rapid decision and a high degree of immediate accuracy are desirable (Fig. 20-13).

Although splenic injuries may be treated with careful observation if all indications are that the bleeding has stopped, hepatic injuries should be explored, debrided, and drained, for the risks of hepatic abscess or late-onset hemobilia after a severe laceration of the liver make expectant treatment of known hepatic injuries unwise.

The third solid organ that is frequently injured is the *pancreas*. Because of its hidden location, injuries to it may be concealed for a period of time; thus, any history suggesting that the child received a direct blow to the epigastrium should make the physician suspect pancreatic trauma. The pancreas can be fractured across the vertebral column. An elevated serum amylase level may be helpful in indicating the presence of pancreatic trauma, but this indicator is useful only if the determination is obtained. Thus, pancreatic trauma must be con-sidered and the amylase level determined. Pancreatic trauma is the most common cause of pancreatic pseudocysts in the childhood age group.[22] If obvious acute trauma to the pancreas is not demonstrated on initial evaluation, careful reevaluation of the patient for the development of a pseudocyst is essential. A baseline ultrasound study and upper GI series with lateral films to show displacement of the stomach should be obtained and subsequent films obtained for comparison if the possibility of a pseudocyst persists (Fig. 20-14).

The same type of trauma that can injure the pancreas can lead to injury to *the duodenum*. Such injury may result in perforation but more often leads to a duodenal hematoma with obstruction, which may lead to unnecessary exploration if it is not understood. The short-term bowel obstruction is usually cleared with expectant treatment, and the patient can be treated with nasogastric suction and intravenous fluid and electrolyte maintenance[63] (Fig. 20-15).

The *kidneys* are fairly well protected in their retroperitoneal position but are frequently injured in major trauma. Two facts about renal injuries are important. First, when mild trauma injures the kidney, an underlying renal tumor or renal anomaly may be present.[51] These were found to

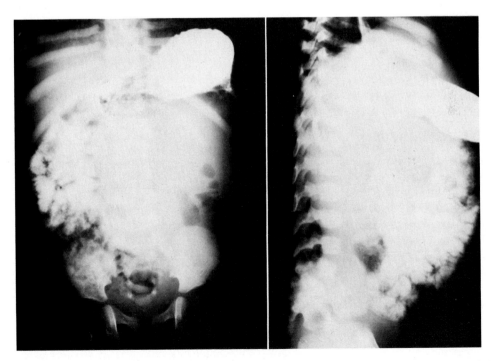

Fig. 20-14. Mass effect on the upper GI series with anterior displacement of the stomach on the lateral film. This finding is consistent with a pancreatic pseudocyst.

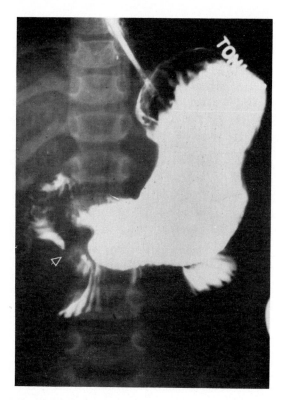

Fig. 20-15. Upper gastrointestinal radiograph showing partial obstruction of the duodenum with a "coiled spring appearance" (arrow) indicative of duodenal hematoma. The child began vomiting 24 hours after sustaining a blow to the epigastrium. (Courtesy Donald Kirks, M.D., Durham, N.C.)

be present in 10% to 23% of children in an emergency room population who sustained renal trauma from seemingly mild injury.[94,105] Second, renal injury may present late and should therefore be looked for subsequent to the initial acute evaluation if it is not found at that time. The initial IVP may show reasonably normal function even though fractures of the kidneys have occurred. Subsequently, the child may develop a perinephric hematoma and leak urine into the same space, resulting in a perinephric abscess.

Although a few years ago there was a burst of enthusiasm for exploration of all renal injuries, the pendulum has recently swung back to a conservative or expectant approach to the initial renal trauma when it is caused by a blunt force, although some centers continue to explore selected patients.

Although blunt trauma rarely produces significant injury to the *intestine,* the possibility does exist and any evidence of peritonitis should be investigated. Trauma in the area of the pelvis should lead to evaluation of the *bladder* and *urethra.* Injuries to the urethra are frequent accompaniments of pelvic fractures. A catheter should be passed into the meatus and a urethrogram obtained and evaluated. A cystogram and voiding cystourethrogram (VCG) should then be obtained to determine if there has been disruption of the bladder or urethra. Finally, a rectal examination should be performed to ensure that there is no evidence of laceration of the *rectum,* particularly in cases involving pelvic fractures. Microscopic evaluation of the urine for hematuria completes the screening modalities.

Stab wounds and missiles

Fortunately, children are not frequently involved in knife and gunshot trauma, but some realization of the differences of these injuries from blunt trauma is important. Injuries with sharp objects are fairly predictable in that their course is straight and it can be fairly well predicted which organs have been injured. The philosophy as to whether or not all stab wounds should be explored has changed back and forth over the years and varies from institution to institution. Nevertheless, it is incumbent on the physician to ensure in one way or another that the stab wound has not penetrated underlying organs to the point of injury. Missiles such as bullets are totally unpredictable and can follow numerous recoiling pathways within body cavities; thus, simply drawing a line from the entrance wound to the point of a projectile located by radiograph does not ensure that that line was the only one followed by the missile.

For both stab wounds and missiles, the fact that organs vary in position depending on the state of inspiration or expiration should be taken into consideration. The liver can descend several centimeters, as can the diaphragm; thus wounds in the upper abdomen may actually involve primarily chest organs—there may be damage to the lungs and heart from what would appear in expiration to have primarily damaged intraperitoneal organs. This fact must be carefully considered in the evaluation of such injuries.

Most authorities believe that all bullet wounds to the peritoneal cavity should be explored. This is not necessarily true of wounds of the thoracic cavities, since these can be evaluated by serial radiographs and vital sign evaluations. Even evidence of intrathoracic bleeding may call for only the placement of a chest tube if such bleeding is quickly controlled.

Major burns

Major burns can obviously affect the child of any age, as they can the adult of any age. Children are burned in house fires, automobile fires, and various other situations in which they are the innocent victims of the fire. Unfortunately, however, as the child enters the early childhood age group, he increasingly becomes the victim of burns that are of his own making. The young child, fascinated by matches and fire in general, may set his clothing on fire or throw matches into explosive liquids such as gasoline or charcoal lighter fluid. Constant vigilance is required on the part of the parents to protect the child of this age from the ravages of major burns.

Therapy of major burns is a topic that has produced volumes of books and journal articles, and a complete treatise on this subject is beyond the scope of this text. Nevertheless, the primary care physician should have some facility with resuscitation of the child with a major burn, since successful resuscitation may depend largely on the rapidity with which it is initiated.

Evaluation of the extent of the burn. The important aspect of this evaluation is to calculate properly the percentage of the body surface that is involved. In the adult and teenage patient, the "rule of nines" provides an easily remembered rough gauge of body surface area to aid in this calculation. According to this rule, the head is 9%, the anterior trunk is 18%, the posterior trunk is 18%, each upper extremity is 9%, and each lower extremity is 18%. This adds up to 99%, and the perineum is usually considered the additional 1%. The extent of the burn is then calculated by estimating the percentage of each of these areas that is burned.

At the other extreme is the young infant, whose head makes up 20% of this body. The anterior and posterior trunk make up 17% each, each upper extremity amounts to 8% of the body, and each lower extremity is 15% of the body.[88] This totals 100%. As the child progresses from infancy toward the teenage years, his body contour changes from the infant contour toward that of the adult. Appropriate changes should be made on the basis of the child's age and body habitus.

Judging the depth of the burn, beyond recog-nizing the first-degree burn, which is mere reddening of the intact epithelium, is extremely difficult. Particularly, differentiating very deep second-degree from third-degree burns may be impossible on initial evaluation. This is of little consequence, however, to the resuscitative efforts, for second- and third-degree burns require the same consideration as to fluid replacement.

Initial treatment. Initial treatment includes fluid replacement, airway involvement, and care of the burn wound.

Fluid replacement. Fluid is lost both externally into the environment through the destroyed epidermis and internally as edema into the subcutaneous tissues. Blistered second-degree burns represent fluid loss into the layer between the destroyed epidermis and the dermis. When the epidermis is totally burned off or the blisters rupture, continuing losses of fluid to the environment occur. It has been shown that most of the fluid shifts take place during the first hour after the burn injury and that almost all shifts occur within 8 hours following the burn.[82] Thus, resuscitative efforts must be initiated rapidly.

Many different regimens have been popularized over the years for replacement of fluids for the burn patient, with the major point of disagreement being the use of colloids in the initial resuscitative efforts. If the primary care physician can achieve a dependable cannula for vascular access, then calculate a 24-hour fluid replacement based on the individual's maintenance fluids plus a replacement based on the calculated percentage of the burn wound, and then begin infusing these fluids at a rate such that half of the 24-hour fluid requirement will be administered in the first 8 hours, he will have made a major contribution to the patient's successful resuscitation. The easiest approach for this initial therapy is to give the patient a maintenance volume of fluid plus 4 ml times the percent of the burn times the weight in kilograms, all this volume being given as 5% dextrose in Ringer's lactate. Again, note that half of this amount should be given in the first 8 hours following the burn. Transportation to a burn center should be arranged and the fluids set to run at the appropriate rate. If rapid transportation cannot be arranged, the rate of fluid administration should be increased to achieve a urine output of 2 ml/kg/hr.

Airway involvement. Another important consideration for the primary care physician in resuscitating the burn victim is that of airway involvement. Burns acquired outdoors rarely involve the airway unless the victim is directly burned around the head and face. However, burns occurring indoors, and especially explosions in closed places, may involve the inhalation of hot gases, which may cause severe edema of the respiratory tract, resulting in respiratory insufficiency. Early recognition of such injury is mandatory so that ventilatory support can be provided. Although this injury may initially appear to be quite benign, it is associated with a high mortality.

Care of the burn wound. Initial care of the burn wound by the primary care physician should consist primarily of protecting it from additional contamination. Wrapping the burn with sterile saline-soaked gauze dressings followed by additional dry sterile dressings is probably the easiest form of management. A topical antiseptic ointment such as silver sulfadiazine can be used if it is available. Mafenide is an excellent topical agent but is associated with carbonic anhydrase inhibition and, particularly if any pulmonary insufficiency exists, may lead to severe acidosis due to interference with excretion of acid by the kidney. Greasy ointments and gauze impregnated with greasy antiseptic compounds should not be used.

Referral. The best care and the highest survival rates for major burns occur in centers where a team approach to burns is utilized and where burns are cared for frequently. Transport to a center can usually be arranged readily. Most major medical centers have burn units, and Shriners hospitals throughout the country have been converting their facilities to burn units since the successful eradication of polio as a major chronic disease state in children.

· · ·

As noted initially, this discussion has not been intended to serve as an exhaustive treatise on major trauma. Obviously, the primary care physician needs the early consultative help and direction of an experienced surgeon or surgeons, depending on the areas of the body involved and the injury.

One area that the primary care physician may contribute considerably to is that of the emotional trauma to the child associated with major trauma. Often children who have been traumatized will have acute personality changes, some of which can be explained by the way the child views the trauma. It is common for parents to make admonitions to the child during the formative years regarding safety. For example, they may tell the child that disobedience of traffic laws will lead to the child being severely injured. When the child is injured, even though the child may not have contributed directly through his own negligence to the injury, the child immediately sees the injury as being the result of some misconduct or failure on his part. Thus, his pain and fear are mixed with guilt and anxiety, and the combination often makes the child withdrawn, fearful, and hostile. The child may expect additional punishment on top of the injury for his presumed misconduct. The parents must be helped to see how the injury looks to the child and to support and reassure him. With time as his injury abates, the child's guilt and anxiety will lessen and his normal personality will be restored. It is important that hospital personnel realize these emotional problems in children and respect their sometimes hostile and uncooperative attitudes. The parents must realize that these changes in the child's personality are acute and explainable and that they will revert back to normal with time and support.

Minor trauma

Minor burns are discussed in connection with the infant-toddler age group (Chapter 15), and their care in the older child is similar.

Lacerations

Lacerations are a common trauma for children and are often caused by falls or by the child being hit by such playground items as a swing. The usual locations are about the face and head, and the extremities are also frequently involved.

Evaluation. Evaluation of any underlying trauma, such as intracerebral trauma in relationship to lacerations about the face and head is essential. Where the possibility of bony injury is present, appropriate radiographic evaluation should be accomplished. In the past, skull x-ray films have been obtained much too thoughtlessly. They are probably unnecessary in any child who has not been unconscious and who has no palpable depression of bone. The injuring object and the extent of the force should be taken into consideration in making this decision, however.

A laceration occurring from broken glass or from a splinter or piece of wood must be investigated for the presence of a foreign body. The other source of foreign body is a laceration occurring through clothing. This evaluation can be accomplished by extensive probing of the well-anesthetized wound. Occasionally, radiographic evaluation is helpful, particularly if there is lead in the glass.

Treatment. Treatment of the laceration requires adequate debridement of any devitalized tissue as well as any foreign matter present in the wound. Extensive irrigation should be achieved. The decision to close the wound primarily immediately rather than use delayed primary closure or open packing with healing by secondary intention depends on the length of time since the injury, the degree of contamination and the ability to clean the wound, and, to some extent, the location of the injury.

Clean wounds seen within 6 to 8 hours from the time of injury may be sutured with the expectation that primary healing will occur. Minor lacerations can often be handled with the use of surgical adhesive strips, avoiding the need for sutures and their removal. More extensive lacerations should be carefully approximated with absorbable deep suture material and very fine, carefully placed sutures in the skin.

Wound healing considerations. It is essential to be familiar with the chronologic steps in wound healing in order to evaluate the time that the wound requires suture stability and immobilization. The following discussion contains the major time factors for the healing of a clean surgical wound.

The most obvious occurrence after a clean incised wound is that of hemorrhage. This is followed by clotting, which forms a fibrin matrix that binds the wound together and eventually seals it. In response to the injury, a polymorphonuclear leukocyte response ensues and lasts for 1 to 2 days. This response is followed and in the later stages accompanied by a macrophage phagocytic response that cleans up the debris in the wound. From approximately 3 to 7 days after the wound occurs, the major activity is that of capillary ingrowth forming granulation tissue. Toward the end of this stage, fibroblasts appear in the wound and soon become numerous. By the seventh day, the wound contains primarily granulation tissue, fibroblasts, and some early collagen formation.[91]

During the next 7 days, lasting until approximately the fourteenth day after wounding, the primary activity is that of continued fibroblast

proliferation and the formation of collagen. From days 14 to 21, this collagen is added to and oriented into fibrils, giving the wound its initial tensile strength.

Over the course of the next several months, additional collagen is laid down in the wound and further orientation of the collagen into fibrils occurs. This phase is one of hypertrophic scar formation, and the metabolic activity in the wound continues at an accelerated pace. During the last 6 months of the year after the occurrence of the wound, the hypertrophic scar formation ebbs and eventually some scar is withdrawn and the wound becomes softer and somewhat more elastic. By the end of the year, there is usually no obvious excess metabolic activity occurring in the wound.

This chronologic scheme is helpful in making decisions about such things as the removal of sutures, the need for splinting, and also the length of time that tubes and drains should remain. (The management of tubes and drains is covered in Chapter 6 in the section on general considerations.) Those wounds that are in an area where cosmesis is important are often handled differently from the average. For the standard wound, the major considerations in removing sutures have to do with balancing the need to hold the wound together against the propensity of sutures to become infected sinus tracts and form epithelialized and collagenized tracts. Since there is little collagen laid down in the wound before the seventh day, most wounds can remain sutured until this time. The longer the sutures remain after the seventh day, however, the more collagen is laid down around them and the more epithelialized the suture tract becomes. Therefore, for most wounds the sutures are removed on the seventh day.

For wounds where cosmetic considerations are of major import, such as on the face, the sutures should be removed earlier, before any collagen formation occurs and before there is any degree of epithelialization of the tract. Thus, these sutures are often removed on the third or fourth postoperative day. The looseness of the skin about the face makes this possible, as does the excellent blood supply, which tends to increase the overall speed with which the wound heals.

Sutures can almost always be replaced by butterfly bandages (Steri-Strips) if adequate splinting is provided. This may take the form of a bulky dressing or, if the wound is in the area of a joint, may require either a half-shell splint or a full cast. With early removal of the sutures and utilization of adhesive strips and splinting to maintain the integrity of the wound, the cosmetic effects are superior and the risk of infection reduced.

Realization that adequate tensile strength is really reached in a wound only after approximately 21 days should lead the physician to maintain splinting of the wound in the area of a joint or major muscle group until such strength is acquired. It is a great disservice to the patient to free him of the burden of the primary wound early only to have the wound dehisce with the possible consequence of secondary infection and a prolonged debility. I have seen children with lacerations of the knee whose sutures were removed on the seventh day and in whom there was instant wound dehiscence. When the primary care physician failed to reclose the wound immediately, it became contaminated and infected, requiring repeated surgical procedures and prolonged dressing care over a period of 2 to 3 months to achieve secondary healing. A simple splint applied for 2 weeks would have avoided this maloccurrence.

Finally, it should be recognized that if a wound does dehisce because of secondary trauma or the forces acting around a joint and there is no evidence of infection in the wound, it can be immediately washed out with antiseptic solution and resutured or taped together. All of the elements necessary to heal the wound are in the immediate vicinity of the disrupted wound, and most often healing will occur at an accelerated pace. Leaving the wound open to become secondarily contaminated and infected is a major mistake.

When a laceration fails to heal, the presence of a foreign body should be suspected. Radiographs should be obtained; and if these prove to be negative, the wound should be carefully reexplored for pieces of glass or foreign debris.

Injuries deserving special consideration

Two injuries that are somewhat unusual but that require special understanding are those of wringer and bicycle spoke injuries. To some extent, they are similar in their complexity and complications.

Wringer injuries[2,104] occur in the population that still uses electric wringer washing machines. The infant and sometimes young child will, out of curiosity, put his hand and arm into the running wringer. What happens next determines to a great extent how serious the injury may be. Children's

tissues are highly elastic and resilient, and if the parent simply turns off the wringer, releases the pressure, and allows the child to remove his extremity, little damage usually occurs. However, if the parent, in a state of panic, pulls the child's arm from the still-running wringer, a counterforce is applied that produces a "degloving" type of force that may cause severe compressive injury to the child's extremity. Fractures are unusual associated injuries but should be sought by radiography. The main injury to be concerned with is that to the antecubital fossa, where compression injury may lead to severe swelling and cause obstruction of the vascular supply to the distal arm and hand. This obstruction produces Volkmann's ischemic contracture, and the resulting edema may lead to a complication that is more serious than the initial injury. There may be little obvious external injury to such an extremity, but hospitalization and observation are essential to prevent the ischemic injury that may follow. On the other hand, there may be obvious damage to the superficial tissues (Fig. 20-16); and if a severe degloving type of force was applied, there may be actual flaps of skin and soft tissue lifted from the extremity.

For the usual wringer injury, simple cleansing and wrapping with a loose wrap and elevation of the extremity will suffice during the 24- to 48-hour period of observation. The distal extremity should be exposed and observed at least hourly to ensure that the blood supply remains intact. The arm should be unwrapped and careful inspection of the entire extremity provided at 24 and 48 hours following the injury. If no complications have developed by that time, the child may be released for routine follow-up of any obvious injuries.

Bicycle spoke injuries[64] arise by a similar mechanism. The increasing popularity of bicycles has led many young parents to carry their young children on the back of the bicycle. Unless the infant seat provided has a flap on each side to protect the child's lower extremities from the rotating wheels, the child may accidentally or intentionally put his foot into the revolving wheel. It is then caught in the revolving spokes and turned until it hits the immovable strut coming down from the frame to the axle. There the child's foot is caught between the rotating spokes and the fixed strut and compressed in a crushing, shearing type of force that produces a typical injury involving a distally based triangular skin flap on the medial

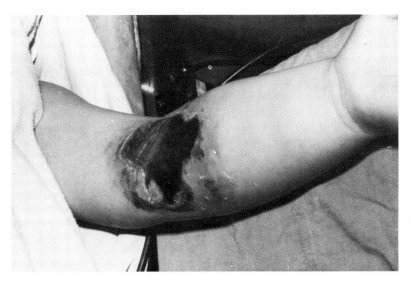

Fig. 20-16. Full-thickness skin loss in the antecubital fossa in a child with a wringer injury who was inadequately followed.

side of the ankle and a severe crush of the under-lying soft tissues.

Rarely is a fracture involved, but radiographs should be obtained. The major considerations are to realize that the distally based flap has a poor blood supply, which must come in by collateral vessels, and to recognize the severity of the un-derlying crush injury. Again, subsequent edema may produce ischemic loss to the tissues distal to the site of the injury, and elevation, soft com-pressive wrapping, and frequent observation, as in the case of the wringer injury, are important aspects of initial care. The distally based flap may fail to survive. The injury should be inspected at frequent intervals and debrided, and eventually skin grafts should be done if necessary. The typical serious bicycle spoke injury will incapacitate the child as far as the use of that extremity for an average of 6 weeks. Discussion of these factors with the parents at the time of the initial injury will avoid a great deal of misunderstanding and animosity if subsequent complications do develop.

FOLLOW-UP ON EARLIER SURGICAL CONDITIONS

Once a child has had surgery, that fact in his history becomes of significance to the examining physician, especially when the surgery was in the abdomen. Rather than being concerned about recurrence of specific entities, the physician should forever keep in mind the common and frequent complication of abdominal surgery: intestinal obstruction due to adhesions. It matters not how simple or complex the original surgical problem was; the mere entry into the peritoneal cavity puts the child at lifelong risk for developing adhesive bowel obstruction. The fact that symptomatic obstruction is frequently brought on by a gastro-intestinal viral syndrome probably is related to the change in anatomic relationships of the loops of bowel that are already adherent one to another. Increased peristaltic activity during an episode of gastroenteritis may cause a loop of bowel to inter-pose itself between already adherent loops or to twist itself about a fibrous band formed from an old adhesion. In addition, the rapid peristalsis associated with many gastrointestinal syndromes may make a partial obstruction more symptomatic because of the inability of the intestinal contents to pass through the narrowed area. The ensuing dilatation of the bowel proximal to the obstruc-tion may lead to kinking and further obstruction of the loop.

Complete obstruction is generally heralded by cessation of stools, abdominal distention, crampy abdominal pain, and vomiting of bile-stained or feculent material. When strangulation obstruction is involved and loops of bowel are ischemic, rapid loss of vascular integrity and a shocklike picture may develop. On the other hand, partial obstruc-tion may present as an episode of crampy ab-dominal pain and distention, following shortly after the onset of what seemed to be a typical gastroenteritis syndrome with diarrhea, fever, and vomiting. Any child who has had previous abdominal surgery and who has symptoms of crampy pain, distention, and vomiting should have an early abdominal radiographic series looking for signs of intestinal obstruction. If complete obstruction can be identified from the plain films, and particularly when the child is severely symptomatic, surgery should be accomplished at once. If complete obstruction is not clearly evident, we favor instilling 2 to 3 ounces of barium into the stomach and obtaining plain abdominal films over the next several hours to follow the course of the barium through the bowel. If the barium passes on through the colon, partial obstruction is proved and the child can be treated with nasogastric decompression, intravenous fluid therapy, and watchful waiting. Often the intestinal obstruction will be resolved as the gastrointestinal syndrome abates. On the other hand, if complete obstruction is demonstrated, surgery can be accomplished expeditiously.

We do not share the fear that many individuals have expressed in the past of putting barium down behind an obstruction. This does not lead to the kind of problems that occur in an adult patient with an obstructing colon carcinoma in whom a barium cast of the colon is formed behind the obstruction, which cannot be cleaned out and which leaves the patient at considerable risk for soilage to occur during the surgical procedure. The use of barium has often resolved what might otherwise have been a worrisome differential diagnosis problem and has led either to the avoidance of additional surgery for the child or to the expeditious accomplishment of indicated surgery.

Although each entry into the peritoneal cavity may cause the formation of additional adhesions, recurrent obstructions are fortunately not usual, probably because the more adhesions there are, the less free bowel there is to become entrapped. Nevertheless, recurrent adhesive bowel obstruction is of concern in the child who has had recurrent abdominal exploration.

What follows is a step-by-step review of the major entities of the newborn and infant-toddler periods; in each of the lesions, the long-term complications to be looked for are pointed out.

Diaphragmatic and hiatus hernias

As with all hernias, recurrence of a diaphragmatic hernia is possible. Proper repair of a diaphragmatic hernia of Bochdalek, with a careful search for the occasionally present peritoneal sac, makes recurrence unlikely, however. A hiatus hernia whose major symptomatic problem is gastroesophageal reflux may recur, but it is a failure of the antireflux procedure rather than a breakdown of the hernia repair that usually leads to the return of symptoms. With the fundoplication procedures, recurrence of gastroesophageal reflux is unusual.

Lobar emphysema

When lobar emphysema is truly a localized isolated entity, it is usually resolved with medical management or leads to urgent surgical excision of the lobe in infancy. When, however, lobar emphysema is part of a generalized congenital adenomatoid degeneration of the lung, further symptomatic changes in additional areas of the lung may occur over time and lead to progressive lung dysfunction.

Chest wall deformities

A small but definite percentage of chest wall deformities recur, and since the original surgery was done both for cosmetic reasons and to correct any impairment of cardiovascular function, recorrection must again be based on the extent of cosmetic deformity and the extent of cardiac compression. The attitudes of the child and the parents toward the deformity should also influence the decision.

Esophageal atresia and gastroesophageal reflux

Although many authorities have described the long-term dysfunction of patients with esophageal atresia repairs, and most functional evaluations of the esophagus show some dysmotility of the repaired esophagus,[106] in our experience most children have had little in the way of symptoms after repair. When primary anastomosis with careful mucosal-to-mucosal apposition of the esophageal segments without tension and with well-vascularized tissue is accomplished, the postoperative course is generally benign and the child requires little in the way of long-term care. It must be recognized however, that the potential for stricture formation and for narrowing of the esophagus with growth is present; thus, if the child has symptoms of dysphagia or frank choking episodes, early reevaluation of the esophagus is indicated. In addition, either all children have a propensity to swallow strange objects or children with esophageal atresia have a greater propensity to do so, because the incidence of foreign bodies lodging above the esophageal atresia repair is significant. Therefore, when the child who has had a remote repair of esophageal atresia and who has had normal functioning suddenly presents with signs of esophageal dysfunction, ingestion of a foreign body should be strongly suspected and the child should be evaluated with a barium esophagogram followed by esophagoscopy if indicated (see Fig. 15-27).

The incidence of gastroesophageal reflux in patients after esophageal atresia repair has been significant.[4,102] Some of this may be due to excessive mobilization of the distal esophageal segment, which may cause the segment to be pulled up into the chest, destroying the normal angle of His at the gastroesophageal junction. Nevertheless, we have had a significant incidence of postoperative gastroesophageal reflux problems with our esophageal repairs despite the fact that we do almost no mobilization of the distal segment whatsoever. Although the child with recurrent aspiration pneumonia after esophageal atresia and tracheoesophageal fistula repair should be evaluated for the possibility of a recurrent tracheoesophageal fistula, the more likely finding will be that the child has gastroesophageal reflux and is aspirating from this entity. When the problem occurs in the early postoperative period, positional therapy may be successful in restoring normal gastroesophageal sphincter function. If the problem persists, if recurrent pneumonia is noted while the child is undergoing positional therapy, or if the reflux is believed to be contributing to recurrent stenosis at the anastomotic site, surgical correction by fundoplication should be accomplished.

Evaluation for a recurrent tracheoesophageal fistula after esophageal atresia and tracheoesophageal fistula repair can be one of the most difficult evaluations in pediatric surgery. Bronchoscopy and esophagoscopy with the Storz infant telescopic endoscope will be 100% successful in demonstrating a primary tracheoesophageal fistula.[53] However, for a recurrent fistula, the tracheal pit representing the location of the previous fistula is expected to be present, and it is necessary to demonstrate that this pit still connects to the esophagus. Demonstrating this connection by endoscopy may be very difficult (see Fig. 15-26), and cinefluorography of the esophagus may show what appears to be a recurrent fistula when what is being seen is actually gastroesophageal reflux with aspiration of small amounts of the contrast medium into the trachea and into the pit. We have found that catheters such as those used for cardiac catheterization passed down the esophagus during fluoroscopy can be used to cannulate the recurrent fistula and demonstrate its presence clearly.[75] Obviously, this technique should be done by a pediatric radiologist experienced in its use.

Pure tracheoesophageal fistula and laryngotracheoesophageal cleft

The pure tracheoesophageal fistula and laryngotracheoesophageal cleft repairs may break down; thus, if recurrent aspiration pneumonia is a problem after these lesions have been repaired, reevaluation for recurrence should be accomplished expeditiously.

Pyloric stenosis

When proper surgical techniques are utilized in performing a pyloromyotomy, persistence or recurrence of pyloric stenosis is extremely unusual and complications occur very infrequently. However, unless the pyloromyotomy is carried proximal enough onto the gastric wall, dividing the oblique muscle of Torgersen,[66] persistence of the obstruction may be expected. Since the procedure involves only a limited area of the upper abdomen, the incidence of postoperative adhesive bowel obstruction is low.

Atresias of the small bowel

Atresias of the small bowel, when properly corrected, are associated only with the routine adhesive bowel obstructions common to any intraabdominal procedure. For high intestinal obstructions, especially those high in the jejunum, where resection of the overly dilated proximal portion of bowel is not possible, an end-to-end anastomosis carefully performed may still turn out to be functionally an end-to-side anastomosis. This is due to the marked disparity in the size of the bowel, which results in an oblique suture line and may lead to a blind loop syndrome typical of the side-to-side anastomoses performed for these lesions in earlier years[55,100] (Fig. 20-17). With constant buffeting of the intestinal contents against the bulbous end of the enlarged proximal segment, stretching of this segment beyond the anastomotic level may occur, forming a blind loop, which may lead to stasis of the intestinal

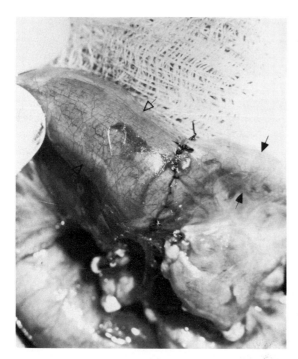

Fig. 20-17. Oblique suture line resulting when a dilated proximal segment (open arrow) is sutured to a narrowed distal segment (closed arrows) after resection of an area of jejunal atresia. This procedure may result in a blind loop syndrome similar to the side-to-side anastomosis complication illustrated in Fig. 20-18.

contents with a change in bacterial flora and a change in the ratio of bile salt to bile acid (Fig. 20-18). The result may be malabsorptive symptoms in the distal ileum, with failure of absorption of those entities, such as vitamin B_{12}, that are absorbed only in the distal ileum. An intestinal hurry syndrome due to the cathartic effect of the bile salts may lead to inadequate absorption of nutrients, which may lead to small stature, growth retardation, and chronic intestinal discomfort. Treatment involves reresection of as much dilated proximal bowel as possible, with tailoring of the new anastomosis to achieve an end-to-end coaptation. Usually this technique can be better accomplished at this later stage of life, when the child's intestine is larger and there is less disparity between the proximal bowel and the now more widely dilated and developed distal segment.

Meconium ileus

Since meconium ileus is the intestinal syndrome associated with cystic fibrosis, which presents in the newborn period, the same combination of events that lead to meconium ileus in utero can present an equivalent picture in postnatal life known as *meconium ileus equivalent*.[24] This entity involves inspissation of intestinal contents in the distal ileum and proximal colon due to inadequate intestinal enzymes and thick intestinal secretions. The use of pancreatic enzymes will lessen the incidence and risks of this entity developing, but frequently patients who are taking these preparations will experience episodes of obstruction when they either fail to take their medication or when other illnesses such as viral syndromes associated with vomiting make it impossible for them to keep the medication down. The physician caring for such patients should be aware of these problems and be prepared to treat any signs of obstruction with enemas, laxatives, and mineral oil early in their course. Usually, with the irrigation of enzymes down from above and the utilization of water-soluble contrast enemas from below, meconium ileus equivalent episodes can be treated without surgery. Occasionally, the obstruction becomes so severe that surgical decompression is necessary. Thus, early vigorous medical therapy is warranted to avoid the need for surgery in these high-risk patients. Great care must be taken to differentiate the acute abdomen of appendicitis or other lesions from meconium ileus equivalent. Too often, the child with cystic fibrosis is readily branded as having another episode of meconium ileus equivalent every time he has abdominal symptoms. With the child receiving chronic antibiotic therapy, the flagrant inflammatory reaction of appendicitis may be aborted, and the child may go on with a low-grade inflammatory process in the appendix for months or years before it is discovered that the episodes thought to be meconium ileus equivalent were, in fact, chronic appendicitis. On the other hand, what we thought was a chronically inflamed appendix in a child with an asymptomatic cecal mass proved to be meconium inspissated in the cecum.

Necrotizing enterocolitis

Necrotizing enterocolitis of the newborn generally takes its greatest toll in that period of life. However, some patients who recover from necrotizing enterocolitis with medical therapy will, weeks or months later, have intestinal obstruction due to stricture formation in areas of the bowel where the damage was significant but not extensive enough to cause perforation.[87,125] These chil-

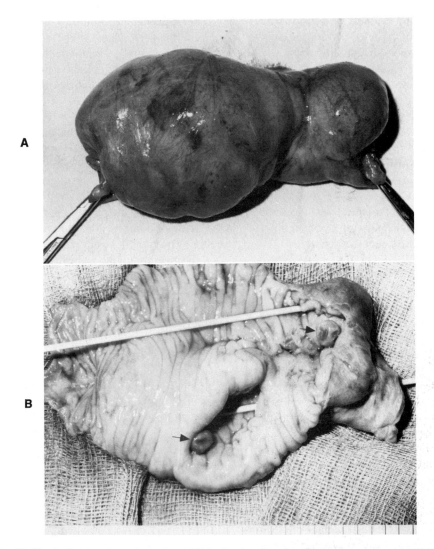

Fig. 20-18. A, Resected specimen in a child who developed a partial obstruction and "blind loop syndrome" from an old side-to-side anastomosis. **B,** The bowel lumen is exposed with the markers passed through the two channels. The stasis that exists in such an entity is suggested by the two peas indicated by the arrows.

dren will have signs of intestinal obstruction and can usually be treated quite readily with a straight-forward excision of the strictured area with primary anastomosis. The morbidity following such procedures is low and the cure rate high.

Of greater concern are those children who are left with a short bowel syndrome. This syndrome may be due to actual intestinal resection at surgery when the bowel is extensively destroyed by the primary lesion, or it may be due to extensive destruction of the mucosal lining with a malabsorption syndrome that may persist over prolonged periods of time. If the child can be maintained on a regimen of total parenteral nutrition without

sustaining episodes of severe sepsis, the bowel will usually adapt by means of villous hypertrophy of the mucosal lining and enable the child to gradually resume a normal diet. However, the child's intestinal tract remains sensitive to any changes in his general health, and with the least little bacterial or viral illness he may develop severely debilitating gastroenteritis. The child should be admitted to the hospital early in the course of the disease so that the bowel can be placed at rest and intravenous fluid support given to avoid excessive challenge to the sensitive intestinal lining.

Probably not enough children have been followed for a long-enough time after severe necrotizing enterocolitis to evaluate any growth retardation or long-term chronic malabsorption syndrome that may result. It certainly is possible, however, that these children will exhibit varying degrees of malabsorption problems, particularly since the disease so frequently destroys the distal ileum with its several unique, localized functions.[70] Therefore, the primary care physician must stay ever alert to the fact that the child had this severe disease in the neonatal period; if any signs of anemia, growth retardation, failure to thrive, or recurrent bowel dysfunction develop, he should investigate the intestines thoroughly. Error should be on the side of overtreating and overprotecting the gastrointestinal tract.

Meconium plug and small left colon syndromes

The neonatal constipation syndromes such as the meconium plug and small left colon syndromes have little in the way of long-term complications except for the usual risk of adhesive bowel obstruction. This risk would be significant only if the child required surgery in the course of treatment. Since most of these patients respond to water-soluble enema evacuation, the incidence of adhesive bowel obstruction should be low.

Hirschsprung's disease

Hirschsprung's disease is usually cured by anastomosis of ganglion-containing bowel to the anus. However, each surgical procedure for Hirschsprung's disease has its own peculiar set of complications.[36,79,112] The Swenson procedure, a pull-through of the full proximal colon for anastomosis to the full anus utilizing an everted cuff of anorectum,[129] has significant complications, especially in the hands of surgeons not trained in the procedure. The major complications are anastomotic leak, anastomotic stenosis, failure to achieve a low-enough anastomosis (resulting in persistence of the constipating symptoms of Hirschsprung's disease), and destruction of the nerve supply to the urogenital structures during the pelvic dissection. All of these problems should be considered in following the child who has had a Swenson procedure. Constipation symptoms should be thoroughly investigated with barium enema evaluation to be sure that the bowel proximal to the anastomosis is not dilated and hypertrophied, suggesting the persistence of an excessively long aganglionic segment.

The Duhamel procedure,[35,92,124] which is popular in many centers, is the simplest operation for Hirschsprung's disease and with the advent of the automatic stapling devices has had a lessened incidence of complications. Originally, the patient was left with a significant flap or septum between the retained proximal aganglionic pouch and the posterior pulled-through normal colon. In this procedure normal colon is pulled down behind a pouch of aganglionic bowel and anastomosed just above the anus in an end-to-side fashion, leaving a double wall made up of the posterior wall of the aganglionic rectal pouch and the anterior wall of the normal pulled-through colon. This double wall was previously crushed with a crushing clamp, and if the clamp failed to achieve adequate destruction of the wall, stool would accumulate in the aganglionic proximal pouch and eventually a large fecaloma would form, pushing the septum backward and occluding the normal colon segment. With the use of the automatic stapling devices, a better and more definitive opening can be accomplished in the conjoined wall so that this flap does not remain. However, the staples are applied in such a way that complete hemostasis may not be achieved, and bleeding episodes in the raw cuff after this procedure may be significant. They may come on many months or years after the original surgery.

The most common operation being performed for Hirschsprung's disease in the United States today is the Boley modification of the Soave procedure.[15,77,124] Based on attempts by Ravitch and Sabiston[111] to save the rectum for patients with ulcerative colitis and familial polyposis, this procedure entails leaving the muscular wall of the rectal segment and denuding it of its mucosal lining. This tunnel is then used to pull the normal proximal ganglion-containing colon through to the anus, where an anastomosis between the full-thickness pulled-through normal colon and the mucosa of the anorectum is accomplished. This tunnel protects the anastomosis, so that leakage into the pelvis cannot occur, and in addition protects the urogenital nerve supply from injury during the dissection.

The disadvantage of the procedure is that normal bowel that contains ganglion cells is pulled through a cuff of abnormal bowel that is aganglionic. If the tunnel, or tube of abnormal bowel, is actually left intact, it will react as a segment of aganglionic bowel and go into spasm around the normal intestine with each stimulus. Thus, the signs of Hirschsprung's disease will persist or recur. A surgeon new at performing this procedure will usually damage the seromuscular tube to an extent that it cannot act any longer in a constricting fashion. However, many surgeons find that as they gain experience with the procedure, their facility with it improves and they are able to strip the mucosa without damaging the seromuscular tube. At this point they will note that their patients are developing recurrent symptoms of Hirschsprung's disease. Realization that the intact tube is the factor involved will lead them to slit it posteriorly down to the anorectal level so that it cannot act in a constricting fashion. However, if a patient after a Soave pull-through procedure has recurrent symptoms of Hirschsprung's disease, intactness of the seromuscular tube should be suspected. In the immediate postoperative period, the anastomosis can still leak into the space between the pulled-through colon and the cuff, producing a cuff abscess. Early drainage will prevent generalized systemic symptoms and avoid damage and destruction of the surrounding tissues. Because the pulled-through segment of colon lacks the accommodation ability of a normal rectum, many of these patients in the postoperative months will have a deficit of reservoir function leading to a pattern of frequent stools. The result may be severe irritation of the surrounding perianal skin with breakdown and superficial lesions. Local care to this area will suffice until the pulled-through segment adapts and the number of stools lessen.

With all the surgical procedures for Hirschsprung's disease, the risk of recurrence of pseudomembranous enterocolitis is present, especially if the patient had this entity before the definitive surgical procedure was done.[77] Some surgeons consider the incidence of enterocolitis after the Soave procedure to be significantly higher than that with other procedures, and I believe the factors discussed above relating to the presence of the intact muscular cuff are the reasons for this. In any case, the significant incidence of recurrent enterocolitis following the Soave procedure in some surgeons' hands has led them to abandon earlier enthusiasm for this procedure and return to the Duhamel procedure. The primary care physician should be aware of the surgical procedure that was performed for Hirschsprung's disease in the patient and be alert to its peculiar complica-

tions. Reevaluation early may prevent the ravages of recurrent enterocolitis for the child. This latter entity carries a high mortality unless vigorous resuscitative care is provided early.

Intussusception

Whether the intussusception was reduced by hydrostatic barium enema or by exploratory laparotomy and surgical reduction, the incidence of recurrent intussusception is approximately 5% to 10%.[37] When reduction is impossible at the time of surgery and resection of the distal ileum and proximal colon with end-to-end anastomosis is accomplished, the incidence of recurrence is lower. It has been the belief of some authorities that recurrence of intussusception indicates the presence of an anatomic leading point such as a polyp or Meckel's diverticulum, but recent reports suggest that this may not be true.[38] When the intussusception recurs within the same period of illness, that is, the next day or before the child is discharged, one must suspect either incomplete reduction or the inability to achieve complete reduction, which does suggest a leading point. However, recurrence of intussusception at some later time may simply be due to the development of another Peyer's patch in response to subsequent illness and not to an anatomic leading point. Other than recurrence and the problem of adhesive bowel obstruction following surgery, there are no other peculiar long-term complications.

Biliary atresia

If a successful reconstructive procedure utilizing either the gallbladder and distal common duct or a Roux-en-Y bowel segment can be achieved, the child's chances of clearing his jaundice by draining significant amounts of bile are approximately 50%; and approximately 50% of these children will have a successful result over a long period of time.[72,86] Thus, the first complication of the Kasai procedure might be its high failure rate. Nevertheless, its success must be measured against almost total failure in the treatment of biliary atresia prior to the use of this procedure.[1]

Among the complications of the Kasai procedure, ascending cholangitis stands out for its frequency and severity.[59,60] This entity may be so devastating as to destroy the duct systems secondarily after what appears to be a successful drainage procedure. Modifications of the original Kasai procedure to provide a vent through which

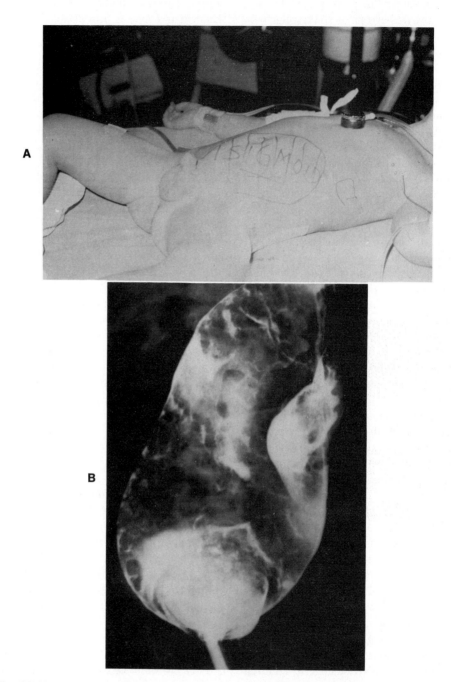

Fig. 20-19. A, Outline of an impacted sigmoid colon behind an obstructed, scarred anal stoma resulting from an inadequate perineal anoplasty. The barium-filled sigmoid is further defined in the radiograph in **B.**

any intestinal contents that are backing up retrograde can escape may lessen the incidence of cholangitis but does not eliminate it completely. Ascending cholangitis is less likely to occur when the gallbladder and distal common duct can be used for drainage.[85] Long-term maintenance antibiotic therapy has also been useful in reducing the frequency and severity of the attacks. The development of fever, malaise, and recurrent jaundice in a child following a successful Kasai procedure should lead to immediate hospitalization, supportive and resuscitative care, and intravenous broad-spectrum antibiotic coverage, usually with ampicillin and gentamycin.

Other complications include stenosis of any of the anastomotic areas and ascites formation, the latter being a sign of progression of the liver disease rather than a complication of the procedure. Progressive liver damage will manifest itself with all the signs of progressive cirrhosis, including ascites formation, nutritional deficiency, liver enzyme elevations, and eventually the development of portal hypertension and esophageal varices. The latter may lead to severe esophageal variceal hemorrhage, which has been the source of demise for many of these patients.

Imperforate anus

Most problems with imperforate anus result from failure of one of the three major management requirements: technically correct surgery performed at the proper time, adequate postoperative dilatation to provide a pliable, adequately sized anus, and physiologically appropriate toilet training.

The major complications following imperforate anus are constipation and soiling, which may exist together or independently. There are basically two types of soiling. One type is due to overflow passage of liquid bowel contents around a huge solid impaction. The other type is the soiling of the underwear with streaks of solid fecal material due to the patient carrying stool in the rectal segment and allowing it to protrude through the patulous anus. If the surgery has been performed correctly and the puborectalis sling is innervated and functioning, these problems will respond to a thorough cleanout, a period of maintained rectal emptiness to allow recovery of tone, and then a bowel training program such as that outlined earlier in this chapter. If the child has an inade-

quately sized anal stoma because inadequate dilatations have left the child with an overly firm, inelastic stoma or because of the child's own tendency to form hypertrophic scar tissue, increasing constipation may result as the child grows and the anus becomes less and less adequate for his size. The result may be marked dilatation and hypertrophy of the proximal bowel segment accompanied by fecal impaction and soiling (Fig. 20-19).

Abdominal wall deformities

Once successful repair of either omphalocele or gastroschisis is accomplished, the complications result from the adhesive scarring that leads to bowel obstruction, as in any other abdominal procedure, and from breakdown of the repair with the resultant formation of ventral hernias.

Sacrococcygeal teratoma

There are few complications after repair of sacrococcygeal teratoma in the early infant age group. There may be some tendency to constipation on a long-term basis, but it need not be severe and can be managed with the usual measures. Ongoing observation and reevaluation for any evidence of persistence, recurrence, invasiveness, or metastases are warranted over the first few years following excision despite the low incidence of metastatic complications following excision in the newborn period.

Airway obstructions and deformities

Airway obstructions and deformities include benign tumors, acquired lesions (such as subglottic stenosis), generalized deformities of the jaw and oropharynx (such as the Pierre Robin syndrome), and inadequate development of the airway structures (such as the omega-shaped epiglottis of laryngomalacia and the misshapen trachea of tracheomalacia). Be aware that with any episodes of airway inflammation, such as croup, these children are at greater risk than the average child and should be placed under adequate medical supervision earlier in the course of the disease.

REFERENCES

1. Adelman, S.: Prognosis of uncorrected biliary atresia: an update, J. Pediatr. Surg. **13:**389, 1978.
2. Allen, J. E., Beck, A. R., and Jewett, T., Jr.: Wringer injuries in children, Arch. Surg. **97:**194, 1968.

3. Altman, R. P., and Margileth, A. M.: Cervical lymphadenopathy from atypical mycobacteria: diagnosis and surgical treatment, J. Pediatr. Surg. **10**:419, 1975.

4. Ashcraft, K. W., and others: Early recognition and aggressive treatment of gastroesophageal reflux following repair of eosphageal atresia, J. Pediatr. Surg. **12**:317, 1977.

5. Athanasoulis, C. A., and others: Angiography: its contribution to the emergency management of gastrointestinal hemorrhage, Radiol. Clin. North Am. **14**:265, 1976.

6. Beal, J. M.: The acute abdomen. In Sabiston, D. C., Jr., editor: Davis Christopher textbook of surgery, Philadelphia, 1977, W. B. Saunders Co., p. 881.

7. Beckwith, J. B., and Palmer, N.: Histopathology and prognosis of Wilms' tumor: results of the National Wilms' Tumor Study, Cancer **41**:1937, 1978.

8. Beiser, G. D., and others: Impairment of cardiac function in patients with pectus excavatum with improvement after operative correction, N. Engl. J. Med. **287**:267, 1972.

9. Belin, R. P., and others: Diagnosis and management of scrofula in children, J. Pediatr. Surg. **9**:103, 1974.

10. Benson, C. D.: Surgical implications of Meckel's diverticulum. In Ravitch, M. M., and others, editors: Pediatric surgery, ed. 3, Chicago, 1979, Year Book Medical Publishers, Inc., pp. 955-960.

11. Bishop, H. C., and others: Survival in bilateral Wilms' tumor: review of 30 National Wilms' Tumor Study cases, J. Pediatr. Surg. **12**:631, 1977.

12. Blackburn, W. W., and Filston, H. C.: Common symptoms in children: routine illness or abdominal lymphoma, Am. J. Surg. **130**:539, 1975.

13. Bloom, D. A., and Fonkalsrud, E. W.: Surgical management of pheochromocytoma in children, J. Pediatr. Surg. **9**:179, 1974.

14. Boles, E. T., Jr., Haase, G. M., and Hamoudi, A. B.: Partial splenectomy in staging laparotomy for Hodgkin's disease: an alternative approach, J. Pediatr. Surg. **13**:581, 1978.

15. Boley, S.: New modification of the surgical treatment of Hirschsprung's disease, Surgery **56**:1015, 1964.

16. Buntain, W. L., Wood, J. B., and Woolley, M. M.: Pancreatitis in childhood, J. Pediatr. Surg. **13**:143, 1978.

17. Cameron, J. L.: Chronic pancreatic ascites and pancreatic pleural effusions, Gastroenterology **74**:134, 1978.

18. Cantrell, R. W., Jensen, J. H., and Reid, D.: Diagnosis and management of tuberculous cervical adenitis, Arch. Otolaryngol. **101**:53, 1975.

19. Carithers, H. A., Carithers, C. M., and Edwards, R. O., Jr.: Cat-scratch disease: its natural history, J.A.M.A. **207**:312, 1969.

20. Clatworthy, H. W., Jr.: Extrahepatic portal hypertension. In Childs, C. G. III, editor: Portal hypertension, Philadelphia, 1974, W. B. Saunders Co.

21. Constantopoulos, A., Najjar, V. A., and Smith, J. W.: Tuftsin deficiency: a new syndrome with defective phagocytosis, J. Pediatrics **80**:564, 1972.

22. Cooney, D. R., and Grosfeld, J. L.: Operative management of pancreatic pseudocysts in infants and children: a review of 75 cases, Ann. Surg. **182**:590, 1975.

23. Copeland, E. M., and Long, J. M., III: Elective appendectomy for appendiceal calculus, Surg. Gynecol. Obstet. **130**:439, 1970.

24. Cordonnier, J. K., and Izant, R. J., Jr.: Meconium ileus equivalent, Surgery **54**:667, 1963.

25. Coupland, G.: Pancreatic ascites: a rare complication of pancreatitis in childhood, Aust. N.Z. J. Surg. **40**:252, 1971.

26. Crane, J. M., Amoury, R. A., and Hellerstein, S.: Hereditary pancreatitis: report of a kindred, J. Pediatr. Surg. **8**:893, 1973.

27. Curci, M. R., and others: Peptic ulcer disease in childhood reexamined, J. Pediatr. Surg. **11**:329, 1976.

28. D'Angio, G. J., and others: The treatment of Wilms' tumor: results of the National Wilms' Tumor Study, Cancer **38**:633, 1976.

29. Davis, G. B., Booksteen, J., and Hagan, P. L.: The relative effects of selective intra-arterial and intravenous vasopressin infusion, Radiology **120**:537, 1976.

30. Dean, R. H., Scott, H. W., Jr., and Law, D. H., IV: Chronic relapsing pancreatitis in childhood: case report and review of the literature, Ann. Surg. **173**:443, 1971.

31. DeCosse, J. J., and others: Subphrenic abscess, Surg. Gynecol. Obstet. **138**:841, 1974.

32. Dehner, L. P.: Pediatric surgical pathology, St. Louis, 1975, The C. V. Mosby Co.

33. Donowitz, M., Kerstein, M. D., and Spiro, H. M.: Pancreatic ascites, Medicine **53**:183, 1974.

34. Douglas, G. J., and Simpson, J. S.: The conservative management of splenic trauma, J. Pediatr. Surg. **6**:565, 1971.

35. Duhamel, B.: A new operation for the treatment of Hirschsprung's disease, Arch. Dis. Child. **35**:38, 1960.

36. Ehrenpreis, T., Livaditis, A., and Okmian, L.: Results of Duhamel's operation for Hirschsprung's disease, J. Pediatr. Surg. **1**:40, 1966.

37. Ein, S. H.: Recurrent intussusception in children, J. Pediatr. Surg. **10**:751, 1975.

38. Ein, S. H.: Leading points in childhood intussusception, J. Pediatr. Surg. **11**:209, 1976.

39. Ellis, E. F., and Smith, R. T.: The role of the spleen in immunity: with special reference to the post-splenectomy problem in infants, Pediatrics **37**:111, 1966.

40. Eraklis, A. J., and Filler, R. M.: Splenectomy in childhood: a review of 1413 cases, J. Pediatr. Surg. **7**:382, 1972.

41. Exelby, P. R.: Method of evaluating children with Hodgkin's disease, Cancer **21**:95, 1971.

42. Exelby, P. R., Filler, R. M., and Grosfeld, J. L.: Liver tumors in children in the particular reference to hepatoblastoma and hepatocellular carcinoma, American Academy of Pediatrics, Surgical Section Survey, 1974, J. Pediatr. Surg. **10**:329, 1975.

43. Feldman, J. M., and others: Alterations in plasma norepinephrine concentration during surgical resection of pheochromocytoma, Ann. Surg. **188**:758, 1978.

44. Filston, H. C., Jackson, D. C., and Johnsrude, I. S.: Arteriographic embolization for control of recurrent severe gastric hemorrhage in a 10-year-old boy, J. Pediatr. Surg. **14**:276, 1979.

45. Filston, H. C., and Johnson, D. G.: Percutaneous venous cannulation in neonates and infants: a method for catheter insertion without "cut-down," Pediatrics **48**:896, 1971.

46. Filston, H. C., and others: Improved management of pancreatic lesions in children aided by ERCP, J. Pediatr. Surg. **15**:121, 1980.

47. Folkman, J.: Appendicitis. In Ravitch, M. M., and others, editors: Pediatric surgery, ed. 3, Chicago, 1979, Year Book Medical Publishers, Inc., p. 1005.

48. Fonkalsrud, E. W., and Longmire, W. P.: Reassessment of operative procedures for portal hypertension in infants and children, Am. J. Surg. **118**:148, 1969.

49. Fonkalsrud, E. W., and others: Management of pancreatitis in infants and children, Am. J. Surg. **116**:198, 1968.

50. Food and Drug Administration: Selection criteria reduce unnecessary skull x-rays, FDA Drug Bull. **8**:30, 1978.

51. Futrell, J. W., Filston, H. C., and Reid, J. D.: Rupture of a renal cell carcinoma in a child: five-year tumor-free survival and literature review, Cancer **41**:1565, 1978.

52. Gaisford, J. C., and Anderson, V. S.: First branchial cleft cysts and sinuses, Plast. Reconstr. Surg. **55**:299, 1975.

53. Gans, S. L., and Berci, G.: Inside tracheoesophageal fistula: new endoscopic approaches, J. Pediatr. Surg. **8**:205, 1973.

54. Grosfeld, J. L., Clatworthy, H. W., Jr., and Newton, W. A., Jr.: Combined therapy in childhood rhabdomyosarcoma: an analysis of 42 cases, J. Pediatr. Surg. **4**:637, 1969.

55. Gross, R. E.: The surgery of infancy and childhood, Philadelphia, 1953, W. B. Saunders, Co., p. 158.

56. Hays, D. M., and others: Laparotomy for the staging of Hodgkin's disease in children, J. Pediatr. Surg. **7**:517, 1972.

57. Heikkinen, E. S., and Akerblom, H. K.: Diagnostic and operative probelms in multiple pheochromocytomas, J. Pediatr. Surg. **12**:157, 1977.

58. Hendren, W. H., Greep, J. M., and Patton, A. S.: Pancreatitis in childhood: experience with 15 cases, Arch. Child. **40**:132, 1965.

59. Hirsig, J., Kara, O., and Rickham, P. P.: Experimental investigations into the etiology of cholangitis following operation for biliary atresia, J. Pediatr. Surg. **13**:55, 1978.

60. Hitch, D. C., and Lilly, J. R.: Identification, quantification, and significance of bacterial growth within the biliary tract after Kasai's operation, J. Pediatr. Surg. **13**:563, 1978.

61. Holton, C. P., and others: Extended combination therapy of childhood rhabdomyosarcoma, Cancer **32**:310, 1973.

62. Huhti, E., and others: Tuberculosis of the cervical lymph nodes: a clinical, pathological, and bacteriological study, Tubercle **56**:27, 1975.

63. Izant, R. J., Jr., and Drucker, W. R.: Duodenal obstruction due to intramural hematoma in children, J. Trauma **4**:797, 1964.

64. Izant, R. J., Jr., Rothmann, B. F., and Frankel, V. H.: Bicycle spoke injuries of the foot and ankle in children: an underestimated "minor" injury, J. Pediatr. Surg. **4**:654, 1969.

65. Jaffe, N., and others: Improved outlook for Ewing's sarcoma with combination chemotherapy and radiation therapy, Cancer **38**:1952, 1976.

66. Javett, S. L., Jackson, H., and Utian, H. L.: Torgersen's muscle and infantile hypertrophic pyloric stenosis, J. Pediatr. Surg. **8**:383, 1973.

67. Jenkins, R. D.: Primary gastrointestinal tract lymphoma in childhood, Radiology **92**:763, 1969.

68. Johnsrude, I. S., and Jackson, D. C.: A practical approach to angiography, Boston, 1979, Little, Brown & Co.

69. Jona, J. Z., Belin, R. P., and Selke, A. C.: Barium enema as a diagnostic aid in children with abdominal pain, Surg. Gynecol. Obstet. **144**:351, 1977.

70. Jones, R. S.: The small intestine: anatomy, physiology. In Sabiston, D. C., Jr., editor: Davis Christopher Textbook of surgery, Philadelphia, 1977, W. B. Saunders Co., pp. 994-1002.

71. Jordan, P. H., Jr.: An interim report on parietal cell vagotomy versus selective vagotomy and antrectomy for treatment of duodenal ulcer, Ann. Surg. **189**:643, 1979.

72. Kasai, M.: Treatment of biliary atresia with special reference to hepatoportoenterostomy and its modifications, Prog. Pediatr. Surg. **6**:5, 1974.

73. Kilpatrick, Z. M.: Scanning in diagnosis of Meckel's diverticulum, Hosp. Pract. **9**:131, June 1974.

74. King, H., and Shumacker, H. B., Jr.: Splenic studies: susceptibility to infection after splenectomy performed in infancy, Ann. Surg. **136**:239, 1952.

75. Kirks, D. R., Briley, C. A., Jr., and Currarino, G.: Selective catheterization of tracheoesophageal fistula, A.J.R. **133**:763, 1979.

76. Kirks, D. R., and others: Myelography in the evaluation of paravertebral mass lesions in infants and children, Radiology **119**:603, 1976.

77. Kleinhaus, S., and others: Hirschsprung's disease: a survey of the members of the Surgical Section of the American Academy of Pediatrics, J. Pediatr. Surg. **14**:588, 1979.

78. Kodesch, R., and DuPont, H. L.: Infectious complication of acute pancreatitis, Surg. Gynecol. Obstet. **136**:763, 1973.

79. Koop, C. E.: The choice of surgical procedures in Hirschsprung's disease (editorial), J. Pediatr. Surg. **1**:523, 1966.

80. Koop, C. E., and Johnson, D. G.: Neuroblastoma: an assessment of therapy in reference to staging, J. Pediatr. Surg. **6**:595, 1971.

81. Kumar, A. P., and others: Combined therapy for malignant tumors of the chest wall in children, J. Pediatr. Surg. **12**:991, 1977.

82. Leape, L. L.: Early burn wound changes, J. Pediatr. Surg. **3**:292, 1968.

83. Leape, L., Breslow, N., and Bishop, H. C.: The surgical treatment of Wilms' tumor: results of the National Wilms' Tumor Study, Ann. Surg. **187**:351, 1978.

84. Likhte, V. V.: Immunological impairment and susceptibility to infection after splenectomy, J.A.M.A. **236**:1376, 1976.

85. Lilly, J. R.: Hepatic portocholecystostomy for biliary atresia, J. Pediatr. Surg. **14**:301, 1979.

86. Lilly, J. R., and Altman, R. P.: Hepatic portoenterostomy (the Kasai operation) for biliary atresia, Surgery **78**:76, 1975.

87. Lloyd, D. A., and Cywes, S.: Intestinal stenosis and enterocyst formation as late complications of neonatal necrotizing enterocolitis, J. Pediatr. Surg. **8:**479, 1973.

88. Lund, C. C., and Browder, N. C.: The estimation of areas of burns, Surg. Gynecol. Obstet. **79:**352, 1944.

89. MacKellar, A.: Diagnosis and management of atypical mycobacterial lymphadenitis in children, J. Pediatr. Surg. **11:**85, 1976.

90. MacKenzie, M., Fordyce, J., and Young, D. G.: Subphrenic abscess in children, Br. J. Surg. **62:**305, 1975.

91. Madden, J. W.: Wound healing: biologic and clinical features. In Sabiston, D. C., Jr., editor: Davis Christopher textbook of surgery, Philadelphia, 1977, W. B. Saunders Co., pp. 271-294.

92. Martin, L. W., and Caudill, D. R.: A method for elimination of the blind rectal pouch in the Duhamel operation for Hirschsprung's disease, Surgery **62:**951, 1967.

93. Maurer, H. M.: The intergroup rhabdomyosarcoma study (NIH): objectives and clinical staging classification, J. Pediatr. Surg. **10:**977, 1975.

94. Miller, R. C., and others: The incidental discovery of occult abdominal tumors in children following blunt abdominal trauma, J. Trauma **6:**99, 1966.

95. Mishalany, H.: Repair of the ruptured spleen, J. Pediatr. Surg. **9:**175, 1974.

96. Moore, K. L.: The developing human: clinically oriented embryology, Philadelphia, 1973, W. B. Saunders Co., p. 192.

97. Moossa, A. R.: Pancreatic pseudocysts in children, J. R. Coll. Surg. Edinb. **19:**149, 1974.

98. Morse, T. S.: Evaluation and initial management. In Touloukian, R. J., editor: Pediatric trauma, New York, 1978, John Wiley & Sons, Inc., pp. 27, 28, 29.

99. Murphy, J. F., and Fred, H. L.: Infectious lymphadenitis or lymphoma? seven lessons, J.A.M.A. **235:**742, 1976.

100. Nixon, H. H.: Surgical conditions in pediatrics, London, 1978, Butterworth & Co. (Publishers), Ltd., pp. 190, 263, 400-402.

101. Oddson, T. A., and others: Acute gastrointestinal hemorrhage: the changing role of barium examinations, Radiol. Clin. North Am. **16:**123, 1978.

102. Parker, A. F., Christi, D. L., and Cahill, J. L.: Incidence and significance of gastroesophageal reflux following repair of esophageal atresia and tracheoesophageal fistula and the need for antireflux procedures, J. Pediatr. Surg. **14:**5, 1979.

103. Parodi-Hueck, L. E., and Koop, C. E.: Subhyoid midline ectopic thyroid tissue in the absence of normal thyroid gland, J. Pediatr. Surg. **3:**710, 1968.

104. Perry, A. W., Reeves, C., and Woolley, M. M.: Wringer arm injuries, Am. Surg. **35:**53, 1969.

105. Persky, L., and Forsythe, W. E.: Renal trauma in childhood, J.A.M.A. **182:**709, 1962.

106. Postlethwait, R. W.: Surgery of the esophagus, New York, 1979, Appleton-Century-Crofts, pp. 23, 24.

107. Ranson, J. H., and Spencer, I. C.: The role of peritoneal lavage in severe acute pancreatitis, Ann. Surg. **187:**565, 1978.

108. Ratner, M. H., and others: Surgical repair of the injured spleen, J. Pediatr. Surg. **12:**1019, 1977.

109. Ravitch, M. M.: Congenital deformities of the chest wall and their operative correction, Philadelphia, 1977, W. B. Saunders Co., pp. 78-205.

110. Ravitch, M. M., and Duremdes, G. D.: Operative treatment of chronic duodenal ulcer in childhood, Ann. Surg. **171:**641, 1970.

111. Ravitch, M. M., and Sabiston, D. C., Jr.: Anal ileostomy with preservation of the sphincter, a proposed operation in patients requiring total colectomy for benign lesions, Surg. Gynecol. Obstet. **84:**1095, 1947.

112. Rehbein, F., and others: Surgical problems in congenital megacolon (Hirschsprung's disease): a comparison of surgical technics, J. Pediatr. Surg. **1:**526, 1966.

113. Rodgers, B. M., and Talbert, J. L.: Distal spleno-renal shunt for portal decompression in childhood, J. Pediatr. Surg. **14:**33, 1979.

114. Rosenkrantz, J. G., and others: Intussusception in the 1970's: indications for operation, J. Pediatr. Surg. **12:**367, 1977.

115. Sankaran, S., and Walt, A. J.: Pancreatic ascites, Arch. Surg. **111:**430, 1976.

116. Schmitt, B. D.: Cervical adenopathy in children, Postgrad. Med. **60**(3):251, 1976.

117. Schuster, S. R., and Gross, R. E.: Peptic ulcer disease in childhood, Am. J. Surg. **105:**324, 1963.

118. Seashore, J. H.: Soft tissue injuries. In Touloukian, R. J., editor: Pediatric trauma, New York, 1978, John Wiley & Sons, Inc., p. 226.

119. Sherman, N. J., and Asch, M. J.: Conservative surgery for splenic injuries, Pediatrics **61:**267, 1978.

120. Sieber, W. K., Dibbins, A. W., and Wiener, E. S.: Retroperitoneal tumors. In Ravitch, M. M., and others, editors: Pediatric surgery, ed. 3, Chicago, 1979, Year Book Medical Publishers, Inc., p. 1082.

121. Silverman, N. A., and Sabiston, D. C., Jr.: Primary tumors and cysts of the mediastinum. In Hickey, C., editor: Current problems in cancer, vol. 2, No. 5, Chicago, 1977, Year Book Medical Publishers, Inc., pp. 51-54.

122. Singer, D. B.: Postsplenectomy sepsis. In Perspectives in pediatric pathology, Chicago, 1973, Year Book Medical Publishers, Inc., p. 285.

123. Sistrunk, W. E.: Technique of removal of cysts and sinuses of the thyroglossal duct, Surg. Gynecol. Obstet. **46:**109, 1928.

124. Soper, R. T., and Figuera, P. R.: Surgical treatment of Hirschsprung's disease: comparison of modifications of the Duhamel and Soave operations, J. Pediatr. Surg. **6:**761, 1971.

125. Stein, H., Kavin, I., and Faerber, E. N.: Colonic strictures following nonoperative management of necrotizing enterocolitis, J. Pediatr. Surg. **10:**943, 1975.

126. Stone, H. H., and others: Prophylactic and preventive antibiotic therapy: timing, duration and economics, Ann. Surg. **189:**691, 1979.

127. Strickland, A. L., and others: Ectopic thyroid glands simulating thyroglossal duct cysts, J.A.M.A. **208:**307, 1969.

128. Sutow, W. W.: General concepts of childhood cancer. In Sutow, W. W., Vietti, T. J., and Fernbach, D. J., editors: Clinical pediatric oncology, St. Louis, 1977, The C. V. Mosby Co., p. 4.

129. Swenson, O., and Bill, A. H., Jr.: Resection of rectum and rectosigmoid with preservation of the sphincter for benign spastic lesions producing megacolon, Surgery **24:**212, 1948.

130. Tawes, R. L., and DeLorimier, A. A.: Thyroid carcinoma in youth, J. Pediatr. Surg. **3:**210, 1968.

131. Tefft, M., Vawter, G. F., and Mitus, A.: Secondary primary neoplasms in children, A.J.R. **103:**800, 1968.

132. Telander, R. L., and Deane, S. A.: Thyroglossal and branchial cleft cysts and sinuses, Surg. Clin. North Am. **57:**779, 1977.

133. Thomas, K. E., and others: Natural history of Gardner's syndrome, Am. J. Surg. **115:**218, 1968.

134. Thompson, N. W., and others: Surgical treatment of thyrotoxicosis in children and adolescents, J. Pediatr. Surg. **12:**1009, 1977.

135. Urakami, Y., Seki, H., and Kishi, S.: Endoscopic retrograde cholangiopancreatography (ERCP) performed in children, Endoscopy **9:**86, 1977.

136. Voorhees, A. B., Jr., and others: Portal-systemic encephalopathy in the non-cirrhotic patient: effect of portal-systemic shunting, Arch. Surg. **107:**659, 1973.

137. Voorhees, A. B., Jr., and Price, J. B., Jr.: Extraheptic portal hypertension: a retrospective analysis of 127 cases and associated complications, Arch. Surg. **108:**338, 1974.

138. Warren, W. D., and Marsh, W. H.: An appraisal of surgical procedures for pancreatic pseudocyst, Ann. Surg. **147:**903, 1958.

139. Warren, W. D., and others: Selective distal splenorenal shunt: technique and results of operation, Arch. Surg. **108:**306, 1974.

140. Welch, K. J.: The pancreas. In Ravitch, M. M., and others, editors: Pediatric surgery, ed. 3, Chicago, 1979, Year Book Medical Publishers, Inc., pp. 868-877.

141. White, J. J., and others: Conservatively aggressive management of bilateral Wilms' tumors, J. Pediatr. Surg. **11:**859, 1976.

142. White, J. J., and others: Letter to the editor, J. Pediatr. Surg. **12:**798, 1977.

143. Williams, T. E., Jr., Sherman, N. J., and Clatworthy, H. W., Jr.: Chronic fibrosing pancreatitis in childhood: a cause of recurrent abdominal pain, Pediatrics **40:**1019, 1967.

144. Williams, W. H., and Hendren, W. H.: Intrapancreatic duodenal duplication causing pancreatitis in a child, Surgery **69:**708, 1971.

145. Wine, C. R., Nahrwold, D. L., and Waldhausen, J. A.: Role of the technetium scan in the diagnosis of Meckel's diverticulum, J. Pediatr. Surg. **9:**885, 1974.

146. Winkelstein, J. A., and Lambert, G. H.: Pneumococcal serum opsonizing activity in splenectomized children, J. Pediatrics **87:**430, 1975.

147. Wrenn, E. L., Jr.: Tubular duplication of the small intestine, Surgery **52:**494, 1962.

CHAPTER 21

Urologic considerations

JOHN W. DUCKETT and HOWARD C. FILSTON

GENERAL CONSIDERATIONS

All of the considerations discussed under evaluation of the infant-toddler age group (Chapter 16) apply to the childhood age group as well. The child who continues to have failure to thrive, recurrent fevers of unknown origin, or intermittent bouts of abdominal pain should be suspected of having a urinary tract abnormality or infection or both and should be evaluated. The likely findings are similar to those of the infant-toddler age group except that long-standing obstructive uropathy may have led to more advanced damage to the upper urinary tract and kidneys in this older age group. Prolonged obstructive uropathy or persistent or repeated urinary tract infections may destroy the renal parenchyma and render the kidney unsalvageable. The goal should certainly be to pick up on such abnormalities in the younger age group; but if the primary care physician is presented with a child not previously diagnosed, all of the considerations discussed for these abnormalities in the infant-toddler section should apply. The standard workup would consist of a voiding cystourethrogram (VCG) followed by an intravenous pyelogram (IVP) and then, if indicated, a renal scan to evaluate the function of the residual renal parenchyma. Following this, further urologic investigation should be undertaken by a knowledgeable pediatric urologist or urologically experienced pediatric surgeon.

ENURESIS

One entity that is common in the childhood age group is enuresis. Total or diurnal enuresis is more likely to be a sign of urinary tract abnormality than is nocturnal enuresis. An ectopic ureterocele or ectopic ureteral orifice entering the urethra beyond the bladder sphincter may present as wetting. This anomaly will usually be demonstrable by the IVP and VCG. It is unusual for enuresis to be the only sign of organic disease; if diurnal enuresis persists, however, further evaluation of the urinary tract is probably warranted.

All enuretics should have a urinalysis and culture, since enuretic girls, particularly, have a 4-to-1 incidence of recurrent or chronic urinary tract infections when compared with nonenuretics.[7] Infection is less common in boys. It is important to differentiate primary enuresis, in which the child is never continent, from secondary enuresis. Primary diurnal enuresis may be associated with structural abnormalities or a neurogenic bladder, whereas secondary diurnal enuresis is more likely to be due to urinary tract infection. Nocturnal enuresis is a common finding and is rarely associated with structural abnormalities. It has been the cause of much emotional upheaval in families as year after year goes by while the child, particularly the male child, is unable to stay dry at night. It is now believed that this is a problem with maturation and has little to do with the integrity of the urinary tract. Ninety-eight percent of enuretics will have spontaneous cures by the age of 15 years.

Treatment. Treatment of enuresis in a child with no structural or neurogenic abnormalities is difficult. Extensive discipline routines, including awakening the child in the middle of the night and providing electrical devices that awaken the child when he wets in an attempt to program him to awaken and void have met with the best success. The drug imipramine has shown a 50% response rate but only a 30% cure; 70% of patients so treated relapse after the drug is discontinued.[2,8] This drug alters the bladder capacity and may affect sleep patterns. The best form of therapy is reassurance to the family and the child that this is not an emotional disorder, although it can be made one by excessive attention. As the child's bladder capacity improves and his sleep pattern changes, he will achieve nighttime continence in most cases.

TORSION OF THE TESTICLE AND APPENDAGES

Swelling of the testicle associated with pain and tenderness on examination must be considered torsion of the testicle until it is proved otherwise. Torsions of the appendices of the testicle and cord occur more frequently than torsion of the testicle itself, and occasionally a hydrocele will acutely fill with fluid, causing some discomfort. Nevertheless, it is best to consider all symptomatic swellings of the scrotum torsion of the testicle. There are two types of torsion: one more common in early infancy and the other more common in later childhood. The infant variety, known as the bell-and-clapper deformity, involves twisting of the testicle within the tunica vaginalis due to inadequate attachment of the testicle to the surrounding membranes. It is similar to the relationship of the clapper to a bell and thus its name. It is characterized by swelling and tenderness without shortening, since the cord itself is not twisted. On the other hand, torsion of the entire cord, which is the common variety in the older child, leads to foreshortening of the cord and a high testicle.

Torsion of the appendices of the testicle can be

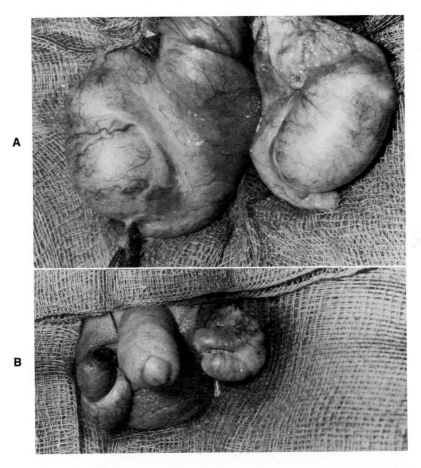

Fig. 21-1. Two examples of torsion of the testicle. **A** shows an older child and clearly demonstrates the torsion of the cord on the right (arrow). **B** shows torsion of the testicle with necrosis in an infant who had only had symptoms for a few hours prior to surgery. Both figures show the normal untwisted left testicle for comparison.

differentiated if the testicle can be cradled within the scrotum and the examining hand and gently probed with the eraser end of a pencil or other soft object. If the main body of the testicle is not tender but exquisite tenderness is elicited at the superior or inferior pole, this suggests torsion of an appendix. Transillumination may show the dark spot of the hemorrhagic strangulated appendix, confirming the diagnosis. Generally, little time need be wasted in differentiating these two entities, since torsions of the appendices of the testes and cord respond best to surgical removal of the appendix. Surgical intervention in all cases will identify patients with torsion of the testis and give an opportunity for correction and preservation of the testicle (Fig. 21-1, *A*). Occasionally, untwisting of the cord can be achieved manually and orchidopexy can then be scheduled electively. Since the testicle does not withstand ischemia for any prolonged period, even in cases where only a few hours have passed since the symptoms began, the testicle may be found to be nonviable (Fig. 21-1, *B*).

Acute enlargement of a hydrocele can usually be differentiated by the ease of transillumination, the identification of the testicle as a discrete entity within the scrotal sac, and particularly the demonstration that the testicle is not tender. A hydrocele should never be "needled" in an attempt to demonstrate its presence, since occasionally an in-carcerated hernia may appear similar to a hydrocele and needle aspiration of such an entity could lead to perforation of the intestine and severe infection.

Medical versus surgical treatment. As noted above, it is not absolutely mandatory to remove the twisted testicular appendages, since they will eventually necrose and undergo autolysis (Fig. 21-2). Nevertheless, this takes considerable time, during which the child is encumbered with a tender, swollen scrotum. The symptoms are resolved more quickly with surgical excision, and this fact together with the possible misdiagnosis of torsion of the testicle make surgical therapy preferable if the child is an average candidate for anesthesia and surgery. Surgical correction of the twisted testicle involves derotation and fixation of the testicle to the surrounding membranes, and this procedure requires elevation of a flap of the tunica albuginea so that adherence of the membrane to the testicle is ensured.[6] Simple suture of the testicle to the surrounding membranes may fail to provide adequate fixation. If the testicle appears severely ischemic, it should not be removed, since parts of it may recover and at least the Leydig cell function may be preserved. Most surgeons believe that the anatomic derangement that led to torsion on one side is probably present on the opposite side, so that orchidopexy should be accomplished electively on the opposite side by simple extension through

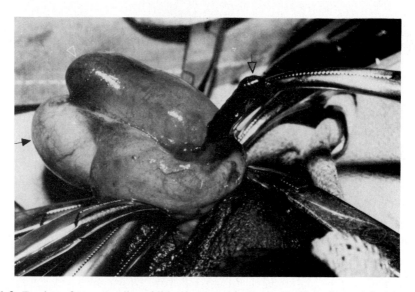

Fig. 21-2. Torsion of an appendix epididymis (open black arrow). Note the testicle (closed black arrow) and the swollen epididymis (open white arrow).

the scrotal raphe or a second small incision on the contralateral side.

Complications. The testicle may go on to atrophy after torsion. All but a nubbin of the testicular tissue may disappear, or the testicle may remain infantile. These observations become important in avoiding subsequent surgery for ''undescended testicle.'' Incarceration of an inguinal hernia may also lead to atrophy of the testicle and subsequent reexploration for ''undescended testicle.'' The primary care physician's clear notation of the earlier presence of a normally descended testicle will avoid this confusion.

UNDESCENDED TESTICLES

The problem of the undescended testicle remains a somewhat controversial and evolving one at this time. Of primary importance is distinguishing the child with the testicle that will not enter the scrotum from the child whose testicle retracts from the scrotum. Of any 100 children found during routine physical examination to have one or both testicles not residing in the scrotal sac, well over 90 of them will have retractile testicles requiring no surgery. These are children with active cremasteric reflexes whose testicles are incompletely attached to the scrotal fascia. With minimal stimulation, such as that of air blown across their thighs when they are undressed, the cremaster pulls the testicle up into the inguinal canal. Usually these testicles can be easily milked back down into the scrotum, but occasionally the differentiation of this problem from the truly undescended testicle is difficult.

Various maneuvers are helpful in achieving descent of the retracted testicle, but the most useful one is to place the child with his back against the wall next to the examining table in the seated position, placing the soles of his feet together and allowing his knees to fall abducted on the examining table. The child's scrotum thus hangs down within the circle formed by his lower extremities, and in this position the testicle tends to return as the cremasteric reflex is negated. Gentle palpation from the upper inguinal area down toward the scrotum will help to milk the testicle back into the scrotum, where it can then be grasped. If it can be demonstrated that the testicle is clearly within the extended scrotum, no surgical maneuvers are necessary. However, inverting the scrotum up into the inguinal canal will often allow an undescended testicle to be grasped, and this does not represent

descent of the testicle into the scrotum. Thus, the scrotum must be stretched out and the testicle demonstrated to be within the extended scrotum before a decision against surgery can be made.

Of those testicles that are not demonstrably retractile, it is helpful to think of three varieties. The truly abdominal cryptorchid testicle is less common and represents a testicle that has never entered the inguinal canal. The more common entities are the canalicular testis, which resides between the internal and external rings, and the ectopic testicle, which has descended from the retroperitoneum through the internal ring and into the inguinal canal. At this point, its descent is interrupted and it may take one of several courses. It may remain at the external ring; it may pass through the external ring and reside in a suprapubic pouch above the scrotum; it may turn back into the subcutaneous tissue over the inguinal canal after passing through the external ring; or it may pass through the external ring and out into the thigh. The latter two variants are easier to repair than the abdominal cryptorchid testicle because there is usually sufficient length of vas deferens and vessels to allow them to be placed into the scrotum. Thus, most undescended testicles can be treated by a procedure described by Koop[4] that is little more complex than a herniorrhaphy.

Because most children with an empty scrotum have merely retractile testicles, evaluation of treatment modalities will be inaccurate if these children are included with those who truly have cryptorchidism. It is because of this that in the past many primary care physicians waited until puberty to refer a child for surgery. If our original group of 100 children noted above are followed through to puberty, it will be found that most of them will have their testicles residing in their scrotal sacs. This is because the child with a retractile testicle, as he enters puberty, will have a lessened cremasteric reflex and the enlarged testicle will remain in the scrotum rather than be retracted into the inguinal canal. However, the children with truly undescended testicles will still have testicles that will not enter their scrotal sacs.

Indications for surgery. As it has gradually been realized that the testicle that resides full time outside of the scrotum is subjected to thermal damage that leads to decreased spermatogenesis, the age at which surgery for undescended testicles has been recommended has been pushed back further into infancy.[5] Once again, however, many primary care physicians have chosen to treat all of these children with testosterone in the belief that it will cause the undescended testicle to migrate into the scrotum. Again, looking at our original 100 children with empty scrotal sacs, the treatment of the 90+ children with retractile testicles with testosterone will indeed cause their testicles to enter the scrotal sac—first, because there is no inhibition to the testicles residing there and second, because the testosterone will cause an enlargement of the testicle and a decrease of the cremasteric reflex, as it will at puberty. Again, however, many authorities believe that the testosterone will have little effect on the truly undescended testicle, particularly if a suprapubic pouch prevents entry into the scrotum. At the time of surgery, forceful dilatation of the scrotal tissues is often necessary to form a passage way into the scrotum for the undescended testicle. In series in which children with definite cryptorchidism rather than retractile testicles have been treated with hormones, 20% to 25% of the testicles have descended.[9] A brief trial of hormone therapy probably is harmless, but prolonged treatment delaying surgical correction is contraindicated. However, for the child in whom the diagnosis between retractile testicle and truly undescended testicle remains difficult after careful physical examination, a short course of testosterone may help to resolve the problem. The main consideration is to accomplish surgery at an age early enough to avoid the thermal damage attendant on prolonged nondescent.

In discussing with parents the indications for surgery, the primary indication is to preserve the sperm-forming function. Secondly, cosmetic appearance of the child is of importance, especially in bilateral nondescent. At least during childhood, the least important reason for orchidopexy is the risk of subsequent malignancy in the undescended testicle. The incidence of malignancy in an undescended testicle has been quoted as being 20 to 30 times that of the normally descended testicle, but the incidence of testicular tumors is so low that even this twenty- to thirtyfold increase makes the incidence in undescended testicles extremely low.[10] Orchidopexy places the testicle into the scrotal sac, where routine physical examination would hopefully identify a developing tumor early enough for successful treatment, and this becomes a third reason for surgery.

Surgical considerations. The age at which the child is referred for orchidopexy has been pushed further and further back from the initial recommendation of puberty. For many years the age of 5 years was held to, but more recent evidence has suggested that after the age of 2, significant damage to the spermatogenic mechanism takes place.[5] There also has been information that an undescended testicle may cause damage to the normally descended testicle on the contralateral side. Others have contested this idea, believing that both testicles in these children are immature. The undescended testicle is generally characterized by an immature stage at which the epididymis is not firmly attached to the testicle and may, in fact, be splayed out along the cord. There are often one or more epididymal or testicular appendages representing the remnants of the müllerian duct system of the female. A hernia sac is found accompanying the undescended testicle in the great majority of cases (85% to 90%). These hernia sacs generally do not become symptomatic prior to orchidopexy, but occasionally they may. The freeing of the hernia sac from the cord often provides the major part of the lengthening of the cord necessary for successful scrotal positioning of the testicle.

The dissection of the hernia sac from the cord of the undescended testicle is one of the most delicate procedures in surgery (Fig. 21-3). Improper technique may lead to serious damage to the lower abdominal wall, may result in a persistent hernia, or may lead to damage to the vascular structures of the cord or to the vas itself. In the hands of an experienced pediatric surgeon or pediatric urologist, orchidopexy should have a very low morbidity and may be accomplished under the same circumstances as those of inguinal herniorrhaphy. Thus, day surgery and minimal postoperative morbidity should be the rule. Modern techniques of orchidopexy rarely include any traction devices to hold the testicle in the scrotum. Most surgeons today utilize a fixation method such as the subdartos pouch technique, in which the surrounding tissues are loosely sutured around the cord to hold the testicle trapped in the scrotum.

Abdominal cryptorchid testicle. When the testicle is truly an abdominal cryptorchid one, a more extensive exploration may be required. This may include division of the abdominal wall muscles requiring repair and an extensive retroperitoneal dissection, for the testicle may reside anywhere in the retroperitoneum up to the kidney level. Occasionally, a transabdominal procedure may be required to locate a testicle.

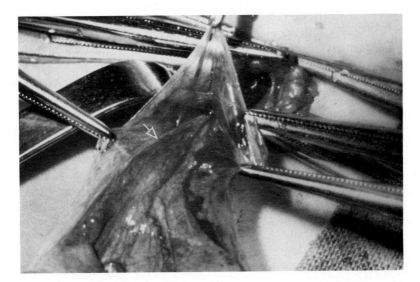

Fig. 21-3. View looking down into the peritoneal cavity through the open hernia sac associated with an undescended testicle. The cord (arrow) appears to be within the hernia sac, but this appearance is due to the close enwrapping of the cord by the posterior wall of the sac.

A limited inguinal operation will result in successful orchidopexy for the majority of patients. Occasionally, one finds a vas ending in a bit of fibrous tissue accompanied by the termination of the spermatic vessels, representing probable loss of the testicle through torsion or other injury in utero or in the early infant period. When it has been determined that the testicle or testicles cannot be found in the inguinal area or that portion of the retroperitoneal space reachable through an inguinal incision, the decision for transabdominal exploration must be made. Once failure to find the testicle is demonstrated, the child should have an IVP to ensure that there is a kidney on that side. Absence of a kidney suggests probable absence of the entire nephrogenic ridge and can be taken as a reasonable assurance that there will be no testicle on that side. If a kidney is present or the child has bilateral undescended testicles that could not be found through inguinal exploration, a more thorough endocrine evaluation should be accomplished to demonstrate the response of the testicle to stimulation. Such evaluation requires the following procedures:

1. Obtain basal testosterone levels, then give human chorionic gonadotrophin (HCG) for 4 days. A testosterone rise of 5 to 10 times represents functional testicular tissue.
2. If no rise in testosterone occurs after HCG has been administered, measure plasma levels of follicle-stimulating hormone (FSH) and luteinizing hormone (LH). Elevation confirms anorchia.
3. If FSH and LH levels are normal, abdominal exploration for testicles is indicated.

When the testicle will not reach the scrotum because of a foreshortened vascular pedicle, the Fowler-Stephens procedure may allow successful scrotal positioning.[1] This procedure requires division of the spermatic vessels leaving the testicle supplied by the delicate vessels that accompany the vas deferens. The procedure is a delicate one requiring planning and meticulous dissection. An 85% success rate is achievable, however.

PRIAPISM

Priapism is a rare condition in children and is mostly seen with sickle cell trait and disease.[3] It is now managed with hypertransfusion or partial exchange transfusion to reduce the sickle cell hemoglobin to below 30%. Shunting procedures are rarely needed for children with this condition.

FOLLOW-UP OF UROLOGIC LESIONS FROM EARLIER YEARS

As the child proceeds through the childhood age group, few new urologic lesions are likely to occur. Obviously, those occurring in the newborn and infant-toddler age groups may have been missed, but consideration in their evaluation is little different at this time. What the primary care physician may be involved with, however, are the surgical results of earlier treatments. Usually the pediatric urologist or pediatric surgeon who has undertaken the surgical procedures will have continued to follow the child closely with the primary care physician, and communication between the two will provide the primary care physician with the support he needs to care for the child. Occasionally, however, the primary care physician is faced with dealing with a new patient with previously treated urinary abnormalities, and some understanding of the problems of these procedures is important to him.

Temporary and permanent diversions of the urinary tract

Most *temporary diversions* of the urinary tract involve pyelocutaneous or ureterocutaneous stomas in which either the renal pelvis or the ureter is sutured to the skin. Although these procedures are used less frequently today, they are usually done to provide drainage of the kidney to avoid the pressure of obstructive uropathies and to allow time for infection to clear before reconstructive procedures are begun. Once the distal obstructions have been surgically repaired, these temporary diversions are usually closed.

The more *permanent forms of diversion* include the anastomosis of one ureter to another or of one or more ureters into a loop of intestine. These procedures are usually performed when the bladder is not useful, such as in severe cases of neurogenic bladder, exstrophy of the bladder, and formerly in some cases of outlet obstruction. Such diversion was also common in patients with abdominal muscle deficiency syndrome. Improved reconstruction techniques today have made permanent diversion unnecessary for many of these conditions, and consideration for undiverting should be offered to all children with a "permanent" diversion.

The most common urinary diversion performed in the past was that of the ileal conduit, or ileal loop. In this procedure a loop of ileum is isolated, one end is closed, the ureters are anastomosed to the ileum, and the other end of the ileum is brought out as an enterostomy stoma. This technique provides a reservoir through which urine can empty into a collecting bag. Recently it has been appreciated that problems with conduit-ureteral reflux

occur and that chronic infection remains a serious problem for these patients. The consequent ongoing destruction of the upper urinary tract has made this procedure less than optimal. The sigmoid colon has become the popular conduit because the ureters can be anastomosed in an antirefluxing fashion similar to that of a ureterovesical reimplantation. Long-term results of this technique, however, may not make it as free of complications as expected.

Formerly the sigmoid colon was used as an intact segment to divert the urinary tract into the intestinal tract (ureterosigmoidostomy). Problems with this procedure included loose, watery stools, hyperchloremic acidosis that resulted from resorption of urinary electrolytes through the colon mucosa, and ascending infection from the gastrointestinal tract. Isolation of the sigmoid loop averts most of these problems.

Nevertheless, urinary tract diversion is not a perfect answer, and continuous reevaluation of the results of these procedures is mandatory. The primary care physician should establish contact for the patient with an experienced surgeon and participate in the lifelong reevaluation that must be part of the overall management of these problems. Enterostomal therapists have added considerably to the overall management of children with permanent diversions.

Although conduits have gone far to protect the upper urinary tract and are socially manageable, no conduit is as functionally dependable or socially acceptable as an intact urinary tract. Urinary undiversion is now possible, and the evolution of newer techniques may increase the chances for reconstructing an intact urinary tract. *Intermittent catheterization* now makes it possible for a child to stay dry even though the normal voiding function is not satisfactory to empty the bladder.

REFERENCES
1. Gibbons, M. D., Cromie, W. J., and Duckett, J. W., Jr.: Management of the abdominal undescended testicle, J. Urol. **122:**76, 1979.
2. Kales, A., and others: Effects of imipramine on enuretic frequency and sleep stages, Pediatrics **60:**431, 1977.
3. Kinney, T. R., and others: Priapism in association with sickle hemoglobinopathies in children, Pediatrics **86:**241, 1975.
4. Koop, C. E.: Technique for herniorrhaphy and orchidopexy, Birth Defects **13**(5):293, 1977.
5. Mengel, W., and others: Studies on cryptorchidism: a comparison of histological findings in the germative epithelium before and after the second year of life, J. Pediatr. Surg. **9:**445, 1974.

6. Morse, T. S., and Hollabaugh, R. S.: The "window" orchidopexy for prevention of testicular torsion, J. Pediatr. Surg. **12:**237, 1977.

7. Perlmutter, A. D.: Enuresis. In Kelalis, P. P., King, L. R., and Belman, A. B., editors: Clinical Pediatric Urology, Philadelphia, 1976, W. B. Saunders Co., p. 166.

8. Poussaint, A. F., and Ditman, K. S.: A controlled study of imipramine (Tofranil) in the treatment of childhood enuresis, J. Pediatr. **67:**283, 1965.

9. Rajfer, J., and Walsh, P. C.: Testicular descent, Birth Defects **13**(2):107, 1977.

10. Woolley, M. M.: Cryptorchidism. In Ravitch, M. M., and others, editors: Pediatric surgery, ed. 3, Chicago, 1979, Year Book Medical Publishers, Inc., p. 1402.

CHAPTER 22

Neurosurgical considerations

W. JERRY OAKES and ROBERT H. WILKINS

POSTERIOR FOSSA TUMORS AND CYSTS

Mass lesions that occur intracranially are usually divided into two anatomic subgroups. Those occurring above the tentorium are supratentorial lesions. Those occurring below the tentorium are infratentorial, or posterior fossa, lesions. Occasionally, a lesion will be found that has both supratentorial and infratentorial components, but its primary clinical effect will usually be restricted to only one of these. Since the clinical presentation, physical findings, and surgical approaches are quite different with lesions in these locations, it is best that they be discussed separately. Supratentorial lesions are discussed in Chapter 27 in the section on the teenager. The current discussion deals with lesions occurring below the tentorium, which is the predominant location for neoplasms and cysts in childhood; more than 60% of such lesions occur in this location.[24,28] This relationship is reversed in adults; 75% of brain tumors are located above the tentorium. It is also important to emphasize that in childhood many commonly found infratentorial masses are benign and readily curable. Malignant tumors certainly do occur, but all is not lost when a mass is discovered in the posterior fossa. Even with malignant tumors, significant progress has been made in lengthening postoperative symptom-free survival, and the occasional patient may be cured.

Routine examination for age. The cerebellum of the child modulates voluntary motor activity. It does not directly control strength, sensation, or consciousness. Abnormalities of cerebellar function cause altered equilibrium or balance. The neonate, for example, may try to suck his thumb, and he may possess the strength to move

the thumb to his mouth. However, the lack of smooth, coordinated movement of the muscles of his arm, expressed as irregular and jerky movement, may prohibit him from accurately placing the thumb in his mouth. With maturation of the cerebellum and its connections, such movement becomes smooth and precise.

Cerebellar function can be tested by observing the child's posture and voluntary movements. When sitting, the child should not have to brace the trunk with the arms to gain stability. The ability of the child to monitor truncal stability can be tested by observing the gait, especially while the child is turning. Movement of the outstretched arms should be smooth without oscillation. Drinking from a cup or threading beads on a stick requires significant coordination and is easily tested in childhood. Cerebellar input also influences muscular tone and the deep tendon reflexes, both decreasing or becoming hypoactive with cerebellar disease. Activities requiring rapid alternating movement, such as hand clapping and foot tapping, are also strongly influenced by the cerebellum. The rhythm or rate of the movement, as well as the force exerted during each movement, are controlled by the cerebellum. The muscles of phonation are affected in a similar manner. Extraocular movements, like other voluntary movements, are affected by cerebellar function, with the development of nystagmus in the pathologic situation.

Possible findings. In general, mass lesions of the posterior fossa obstruct cerebrospinal fluid (CSF) flow early in the course of the illness, resulting in hydrocephalus. This occurs secondary to the small size and the location of the CSF path-

382

ways that are present in the posterior fossa. The block of flow most frequently occurs at the level of the aqueduct of Sylvius. Infratentorial mass lesions are predominantly located behind or lateral to the aqueduct and will displace its caudal portion ventrally, resulting in angulation or kinking of the central portion of the aqueduct and obstruction to CSF flow at that point. An additional factor that leads to the development of symptoms early in the course of the disease is the relative inability of the posterior fossa to expand in response to a growing mass. In the area of the aqueduct a small, strategically located tumor can easily result in hydrocephalus and yet be difficult to identify by screening radiographic techniques. Because of this, every case of hydrocephalus must be carefully evaluated for the site of obstruction of CSF flow and the cause of that obstruction. If new, unexplained symptoms appear in a patient with hydrocephalus of unknown cause, the patient must be reevaluated to ensure that the new symptoms are not a sign of a previously unrecognized posterior fossa mass.

When a posterior fossa mass lesion is present, symptoms and signs occur that can help the clinician differentiate which structures are predominantly affected by the mass. These findings will help localize the mass in the middle cerebellar structures, in one of the cerebellar hemispheres, in the substance of the brain stem, or in the cerebellopontine angle.

A mass lesion that occurs in the midline portion of the cerebellum expands locally, and the patient will frequently have only complaints referable to hydrocephalus. The classic triad of headache, nausea and vomiting, and papilledema implies increased intracranial pressure and is seen with the development of hydrocephalus. A careful history may reveal transient or episodic cerebellar dysfunction associated with a minor head injury, a febrile illness, or other nonspecific insult. The cerebellar dysfunction is usually nystagmus or truncal ataxia with gait and equilibrium difficulties or symptoms referable to increased intracranial pressure. The clinical symptoms may last for several hours or even a few days before they disappear. These findings frequently will be unnoticed because the child recovers spontaneously and is left with no recognizable deficit. It may then be weeks or months before any new symptoms occur. These may simply be irritability, excessive fatigue, or vomiting. None of these findings are specific, and

all are easily passed over in the initial stages of the disease. The complaints then become more constant with less fluctuation until finally they become constant. The headache may begin in the early morning on awakening or, more significantly, may awaken the child from sleep. There is no characteristic location for the headache; it may occur anteriorly, posteriorly, over the vertex, or over the entire head. Vomiting may occur spontaneously without abdominal pain and, occasionally, without complaint of headache. The vomiting may occur at any time, but it is particularly characteristic in the early morning on arising and in the afternoon after a brief rest or nap. The child will also tend to develop malaise, going to bed early without being asked or not playing actively with his peers. Fine nystagmus may be seen on lateral gaze, and the child will become unsteady on his feet. Skills requiring truncal coordination and balance are affected first, resulting in inability to ride a bicycle or walk on top of a wall. Difficulty in maintaining balance increases, so that the normal gait is affected; it becomes wide based, and the child has particular difficulty during turning. Usually the fine movements of the hands and legs are not affected initially. In extreme cases, the central or truncal ataxia is so severe that the child has difficulty sitting without using his arms to support or brace his trunk. If left unsupported while sitting or standing, the child may sway to and fro, as if in a wind that is rapidly changing direction. This finding may be brought out during the examination by narrowing the child's base and having him stand with the feet in tandem. Diplopia develops, usually due to a sixth nerve palsy with weakness of the lateral rectus muscle. If left unattended, the child may develop "cerebellar fits" with episodic altered consciousness, bilateral extensor posturing of the extremities, arching of the back, dilatation of the pupils, bradycardia, and respiratory irregularities. These are thought to represent periodic rapid rises in intracranial pressure, resulting in medullary dysfunction. During these attacks, respiration may stop altogether, resulting in the child's death. Typical epileptic seizures do not occur with lesions of the posterior fossa.

Lesions that primarily affect one cerebellar hemisphere may have a similar early history with transient symptoms that occur in response to minor trauma or systemic illness. Symptoms of raised intracranial pressure are also common and are similar to those occurring with midline cerebellar masses, but they may appear somewhat later in the course of the illness. The ataxia that develops from laterally placed lesions, however, is not truncal but appendicular initially, involving fine, coordinated movements of the ipsilateral hand, arm, leg, and foot. Demanding motor skills, such as threading beads on a string or stacking blocks, become impossible. The child learns to compensate for his disability by bracing his arm at the elbow and wrist to maximize the stability of his hand. Progressive oscillations of the hand as it approaches the target (dysmetria) during the finger-to-nose test also become apparent on the side of the lesion. Rapid alternating movements also become difficult; rapid clapping of the hand or tapping of the foot has an irregular rhythm and force. Nystagmus occurs that is no longer fine but very coarse, with the fast component of the nystagmus to the side of the lesion. A head tilt becomes apparent, with neck pain developing if a normal head posture is assumed. The tilt may occur toward or away from the involved cerebellar hemisphere. Pain on movement helps to differentiate this head tilt from that seen with compensation for diplopia. Tone in the ipsilateral extremities is decreased, as are the ipsilateral deep tendon reflexes. Strength and sensation are usually not affected. If pathologic reflexes do develop, this implies compression or invasion of the brain stem and occurs late in the course of the disease.

Tumors that infiltrate the brain stem will initially involve cranial nerve and pyramidal tract function. Most commonly affected are the sixth and seventh cranial nerves, either unilaterally or bilaterally. The lower cranial nerves may also be involved, resulting in the complaint of hoarseness, difficulty with swallowing liquids, or regurgitation of fluid into the nasal cavity. The speech may become nasal in quality, and the gag reflex is depressed on the involved side. The uvula may not elevate in the midline but may be pulled to the normal side. Internuclear ophthalmoplegia may also be seen and when present strongly suggests a lesion within the substance of the brain stem, as opposed to an extra-axial lesion compressing the brain stem. This condition is characterized by limitation of movement of the adducting eye on lateral gaze, but with preservation of adduction during convergence. Usually the abducting eye on lateral gaze will demonstrate coarse nystagmus. The corticospinal tracts are commonly involved, resulting in complaints of stiffness and weakness of the legs.

As opposed to the other mass lesions found in the posterior fossa, intrinsic brain stem tumors cause hydrocephalus later in the course of the disease.

Lesions in the cerebellopontine angle are quite unusual in childhood. When they do occur, they may involve hearing and facial sensation. The corneal reflex is the best method of assessing facial sensation in childhood. At a later time, the ipsilateral face may become weak. Abnormalities of lower cranial nerve function may follow. Hydrocephalus occurs early, resulting in obstruction to flow at the level of the aqueduct of Sylvius. With large lesions, brain stem and cerebellar compression result. Depending on the degree of involvement of these structures, other findings will then occur as described above.

Common occurrences. There are four types of neoplasms that occur with some frequency in the posterior fossa in children. In order of their occurrence, they are the cerebellar astrocytoma, medulloblastoma, brain stem glioma, and ependymoma. In addition, arachnoid cysts are common, particularly in patient with symptoms within the first 5 years of life. Other, less common lesions include dermoid cysts, cerebellar sarcomas, mixed gliomas of the cerebellum, choroid plexus papillomas, chordomas, hemangioblastomas, and acoustic neuromas.

Cerebellar astrocytomas are neoplasms occurring in the cerebellar hemisphere or vermis. They are the commonest neoplasm in the posterior fossa and carry a favorable prognosis. The peak age of presentation is the second half of the first decade. There is an equal occurrence rate in boys and girls. The clinical presentation is one of hydrocephalus without any findings localized to the cerebellum or hydrocephalus combined with truncal or appendicular ataxia. Characteristically, the neoplasm will be associated with a cyst that expands into the substance of the cerebellum. It is not unusual for the cyst to have several times the volume of the actual neoplasm. The cyst lining will frequently be seen to be a glistening surface with little irregularity. In one area of the cyst wall, a mural nodule will be found, which represents the neoplasm. Within the cyst is xanthochromic proteinaceous fluid, which is relatively hypocellular. A minority of the tumors remain solid without significant cyst formation. If the lining of the cyst is not smooth and glistening, the possibility exists that the tumor is diffusely located around the cyst wall rather than solely in a mural nodule.

By the time of presentation, only 10% to 15% of cerebellar astrocytomas will have grown into surgically nonresectable areas such as the cerebellar peduncles or brain stem.[30]

The *medulloblastoma* occurs only slightly less frequently than the cerebellar astrocytoma.[28] Each represents between 30% and 35% of the posterior fossa neoplasms seen in children. This tumor tends to occur earlier in life, and the peak age of presentation is between the third and sixth year.[28] Boys are affected significantly more commonly than girls, with a ratio of 2½ to 1. The tumor characteristically originates in the midline in the anterior medullary velum and expands locally. The vermis and more medial cerebellar structures are involved first. As the tumor then expands into the fourth ventricle, it may completely occupy and expand this structure. Hydrocephalus with a midline cerebellar syndrome is the characteristic presentation. The length of clinical symptoms is usually only 1 to 3 months, which is significantly shorter than the clinical history for cerebellar astrocytomas. Cyst formation with medulloblastomas is unusual. The tumor has a strong tendency to spread within the CSF pathways, causing subarachnoid seeding over the surface of the cerebellum and around the spinal cord. In addition, seeding may take place over the surface of the brain or within the ventricular system. Occasionally, the metastatic seeding of the tumor may result in the initial symptoms being referable to the spinal cord or cerebrum. The medulloblastoma is a malignant tumor with rapid growth characteristics. However, its sensitivity to radiotherapy and chemotherapy makes long-term survival a realistic possibility.[6,14,50]

Brain stem gliomas vary slightly in their presentation from other tumors of the posterior fossa. The age of presentation is similar, peaking at 7 years.[28] Hydrocephalus and increased intracranial pressure are unusual; when they do occur, it is late in the course of the disease. The tumor is seen to be composed of benign-appearing glial cells, predominantly astrocytes, which initially separate and infiltrate the structures of the brain stem without causing clinical symptoms. The majority of these tumors begin in the pons with involvement of the mesencephalon, medulla, and cerebellar peduncles occurring later in their course. The pons simply enlarges to accommodate the expanding mass until a critical size is reached, at which time symptoms begin. By this time, the brain stem is usually massively enlarged.

Cranial nerve dysfunction frequently begins with weakness of the lateral rectus muscle (secondary to sixth nerve paralysis) and peripheral facial weakness. As the lesion continues to expand, other cranial nerves become involved, including those of the medulla, causing difficulty with speech and swallowing. Involvement of the trigeminal nuclei and nerves at the upper aspect of the pons causes loss of facial sensation and weakness of mastication. Motor function is involved early, resulting in the development of spastic weakness of the extremities, increased tone, and exaggerated deep tendon reflexes and extensor plantar responses. The cranial nerve abnormalities commonly occur bilaterally. The clinical picture of multiple cranial nerve abnormalities, spastic weakness of the extremities, and absence of increased intracranial pressure are so characteristic that a presumptive diagnosis can be made on clinical findings only. Late in the course, hydrocephalus with obstruction of the aqueduct of Sylvius may be seen.

Ependymomas make up only 10% of posterior fossa tumors in children. They frequently originate in the floor of the fourth ventricle and expand locally to occupy this cavity. Like cerebellar astrocytomas and medulloblastomas, they cause hydrocephalus early in their clinical course. The site of origin is frequently near the facial colliculus, and the tumors cause peripheral facial and lateral rectus weakness. Their attachment to the floor of the fourth ventricle and local invasion of the brain stem make their total resection ill advised. These tumors occur at a significantly earlier peak age (2 to 4 years) than other tumors of the posterior fossa.[28] Ependymomas are rarely cystic but do calcify with some frequency. Although most of the tumor can be surgically excised and a high dose of radiation given postoperatively, these patients have a poor prognosis.[33,46] Seeding of the CSF pathway may be seen but with less frequency than with medulloblastomas.

A much more positive approach can be applied to *arachnoid cysts,* which occur in the posterior fossa. These mass lesions are congenital collections of fluid between two layers of arachnoid.[41] They are found over the cerebellar hemispheres and vermis, over the quadrigeminal plate, and in the cerebellopontine angle. Below the age of 18 months, they are the most common of the posterior fossa masses.[29] These lesions do not have free communication with the CSF pathways, and they enlarge slowly, compressing the surrounding brain structures. Fluid within the cyst is slightly xanthochromic but is otherwise similar to CSF. The presentation of these tumors may be acute (following minor head injury with bleeding into the cyst) or chronic (with symptoms resulting from compression of the surrounding brain structures). Hydrocephalus is frequently seen in association with the posterior fossa arachnoid cyst, and the symptoms are indistinguishable from those of neoplasms occurring in this area.

Evaluation. Following a thorough clinical evaluation, routine skull x-ray films are obtained. These often are of little localizing value, but they may indicate calcification within the posterior fossa or thinning and expansion of the occipital squamosa over the cerebellar hemisphere on the involved side. Evidence of suture separation may also be seen, along with signs of chronically elevated intracranial pressure (amputation of the posterior clinoids or a beaten silver appearance of the cranial vault) (Fig. 22-1). Calcification is seen occasionally in ependymomas and only rarely within other tumors of the posterior fossa. Expansion of the occipital squamosa implies an expanding mass laterally placed in the posterior fossa. Following routine skull x-ray films, a computerized tomographic (CT) brain scan with enhancement is obtained. This scan will frequently give all the radiographic information that is necessary prior to surgical exploration. With the use of this modality, arachnoid cysts are well seen, as is the position and shape of the fourth ventricle. When questions arise as to whether a cyst is in communication with the normally circulating CSF and not acting as a mass lesion or is loculated and compressing brain tissue, two findings are useful. Mass lesions shift normal brain structures away, and this phenomenon can be appreciated on the CT scan. To determine if the cyst is in communication with CSF circulation, metrizamide is injected into the lumbar subarachnoid space or the lateral ventricle and allowed to circulate. If opacification occurs in the CSF adjacent to the cyst but not within the cyst, it can be presumed that the cyst is excluded from the CSF circulation. This finding raises the likelihood that the cyst will act as a mass, and such a cyst should be treated (Fig. 22-2).

In smaller children and infants, the detail of the structures in the posterior fossa may not be clear because of movement artifact. Rather than using an invasive radiographic modality, it is wise to repeat the CT brain scan, with a general anesthetic if necessary, to obtain maximal information from this study. Overlapping sections may be of help in demonstrating small structures and in confirming or denying abnormalities seen in only one slice.

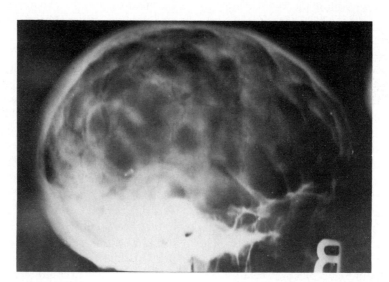

Fig. 22-1. Radiograph of a patient with chronically increased intracranial pressure and a beaten metal appearance of the cranial vault. The cranial sutures are not separated in this teenager, because the sutures have physiologically fused before the intracranial pressure became raised. The sella turcica is expanded, and the posterior clinoids have been amputated from the dilated third ventricle.

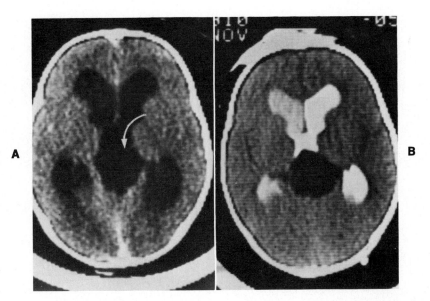

Fig. 22-2. A, CT brain scan demonstrating moderate enlargement of the frontal and occipital horns of both lateral ventricles in a young child with an acclerated rate of head growth and macrocrania. Within the dilated third ventricle a horizontal septation can faintly be seen (arrow). **B,** Repeat scan following the injection of contrast medium (metrizamide) into the right lateral ventricle. The contrast medium diffuses through the ventricular system but fails to opacify the CSF attenuation in the area of the posterior third ventricle and quadrigeminal plate. The cyst compressed the aqueduct of Sylvius, causing the internal, or noncommunicating hydrocephalus.

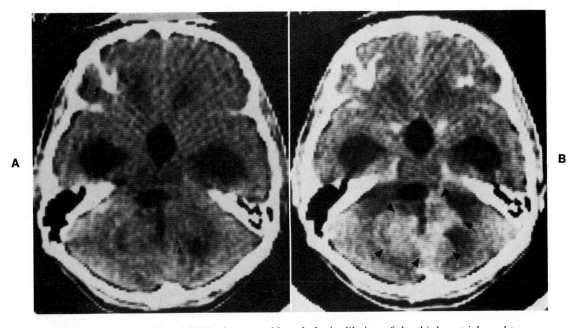

Fig. 22-3. A, Unenhanced CT brain scan with pathologic dilation of the third ventricle and temporal horns in a 14-year-old boy whose complaints included headaches, ataxia, and bilateral papilledema. The fourth ventricle is enlarged, irregular, and anteriorly placed. **B,** Following contrast enhancement, a large midline cerebellar tumor can be seen (medulloblastoma) (arrows).

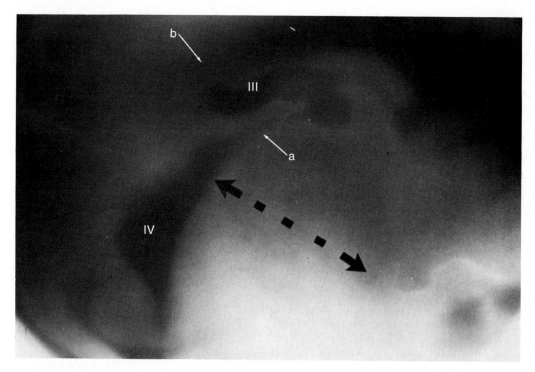

Fig. 22-4. Lateral skull radiograph during a pneumoencephalogram. Visualized are the triangular fourth ventricle *(IV)*, the aqueduct of Sylvius *(a)*, and the posterior third ventricle *(III)* with a large suprapineal recess *(b)*. The distance between the floor of the fourth ventricle and anterior surface of the brain stem (arrows) is increased, indicating an expanding lesion of the brain stem.

Without visualization of the fourth ventricle in its normal position, and with a normal configuration, no scan may be called normal. Intravenous enhancement may bring out the location and extent of neoplasms that are of similar attenuation to brain on the unenhanced study (Fig. 22-3). The size of the third and lateral ventricles may also be seen, along with any evidence of distally placed intracranial metastases. Angiography may occasionally be employed when the CT appearance of an abnormality is consistent with a vascular malformation or aneurysm. Some surgeons feel more secure when they have evaluated the position of the major vascular structures in the posterior fossa preoperatively and for that reason will obtain an angiogram. It is our opinion that this is only necessary in a minority of patients.[7] The use of ventriculography and pneumoencephalography, which were so frequently employed in the past to localize posterior fossa lesions, has been greatly restricted since the introduction of CT scans. They are still periodically necessary for the evaluation of brain stem gliomas. In combination with tomography, these studies are occasionally used

in difficult diagnostic situations to outline the fine anatomy of the posterior fossa in more detail than is possible with current CT scans (Fig. 22-4). Brain stem gliomas are somewhat more difficult to diagnose from the CT scan alone because of their tendency to have an attenuation similar to normal brain, even with intravenous enhancement. This fact leaves the diagnosis by CT scan based on compression of the surrounding CSF-containing structures, such as the fourth ventricle and basal cisterns (Fig. 22-5). These structures are small and are frequently difficult to visualize. Since the usual therapy recommended for this lesion is nonsurgical and no histologic confirmation is obtained, further detail of the fine structures of the posterior fossa can be obtained by pneumoencephalography before the child is submitted to radiation therapy. One indication for surgery in brain stem gliomas is the presence of a symptomatic cyst within the tumor.[30] These can only be diagnosed by CT scan (Fig. 22-6). A small group of patients will have typical complaints of a posterior fossa mass with no demonstrable abnormalities by CT scan, angiography, or

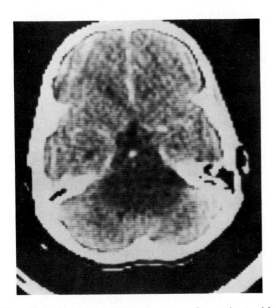

Fig. 22-5. Enhanced CT brain scan of a patient with low-attenuation enlargement of the brain stem. The fourth ventricle and posterior fossa CSF cisterns cannot be visualized because of the expanding mass. The white dot ventral to the expanded brain stem represents the contrast-filled basilar artery.

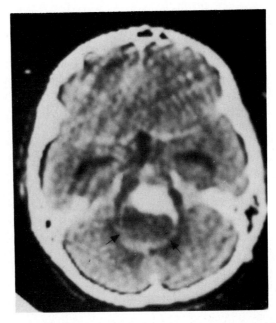

Fig. 22-6. Enhanced CT brain scan of a patient with bilateral cranial nerve abnormalities from a brain stem glioma. A ringlike enhancement can be seen within the posterior fossa (arrows). The more solid portion of the tumor is located anteriorly and is enhanced homogeneously.

pneumoencephalography. It is helpful in such cases to search carefully and repeatedly in the CSF by cytologic techniques for the presence of malignant cells. If this search proves negative and no other diagnosis becomes obvious, the CT scan should be repeated and used to follow the child in addition to frequent clinical assessments. It should also be emphasized that lumbar puncture in the presence of a posterior fossa mass may precipitate a rapid clinical deterioration.[9,16] Because of this possibility, lumbar puncture should be avoided until the CT scan has demonstrated no hydrocephalus or evidence of a mass in the posterior fossa. The lumbar puncture necessary for the pneumoencephalogram and the repeated CSF cytologies should be performed with a neurosurgeon available should clinical deterioration develop.

Referral. In general, the smaller the neoplasm and the fewer the clinical signs at the time of diagnosis of the posterior fossa mass, the better the chances of cure or prolonged palliation. Children who arrive on referral in a morbid condition, even with benign neoplasms and cysts, have a much more guarded prognosis than those who ar-

rive in good clinical condition. The ability of surgery to reverse a neurologic deficit once it has developed fully is limited. Early referral is indicated, particularly since evaluation is noninvasive in the majority of cases. This is not to say that every child with headache or protracted vomiting should be evaluated for a posterior fossa mass. However, this evaluation is indicated if even subtle neurologic findings can be found on the screening physical examination.

Medical versus surgical treatment. Many tumors found in the posterior fossa can be cured readily by surgical removal (cerebellar astrocytomas, dermoids, epidermoids). Other tumors occurring in the same location (medulloblastomas, ependymomas) cannot be accurately differentiated from the more benign tumors on clinical or radiographic grounds. Therefore, mass lesions occurring in the cerebellum or in the cerebellopontine angle should be explored surgically for histologic verification, reestablishment of the CSF pathway, and tumor removal where possible. Patients with tumors that are unequivocally found to be located within the substance of the brain stem by clinical and radiographic evaluation are obviously not candidates for radical tumor resection. Occasionally, these lesions will demonstrate a superficially placed cystic component or localized hemorrhage. With symptoms related to the cyst or hemorrhage, a limited surgical procedure to drain the involved area may be beneficial. If a clinical or radiographic question is raised regarding the diagnosis of a brain stem tumor, these patients are considered for posterior fossa exploration and biopsy of exophytic portions of the mass. Tumors that are malignant or only partially removed may then be considered for other forms of treatment, including radiation therapy and chemotherapy. Radiation therapy is routinely employed in medulloblastomas, ependymomas, and brain stem gliomas. The role of chemotherapy is still not totally defined. Many clinical trials are underway, and in the next few years the role of this form of therapy may become clearer.

A more controversial issue than whether posterior fossa tumors should have surgical exploration is whether those associated with hydrocephalus should routinely have placement of a ventriculoperitoneal or ventriculoatrial shunt prior to surgery on the posterior fossa tumor. Some recent data have shown a decreased mortality associated with the placement of a shunt prior to the removal of the posterior fossa tumor.[1] This technique, however, requires a second procedure and carries with it all the risks and hazards already described with shunt placement. We currently advise shunting in selected cases with clinical evidence of markedly increased intracranial pressure and hydrocephalus, but not on a routine basis. As a consequence of the shunt and decompression of the supratentorial compartment, the patient may demonstrate evidence of upward transtentorial herniation. Clinically, this herniation may be recognized by symptoms similar to those seen with central transtentorial herniation associated with supratentorial mass lesions. Initially the patient becomes lethargic; unilateral pupillary dilatation then follows, progressing to a complete third-nerve palsy. Decorticate posturing develops and is succeeded by decerebrate posturing. If such posturing occurs following shunting of the lateral ventricle, it is an indication for immediate infratentorial decompression. Congenital arachnoid cysts occurring in the posterior fossa, causing hydrocephalus and mass effect, are most simply treated by shunting the cyst into the peritoneal cavity. When hy-

drocephalus is present, it may be necessary to include the lateral ventricle in the shunt system. In this case, catheters will be placed in both the lateral ventricle and the posterior fossa cyst and subsequently will be attached to a peritoneal catheter. This method of treatment is preferred over exploration and resection of the posterior fossa cyst wall because of the frequent failure seen with the latter method.

Surgical options. If shunt placement prior to posterior fossa exploration is advised, it is performed in a routine fashion with the insertion of a valve-regulated ventriculoperitoneal shunting system. A millipore filter system has been developed to decrease the incidence of intraperitoneal metastasis through the shunt.[22] However, this filter system is also associated with a higher rate of shunt blockage than that with unfiltered shunts.[7]

CT scan localization of the extent of the tumor has greatly aided the surgeon in accurately placing the bony opening over the neoplasm. Following the incision of the dura, the subarachnoid space is inspected. Discrete tumor implants are sometimes seen over the surface of the cerebellum. Occasionally, the arachnoid will simply appear thickened or cloudy because of metastatic spread. Midline tumors may actually be seen to protrude through the foramen of Magendie and overlie the medulla and upper cervical spinal cord. The cerebellar folia will sometimes be seen to be widened and pale over the intraparenchymal mass. If no abnormality is seen over the exposed surface of the cerebellum, a cortical incision is made, guided by the previous CT scan localization of the tumor. Lateral hemisphere cysts may be verified by needle aspiration prior to cortical incision. Frozen section diagnosis is helpful in guiding the surgeon at the time of tumor removal. In the presence of a cerebellar astrocytoma, every effort is made to resect the tumor radically without embarrassing vital neural structures. This is possible in more than 80% of patients.[28] Medulloblastomas and ependymomas are removed as completely as possible without purposefully risking increased neurologic deficit. Residual tumor with both these lesions can be treated effectively with radiation and chemotherapy. Postoperative recovery is enhanced by watertight closure of the dura with a pericranial or fascial graft.

As previously described, shunting of posterior fossa cysts has proved very effective. The common occurrence of hydrocephalus with these cysts may necessitate a system with two proximal catheters—one in the posterior fossa cyst and one in the dilated ventricular system. These catheters are then joined proximal to the pressure-regulating valve.

Postoperative course. Following posterior fossa exploration, children will need careful medical attention and supervision for several days. They are best managed in a surgical intensive care unit accustomed to dealing with children. The children are nursed head up 30 degrees from the horizontal. This position enhances intracranial venous return and thereby decreases the intracranial volume and pressure. The endotracheal tube is left in place until the patient is fully conscious and has a stable respiratory pattern. Oral feeding is withheld until a vigorous gag response is shown to be present. An intra-arterial monitoring catheter is of great help in maintaining blood gases, serum electrolytes, and hemoglobin within the normal range. Hyperpyrexia is commonly seen following posterior fossa craniectomy and is managed by vigorous measures to lower the temperature to the normal range. Antipyretic medications, including aspirin or acetaminophen, are routinely given rectally. Exposure of large skin surfaces to the environment with cooling air as well as the use of a cooling blanket under the child may be necessary to maintain the temperature in the normal range. Hyperpyrexia is thought to be due to chemical meningitis from the blood released into the subarachnoid space at the time of surgery. Dural closure will prevent further tissue fluids of the paraspinal muscles from gaining access to the subarachnoid space and worsening this problem. The skin sutures are left in place for 5 to 7 days. Patients are routinely discharged on about the tenth postoperative day if no further therapy is planned.

Patients with posterior fossa cysts that have been shunted are usually nursed flat for 12 to 24 hours following the procedure. The head is gradually elevated over the next 3 to 4 days until finally the child is able to assume the erect position without becoming pale or diaphoretic. Once the child is able to assume the erect position and remain asymptomatic, he is eligible for discharge.

Prognosis. Posterior fossa cysts have an excellent prognosis, although attention should be directed to maintaining a continually functioning shunt system. Neurologic deficits that have developed prior to surgery may reverse. However, long-standing deficits usually remain unchanged,

which underscores the necessity for early detection and therapy.

The outcome of patients with posterior fossa tumors is very much a function of tumor histology. As previously stated, the cure rate for cerebellar astrocytomas is greater than 80%.[30] These patients are treated with surgical resection only and no adjunctive therapy. Operative mortality and morbidity are low. Matson[28] reported 98 consecutive cases without an operative death. Patients in whom the tumor cannot be totally excised may show a symptom-free survival of several years. Even with recurrent symptoms, a careful evaluation is necessary to decide whether the deterioration is due to brain stem invasion, hydrocephalus, surgically accessible regrowth of tumor, or cyst formation within the resection site. The treatment of each of these problems is different, as are the implications for the patient.

Medulloblastomas are deceptive at the time of surgery; they frequently demonstrate a well-developed cleavage plane between the tumor and the surrounding brain structures. It is now known that distal subarachnoid metastases at the time of initial diagnosis are relatively common.[40] The surgical resection of the tumor itself carries a 5% to 7% mortality, although improvement of this figure has been seen with early ventriculoperitoneal shunting. In addition to high-dose radiation directed to the posterior fossa, lesser doses are administered to the spinal cord and supratentorial compartment. With the use of this regimen, some success has been reported in long-term survival.[6] Various chemotherapeutic regimens are also being employed. The long-term effect of these agents is yet to be determined. With the use of these multiple forms of therapy, current survival statistics show a 5-year-survival of 40% and a 10-year survival of slightly more than 20%.[5]

Recent surveys of fourth ventricular ependymomas are less encouraging; fewer than 10% of the patients survive for 5 years.[33,46] Again, the operative mortality is in the range of 5% to 10%. Whole-brain radiation in a young child is frequently associated with mental retardation. This has been seen not only with posterior fossa tumors, but also with vigorous treatment regimens employed in controlling childhood leukemia.[29,38] It is still our practice to employ radiation as an integral part of therapy for these children; however, the exact dose and ports employed may need adjustment when follow-up data are analyzed.

Our level of confidence in analyzing the statistics for brain stem glioma is low. Long-term survivors have been reported; however, the vast majority of these cases have not had histologic confirmation. It is well recognized that there are many causes of brain stem enlargement, only one of which is brain stem glioma. There is little doubt, however, that true cases of brain stem glioma have a dismal prognosis; death usually occurs within 4 years.[36] If no radiation is administered, this process is hastened, so that survival is usually no longer than 9 to 12 months following the onset of symptoms.[30] Again, the occasional patient may survive years or decades without symptomatic progression.

Important aspects of follow-up. At the time of the child's discharge from the hospital, his neurologic recovery will frequently not be complete. Over the next few weeks to months, return of neurologic function will usually continue. The exact level of function that the child may eventually achieve is difficult to predict. It is, however, greatly influenced by the extent and duration of symptoms prior to therapy and the effectiveness of the particular therapy. Deterioration of neurologic function should always be reinvestigated; therefore, a baseline examination, including not only a neurologic examination but a postoperative CT scan as well, before hospital discharge is of critical importance.

Complications. Since many of these patients will have preoperative or postoperative shunts placed to control hydrocephalus, careful monitoring of the intracranial pressure and ventricular size is important. Late complications from infection or hemorrhage in the operative site are unusual. As mentioned earlier, evidence of neurologic deterioration need not necessarily mean regrowth of the tumor. It may be related to a more benign process that can be readily corrected, such as shunt malfunction or cyst formation at the operative site.

Other, less common lesions. Many other types of tumors may be found in the posterior fossa of children. Of particular importance is the dermoid tumor, which characteristically occurs in the midline and may be associated with a *dermal sinus tract* over the occiput. These tumors may present with recurrent meningitis, symptoms of truncal ataxia from midline cerebellar compression, or hydrocephalus. They are of particular importance because of their benign nature and favorable re-

sponse to therapy. Epidermoid tumors, which characteristically occur in the cerebellopontine angle of the posterior fossa, also have a favorable outlook. These tumors, however, are unusual in childhood despite their congenital nature.

The *hemangioblastoma* is a benign, frequently cystic tumor, found in the cerebellar hemisphere. Approximately one fifth of the cases of hemangioblastoma are associated with von Hippel-Lindau disease, in which the central nervous system tumor occurs with concomitant retinal angiomas; cysts of the pancreas, liver, and kidney; and polycythemia.[26,30] Occurring in the cerebellum and in the substance of the brain stem and spinal cord, hemangioblastomas may be multiple.

Another benign tumor that can occur in the posterior fossa is the *choroid plexus papilloma*. However, this location is an unusual one for this tumor in childhood. It is more characteristically found in the fourth ventricle in adults; in childhood the usual location is the atrium of the lateral ventricle. Within the posterior fossa the tumor may be found solely within the fourth ventricle, or it may grow laterally through the foramen of Luschka and present as a mass in the cerebellopontine angle. Although they are histologically benign, these tumors represent a major surgical challenge because of their location.

The *acoustic neuroma,* which is not uncommonly seen in adult life, is rarely seen in childhood. When it is encountered, it is frequently associated with von Recklinghausen's disease, and bilateral tumors may be found.

LOCALIZED INTRACRANIAL INFECTIONS

With the advent of antibiotics the occurrence of intracranial abscesses has decreased dramatically. Despite this decrease in incidence, a 40% mortality continued to be the rule until CT brain scanning was introduced.[34,48] Recent reports have shown that with exact localization of abscess cavities, surgical therapy can be accurately directed and the effect of therapy more easily followed. This is reflected in a recent decrease in the mortality rate.[34,42,47] Because of the noninvasive nature of the CT brain scan, physicians are more willing to survey patients at risk of abscess formation. As a result, patients with localized intracranial infections are being detected earlier and treated before major neurologic sequelae develop. It should also be borne in mind that 20% of patients with brain abscesses will not have a history of factors that would predispose them to abscess formation. That, together with the fact that the patient with a brain abscess usually does not show evidence of acute infection with hyperpyrexia or elevation of the peripheral leukocyte count, makes brain abscess an important differential diagnosis in any patient with a localized intracranial mass.

Possible findings. Localized infection in the brain may occur by direct extension from a parameningeal focus or by hematogenous seeding. The parameningeal source may be found to be a paranasal sinus, middle ear or mastoid sinus, transcranial venous channel, or comminuted depressed skull fracture. A patient with one of these sources will initially demonstrate acute evidence of infection with fever, leukocytosis, malaise, irritability, localized tenderness, and purulent drainage. Involvement of the brain is usually not clinically apparent at this point. As the infection reaches the dura and involves the brain, cerebritis develops and may be manifested by focal neurologic compromise. At this point, abscess formation is not assured.

Cerebritis may be treated effectively with appropriate antibiotics, resulting in complete resolution of the infectious process. If foreign material (depressed bone fragments, wood fragments, cotton wadding) remains within the brain parenchyma, the likelihood of abscess formation is markedly increased.[18,31] If cerebral infarction has occurred, either as a consequence of embolization or venous occlusion, the incidence of abscess formation is also increased.[3,32]

In 10 to 14 days localized infection in the brain will begin to develop into an abscess capsule. With additional time the capsule will thicken and become more fibrous. This process is slowed if the patient is immunologically suppressed. As the abscess encapsulates, focal neurologic signs may be lacking. Over a period of weeks to months, the abscess enlarges and signs of focal neurologic compromise develop.

In young children and infants the only sign of abnormality may be the development of increased intracranial pressure and macrocrania.[21,44,45] Fever and leukocytosis characteristically are resolved, as are other signs of localized infection prior to the presentation of the abscess. Children whose infections have a hematogenous source will frequently be found to have congenital cyanotic heart disease (tetralogy of Fallot, truncus arteriosus, ven-

tricular septal defects), subacute bacterial endocarditis, a lung abscess, or bronchiectasis. Meningitis is rarely associated with brain abscess formation except in the case of a dermal sinus tract and intracranial dermoid where the abscess formation occurs within the tumor.

Common occurrences. Brain abscesses occur in characteristic locations, depending on the source of the infection. Lesions associated with penetrating trauma will occur adjacent to the point of dural penetration. The bone fragments or other bits of foreign material that are driven into the brain are contaminated and are likely sources of potential infection. High-velocity bullet fragments are sterile and possess a low likelihood of being associated with abscess formation. Paranasal sinus infection characteristically causes abscess formation in the undersurface of the frontal lobe with attachment to the floor of the anterior fossa. Middle ear disease may be associated with a temporal lobe or cerebellar abscess. The temporal lobe abscess is based on the petrous ridge and the floor of the middle fossa. Cerebellar abscess formation occurs anteriorly and laterally within the posterior fossa, based on the posterior portion of the petrous ridge. In patients with metastatic abscess formation, the abscess is not based on the inner aspect of the skull but lies free within the brain parenchyma, usually in the distribution of the middle cerebral artery. These abscesses are thought to originate at the junction of the gray and white matter. With growth they will expand into the white matter.

The organisms frequently responsible for abscess formation in childhood are anaerobic or microaerophilic bacteria; streptococci are the most frequent group. Thus, when material is being obtained for culture, anaerobic transfer media should be provided in the operating room. Previously, large numbers of brain abscesses were considered sterile. However, more effective culturing techniques have shown these to probably represent anaerobic or microaerophilic bacterial infection.[8,15,20,43] Other organisms that can be involved include staphylococci, *Haemophilus influenzae,* and gram-negative bacteria. In young infants gram-negative bacteria are the most common cause of brain abscess. In the immunologically suppressed, unusual organisms can be found, including *Nocardia, Aspergillus,* and *Candida,* as well as other fungi. This fact necessitates that brain abscesses be cultured for aerobic and anaerobic bacteria and fungi. Localized tuberculous disease (tuberculoma) occurs rarely in the United States today. When it is seen, it is easily confused with other infections or neoplastic processes. The granulomatous material within the tuberculoma may be indistinguishable from bacterial or fungal pus. In addition to those cultures previously mentioned, cultures for *Mycobacterium tuberculosis* should be submitted.

It should again be emphasized that 20% of brain abscesses will have no predisposing factors. These patients are thought to have had hematogenous spread of infection resulting from previous septicemia. Clinically silent right-to-left cardiac shunts may allow poorly oxygenated venous blood to bypass the filtering capillaries of the lung and be distributed in the systemic circulation. During a bout of septicemia, a small focus of septic infarction will grow into a brain abscess.

Evaluation. Following a careful history with particular reference to previous penetrating head injury, sinusitis, ear infection, or systemic illness, a detailed physical examination is performed. Evidence of paranasal sinus infection, chronic middle ear or mastoid infection, or a remote focus of infection capable of metastasizing to the head is sought. Skull x-ray films are of importance in evaluating the radiographic appearance of the paranasal sinuses, the middle ear, and the mastoid, as well as in providing evidence of previous skull trauma. Rarely, gas-forming organisms may produce enough gas within the abscess to be visualized on routine skull x-ray films. The presence of a foreign body or bone spicules within the brain strongly raises the possibility of abscess formation. X-ray films of the chest are important to support the clinical suspicion of localized pulmonary disease or congenital heart disease, both of which are strong predisposing factors to hematogenous spread as the source of an abscess.

The procedure of choice, as outlined previously, is a CT scan of the brain. Both enhanced and unenhanced studies are necessary (Fig. 22-7). Serial CT scans may be used to follow the scan appearance of localized intracranial infection, beginning with cerebritis prior to the development of an abscess capsule and following through to the formation of the capsule with central liquifaction necrosis. CT scanning has many advantages, including its noninvasive nature and exact localization of surgically important brain abscesses. Abscesses that are less than 1 cm in diameter and located near large bony prominences may occa-

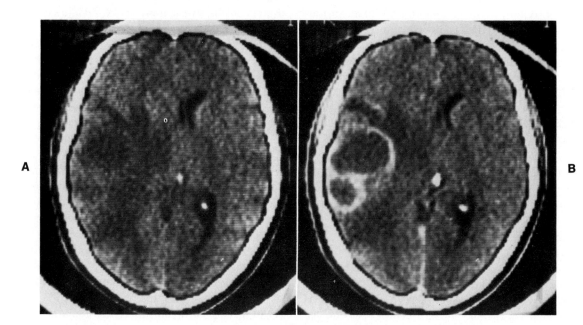

Fig. 22-7. A, Unenhanced CT brain scan of a patient with a left temporoparietal mass effect with surrounding edema. **B,** With enhancement the lesion is seen to be composed of two well-defined circular densities with a rather uniform thickness of the enhancing rim. The lesion proved to be a cerebral abscess with a posteriorly placed daughter abscess.

sionally be missed. Typically, the well-developed abscess will have a central area of low attenuation surrounded by a regular thin rim of enhancement. Outside the area of enhancement, the abscess is frequently surrounded by a large amount of vasogenic cerebral edema. The ventricular system may be shifted away from the mass. The presence of foreign material and bony spicules within the brain also can be evaluated easily with the CT scan. Another helpful aspect of the scan is the ability to determine if daughter abscesses are present. These offshoots from the main abscess cavity are usually loculated and result in clinical recurrence unless they are recognized and treated appropriately.

In the presence of increased intracranial pressure secondary to a brain abscess, lumbar puncture is not advised. The risk of precipitating brain herniation is large, and the information to be gained from the lumbar puncture is minimal. CSF that has been obtained in the presence of a well-encapsulated brain abscess will show a limited increase in the number of leukocytes (usually lymphocytes) and a slight elevation of protein content. CSF cultures are characteristically sterile. Arteriography, pneumoencephalography, and ventriculography add very little to the localization of the brain abscess, and all carry some risk to the patient. Because of this, they are rarely employed in current practice. The CT scan appearance of some gliomas and some metastatic neoplasms may be similar to that of brain abscesses. Angiography may be of some help in differentiating an abscess from these neoplasms.

Referral. If a brain abscess is suspected, immediate neurosurgical evaluation is indicated. It is clear that delay in diagnosis and localization of the infection is accompanied by a marked rise in mortality. Because of this, early evaluation and therapy are required to keep mortality figures to a minimum. This is particularly true in the younger child because of the lack of focal neurologic signs associated with large mass lesions in this age group. The accuracy of CT scanning is such that rapid evaluation and assessment of the patient can be made within a period of hours.

Medical versus surgical treatment. The prompt administration of appropriate antibiotics and aspiration or excision of the abscess remain the standard care for this problem. In the cerebritis phase of the illness prior to encapsulation, antibiotic therapy alone may be indicated. This is be-

cause surgical attack on the swollen brain does not allow accurate definition of permanently diseased tissue from tissue that is simply edematous and reactive. Resection of areas of cerebritis, except in the setting of transtentorial herniation, is unwarranted. Antibiotic therapy without surgical aspiration of the abscess is also unwise. The recent improvement in mortality statistics has resulted not from more effective antibiotics, but from increased accuracy in our ability to localize and follow the abscess and its daughter cavities radiographically, which in turn facilitates surgical treatment.

Surgical options. There are currently three methods of surgical treatment for a brain abscess: excision of the abscess cavity, drainage of the abscess cavity through a catheter, and simple aspiration of the cavity. It is our opinion that mature abscess cavities that are located in relatively silent areas of the brain in patients who are not critically ill should be treated by excision of the entire abscess. Abscesses that are located deep within the substance of the brain or in clinically strategic locations are handled more successfully by aspiration of purulent material, instillation of antibiotics within the cavity, and constant catheter drainage (Fig. 22-8). For the child who comes to the hospital critically ill, for whom prolonged anesthetic and surgical manipulation would be ill advised, simple aspiration of the abscess cavity is appropriate; it will establish the diagnosis, provide material for culture, and relieve the increased intracranial pressure. After several aspirations and stabilization of the patient's clinical condition, reassessment regarding excision of the abscess cavity can be made. Following the size and location of the abscess cavity has been so simplified by CT scanning that many surgeons are now tending to employ aspiration and catheter drainage with careful follow-up rather than excision in most patients.

Postoperative course. Antibiotics are routinely administered for 4 to 6 weeks. Abscess cavities that are treated by aspiration or catheter drainage should be followed closely by serial CT scans, which should demonstrate progressive diminution in the size of the cavity. If persistent accumulation of pus occurs, reaspiration is indicated. With excision of the abscess cavity and a benign postoperative course, the child will frequently be discharged (after 10 to 14 days) with continued oral antibiotic therapy. Aspiration and catheterization require hospitalization for 3 to 6 weeks, depend-

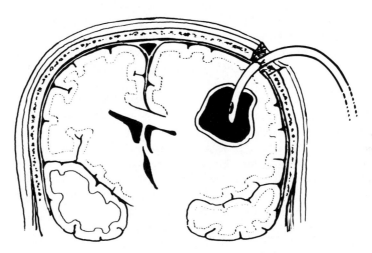

Fig. 22-8. Brain abscess being treated by catheter drainage. The catheter is left in place until purulent drainage is eliminated or markedly decreased and the CT brain scan confirms the diminishing size of the cavity. (From Milhorat, J. H.: Pediatric neurosurgery, Philadelphia, 1978, F. A. Davis Co.)

ing on the patient's response to therapy and the antibiotic and route of administration chosen. With parameningeal infections, consultation with an otolaryngologist is necessary to eliminate the source of infection and prevent recurrent disease. In the presence of cyanotic heart disease or serious lung infection as a source of hematogenous spread of the brain abscess, care should be taken to treat coexisting bacterial endocarditis and suppurative lung disease.

Prognosis. Until recently the mortality for brain abscess had been stable at approximately 40%.[17,25] This included lesions in both the supratentorial compartment and the posterior fossa. Two recent series using a combination of surgical incision, aspiration, and catheter drainage after CT localization have shown no mortality, but larger series are necessary before it is clear that progress has been made in this area.[42,47] Children brought to the hospital in a coma or with marked neurologic compromise continue to be at risk of having permanent neurologic deficits. Another group at high risk of permanent injury, including mental retardation, are infants with giant abscesses associated with massive brain destruction.[21] Even though the abscess is successfully treated, the amount of cerebral tissue that has been destroyed by the time the child comes to clinical attention may result in permanent and severe neurologic compromise.

Important aspects of follow-up. The serious late complications from a brain abscess are pri-

marily re-formation of the abscess cavity or the onset of seizures. Pus will reaccumulate in the abscess cavity in approximatley 8% of cases when the capsule has not been excised.[35] Because of this relatively high recurrence rate, patients undergoing aspiration or catheter drainage should be followed carefully for months to years with serial CT scans. This high rate of recurrence is an argument that is frequently given to support the excision of abscesses rather than their simple aspiration or drainage.

Prophylactic anticonvulsants are administered for 6 months to children with brain abscesses. At the end of that time, an electroencephalogram (EEG) is repeated. If no epileptic activity appears, the anticonvulsants are slowly tapered. Absence of epileptic activity on the EEG does not ensure that seizures will not occur. Anticonvulsants are simply resumed if they do. Physical therapy of weakened extremities is of help in preventing contracture formation and in maximizing rehabilitation.

Other, less common lesions. Localized subdural and epidural infection occur uncommonly, but when present occur following trauma, paranasal sinus infection, meningitis, and middle ear infection. Occasionally, epidural or subdural empyemas thought to originate from a hematogenous source are encountered in association with osteomyelitis of the skull. The disease frequently presents acutely with fever, luekocytosis, and pain

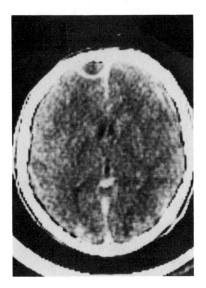

Fig. 22-9. Enhanced CT brain scan of a patient with an epidural abscess. The enhancing lesion is visible in the left frontal area. There is minimal ventricular displacement, although the child showed evidence of having acutely raised intracranial pressure.

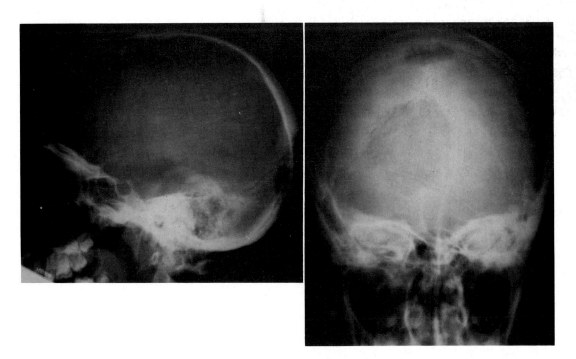

Fig. 22-10. Skull films of a child with osteomyelitis. The bregma and occiput are involved with the destructive process. Soft tissue swelling occurred over both areas, indicating the acute nature of the infection. (Courtesy Donald Kirks, M.D., Durham, N.C.)

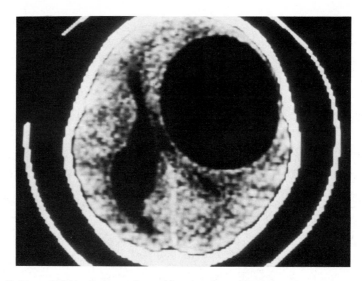

Fig. 22-11. Enhanced CT brain scan of an echinococcal cyst demonstrating a spherical right frontal mass with marked displacement of structures to the left and enlargement of the left lateral ventricle from compression of the foramen of Monro. There is no peripheral enhancement of the mass. (Courtesy Kenneth Till, Hospital for Sick Children, London, Eng.)

over the area of the infection. With extension of the infection from the involved sinuses into the epidural or subdural space, the child becomes lethargic and irritable and frequently demonstrates evidence of increased intracranial pressure with papilledema. The diagnosis is confirmed by a CT scan (Fig. 22-9). Treatment consists of the administration of appropriate antibiotics and drainage of the pus through multiple burr holes. Intraoperatively the extradural or subdural space is irrigated until all free pus has been removed. A catheter is placed in the infected space and left until all drainage ceases.

Osteomyelitis of the skull results from contiguous spread of infection from a parameningeal source, from direct trauma, or by hematogenous dissemination. Patients show acute evidence of infection. The scalp overlying the involved skull becomes warm, red, tender, and boggy to palpation. The diagnosis is confirmed by x-ray films of the skull, although the radiographic changes are known to lag behind the clinical disease (Fig. 22-10). The extent of involvement can be more accurately determined from isotopic bone scanning than from routine x-ray films. The infection is cultured to determine the offending organism and its antibiotic sensitivities. Parenteral antibiotics are begun, and the area of bony involvement is removed by craniectomy. The craniectomy site is

left without a cranioplasty for at least 12 months for fear of infecting the cranioplasty plate from residual infection in the wound. Antibiotics are continued for 3 to 6 weeks, depending on the extent of the infection.

Localized epidural infection of the spine is treated in a manner similar to that for epidural infection in the head. Antibiotics are begun, and adequate drainage is secured immediately to relieve pressure on the spinal cord and to establish the diagnosis. The laminectomy site is left open and allowed to drain into an absorbent dressing. The wound is allowed to close by secondary intention. Antibiotics are administered for 4 to 6 weeks, and physical therapy is advised, depending on the degree of weakness that persists after the recovery phase.

Several other infections can occur in the brain but are exceedingly rare in the United States. Localized tuberculous infection, which is common in some Asian and African populations is seen very rarely. When encountered, tuberculomas are treated as mass lesions and are excised if they are located in a surgically accessible area.

Brain cysts caused by the larvae from *Echinococcus granulosus* are likewise rarely seen in the United States. However, this lesion should be suspected in any child with increased intracranial pressure and a CT scan demonstrating a well-

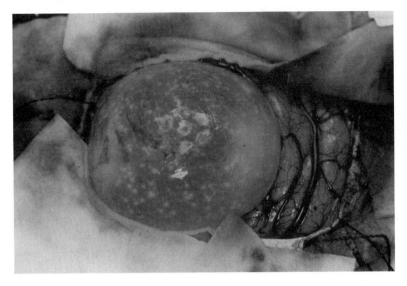

Fig. 22-12. Intraoperative photograph of the same patient as the cyst is being delivered. Of note is the lack of adhesions from the cyst to the surrounding brain. (Courtesy Kenneth Till, Hospital for Sick Children, London, Eng.)

circumscribed mass of CSF attenuation without peripheral enhancement (Fig. 22-11). The surgical treatment of a brain cyst is significantly different from the treatment of a brain abscess. During the surgical removal of the cyst, every effort is made to keep the cyst intact and prevent it from rupturing. The cyst is easily separable from the surrounding brain structures; with patience and gentle pressure on the surrounding brain, the cyst will be delivered intact (Fig. 22-12).

Intracranial cysts caused by *Taenia solium* (cysticercosis cerebri) also occur rarely. Children with this disease will characteristically have increased intracranial pressure and hydrocephalus. The cysts are frequently calcified; they may be solitary or multiple. There is currently no specific therapy for this disease.

SPINAL CORD TUMORS

Although spinal cord tumors are quite uncommon, they are of particular importance because of the devastating effects they can have on the patient. Some 70% of lesions are benign and amenable to therapy. Survival for years or decades is the rule rather than the exception. For this reason, it is important that these children be recognized as early as possible in their clinical course before neurologic sequelae become severe and resistant to therapy.

Routine examination for age. By early childhood, walking without support should be well established and voluntary control of bladder and bowel quickly follow. Once ambulation without support is achieved, the child should begin to run and then hop. His movement should be spontaneous and occur without a fixed posture to the spine. The ages at which the child develops motor milestones are important. Of equal if not more importance, however, is a history of progressive development of motor skills without evidence of plateaus or regression. If a plateau is reached and maintained, or if regression occurs, the interference with nervous system development must be significant and should always be investigated.

Possible findings. The most common problem encountered by patients with spinal cord tumors is difficulty in ambulation. This may take the form of walking with a limp or simply frequent falls because of weakness. The legs may be described as being stiff when, in fact, there is spastic paraparesis. The child with mild weakness may not complain of weakness at all, but observation may show him to be unable to maintain the activity level of his peers. The child may voluntarily come in from playing, either because of pain or leg weakness. Young children localize pain poorly and will simply become irritable and easily distressed. The older child may be able to describe pain and its radiation into an extremity or as a band around the chest in a dermatomic distribution. Of particular importance is pain that is always in the same location or pain that awakens a child. Spinal or extremity pain in a child should never be dismissed as simply "growing pain"; pain is a presenting complaint in 55% of children with spinal cord tumors.[27] Not infrequently the child will be brought to medical attention because of orthopedic complaints referable to the spine. Torticollis may be caused by cervical spinal cord involvement. Likewise, scoliosis and kyphosis are complaints requiring careful neurologic examination, since a spinal cord tumor may be associated with the spinal deformity. Infants and children with a neurogenic bladder or a lax anal sphincter should also have neurologic causes sought.

It should be emphasized that early in the course of a patient with a spinal cord tumor, the clinical signs may be minimal and the diagnosis elusive. Weakness in a young child may be difficult to determine when the child is asked to perform specific isolated muscle tests at the examining table. It is often more helpful to unclothe the child and watch him play about the room with various toys. Of particular note is the ease with which the child is able to change position and the posture of his spine and extremities. The child should be observed while walking without support and his gait analyzed in detail. Abnormalities that are thought to be present in the gait are confirmed by the presence of associated neurologic findings. Increased muscular tone and deep tendon reflexes, loss of superficial reflexes, and the presence of pathologic reflexes imply a lesion of upper motor neurons. Muscle wasting, absent deep tendon reflexes, and fasciculations imply lower motor neuron involvement. Palpation and percussion of the spine are performed to reveal anomalies of the posterior spinal elements and to elicit pain that is reproducible and localized to a specific spinal area. Evidence of metastatic disease elsewhere may be present as abdominal masses, liver or spleen enlargement, or significant lymphadenopathy.

Acute onset of spinal cord dysfunction occurs in a minority of patients; when there is sudden deterioration of neurologic function, however, emergency action is indicated. The patient when first seen may be in a phase of spinal cord shock. His examination will show no reflexes below the level of the spinal lesion, the bladder will be hypotonic and enlarged with overflow incontinence, a dis-

crete sensory level may be appreciated, and the legs will be flaccid. Within a period of hours to weeks, the phase of spinal cord shock leaves. The deep tendon reflexes below the lesion become exaggerated and the legs spastic.

Common occurrences. Spinal cord tumors can best be understood as occurring in specific anatomic compartments within the spine. These include the extradural space, the intradural extramedullary space, and the intramedullary space.

Extradural tumors make up approximately 30% of spinal neoplasms in children.[30] As in adults, this group is composed primarily of malignant tumors that are either metastatic to the epidural space or show direct extension from a primary neoplasm of the spine or in the paraspinal area. The two most common extradural tumors are neuroblastomas that originate in the paraspinal area and extend into the epidural space by direct extension through an intervertebral foramen and sarcomas that metastasize to the epidural space.[39] Occasionally, primary bone tumors located in the spine may compress the spinal cord and cause neurologic dysfunction (these include both malignant and benign processes, such as osteosarcoma, giant cell tumors of bone, and aneurysmal bone cyst).

Intradural tumors may be within the substance of the cord (intramedullary) or lie in the subarachnoid space and compress the cord from without (intradural extramedullary). *Intradural extramedullary tumors* are usually benign. In the child the most common types are dermoid and epidermoid tumors. Another group of tumors present within the subarachnoid space as metastases (seeding) through the CSF pathways from an intracranial primary tumor; these include medulloblastomas, pinealoma, and ependymomas. *Intramedullary tumors* in children make up the most common subgroup (some 35% of patients).[30] These are intrinsic tumors of the substance of the spinal cord. The most common tumor type seen is a benign, slow-growing astrocytoma. However, lipomas, dermoid tumors, epidermoid tumors, and teratomas may also occur. Included in this group is a histologically distinct tumor that occurs only in the area of the filum terminale and conus medullaris and is a myxopapillary ependymoma. Ependymomas within the substance of the spinal cord are rare in children.[30,46]

The anatomic subgroups just described are of little help in predicting the patient's symptoms or signs. Patients with tumors in all three locations may have progressive spinal cord dysfunction. Localized back pain is somewhat more common with extradural tumors, and radicular pain is more commonly seen in intradural extramedullary tumors. The tumors are relatively evenly distributed throughout the areas of the spinal cord from the cervical through the cauda equina areas. The lumbar and high cervical regions are the preferred sites for the occurrence of developmental tumors, including dermoid tumors, epidermoid tumors, lipomas, and teratomas. These areas correspond to the embryonal posterior and anterior neuropores. Occasionally, tumors will present with increased intracranial pressure and papilledema secondary to communicating hydrocephalus. This may be on the basis of the high protein content of the CSF associated with some spinal cord tumors which is thought to obstruct the arachnoid granulations and cause communicating hydrocephalus secondarily.[3] These patients are particularly difficult to diagnose unless there are spinal cord symptoms in addition to the communicating hydrocephalus. In the presence of neurofibromatosis, there is a statistical increase in the incidence of many tumors that occur within the spine. These include neurofibromas, meningiomas and gliomas.[11]

Evaluation. Following a detailed history and physical examination, plain x-ray films of the spine are obtained in the anteroposterior (AP) and lateral projections. Oblique views may be necessary to evaluate the intervertebral foramina depending on which area of the spine is being surveyed. Routine x-ray films are abnormal in 50% to 60% of patients with a neoplasm of the spine or spinal cord; however, the abnormality is usually nonspecific. Extradural tumors are associated with abnormal x-ray films commonly.[19] These changes include bony destruction of the vertebral body and pedicle(s), along with evidence of a paravertebral mass (Fig. 22-13). The disc space is characteristically spared, and this fact helps to differentiate neoplastic involvement of the spine from infection, which frequently involves the disc space and cartilaginous end-plate of the vertebra primarily. Intramedullary tumors produce subtle changes, which may be detectable on plain x-ray films only in retrospect (in about 10% of patients). The primary radiographic changes associated with intramedullary spinal cord tumors are those relating to focal enlargement of the spinal canal

(Fig. 22-14). This enlargement may be appreciated on the projection by an increase in the interpedicular distance at the involved level(s) and by flattening of the medial aspects of the pedicles, or on the lateral projection by an increased sagittal diameter of the spinal canal and scalloping of the posterior surface of the appropriate vertebral body. Spinal deformity with kyphosis, scoliosis, or torticollis may be seen in the presence of a spinal cord tumor and when present makes the assessment of other bony and soft tissue changes more difficult. If foraminal enlargement is present (Fig. 22-15), an "hourglass" or "dumbbell" tumor should be suspected. These intradural extramedullary tumors characteristically have a relatively small but important intraspinal component connected to a larger paravertebral or mediastinal component. These two segments are joined together by a neck of tumor tissue that enlarges the intervertebral foramen (Fig. 22-16). This is a characteristic change seen with neurofibromas. Radiographic changes associated with intradural extramedullary tumors are usually confined to one or two spinal segments. Routine x-ray films may be supplemented by tomography if added bony detail would be helpful or should spinal deformity make evaluation difficult.

Myelography remains the best diagnostic tool in cases of suspected spinal cord tumor. In children, it is performed under general anesthesia. As opposed to myelograms in patients with occult spinal dysraphism, myelography in the presence of a spinal cord tumor carries a risk of increasing the patient's neurologic deficit. This occurs in the presence of a high-grade subarachnoid block, where lowering of the pressure through the lumbar puncture below the level of the block may cause further vascular or mechanical compromise of the spinal cord. Because of this, neurosurgical consultation and availability should be sought before the myelogram is performed. If there is clear evidence of rapid clinical deterioration prior to the myelogram, it may be advantageous to move directly from the x-ray department to the operating room if a complete block is found. In this way, the risk of further deterioration resulting from the myelogram is minimized by immediate surgery and decompression of the spinal cord. Lumbar puncture prior to the myelogram should be avoided. It too can lead to clinical deterioration without providing a radiographic localization of the site of the lesion. In addition, lumbar puncture within the 2 to 3

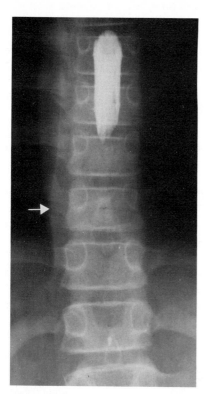

Fig. 22-13. Radiograph of a patient 6 months following a hip disarticulation for osteogenic sarcoma. The patient had progressive weakness of the remaining leg and urinary retention. The only pathologic change on routine films of the spine is an unexplained paraspinal soft tissue density that widens somewhat near the T-10 vertebral body (arrow). The pedicles and vertebral bodies remain intact. Contrast medium was introduced through a cisternal puncture and demonstrates the upper end of a total myelographic block from metastatic epidural osteogenic sarcoma.

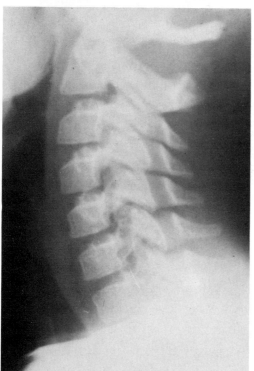

Fig. 22-14. Cervical spine film of a child with expansion of the spinal canal. The sagittal diameter of the canal is increased, and the posterior aspect of the vertebral bodies are scalloped or scooped out from pressure of the adjacent neoplasm.

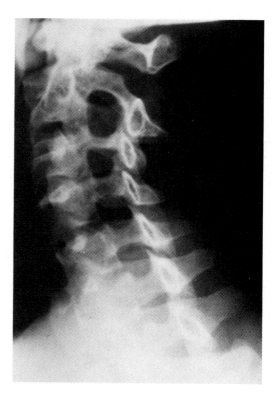

Fig. 22-15. Oblique view of the cervical spine demonstrating enlargement of all of the intervertebral foramina in a patient with neurofibromatosis and mild, spastic quadriparesis.

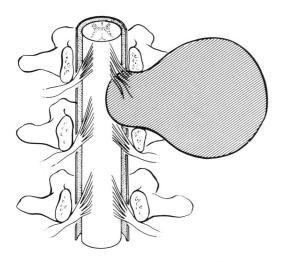

Fig. 22-16. ''Dumbbell'' neurofibroma with bony erosion of the exiting intravertebral foramen. The spinal portion of the tumor is much smaller than the extraspinal portion. Therapy is initially directed toward the intraspinal portion of the tumor to prevent traction on the spinal cord during removal of the extraspinal tumor.

days preceding a myelogram makes the myelogram technically more difficult by collapsing the subarachnoid space and allowing the accumulation of fluid in the subdural space through one or more openings in the arachnoid. The contrast agent usually used is an immiscible oil (Pantopaque). Recent experience with a water-soluble contrast medium (metrizamide) has been promising.

At the time of the myelographic lumbar puncture, a Queckenstedt maneuver is performed by compression of the jugular veins. This raises the intracranial pressure by acutely limiting the venous outflow from the brain. The increased pressure in the intracranial subarachnoid space is quickly transmitted down the spinal subarachnoid space to a manometer attached to the lumbar puncture needle. The fluctuation in the height of the fluid column in the manometer should occur briskly in response to occlusion and release of the internal jugular veins. If there is obstruction to the flow of CSF down the spinal subarachnoid space, as from a spinal cord tumor, there will be a blunting or elimination of the response seen in the manometer. If the column is seen to rise slowly in response to jugular compression, this indicates a partial block to CSF flow, whereas no response indicates a total block in the spinal subarachnoid space. Accuracy of the needle placement should be tested before and after jugular compression by

gently compressing the abdomen and watching a similar rapid rise indicating that the needle is in free communication with the subarachnoid space and in the proper position. It should also be remembered that even in the presence of a total subarachnoid block there will normally be a gentle fluctuation of the pressure seen in the manometer, reflecting respiratory and circulatory excursions. Anxiety and the Valsalva maneuver will also increase the pressure measured in the manometer; thus, it is important that the patient be totally relaxed throughout the examination.

By evaluating the myelographic pattern of the obstructed subarachnoid space, an anatomic localization of the mass can be made (Fig. 22-17). In general, extradural defects cause a tapering of the contrast column, which is suggestive of the narrowing at the tip of a paint brush. The compression may be from a dorsal or ventral direction, depending on where the neoplasm is located. Intradural extramedullary tumors will demonstrate a shift of the spinal cord away from the tumor with a meniscus around the lower pole of the tumor (Fig. 22-18). Widening of the spinal cord with obliteration of the subarachnoid space is indicative of an intramedullary tumor (Fig. 22-19). In the presence of a total myelographic block, it is frequently advisable to perform a cisternal or high lateral cervical puncture and inject the contrast medium, which will allow assessment of the subarachnoid space above the myelographic block previously demonstrated from below. This procedure is done to outline the longitudinal extent of the tumor and to help eliminate the possibility of other partial obstructions at a higher level, which may imply metastatic disease in the subarachnoid space. It will also help to confirm the type of myelographic defect present and the precise anatomic location. If the prone myelogram is normal, it is then important that the child be turned over and the subarachnoid space examined with the child in the supine position if Pantopaque is used. Spinal arteriovenous malformations, dorsal meningoceles, tethered spinal cords, and other lesions frequently may be seen only in this manner.

Occasionally, air is used as the contrast agent to be injected in the subarachnoid space. This agent is particularly helpful if syringomyelia is suspected. In the presence of a communicating syrinx, the enlarged spinal cord may collapse with a change in the patient's position. Cystic cavities

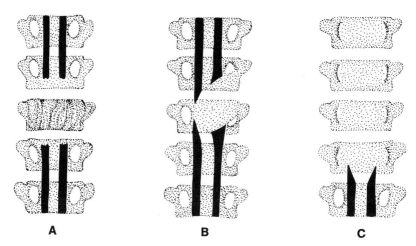

Fig. 22-17. Myelographic patterns seen with neoplastic occlusion of the subarachnoid space. **A,** Extradural tumor—abrupt cutoff of the dye column centered over an abnormal vertebral body with absent pedicles and partial collapse from neoplastic infiltration of the vertebral body. **B,** Intradural extramedullary tumor—spinal cord displaced away from the mass. The intravertebral foramen enlarges as the tumor exits laterally. **C,** Intramedullary tumor—flattening of the medial aspect of multiple pedicles with enlargement of the intraspinal canal. The spinal cord itself is seen to be widened from the infiltrative tumor.

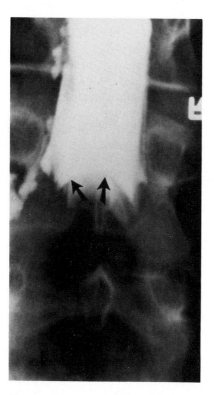

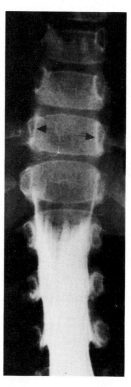

Fig. 22-18. Myelogram of a large intradural extramedullary schwannoma in the lower lumbar spine. Tumor forms a meniscus (arrows) from contrast medium around the upper pole of the tumor. The patient, a teenage boy, had low back pain and limited mobility of the spine without other abnormality of the neurologic examination.

Fig. 22-19. Myelogram of a patient with spinal cord astrocytoma. There is complete obstruction to the flow of the contrast medium because of the obliteration of the subarachnoid space by the tumor. (The medial aspect of the involved pedicles is flattened [arrows].)

associated with neoplasms, however, are not typically in communication with the subarachnoid space and will not collapse with a change in the patient's position.

CSF is obtained at the time of the myelogram for protein and sugar analysis, bacterial and fungal cultures, total and differential cell count, and cytology. Over 90% of tumors that compress the spinal subarachnoid space will be associated with an elevated protein value.[28] This is the most sensitive chemical indicator of the presence of an abnormality.

A radionuclide bone scan of the spine may be helpful to evaluate localized spinal pain in the presence of normal x-ray films and a normal myelogram. Localized bony tumors or inflammatory processes may be seen in this way, even when other studies are normal.

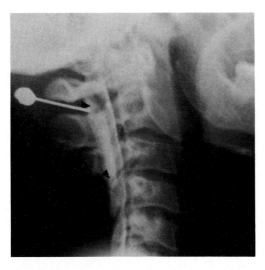

Fig. 22-20. Endomyelogram of a child with a cervicomedullary astrocytoma that had been partially resected and irradiated. The child returned to medical attention following rapid loss of neurologic function. A noncommunicating syrinx was suspected and confirmed during this procedure. The spinal needle penetrated an intramedullary syrinx, and 15 ml of dark yellow fluid was drained. A small amount of contrast medium was introduced into the cavity to outline its extent (arrows). Contrast medium can also be seen outlining the expanded spinal cord. Following the drainage of the noncommunicating syrinx, the patient had a marked improvement in his neurologic examination. This improvement was maintained for more than a year. The child then returned with new symptoms and again improved with drainage. (Courtesy E. Ralph Heinz, M.D., and Leroy Roberts, M.D., Durham, N.C.)

Percutaneous endomyelography is an uncommon procedure used to evaluate cystic cavities within the spinal cord.[23] In this procedure, a needle is introduced through the dura and into an intramedullary cavity. Fluid is withdrawn from the cyst, and a small amount of contrast medium is introduced (Fig. 22-20). This technique may be helpful therapeutically as well as diagnostically. The extent of a cyst within the spinal cord and the location of an intramedullary tumor may be more clearly outlined with this technique. In addition to radiographic evaluation of the spine and spinal cord, a routine chest x-ray film may give evidence of metastatic spread of the tumor. The diagnosis of neuroblastoma may be confirmed by the finding of an elevation of the urinary excretion of catecholamines and their metabolites. The complete blood count, platelet count, or findings on bone marrow aspiration may give clear evidence of either primary hematopoietic malignancy (leukemia), lymphoreticular malignancy (lymphoma), or secondary invasion of the bone marrow by a disseminated neoplasm. In the face of acute spinal cord compression and rapid neurologic deterioration, complete and thorough medical evaluation may by necessity be postponed until the spinal cord has been decompressed.

Referral. Evidence of acute spinal cord compression needs urgent evaluation and, if function is to be returned, therapy. Patients without evidence of spinal cord function for greater than 24 hours almost never have function return. The faster the evaluation is completed and therapy begun, the more complete is the neurologic return. As pointed out earlier, the diagnosis of spinal cord tumors may be elusive. In any child with unexplained neurologic complaints referable to the spinal cord combined with findings of scoliosis, kyphosis, torticollis, or a neurogenic bladder, a neurologic evaluation is required. For long-standing lesions that are slowly progressing, this evaluation can be made on an elective basis.

Medical versus surgical treatment. The therapy of spinal cord tumors can best be discussed by anatomic location. Extradural tumors with evidence of bone destruction are presumed to be malignant. Seventy percent of patients with metastatic tumors already have a known primary neoplasm and need no further histologic confirmation.[4] If the loss of neurologic function has been rapid and the tumor type is unknown or has been shown to be radioresistant in the past, immediate decompressive laminectomy is the therapy of choice. If tissue verification is not needed, if the tumor has been proved to be radiosensitive, and if the neurologic deficit is small and slowly progressive, radiation therapy may be the therapy of choice. Radiation therapy without histologic confirmation is ill advised. If radiation therapy is chosen, the closest possible monitoring of neurologic function must be maintained. If the child deteriorates while radiation is being given, immediate decompressive laminectomy is performed. It is also important if radiation is chosen that it begin immediately after the diagnosis is made and not be delayed for convenience.

Tumors that are within the dura and displace the spinal cord are assumed to be benign and totally resectable until proved otherwise. No consideration is given to other forms of therapy until histologic diagnosis has been made and resection attempted. Tumors within the substance of the spinal cord and originating from the filum terminale should be approached in the same way. The relatively high proportion of developmental tumors that can be effectively cured makes surgery the procedure of choice when a tumor of this type is considered in the differential diagnosis. In addition, radiation to low-grade astrocytomas of the spinal cord is of questionable benefit; thus, surgical removal should be attempted before radiation therapy is considered. If the myelogram demonstrates multiple subarachnoid seedings or multiple extradural impressions, radiation therapy is the therapy of choice; surgery in these debilitated, seriously ill children is of little long-term benefit. In association with surgical resection or radiation therapy, cortical steroids are frequently used in the treatment of acute spinal cord compression.

It should be emphasized that the ''wait and see'' attitude is inadvisable with a fixed or progressive neurologic deficit. Once neurologic function is lost, it frequently will not return. This fact is particularly true with bladder dysfunction, which in the long run remains the life-threatening aspect of any spinal cord disorder.

Surgical options. Once a decision has been made that surgery is the treatment of choice, it should not be delayed. Ideally, it should be performed immediately after the myelogram. Blood must therefore be crossmatched prior to the myelogram to be ready at the time of operation. In these patients the usual firm bony barrier between the surgeon's instruments and the spinal cord may be totally or partially infiltrated by tumor, reducing the resistance of the bone. It is frequently advisable outside the setting of malignant disease that an osteoplastic laminotomy be performed rather than a laminectomy. In this way, postoperative stability of the spine is enhanced.[37] This is particularly important with intramedullary tumors in the cervical and thoracocervical areas and also in the presence of preexisting spinal deformity such as scoliosis or kyphosis. In young children the periosteum is well developed and easily confused with the underlying dura. Epidural fat, which is usually abundant, is frequently diminished or absent in the area of a myelographic block. The spine is opened in such a way that the entire length of the tumor is exposed. If a dermal sinus tract is present, it is dissected and followed cephalad to its termination. If extradural tumor is present, all tumor that can safely be removed is removed. If the tumor is intradural, microsurgical technique will aid in the removal of benign tumors outside the spinal cord and in the dissection of intramedullary gliomas. With a widened spinal cord and no tumor apparent on the surface, a midline myelotomy is made. Tumor will usually be present within the first 1 to 2 mm from the dorsal surface of the cord. Some authors emphasize the resectability of intramedullary astrocytomas.[27] Although we agree that this should be attempted as long as functioning neural tissue is not compromised, the infiltrative nature of this tumor will frequently not lend itself to total resection.[10]

''Hourglass'' tumors with extension outside the spinal canal are best managed by primary spinal resection followed by the removal of the extraspinal portion of the tumor in a subsequent procedure.

Postoperative course. Following laminectomy, where the dura has been opened, the child is nursed horizontally and prone as much as possible. With small children it is difficult to maintain this position, but with the parents' assistance the task is made easier. The more caudal the dural opening, the more pressure there is on the dural closure when the child assumes the erect position. The child is maintained in the horizontal position for 5 to 7 days, after which time he is allowed up at his own rate.

Patients who had a neurogenic bladder preoperatively will continue to have a poorly functioning bladder postoperatively. If recovery of function does occur, it usually requires weeks to months before adequate voluntary emptying is seen. In addition, there are patients with borderline bladder function preoperatively who, with the stress of surgery and horizontal position, are unable to void postoperatively. In these situations catheter drainage, either intermittent or constant, is used. Postoperatively, one should not wait more than 8 to 10 hours before deciding on catheter drainage. Broad-spectrum urinary antibiotics or antiseptics are employed during this period of catheter drainage.

Physical therapy is helpful in helping the child to obtain return of strength to the lower extremities and to ambulate. Children who had preoperative contractures need frequent stretching exercises to prevent further contracture development in the immediate recovery phase. Sutures are routinely removed on the seventh postoperative day; and if the child is ambulatory at that point and no further therapy is planned, he is allowed to return home.

Radiation therapy to malignant tumors is begun on the third or fourth postoperative day if adequate wound healing is present. Suture removal may then be delayed until the tenth postoperative day. The first five to seven radiation treatments require hospitalization to permit observation for further worsening of the neurologic condition. After this time and after the neurologic findings have become static or are improving, further therapy can be administered on an outpatient basis.

Radiation to benign gliomas of the spinal cord is controversial. If adequate subtotal decompression has been performed, radiation is not given. If a simple biopsy has been done and there still exists a significant mass within the cord, radiation can be considered. Long-term survival of cases without radiation and a stable neurologic picture make the necessity for radiation in this setting questionable.

Prognosis. The prognosis for children with spinal tumors depends on several factors, including the histologic type of the tumor, the extent of the tumor, the neurologic status of the patient before and after surgery, and the ability of the surgeon to resect benign tumors. Lipomas, epidermoids, dermoids, teratomas, and neurinomas that are thought to be totally removed are associated with an excellent outlook. Recurrence in this group is unusual. The prognosis for children with malignant tumors is that of the primary disease process; obviously, evidence of spinal metastasis

is a negative factor. Neuroblastomas, however, have a generally favorable outlook with combined radical surgery, radiation, and chemotherapy. With time, some neuroblastomas appear to undergo maturation into ganglioneuromas. In general, with neuroblastoma, the younger the patient at the time of presentation, the higher his chances of cure.[30] Infants will routinely have their disease stop despite widespread dissemination at the time of diagnosis, whereas children more than 2 years of age have an outlook that is much less promising. Subtotally resected developmental tumors and benign gliomas of the spinal cord have an unpredictable course. Following therapy, stabilization of the neurologic picture for years to decades is not unusual. Whether this represents the natural history of the disease or a response to therapy is not known. Further long-term follow-up of large numbers of patients is necessary before an accurate assessment of prognosis can be made. The myxopapillary ependymoma, which occurs in the filum terminale will frequently show recurrence. These tumors occur as two separate types: one is encapsulated and readily removed, and the other is not encapsulated and appears diffusely spread among the nerve roots of the cauda equina. The encapsulated lesions that are totally resected have a much better prognosis than do the disseminated

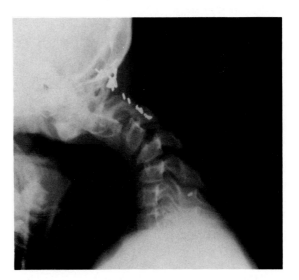

Fig. 22-21. Radiograph of a child with an astrocytoma of the upper cervical spinal cord and medulla. The child had undergone partial resection and radiation several years earlier. The patient then returned with progressive spinal cord dysfunction and was found to have swan neck deformity.

tumors. Radiation therapy is recommended for the disseminated group only. Encapsulated ependymomas that are extirpated radically have an excellent long-term prognosis with a 10-year survival of at least 75%.[33,49]

Important aspects of follow-up. Following surgical removal of a spinal tumor, careful attention must be paid to the neurologic examination. Worsening of the neurologic condition or occurrence of new symptoms must be investigated. As with myelomeningoceles, orthopedic and urologic evaluation is important in the total care of the patient.

Complications. An increase in neurologic deficit following the resection of a spinal tumor need not always represent regrowth of the tumor. Cystic dilatations within the spinal cord can re-form and cause a worsening neurologic condition. Patients may also develop kyphosis or scoliosis, which can cause bony compression of the spinal cord and a worsening of the neurologic condition[13] (Fig. 22-21). Both syringomyelia and spinal deformity can and should be diagnosed and treated to maximize the patient's neurologic function.

REFERENCES

1. Albright, L., and Reigel, D. H.: Management of hydrocephalus secondary to posterior fossa tumors, J. Neurosurg. **46:**52, 1977.
2. Arseni, C., Horvath, L., and Dumitrescu, L.: Cerebral abscesses in children, Acta Neurochir. **14:**197, 1966.
3. Arseni, C., and Maretsis, M.: Tumors of the lower spinal cord associated with increased intracranial pressure and papilledema, J. Neurosurg. **27:**105, 1967.
4. Baten, M., and Vannucci, R. C.: Intraspinal metastatic disease in childhood cancer, J. Pediatr. **90:**207, 1977.
5. Bell, W. E., and McCormick, W. F.: Increased intracranial pressure in children: diagnosis and treatment, Philadelphia, 1978, W. B. Saunders Co.
6. Bloom, H. J. G., Wallace, E. N. K., and Henk, J. M.: The treatment and prognosis of medulloblastoma in children, A.J.R. **105:**43, 1969.
7. Boltshauser, E., and others: Impact of computerized axial tomography on the management of posterior fossa tumors in children, J. Neurol. Neurosurg. Psychiatry **40:**209, 1977.
8. Bradue, A. I.: Anaerobic brain abscess, Med. Times **95:** 29, 1967.
9. Brown, J. K.: Lumbar puncture and its hazards, Dev. Med. Child Neurol. **18:**803, 1976.
10. Burger, P. C., and Vogel, F. S.: Surgical pathology of the nervous system and its coverings, New York, 1976, John Wiley & Sons, Inc.
11. Canale, D. J., and Bebin, J.: Von Recklinghausen disease of the nervous system. In Vinken, P. J., and Bruyn,

G. W., editors: Handbook of clinical neurology. Vol. 14. The phakomatoses, Amsterdam, 1972, North Holland Publishing Co.
12. Carrea, R., Dowling, E., and Guevara, A.: Surgical treatment of hydatid cysts of the central nervous system in the pediatric age (Dowling's technique), Child's Brain **1:**4, 1975.
13. Cattell, H. S., and Clark, G. L.: Cervical kyphosis and instability following multiple laminectomies in children, J. Bone Joint Surg. **49A:**713, 1967.
14. Crafts, D. C., and others: Chemotherapy of recurrent medulloblastoma with combined procarbazine, CCNU and vincristine, J. Neurosurg. **49:**589, 1978.
15. DeVivo, D. C.: Cerebral abscess in children, Dev. Med. Child Neurol. **13:**800, 1971.
16. Duffy, G. P.: Lumbar puncture in the presence of raised intracranial pressure, Br. Med. J. **1:**407, 1969.
17. Garfield, J.: Management of supratentorial intracranial abscess: a review of 200 cases, Br. Med. J. **2:**7, 1969.
18. Hammon, W. M.: Retained intracranial bone fragments: analysis of 42 patients, J. Neurosurg. **34:**142, 1971.
19. Harwood-Nash, D. C., and Fitz, C. R.: Neuroradiology in infants and children, St. Louis, 1976, The C. V. Mosby Co.
20. Heineman, H. S., and Braude, A. I.: Anaerobic infection of the brain, Am. J. Med. **35:**682, 1963.
21. Hoffman, H. J., Hendrick, E. B., and Hiscox, J. L. Cerebral abscesses in early infancy, J. Neurosurg. **33:**172, 1970.
22. Hoffman, H. J., Hendrick, E. B., and Humphreys, R. P.: Metastasis via ventriculoperitoneal shunt in patients with medulloblastoma, J. Neurosurg. **44:**562, 1976.
23. Kendall, B., and Symon, L.: Cyst puncture and endomyelography in cystic tumours of the spinal cord, Br. J. Radiol. **46:**198, 1973.
24. Koos, W. T., and Miller, M. H.: Intracranial tumors of infants and children, St. Louis, 1971, The C. V. Mosby Co.
25. Krayenbuhl, H. A.: Abscess of the brain, Clin. Neurosurg. **14:**25, 1966.
26. Lindau, A.: Discussion on vascular tumors of the brain and spinal cord, Proc. R. Soc. Med. **24:**363, 1930.
27. Malis, L. I.: Intramedullary spinal cord tumors, Clin. Neurosurg. **25:**512, 1978.
28. Matson, D. D.: Neurosurgery of infants and children, ed. 2, Springfield, Ill., 1969, Charles C Thomas, Publisher.
29. McIntosh, S., and others: Chronic neurologic disturbance in childhood leukemia, Cancer **37:**853, 1976.
30. Milhorat, T. H.: Pediatric neurosurgery, Philadelphia, 1978, F. A. Davis Co.
31. Miller, C. F., Brodkey, J. S., and Colombi, B. J.: The danger of intracranial wood, Surg. Neurol. **7:**95, 1977.
32. Molinari, G. F., and others: Brain abscess from septic cerebral embolism: an experimental model, Neurology **23:**1205, 1973.
33. Mork, S. J., and Loken, A. C.: Ependymoma: a follow-up study of 101 cases, Cancer **40:**907, 1977.
34. Moussa, A. A., and Dawson, B. H.: Computed tomography and the mortality rate in brain abscess, Surg. Neurol. **10:**301, 1978.

35. Northfield, D. W. C.: The surgery of the central nervous system, Oxford, 1973, Blackwell Scientific Publications, Ltd.

36. Panitch, H. S., and Berg, B. O.: Brain stem tumors of childhood and adolescence, Am. J. Dis. Child. **119:**465, 1970.

37. Raimondi, A. J., Gutierrez, F. A., and DiRocco, C.: Laminotomy and total reconstruction of the posterior spinal arch for spinal canal surgery in childhood, J. Neurosurg. **45:**555, 1976.

38. Raimondi, A. J., and Tonita, T.: The advantages of "total" resection of medulloblastoma and the disadvantage of full head postoperative radiation therapy; presented at the Seventh Scientific Meeting of the International Society for Paediatric Neurosurgery, Chicago, September 1979.

39. Rand, R. W., and Rand, C. W.: Intraspinal tumors of childhood, Springfield, Ill., 1960, Charles C Thomas, publisher.

40. Reigel, D. H.: Early myelography of children with medulloblastoma; presented at the Seventh Scientific Meeting of the International Society for Paediatric Neurosurgery, Chicago, September 1979.

41. Robinson, R. G.: Congenital cysts of the brain: arachnoid malformations, Prog. Neurol. Surg. **4:**133, 1971.

42. Rosenblum, M. L., and others: Decreased mortality from brain abscesses since advent of computerized tomography, J. Neurosurg. **49:**658, 1978.

43. Salibi, B. S.: Bacteroides infection of the brain, Arch. Neurol. **10:**629, 1964.

44. Samson, D. S., and Clark, K.: A current review of brain abscess, Am. J. Med. **54:**201, 1973.

45. Schurr, P.: Brain abscess in childhood, Dev. Med. Child Neurol. **7:**433, 1965.

46. Shuman, R. M., Alvord, E. C., and Leech, R. W.: The biology of childhood ependymomas, Arch. Neurol. **32:** 731, 1975.

47. Stephanon, S.: Experience with multiloculated brain abscesses, J. Neurosurg. **49:**199, 1978.

48. Unfulfilled expectations in cerebral abscess (editorial), Br. Med. J. **2:**1, 1969.

49. van Duinen, M. T. A.: The ependymoma of the cauda equina, The Hague, 1976, N.V. Druk Kerij Trio.

50. Venes, J. L., and others: Chemotherapy as an adjunct in the initial management of cerebellar medulloblastomas, J. Neurosurg. **50:**721, 1979.

CHAPTER 23

Orthopedic considerations

ROBERT J. RUDERMAN and PETER W. WHITFIELD

EXAMINATION: GENERAL CONSIDERATIONS

The basic elements of the orthopedic examination are covered in the sections on the newborn (Chapter 13) and the infant and toddler (Chapter 18). The need to understand and assess growth and development is what makes the examination during childhood unique. The changes in torsion and alignment, which are detailed in the discussion of the examination of the infant and toddler, continue during the years from 2 to 12 and occupy a great deal of the pediatric orthopedist's time. As the child gains neuromuscular control, learns to walk, and establishes a gait pattern, the issues of gait, gait deviations, and limping come to the foreground. Two other elements of the orthopedic examination are increasingly important during these years: the evaluation of limb length inequality and the evaluation of scoliosis.

GAIT

Until the toddler learns to walk, it is difficult for one to assess his gait. Many children may not cruise or stand unassisted until 9 to 12 months of age and may not walk unassisted until 10 to 14 months of age, although others are more precocious. It may not be until 24 to 36 months that the child can balance on one foot for longer than 1 second.[150]

A toddler's gait, in contrast to an adult's gait, is that of a wide base with increased flexion at the hip and knee. A firm heel strike does not occur, and the knee remains in flexion throughout the stance phase. The arms are abducted, the elbows are extended, and reciprocal arm swing is absent. The entire process is somewhat halting and has been described as being staccato in charac-

ter.[102] At about the age of 18 months, and certainly by 3 years of age, reciprocal arm swing and heel strike (adult heel-toe pattern) are usually present and are the initial determinants of a mature gait. Almost all adult gait parameters are present by the age of 7.[148,150]

A practiced eye may identify as a unit the source and nature of gait deviation; but until one has achieved that practice, it is useful to break down the normal gait pattern into components and analyze those components separately. A full discussion of gait is well beyond the scope of this book; in its simplest elements, however, normal gait can be broken into the stance phase—heel strike, foot-flat, midstance, and toe-off—and a swing phase that has three components: acceleration, mid-swing, and deceleration (Fig. 23-1). The important general characteristics of gait are the cadence (or speed of walking), the vertical and lateral displacement of the center of gravity, the width of the walking base, the horizontal dip of the pelvis, and the knee flexion–stance phase[150] (Fig. 23-2).

The time distribution in gait is important. The stance phase normally accounts for 60%, the swing phase for 40%. There is support from both extremities 11% of the total gait time. As the cadence is increased, the percent spent in the swing phase will increase. Deviations in time distribution can be seen in such conditions as a stiff hip, where limited excursion will shorten the swing phase, or in the short stride of children with hamstring tightness, which may be seen with occult spinal dysraphism or spondylolisthesis. The stance phase is shortened when it is painful to spend time on the extremity, hence the antalgic, or "sore foot," gait.

When one is confronted with a limping child, an

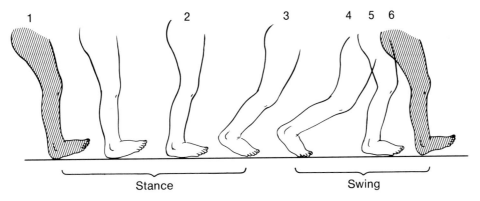

Fig. 23-1. Elements of normal gait: *1,* heel strike; *2,* midstance; *3,* toe-off; *4,* acceleration; *5,* midswing; *6,* deceleration.

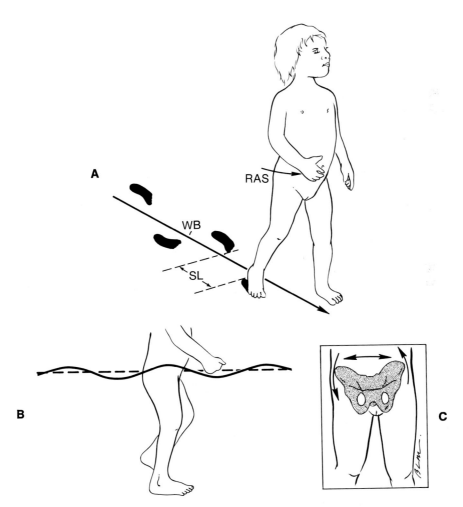

Fig. 23-2. Observation of gait. **A,** When the child is viewed from the front, the presence or absence of reciprocal arm swing *(RAS),* the width of the walking base *(WB),* and the stride length *(SL)* can be observed. **B,** When the child is viewed from the side, vertical displacement of the center of gravity is evident. **C,** In the frontal plane there is a side-to-side oscillatory motion of the center of gravity as well as an alternate dip about the hip joint.

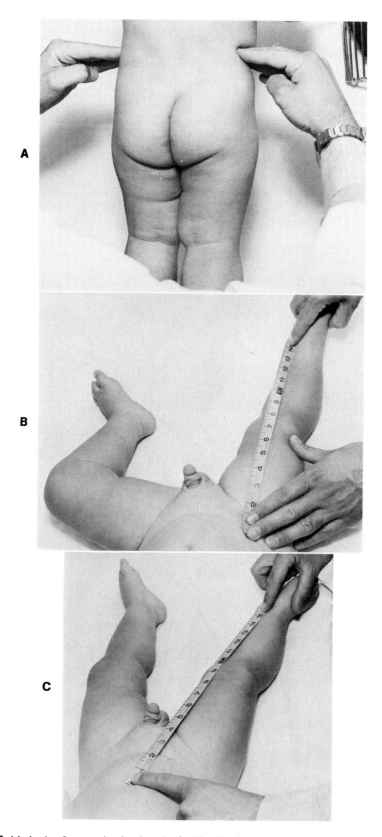

Fig. 23-3. Methods of measuring leg length. **A,** The simplest and most accurate method is to place the hands parallel to the floor and at the level of the iliac crests. Any discrepancy noted is confirmed by remeasuring after appropriate-size blocks are placed beneath the short limb. **B,** The so-called true leg length is measured from the anterosuperior iliac spine to the medial malleolus. **C,** The so-called apparent leg length is measured from the umbilicus to the medial malleolus. Tape measure techniques are useful for confirmation but should not be substituted for the standing test.

accurate diagnosis is mandatory. A limp may result from altered joint mechanics, altered muscle and nerve physiology, or pain. The problem is in localizing the source. An accurate analysis of the gait deviation may be quite useful. Many important problems, particularly about the hip, present as a limp without pain. This presentation is classic in Legg-Calvé-Perthes disease. Finally, hip disorders in children often may present as thigh and knee pain. Unless a specific abnormality can be identified about the knee, careful investigation of the hip is always required.

LEG LENGTH MEASUREMENTS

In *Pediatric Orthopaedics*, Tachdjian[151] introduces the section on leg length inequality by listing over 20 common causes. Some of these are dealt with in more detail later in this chapter. The routine estimation of relative limb lengths should be part of every pediatric examination (Fig. 23-3). The simplest and probably the most accurate method is to observe, from behind, the child standing erect with the feet together and the arms at the side. The examiner places his hands parallel to the floor and at the level of the iliac crests. The height of each iliac crest is estimated and any discrepancy noted and confirmed by remeasuring after appropriate-size blocks are placed beneath the short limb. This method is remarkably accurate and, in the hands of an experienced observer, easily detects differences as small as a quarter of an inch. This standing technique is superior to direct tape measure estimations of leg length, either from the anterosuperior iliac spine to the medial malleolus, the so-called true leg length, or from the umbilicus to the medial malleolus, the so-called apparent leg length. It accounts for variations in the size of the hemipelvis or of the foot, either of which will contribute to any overall difference in limb length. Tape measure techniques, however, are useful for confirmation and do enable one, by using landmarks such as the adductor tubercle or the proximal tibial metaphysis, to separate the measurements into femoral and tibial lengths.

These clinical techniques will suffice for most routine evaluations. Sophisticated radiographic techniques for direct measurement of limb length inequality include the orthoroentgenogram and the scanogram.[12,56] Both theoretically offer the advantage of a direct and accurate measurement of actual and relative bone length. Neither radiographic method accounts for the contribution that a small foot makes to the short leg and

must be complemented by the clinical examination or by a standing x-ray examination of the pelvis. Both methods demand exacting radiographic technique and rigid standardization from examination to examination; otherwise, they are unlikely to be any more accurate than the clinical examination. Such standardization will probably not be achieved outside of children's orthopedic centers.

LIMB LENGTH DISCREPANCIES

Limb length inequality is a symptom, not a disease. Any process that directly affects a major physeal plate will have a significant impact on the longitudinal growth of the long bone in question. This problem is particularly severe when it occurs in early infancy because of the magnitude of the subsequent discrepancy.

Infection or tumor may involve the physeal plate directly, with resultant premature fusion and shortening.

Congenital anomalies commonly produce shortening, particularly when entire segments of major long bones are absent, such as in proximal focal femoral deficiency.

Obviously, *trauma* can produce shortening as well, either indirectly by affecting the physis or directly as a result of malposition or shortening of the fracture fragments. The same disease processes that produce shortening may lead to overgrowth when they serve as a stimulus to increased blood supply and subsequent accelerated growth. This process is particularly true in long bone fractures that occur between the ages of 2 and 10 years.[59] Altered vascularity may result from such *vascular malformations* as an arteriovenous fistula or hemangiomatosis, and these conditions frequently produce overgrowth not only of the long bones (Fig. 23-4), but also of the surrounding soft tissues (Fig. 23-5).[83] Presumably, similar vascular mechanisms result in the overgrowth common in *neurofibromatosis*[79] (Fig. 23-6). The complex interaction of muscle bulk, trophic supply of the nerves, and blood supply is evident in the shortening and atrophy that occur with such *neuromuscular conditions* as polio, meningomyelocele, or peripheral nerve injury.

Congenital hemihypertrophy is worthy of special notice.[24] In its most common form, hemihypertrophy is expressed as a mild asymmetry that often presents as a leg length inequality. With careful measurement, asymmetry of the entire side of the body, including the facial asymmetry that is frequently present, can often be documented.

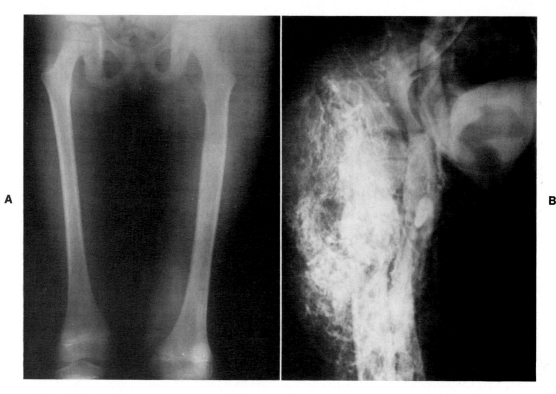

A

B

Fig. 23-4. A, Plain x-ray film of a child with a vascular malformation of the left thigh. The soft tissue mass can be seen, as well as the discrepancy in lengths of the femurs. B, This x-ray film, taken during the venous phase of an arteriogram, demonstrates the extent of the lesion.

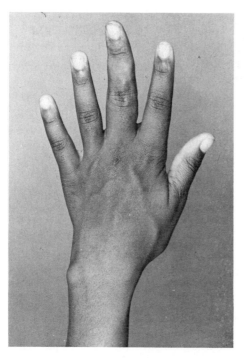

Fig. 23-5. Overgrowth of the soft tissues is apparent in this photograph of the long finger of a child with an arteriovenous malformation.

Often the asymmetry has not been apparent to the patient or the family prior to the time of detailed evaluation. The disparity in size does not disappear spontaneously but only infrequently reaches a degree that requires treatment.

Growth (normal patterns). In all deviations of growth, the longitudinal pattern is most important. Because the chronologic age may not accurately reflect the true skeletal age, bone age should be determined radiographically. The most commonly used technique is a comparison of the development of the hands and wrists utilizing the atlas compiled by Greulich and Pyle.[57]

The general pattern of growth is important. The skull, spine, and long bones do not share equally in growth following birth. In terms of height, the head is closest to its adult size at birth; and while it continues to grow, it does so at a much lower rate than the spine. The spine, in turn, contributes less to ultimate growth in height after birth than do the legs. The incremental increase in growth of the extremities is greatest from birth to 2 years of age. In terms of absolute rate, there is a decline from the years 2 to 10, but this is small and growth

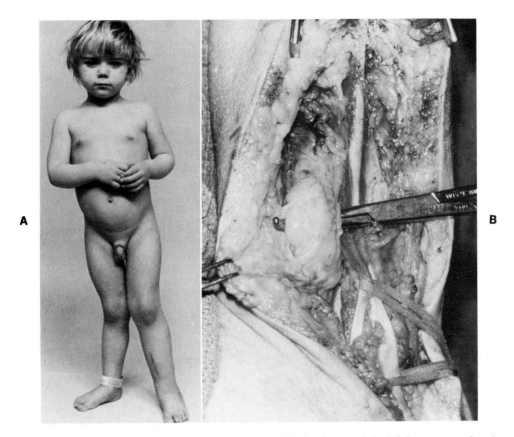

Fig. 23-6. A, Four-year-old child with hypertrophy of all the tissues of the left lower extremity. A previous biopsy had confirmed the diagnosis of plexiform neurofibroma. **B,** Photograph taken at the time of surgical exploration. The massively enlarged posterior tibial nerve is draped over the dissecting clamp. The nerve and surrounding tissues are infiltrated with the wormlike tumorous tissue.

continues at a relatively steady rate until the adolescent growth spurt is reached. Girls reach their growth spurt earlier than boys, beginning at about 10½ to 11 years of age and continuing to approximately 13½ to 14 years of age. (Some small growth will continue up to the age of 15½ to 16.) Boys, on the other hand, do not begin their growth spurt until 11½ or 12 years of age; they continue their spurt longer than girls, until the age of 15½ to 16, and have some growth until 18 years of age.

The major portion of lower extremity growth occurs in the femur (54%), and most growth occurs about the knee: the distal femur contributes 70% to the individual growth of the femur and 37% to the growth of the entire leg, and the proximal tibia accounts for 60% of tibial length and 28% of total extremity length. A similar relationship exists in the upper extremity, where most growth occurs about the elbow.

When growth has completely ceased at a particular site, the calculation of ultimate discrepancy relies only on estimating the rate of growth at the contralateral normal physis as well as the time remaining for that physeal plate to grow. In the more complex situation, where growth has not completely ceased but is rather inhibited or exaggerated by a disease process, one must calculate the percent of inhibition or exaggeration of growth and estimate its relative effect over time. Since limb length discrepancy is a dynamic process, the timing of intervention is crucial. Referral to a pediatric orthopedist is indicated as soon as the potential for inequality is identified, even if no disparity has yet occurred.

Treatment. The comments that follow presume that, whatever the cause of limb length inequality, it has been identified and treated and is a relatively static factor. In general, treatment is predicated on the extent and aggression of the inequality and on the age of the child. The decision to treat inequality actively will depend on many factors and requires both a good understanding of normal growth and development and a careful analysis of each individual child. Small discrepancies require no treatment, and mild discrepancy may be solved by a small shoe lift. Severe inequalities, such as might occur with proximal femoral focal deficiencies, might best be managed with amputation and prosthetic limb replacement. It is in those conditions, which fall between the extremes, that careful study and judgment come into play. Up to ½ inch in limb length discrepancy is easily accommodated without any special procedures or shoe modifications. Even larger discrepancies need not be treated immediately. Rarely is there harm in allowing a child to ambulate without compensatory lifts, at least while one is deciding on the nature and timing of definitive treatment. The child may limp; but, for the most part, the limp will be painless and will not produce secondary deformity. A fixed scoliosis does not result from ambulating with a limb length inequality.

There are basically four treatment options available. Stimulation of the short side has not been practical because of unpredictability. The long extremity may be shortened, if growth remains, by local fusion of the physes (epiphysiodesis). Fusion of more than one physis may be necessary. If one is dealing with an angular deformity, stapling of an epiphysis may provide temporary epiphysiodesis, which can be reversed once the deformity has been corrected. This procedure has its greatest application in malunion of fractures or in localized growth disturbances and is less useful where overall limb length inequality is the problem.

When a child reaches the age wherein inadequate growth remains at the physes or they are closed, moderate limb length discrepancies can be equalized by extracting a segment of bone from the long extremity. If the discrepancy is so great that shortening will produce significant disproportion, surgical lengthening of the short limb can be considered. Lengthening is a formidable procedure, to be undertaken only in severe circumstances. The problems come in the postoperative period, when the limb is gradually lengthened, usually 0.5 to 1 mm per day. It is during this period of time that major complications can occur: joint dislocation, joint stiffness, or neurovascular embarrassment. Unfortunately, these complications are quite frequent. Lengthening must be performed under the careful surveillance of an experienced team. The amount of lengthening that can be achieved in any one procedure is limited.[85] Lengthening can be repeated every few years, and several inches in length can ultimately be gained. After lengthening is completed, secondary stages of bone grafting and plating are often required. Although there is a reasonable success rate at each stage, the possibilities of infection or malunion exist. The referring physician must be aware of these difficulties. The casual implication that the leg can simply be stretched may stimulate inappropriate optimism from the patient and the family. Usually there are far simpler ways to manage length discrepancies.

· · ·

In summary, limb length inequality is a common problem and may result from any number of traumatic or congenital abnormalities. Where the discrepancy is mild, no treatment may be required. The child may walk with a mild limp and stand with a mild degree of scoliosis, but no long-term structural abnormalities will result. When the discrepancy becomes a mild cosmetic or functional problem, it is most simply handled with a small shoe lift. If the problem is progressive, or if the discrepancy is great, multiple surgical options exist. The timing of application of these options is crucial. Since delay in referral may result in eliminating the simplest options, it is apparent that referral should be made early.

COMMON INFECTIOUS PROCESSES
Osteomyelitis

The question of pyogenic infection of bone is partially covered in the section on the infant and toddler (see Chapter 18) in order to emphasize the special anatomic considerations that make the management of pyogenic osteomyelitis in that age group somewhat different from management of the same disease in the older child. Since osteomyelitis has its peak incidence between the ages of 2 and 12, it is appropriate to consider pyogenic osteomyelitis in more detail here.

Bacteria may invade a bone from an external source, producing a so-called exogenous osteomyelitis, the most frequent causes being open fractures and contamination from penetrating wounds. Hematogenous osteomyelitis, on the other hand, is blood borne, affects boys two or three times more frequently than girls, and may result from indolent infections or occult penetrating injuries.[161] Localization of hematogenous osteomyelitis is naturally in those areas of greatest blood supply. In the growing child the largest blood flow is to the metaphyseal end of the long bones.

As the vessels approach the level of the physis, they diminish in size to the arteriolar level, take hairpin turns, and join large sinusoidal veins.[156] At this juncture there is a marked diminution in the *rate* of flow, and it is this high-volume, sluggish flow setting that provides the ideal environment for establishing a nidus of infection. Below the age of 1 year, the physeal plate is traversed by blood vessels and does not serve as a barrier to the spread of infection.[155] Thus, the epiphysis, and through it the joint, may be directly involved. In the older child no blood vessels traverse the physeal plate, which becomes a barrier to the spread of infection and limits the process to the metaphysis or, by extension, the diaphysis of the long bone. In certain joints—proximal femur, proximal humerus, proximal ulna, and distal fibula—the metaphysis of the long bone is intra-articular. Thus, at these sites extension through the metaphyseal cortex can lead to direct involvement of a joint.

Pathophysiology. Once the bacteria have established themselves, the inflammatory process is similar to that in any other organ.[84] The initial cellulitis and subsequent abscess formation develop within the rigid bony container. Thrombosis of vessels and loss of circulation may ensue. Increasing pressure within the rigid container accounts for the initial pain. This process occurs within the first 24 to 72 hours. If the pressure is not relieved, either by surgical intervention or by rupture of the abscess through the cortex and beneath the periosteum, infarction of metaphyseal trabecular bone and the formation of isolated islands of necrotic bone *(sequestrum)* may occur.

In this early stage of osteomyelitis, there will be no observable radiographic changes. If the inflammatory process is widespread, interstitial edema in the surrounding soft tissues blurs the tissue planes seen in the soft tissue portions of the x-ray film.

As the infection continues over the course of 10 to 14 days, further granulation tissue, abscess formation, and infarction occur. In the areas surrounding the infection, increased blood supply and attempts at control and repair will lead to osteoclastic resorption of the living bone. Pain and diminished activity result in disuse osteoporosis of

the infected extremity. This combination of peripheral resorption and osteoporosis yields an apparent increase in density of the central infarcted bone, which remains at its normal density because of the failure of active metabolic processes. Radiographically, this sequence accounts for the patchy sclerosis and osteoporosis characteristic of the early radiographic changes in this disease. In these early stages of osteomyelitis, if appropriate medical intervention occurs or the host is able to combat the infection, one could expect resorption and remodeling, resulting in resolution of all radiographic changes.

If the infection continues, it spreads within the long bone. Pus penetrates Volkmann's canals, traverses the cortex, and reaches the subperiosteal space, elevating the periosteum. Thus, the abscess decompresses itself subperiosteally. If the periosteal plane remains reasonably intact, the pus may dissect throughout the entire length of the cortex. Attempts at repair and periosteal irritation as a result of stripping and inflammation result in the formation of new periosteal bone *(involucrum)* (Fig. 23-7).

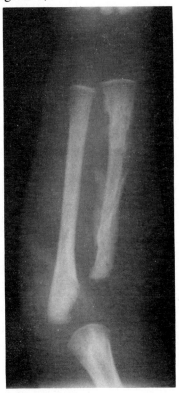

Fig. 23-7. Osteomyelitis affecting the entire radius. There is extensive periosteal new bone formation (involucrum).

In extensive infection, the involucrum completely surrounds the cortex. At this point, the entire cortex may be isolated from its blood supply and become a sequestrum. This advanced stage of chronic osteomyelitis is rarely seen now, but it is well documented in the medical museums. If the infection continues unchecked, rupture through the soft tissues will produce draining sinus tracts and all the long-term sequelae associated with advanced disease. In the modern era this sequence is preventable, given early recognition and immediate intervention.

Clinical presentation and evaluation. The initial clinical presentation of osteomyelitis may be subtle. Fever may or may not be present. In the younger child the only symptoms may be malaise, irritability, and perhaps diminished use of the involved extremity. Swelling of the extremity may be mild enough to be difficult to detect. Careful palpation along the long bones will reveal point tenderness in the region of the metaphysis.

If an area of maximal tenderness can be localized, an attempt at aspirating the subperiosteal space should be made. If possible, a large-bore needle should be advanced into the metaphysis to obtain an aspirate for culture. Great care must be taken not to traverse a joint space that is uninvolved with infection. The cultures are negative 50% of the time, even when they are obtained prior to any antibiotic intervention.

More than 80% of hematogenous osteomyelitis in the otherwise normal child is due to staphylococcus aureus. Since a vast majority of these organisms will be resistant to penicillin,[33] methicillin or its appropriate analog should be begun as initial intravenous therapy. Blood cultures should be obtained. In the younger age groups one must, of course, be aware of the possibility of *Hemophilus influenzae,* and occasional cases of tuberculous or fungal osteomyelitis are seen.[74] In the black population the possibility of a salmonella infection in a child with sickle cell disease should be considered, though even in these patients staphylococcus is still the leading cause of bone infection. Increasingly, we are seeing hematogenous osteomyelitis in children who have diabetes or some other systemic illness. In these special groups a variety of organisms may be present.

Bone scanning utilizing technetium 99 polyphosphate has recently been utilized in the detection and localization of osteomyelitis at the early stage, when radiographic changes are not yet ap-

parent.[45] When the disease is established and radiographic changes are already present, localization is then obviously easy. A bone scan may be useful at this point in finding other sites of involvement; multifocal disease is common.

Differential diagnosis. The differential diagnosis includes any inflammatory process that may affect an extremity. In particular, one must differentiate pyarthrosis. When one is dealing with a joint where the metaphysis is intra-articular, pyarthrosis and osteomyelitis may, and commonly do, coexist. Aspiration of the joint and appropriate workup for other inflammatory processes should clarify this issue. In black children the dactylitis of sickle cell disease may produce a confusing picture (Fig. 23-8). Malignancies, particularly leukemia and Ewing's sarcoma, may simulate acute osteomyelitis.

Treatment. The choice of treatment depends on the stage at diagnosis. During the first few days, prior to the formation of a sequestrum or x-ray changes, the diagnostic measures outlined above are undertaken and the child is immediately begun on a regimen of intravenous antibiotics. It is unusual in osteomyelitis to see a rapid lysis of temperature, but one should see a clinical response within 24 to 36 hours. If improvement fails to occur, or if the temperature persists for 48 to 72 hours without a suggestion of defervescence, surgical decompression should be considered. The goal is to prevent pressure necrosis of the metaphyseal bone and sequestrum formation. If the abscess ruptures subperiosteally, the metaphysis is decompressed. A subperiosteal abscess will be detected by the persistence of fever, toxic symptoms, localized pain, erythema, and swelling. Incision and drainage of a subperiosteal abscess are as appropriate here as in any other area of the body. If the infectious process ruptures into the joint, the joint must be managed as in pyarthrosis (see p. 419). The limb is immobilized, because immobilization controls local pain, swelling, and muscle spasm and has a beneficial effect on the inflammatory process.

Children with acute osteomyelitis may be systemically quite ill. Attention to fluid and electrolyte balance and correction of anemia are mandatory and should be undertaken before any surgery is planned.

In the later stages of the disease process, should a sequestrum be present it will interfere with resolution of the infectious process. The dead bone is

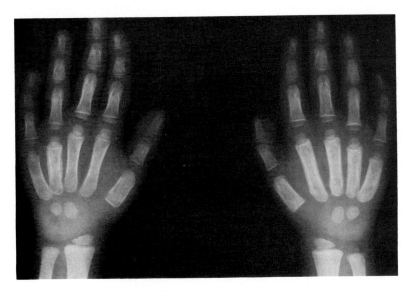

Fig. 23-8. Sickle cell dactylitis.

surgically excised (sequestrectomy), the cortex is windowed, and necrotic tissue and bone are debrided. The wound is left widely open (saucerization). Protection of the extremity must continue until adequate resolution of the infection occurs. A pathologic fracture through an area of osteomyelitis may be a disaster. If the limb is extensively involved, the period of time during which external protection and non-weight bearing are needed may extend for several weeks or even months.

If the acute infection responds to antibiotic treatment, one can begin to move the limb as soon as the local symptoms are under control. Within a few weeks, weight bearing is allowed. The intravenous antibiotics must be continued, at least until control of all local and systemic toxic signs is achieved. One way of monitoring the response to therapy is provided by the erythrocyte sedimentation rate (ESR). The ESR normalizes more slowly than fever and the white blood cell count.

There is much debate in the literature about when (or if) oral antibiotic therapy can supplant intravenous therapy.[153] It may begin quite early in the appropriate setting, which requires identification of an organism and maintenance of the organism in the laboratory so that appropriate kill levels can be established. The patients are monitored to confirm that proper levels are being achieved with the oral medication. Some children can be discharged home on a regimen of oral antibiotics; others may be best maintained in a protective environment until the full course of anti-biotic therapy is completed, that is, 4 to 6 weeks.

Following this treatment plan, one can expect eradication of the infection in most cases. If the infection is treated very early, radiographic changes may never develop. If the infection is not controlled, chronic osteomyelitis develops with sequestrum formation and draining sinuses. The infection may become quiescent, only to flare up later with periodic drainage, fever, and swelling. In such chronic cases, amputation may ultimately be the only solution, underlining the need for early, aggressive management of osteomyelitis.

Pyarthrosis

As with osteomyelitis, the infection of a joint with bacterial organisms may occur by hematogenous spread or by direct involvement from penetrating wounds or foreign bodies. Pyarthrosis may coexist with osteomyelitis; and when the metaphysis is intraarticular, it may be difficult to distinguish isolated pyarthrosis from adjacent osteomyelitis. Immediate attention must be directed to the joint, since the fate of the articular cartilage is probably a more crucial consideration than the possible involvement of bone. Hematogenous pyarthrosis occurs most commonly in younger children. The responsible organism is most frequently *Staphylococcus aureus;*[61] but below the age of 4 years, *Hemophilus influenzae* is frequent.[162] In the neonatal period, non–group A beta hemolytic streptococcus has become increasingly frequent.[103]

The synovial membrane responds to the inflammatory process within the joint by producing increased synovial fluid, an effusion that will be laden with neutrophils and bacteria (Fig. 23-9). The combination of the toxic products of the bacteria and the lysosomal enzymes of the inflammatory cells will result in the destruction of the articular surface and lead to secondary degenerative arthritis.

Clinical presentation and evaluation. In addition to the usual signs of inflammation, there is splinting of the affected part and the child will refuse to move the joint. Even if there is no overlying erythema, swelling, or warmth, there is usually exquisite joint tenderness on palpation and the child will show marked apprehension at any attempt at joint motion. Depending on the stage of the disease, there will be fever, an elevated white blood cell count, and an elevated ESR. The diagnosis is confirmed by aspirating the infected joint with a large-bore needle and obtaining a turbid synovial fluid with a white blood cell count ranging from 50,000 to 200,000/ml[3]. A markedly elevated white blood cell count may be seen in such

noninfectious inflammatory conditions as juvenile rheumatoid arthritis, but a gram stain that shows organisms will confirm the presence of pyarthrosis. Counter-immunoelectrophoresis (CIE) offers a powerful tool for the identification of certain organisms in joint fluid or blood that are difficult to see on gram stain. Since CIE does not rely on viable organisms, one may be able to identify the infectious agents, even in partially treated cases. The results from CIE are available within an hour or so, making this study useful in the emergency situation.

If needle aspiration is unsuccessful, the aspiration should be performed under fluoroscopic control, with injection of a small amount of a radiodense material to confirm that the needle is intraarticular.

Medical versus surgical treatment. Treatment must be instituted immediately. Systemic antibiotics are begun intravenously as soon as the appropriate cultures are obtained. Our preference in the younger age group is to begin a methicillin analog and chloramphenicol intravenously until we can ascertain whether or not the organism is

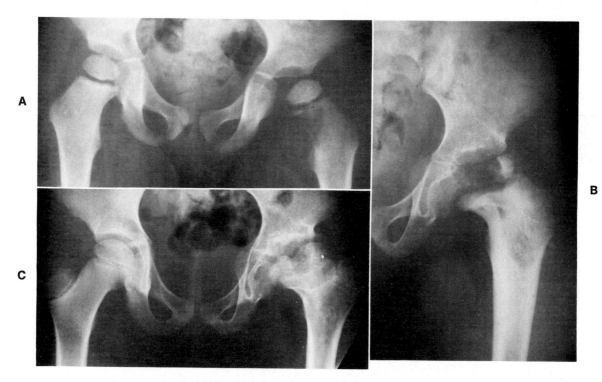

Fig. 23-9. Staphylococcal pyarthrosis of the left hip. The initial x-ray film (**A**) shows lytic changes in the metaphysis, indicating associated osteomyelitis. The marked widening of the joint space is a result of purulent effusion. Despite aggressive treatment, this hip went on to severe destruction (**B** and **C**).

Staphylococcus aureus or *Hemophilus influenzae*. Chloramphenicol is utilized until it can be determined that the *Hemophilus influenzae* is susceptible to ampicillin. Supportive measures including fluids and antipyretics are also begun. The joint should immediately be immobilized with traction or a cast.

Controversy arises as to whether joint aspiration or surgical drainage is the appropriate management of pyarthrosis.[61,141] It is our opinion that open drainage of the joint is the conservative approach and should never be done reluctantly. However, some infections can be managed without surgical drainage, and a trial of medical therapy is appropriate. This will depend, in part, on the organism present and the nature of the joint effusion.[68] Staphylococcal infections commonly loculate themselves within the joint space; repeated aspirations in this setting are bound to fail. On the other hand, some organisms such as streptococcus or gonococcus produce a joint effusion that can be aspirated more successfully. *Hemophilus* seems to be intermediate and produces joint fluid of varying viscosity. Other factors are the sensitivity of the organism to specific antibiotics and the specific joint in question. A knee is readily accessible to the needle, but a hip is not. Furthermore, the hip, because of the peculiarities of its circulation, is quite prone to damage from intra-articular pressure; and this pressure must be relieved. Although drainage of an infected hip is mandatory, in joints such as the knee there is room for discretion.

TRAUMA

"Children are not just small adults" was selected by Rang[128] as the title for the first chapter in his excellent and very readable monograph on children's fractures. It is important to understand the skeletal differences between children and adults because they explain the nature of certain fractures in children and their healing response. While "children's fractures are usually easy to treat, . . . they do not always remodel. There are bad results."[128]

The child's bone is relatively less dense than the adult's, has larger haversian canals, and is thus more porous. This increased porosity and decreased density account for the ability of children's long bones to fail in compression, as in the torus or buckle fracture in a young child (Fig. 23-10), a mechanism that is unusual in normal adults. Children's bones may actually bend without grossly identifiable fracture. Bending may be a clinically important, unrecognized cause of deformity following injury (Fig. 23-11). When the bending extends beyond the plastic limits of the bone, a greenstick fracture is produced. Complete reduction of a greenstick fracture requires momentary overreduction with completion of the fracture. The thicker and stronger periosteum of the child as compared to that of the adult is another important anatomic difference with physiologic implications. The strong periosteum may serve as a hinge and act as an important ally in obtaining a satisfactory reduction, but it may also account for persistent angulation and loss of reduction.

The most important difference between immature and adult bone is the presence of the growth center. The physeal plate is responsible for the longitudinal growth of the long bone. The cartilaginous plate is radiolucent on macroradiographs. Injury to the physis is only inferred by displacement of the epiphysis in relation to the metaphysis.

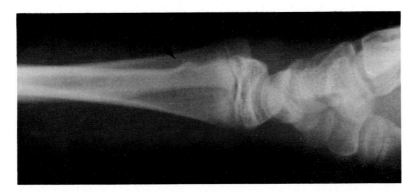

Fig. 23-10. Buckle or torus fracture (arrow) of the distal radius.

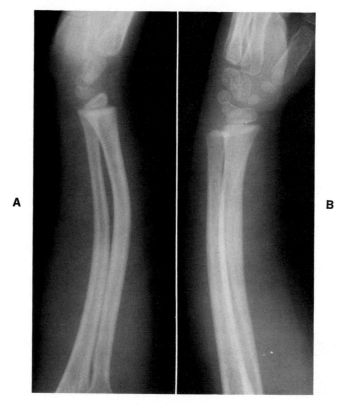

Fig. 23-11. Children's bones may bend without breaking. The x-ray film seen in **A** shows the initial deformity. Only 3 weeks later, a follow-up x-ray film (**B**) shows periosteal new bone being formed in the concave side of the deformity. This is the process of fracture remodeling.

Injury to the growth plate has severe implications for the subsequent development of the bone.

The combination of these anatomic and physiologic differences between child and adult bone results in certain features of fracture healing in children that are not common in adults. First, the fractures heal with much greater speed. This means that reduction cannot be delayed if malunion is to be avoided. After reduction, even of a simple fracture, follow-up x-ray films should be obtained on an early basis, perhaps even weekly. Otherwise, if displacement occurs within the plaster, healing may have progressed to such a point that the opportunity for rereduction or alteration in treatment is lost. Nonunion is unusual in children, but nonunion does occur and may be an indication of interposed soft tissue.

Once healing has occurred, the problems may not be over. A significant degree of angulation will remodel in children; bones remodel best when the fracture is close to an adjacent joint, and they tend to remodel only in the axis of motion of that

joint. Severe varus or valgus angulation may not remodel, nor does malrotation. If the growth center has been injured in the fracture, loss of linear growth may occur. If the damage to the growth plate has been asymmetric, progressive angular deformity may ensue. Finally, massive vascular reorganization and remodeling occur in the entire limb after a fracture of a long bone, which, although necessary to healing of the fracture, may result in stimulation of adjacent physeal plates with a subsequent increase in growth of as great as 1 to 2 cm.[59]

Principles of fracture management

Bad results in management of children's fractures are usually avoidable with due care, diagnostic experience, and proper selection and application of treatment. For these reasons, even fractures that are apparently minimal should be referred to an orthopedic surgeon.

Evaluation. Accurate diagnosis requires appropriate x-ray films. Oblique views are commonly necessary in addition to anteroposterior (AP) and lateral x-ray films and are obligatory in certain joints such as ankles and elbows. The films should routinely include both proximal and distal adjacent joints. Comparative x-ray films of the opposite, uninvolved side are often useful in identifying the specific injury but are *not* obligatory. Many fractures require special views, and in fractures involving unossified epiphyses only alteration of the relationship of the shaft to the remainder of the body will suggest an injury. Direct consultation with the radiologist affords him the benefit of your clinical exam and associated findings, enabling him to order the appropriate special views to identify an occult injury.

Treatment. Anatomic reduction is not necessary in most fractures. What may look appalling to the family on an x-ray film may be a perfectly satisfactory alignment with adequate apposition of bone to ensure satisfactory healing. This does not mean that all forms of malposition can be accepted. One can utilize natural remodeling to a great extent; but remember that remodeling does not occur with rotary displacement, an axis of displacement of the fracture that is not in the plane of motion of the adjacent joint, intra-articular fractures, or fractures that traverse the physeal plate at right angles. Some fractures that might otherwise satisfactorily remodel may be simply reduced with minimal difficulty. For example, reduction of a fracture of the distal radius might be physiologically unnecessary but is relatively easy to accomplish and will decrease some of the parents' anxieties. Such optional reductions must be balanced against any risks and discomfort for the child. Forceful reduction of fractures without anesthesia is inappropriate and inhumane. Intramuscular or intravenous analgesia or sedation can be used for simple reductions; in some instances, general anesthesia is required. The risks of general anesthesia in an otherwise healthy child are exceedingly small in the hands of an experienced anesthesiologist[42] except when recent food ingestion makes aspiration a significant risk.

Cast treatment. It takes a fair amount of practice to apply a good cast, and someone who treats only a very occasional fracture should probably not undertake cast treatment. A poorly applied cast does more harm than good, inadequately immobilizing the fracture while risking skin necrosis or vascular damage.

Whenever a cast is applied to an acute injury,

a written "cast sheet" must be given to the parents in addition to verbal instructions (Fig. 23-12). The anxious parents may not remember everything they are told in the emergency room. The nature of the injury, the date of treatment, and the name or initials of the treating physician should be recorded on the cast with an indelible pencil.

The casted part should be elevated. Ice can be applied directly through the plaster to help reduce swelling. All acute injuries should be seen the next day for a cast check to ensure that the patient is comfortable and that the neurovascular status of the extremity is satisfactory. At least 36 to 48 hours is required for final maturation of a plaster cast before it will be strong enough for weight bearing. A sling should not be provided for upper extremity injuries during the first day, because it encourages dependency; and elevation to retard swelling is mandatory for the first 24 to 48 hours. A cast on the upper extremity should allow satisfactory mobility of the fingers, but to prevent edema it should extend dorsally at least to the level of the metacarpophalangeal joints and a compressive bandage should be applied to the hand and maintained for 24 to 48 hours.

Aftercare is an important part of fracture management. Repeated x-ray films at early intervals are necessary so that loss of reduction can be identified and rereduction obtained. On each occasion, the neurovascular status of the extremity must be carefully assessed. Associated nerve injuries must be identified and corrected immediately when possible. Follow-up visits may be as frequent as weekly for the first 2 to 3 weeks of fracture care, depending on the injury.

A loose cast needs to be replaced. Retraction of the extremity within the cast may represent either an inadequate cast or a loss of reduction with foreshortening of the extremity. Sedation and analgesia are not the proper response to pain. If the child is having pain, that may mean that there is underlying compression and impending vascular compromise or compartment ischemia. The cast must be immediately split widely down to and including the underlying sheet cotton. Volkmann's ischemic contracture is a catastrophic complication that usually can be avoided. If local pain resolves, that may mean that the underlying skin and nerve endings have died.

Traction. Some fractures cannot be manually manipulated because of their nature or the asso-

16873B

MAJOR BUSINESS FORMS, INC.
HILLSBOROUGH, N. C. 27278

FORM
M-1902
rev, 5-71

DUKE UNIVERSITY MEDICAL CENTER

ORTHOPAEDIC SERVICE

Name _____

History # _____

INSTRUCTIONS FOR PATIENTS

Date _____

WITH FRACTURES AND/OR
OTHER INJURIES

THE COLOR OF YOUR FINGERS, THE MOTIONS AND THE FEELINGS OF YOUR FINGERS GIVE IMPORTANT INFORMATION ABOUT THE CONDITION OF BLOOD, MUSCLES AND THE NERVES IN YOUR HAND AND ARM. THE FINGERS AND/OR TOES ARE UNCOVERED SO YOU CAN DETERMINE THEIR COLOR AND MOTION. DO THIS SEVERAL TIMES A DAY FOR THE FIRST FEW DAYS AFTER INJURY.

IF THE FINGERS OR TOES BECOME NUMB, PAINFUL, COLD, PALE, BLUE, OR PROGRESSIVELY LARGER, YOU SHOULD REPORT TO THE EMERGENCY ROOM AT DUKE MEDICAL CENTER IMMEDIATE-LY.

YOU MUST RETURN TO THE EMERGENCY ROOM OR ORTHOPAEDIC CLINIC ON THE DAY AFTER YOUR INJURY. BE CERTAIN THAT YOU KNOW EXACTLY WHEN TO RETURN TO THE ORTHOPAEDIC CLINIC OR DOCTOR'S OFFICE ON YOUR RETURN VISIT.

I HAVE RECEIVED A COPY OF THE ABOVE INSTRUCTIONS, I UNDERSTAND THEM AND I SHALL FOLLOW THEM.

_____
Patient's Signature.

_____
Physician

X-RAYS TO BE ORDERED AT PATIENTS FIRST CLINIC VISIT ARE: _____

_____

_____

DIAGNOSIS:_____

_____
OPC or PDC to be available when patient arrives following day.

Copy to: PATIENT

Fig. 23-12. "Cast sheet." (Courtesy Duke University Medical Center, Durham, N.C.)

ciated injuries. These fractures may be managed best with some form of traction. One example might be a femoral shaft fracture. Traction can be applied to the skin through application of adhesive straps. There is a limit to how much traction skin can tolerate over a period of time without injury and necrosis. Traction usage requires experience and alertness to its dangers. When greater weight is required, or if traction is necessary for prolonged periods of time, the force is applied directly to the skeleton with appropriately placed pins. Special mention should be made of Bryant's or Gallow's traction,[25] a popular form of longitudinal skin traction that treats the small child in extension of both knees with the hips flexed at 90 degrees. Its significant risk of ischemic necrosis and amputation of the uninjured leg overrides its advantages.[154] There are perfectly acceptable alternative methods that carry no risk of vascular embarrassment.

Compartment syndromes and Volkmann's ischemic contracture

Vascular injury to an extremity can occur in several ways. Direct injury to the blood vessel may result from a displaced fracture or a dislocated joint. If there is associated hypotension or a compressive dressing is used, the injury is magnified. The diagnosis of ischemia does not rely only on the absence of peripheral pulses; some pulses may reconstitute from collateral circulation. Distal capillary refill, at least, may be present from such collateral circulation. In the modern era of surgery, with arterial reconstruction readily available and highly successful, there is little excuse for ignoring vascular injury just because collateral circulation will keep most of the remaining limb viable. Relative ischemia of the extremity does occur in children and can be symptomatic. Mild degrees of ischemic contracture may leave one with a relatively functional extremity, but a less than optimal result should not be accepted when it is preventable.[46]

A short period of careful observation may be appropriate in some settings. The vascular embarrassment may be the result of kinking of a vessel or vascular spasm, which will improve with reduction and immobilization. However, there is a time period of only 4 to 6 hours before irreversible muscle damage occurs.[110] If there is any suspicion of vascular injury, referral to an appropriate spe-

cialty treatment center must be initiated immediately.

More subtle, but just as dangerous, is the vascular compromise that comes with small-vessel injury and elevated compartment pressures, resulting from any combination of arterial or venous injury or tissue swelling. This compromise can produce ischemia of the muscle, fibrosis, and contracture, a calamitous complication that may lead to severe functional loss, even after a prolonged period of reconstruction and rehabilitation (Fig. 23-13). The classic symptoms of ischemia are the five "Ps": pulselessness, pallor, pain, paresis, and paresthesia.

The presence of a pulse is not in itself assurance against impending proximal ischemia. Only 30 to 40 mm of mercury of external compression are necessary to occlude small arterioles and

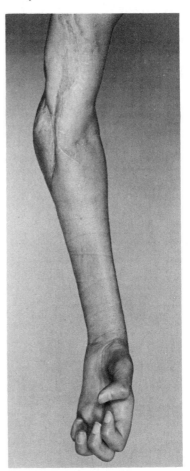

Fig. 23-13. Despite multiple surgical procedures and prolonged rehabilitation, the end result of Volkmann's ischemic contracture is calamitous.

venules (Fig. 23-14). Pallor, an ominous sign of reduced flow, and paresthesia or loss of muscle power resulting from neural compromise are important findings as well. Pain on passive extension of the fingers may be the earliest and most subtle sign of impending ischemia. The discomfort

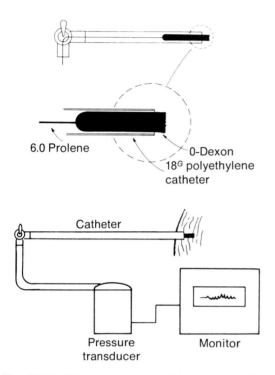

6.0 Prolene   0-Dexon
                     18ᴳ polyethylene
                     catheter

Catheter

Pressure   Monitor
transducer

Fig. 23-14. Schematic representation of one technique available for measuring fascial compartment pressures.

comes from stretch of the underlying muscle. Techniques are now available for the direct measurement of compartment pressures and are useful guides in the questionable situation.[116,164]

When there is a suspicion of ischemia, treatment must be undertaken as an emergency. There is a critical period of only a few hours during which permanent damage can be avoided. Casts must be split, dressings relieved, traction reduced, and all other appropriate measures taken to alter any external compression that may be complicating the issue. When these measures do not suffice, or when local tissue pressures are obviously elevated, adequate fasciotomy should be effected as an emergency even if skin grafting is required for closure.

The battered child

No one knows the true incidence of battering, but there are at least 500,000 episodes in the United States each year and as many as 2,000 mortalities.[44] A great deal has been written about, and most physicians are now familiar with, the social and economic situations that produce battering.[87,133] Battered children are often the children of parents who have themselves been battered.

Physicians treating injuries in children have an obligation to maintain a high index of suspicion. Whenever an explanation of the mechanism of injury is not clearly satisfactory, investigation is mandatory. Any skeletal injury in a child below the age of 1 year must be viewed with misgiving.

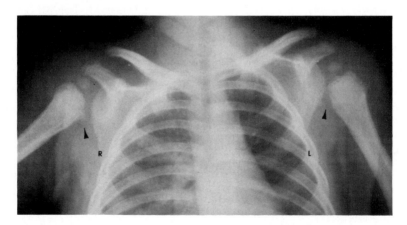

Fig. 23-15. Metaphyseal fleck fractures (arrows) are said to be pathognomonic of battering. The other characteristic skeletal findings are multiple fractures at different stages of healing and multiple posterior rib fractures. There are other suggestive findings, but most long bone fractures, in and of themselves, cannot be distinguished from injuries that occur with routine trauma.

The majority of skeletal injuries that occur from battering are indistinguishable from those that are produced by otherwise incidental trauma. It is the setting that varies. Children who cannot walk are not likely to sustain long bone fractures. Be wary of multiple fractures, particularly those that are at different stages of healing. The incidence of battering is much increased in handicapped children.[144] The classical metaphyseal fleck avulsion fracture is said to be pathognomonic[26] (Fig. 23-15).

The overriding obligation of the physician is to protect the patient. There are not many instances when proper management of simple fractures is lifesaving. Battering is one such instance. Most states have laws that not only protect the physician who refers a child for investigation, but also require that an investigation be initiated whenever suspicion of battering has occurred. Litigation has become so pervasive in our society that even the most responsible practitioner finds it difficult not to be hesitant. The physician is fully pro-tected in initiating an investigation, even if, subsequently, battering is not confirmed. Legal exposure lies in failing to report a suspicious incident.[120]

Pathologic fractures

The most common pathologic fracture is probably that which occurs through a benign uni-cameral bone cyst of the proximal humerus. Certain diseases make the bones of children particularly vulnerable to fractures; these include such metabolic bone diseases as renal osteodystrophy and such systemic diseases as osteogenesis imperfecta and muscular dystrophy, in which the disuse osteoporosis occurs. The only symptom of a fracture in a neurologically impaired child may be fever. There may be local findings of erythema and warmth, otherwise suggestive of infection.

Fat embolism

Fat embolism, so common in adults after long bone fracture or crushing injuries of the extremi-

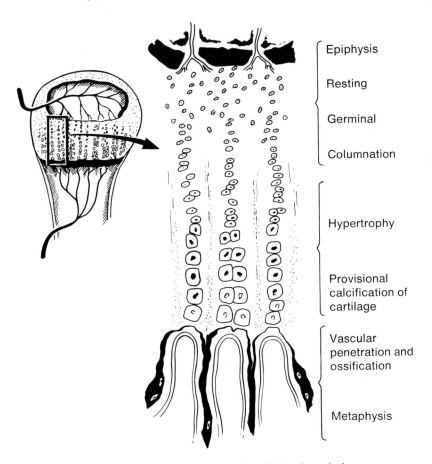

Epiphysis

Resting

Germinal

Columnation

Hypertrophy

Provisional calcification of cartilage

Vascular penetration and ossification

Metaphysis

Fig. 23-16. Schematic representation of the physeal plate.

ties, is extremely rare in children; but it has been reported in children with significant osteoporosis. Children at risk include those with spina bifida, collagen vascular disease, and those receiving steroid therapy.[93] Unexplained respiratory compromise or mental confusion may be symptoms of fat embolism.

Management of specific fractures
Growth plate injuries

The secondary ossification center at the end of a long bone is properly called the epiphysis. The physeal growth plate is the transverse zone of growing cartilage at the junction of the epiphysis and the metaphysis. The epiphysis can be injured without damage to the physeal plate. The best example of this process might be an avulsion of an osteochondral fragment, such as occurs with a typical bicycle injury and tibial spine fracture. More typically, so-called epiphyseal fractures are actually injuries that involve the physeal plate.

Understanding the microanatomy of the physeal plate is important for appreciating why these injuries may interfere with subsequent growth and which injuries are prone to do so. Fig. 23-16 is a schematic representation of the physeal plate. The germinal, or growth, layers are at the epiphyseal end of the plate. At the zone of hypertrophy and provisional calcification, the physeal plate is weakest. It is through this area that fractures commonly occur. With reduction and healing, however, there may be no damage to subsequent growth as long as the area of germination is not traversed. In their classic article entitled ''Injuries Involving the Epiphyseal Plate,'' Salter and Harris[138] demonstrate this important point and classify epiphyseal

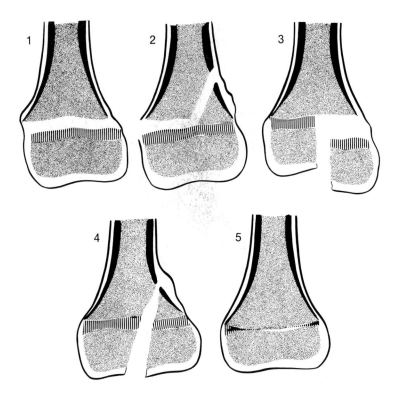

Fig. 23-17. Salter-Harris classification of physeal fractures. In type *1* fractures there is a complete separation through the physeal plate. The articular surface is intact. In type 2 injuries the cleavage plane of the fracture includes a fragment of the metaphysis. The metaphyseal fragment may be only a small fleck of bone or a rather large segment. Again, the articular surface is intact, and the growth portion of the physeal plate is not disturbed. In type *3* injuries the transverse plane through the hypertrophic zone of the physis is incomplete and there is a vertical component that enters the joint. The linear component with type *4* fractures extends through the articular surface into the metaphysis. Type *5* injuries crush the physeal plate. (Modified from Salter, R. B., and Harris, W. R.: J. Bone Joint Surg. **45A:**587, 1963.)

fractures. The Salter-Harris classification has become standard and is useful in both description of and prognosis for the injury. Fig. 23-17 is modified from an illustration in that article, which should be consulted by anyone interested in further details regarding these injuries.

Physeal fractures heal quite rapidly, and periods of immobilization of 3 to 6 weeks are all that are usually required. Because of this rapid healing, malposition may not be correctable much later than 10 days after the initial injury. Early and repeated follow-up evaluation and x-ray films are necessary.

Individual fractures and dislocations

Innumerable individual fractures and dislocations can occur, and each has specific therapeutic requirements. The following is a brief discussion of the more common types of fractures and dislocations with a few words about common complications and follow-up. It is presented to provide information to guide the primary care physician in judging the seriousness of the problem and in supporting the family.

CLAVICLE FRACTURES

Clavicle fractures are the most common long bone fractures of childhood. Occasionally, severe displacement of the fracture produces neurovascular compromise; but, for the most part, the injury is painful only. Anatomic reduction is unnecessary and almost impossible to achieve in a completely displaced fracture. A figure-of-eight bandage worn for 3 to 6 weeks is provided primarily for comfort and general alignment. Care must be taken not to make the bandage so tight as to produce axillary compression. Callus will create a palpable mass at the fracture site, which remodels over the course of a year, correcting any residual angulation and displacement.

RECURRENT DISLOCATIONS OF THE SHOULDER

In the very young child dislocation of the shoulder almost never occurs except in association with pyarthrosis. When recurrent subluxation of the shoulder is seen in the younger child, it is often posterior and there may be evidence of hypermobility of the joints or, perhaps, a systemic disease process such as Ehlers-Danlos syndrome. Repeated subluxation of the joint may be a voluntary maneuver and often is utilized as a parlor or party trick.[134] Although there are surgical procedures that can correct these anatomic aspects of the problem, the primary difficulty is behavioral and attention should be directed there first.

PROXIMAL HUMERAL EPIPHYSEAL FRACTURES

The proximal humeral epiphyseal fracture is a not uncommon birth injury and represents a complete separation of the upper humeral epiphysis, which is not apparent, because the ossification center has not yet presented. In the slightly older child this fracture may be the result of battering.[108]

Because of the excellent range of motion and the rapid growth of the proximal humerus, remodeling in this region is rapid and extensive. Therefore, only fractures with significant displacement need reduction.[118] General anesthesia may be required.

Treatment of these fractures is almost invariably successful because of the remodeling and motion available at the shoulder joint.

FRACTURES OF THE HUMERAL SHAFT

The radial nerve passes posterior and in close approximation to the shaft of the humerus in the spiral groove. At approximately the junction of the middle and distal thirds of the humerus, the nerve passes into the anterior compartment of the arm and is closely approximated to the cortex of the bone. Fractures in this region, as well as supracondylar fractures of the humerus, may produce radial nerve injury. It is important to identify a radial nerve injury before any attempts are made at reduction or immobilization. The injury to the nerve at the time of fracture is usually a contusion, which will recover. When the radial nerve palsy appears after manipulation, there may be entrapment between the fracture fragments, necessitating immediate exploration.

SUPRACONDYLAR FRACTURES OF THE HUMERUS

Supracondylar fractures of the humerus are difficult to manage. At the level of the fracture, the humerus is flattened and may be difficult to reduce and hold. More worrisome is the swelling that occurs in the antecubital fossa that may lead to compression of the anterior neurovascular structures. The brachial artery may be impaled or compressed by the anteriorly displaced, ragged edge of the proximal fragment. Reduction of the fracture usually relieves the vascular compression, but occasionally there is direct injury to the blood vessel, which requires repair. The fracture can be reduced with either traction or with manual manipulation.[40] Traction is safe and allows continued observation of the neurovascular status but requires more prolonged hospitalization. The elbow will be immobilized for a period of 3 to 4 weeks, but it may be as long as 3 months before full motion of the elbow is regained. Some children will have mild, permanent loss of motion. Malunion is not unusual.

Fifteen to twenty percent of children with supracondylar fractures injure one of the major peripheral nerves. The vast majority of these nerve injuries recover without any specific therapy.[100]

FRACTURES OF THE DISTAL HUMERUS

The key to proper diagnosis of fractures of the medial epicondyle or lateral condyle (capitellum) is knowing the timing and order of appearance of the secondary ossification centers of the distal humerus. Fractures that occur prior to the appearance of the ossification centers can be diagnosed only by conjecture. Comparison x-ray films are very helpful.

Closed reduction of a medial epicondylar fracture may be satisfactory. However, if the elbow is unstable with valgus strain, or if the fragment is widely displaced, nonunion and deformity can occur. In these latter circumstances, open reduction is necessary. The prognosis is good; but, as with all injuries about the elbow, a full range of motion may not return.

The more common fracture on the lateral side of the elbow is that of the lateral condyle, or capitellum. A fracture of the lateral condyle not only extends through the distal physeal plate of the humerus but also divides the articular surface. Open reduction is mandatory to achieve anatomic reduction.[66] Although premature closure of the physis is not unusual, it is rare for a significant late deformity to develop.

PROXIMAL RADIUS FRACTURES
AND DISLOCATIONS

Children rarely fracture the radial head. Injury is usually through the metaphysis, physis, or radial neck, leaving the articular surface intact. The goal of treatment is to maintain a full range of motion. Once reduced, the fracture is stable and can be maintained by a cast. Loss of motion is much more frequent after open reduction; and while this probably reflects the severity of the initial injury, it also testifies to the advantages of closed reduction.[130]

NURSEMAID'S ELBOW (PULLED ELBOW, SUBLUXATION OF THE RADIAL HEAD)

When longitudinal traction is applied with the forearm in pronation, the immature radial head subluxes within the annular ligament, which maintains the radius in its normal relationship to the proximal ulna and distal humerus.[139] After the age of 4 or 5 years, the radial head becomes large enough that this injury does not occur. The history is entirely characteristic: the child's arm is pulled by a parent or older sibling. The child cries and immediately stops using the arm, which is then held adducted to the side with the elbow flexed and the hand pronated. Reduction is simply accomplished by flexing and supinating the forearm, resulting in almost immediate restoration of function. For the most part, no immobilization is required. Explaining the mechanism of the injury to the parent should prevent recurrence. The elbow joint (humeral-ulnar joint) does dislocate in children. Dislocation of the elbow is commonly associated with such fractures as that of the medial epicondyle.

FRACTURES OF THE FOREARM[72]

The forearm is a common place to develop the torus and Greenstick fractures that are unique in children. Greenstick fractures should be completed in order to prevent recurrence or progression of the deformity. Complete fractures may tear the periosteal sleeve, making reduction difficult to maintain. The parents should always be prepared for the possible need for rereduction or, on rare occasions, even open reduction. Fractures of the distal radial epiphysis are common and are usually easily reduced, but occasionally general anesthesia may be needed. There is a fairly high incidence of postinjury growth disturbance. Sprains are unusual in young children; one should suspect a minimally displaced epiphyseal fracture or a small buckle fracture when the wrist is traumatized.

Since the two bones of the forearm are intimately bound together by ligamentous structures and the interosseous membrane, fracture of one will usually result in fracture of the other or in dislocation of the proximal or distal joint. Monteggia's fracture dislocation is a proximal ulna fracture with a dislocation of the proximal radioulnar joint. Galeazzi's or the Piedmont fracture occurs in the distal radial shaft and is associated with subluxation of the distal radioulnar joint. In children both Monteggia's and Galeazzi's fractures can be managed satisfactorily by closed reduction. Unsatisfactory results occur when the associated dislocation is not identified.

FRACTURES OF THE HAND

Important fractures and dislocations of the hand are discussed later in this chapter.

FRACTURES AND DISLOCATIONS OF THE
PELVIS AND LOWER EXTREMITY

Rang[128] points out that "the pelvis is like a suit of armor: when it is damaged there is much more concern about its contents than about the structure itself." Pelvic fractures in children are usually the result of vehicular injuries. There is a significant incidence of major associated injuries, and these associated injuries are usually more of a problem than the pelvic fractures themselves. However, gross displacement may lead to late deformity and, in the female, dystocia.[88] If the triradiate cartilage of the acetabulum is disturbed, growth arrest and secondary hip dysplasia can occur. Symptomatic treatment of the fracture gives good to excellent results in the vast majority of children.

FRACTURES AND DISLOCATIONS
ABOUT THE HIP

Fractures of the proximal femur are uncommon but difficult injuries. Nonunion in children is unusual, but malunion is not.[90] Even when internal fixation is utilized, body spica cast immobilization for 6 to 12 weeks is usually necessary.

Traumatic dislocation of the hip can occur in children below the age of 5 years as the result of relatively mild trauma. In the older child more of the articular structures are ossified, so that greater violence, such as that from contact sports and vehicles, is required to produce dislocation. The dislocation is usually posterior, and the extremity is flexed, adducted, and internally rotated, in contradistinction to the externally rotated and shortened position of the fractured extremity. Immediate reduction is mandatory to protect the vascular supply of the proximal femur. Avascular necrosis occurs in about 10% of hip dislocations[124] and in some fractures. One should always be aware of the possible occult epiphyseal fracture in these injuries, which may require an open reduction.

FRACTURES OF THE SHAFT OF THE FEMUR

Fracture of the femur commonly results from bumper injuries. Radiographs must include the knee and hip in the search for unrecognized dislocations of either of these joints. Because significant trauma is involved in producing a fracture of the femur, one should always be aware of other associated injuries. (Be wary of blaming shock on the blood loss that occurs with a fracture of the femur.) In the younger age group immediate spica casting provides satisfactory management because anatomic reduction is not necessary.[80] In the older, larger child initial skeletal traction through a tibial or femoral pin is usually followed by application of a body spica cast. Internal fixation for femoral shaft fractures in children is rarely necessary. The most common late problem in a femoral shaft fracture is inequality of limb length due to failure of overgrowth to compensate for poor reduction.

DISTAL FEMORAL EPIPHYSEAL FRACTURES

Distal femoral fractures occur most commonly with such varus or valgus stress as may occur in a football injury. The major stabilizing external ligaments about the knee are attached to the distal femoral epiphysis, and the physis is weaker than the ligaments. Thus, the result of this football injury is quite different in the child than it is in the adult. There is a high incidence of redisplacement, even after anatomic reduction of a distal femoral fracture. Even with maintenance of reduction and adequate stabilization by pins or plaster, there is a frequent incidence of growth disturbance. Because the distal femur accounts for a major portion of the overall limb length of the child, complete closure of the distal femoral physis will result in significant limb length discrepancy and partial closure may lead to angular deformity. Careful early follow-up is required following fracture to provide intervention as soon as complete or partial closure of the physis is recognized.

FRACTURES ABOUT THE KNEE

The most common fracture within the knee of a child is an avulsion injury of the anterior tibial spine; this injury so frequently occurs during a fall from a bicycle that the injury has earned the title "bicycle fracture."[109] The symptoms are hemarthrosis, pain, and limitation of motion. Radiographs may be negative or show a small ossified fleck or a large osteochondral fragment. The fragment is always larger than is apparent on the x-ray film, and a large segment of the articular surface of the proximal tibia may be attached. Detached fragments require an open reduction followed by immobilization in a cylinder cast for 3 to 6 weeks.

PROXIMAL TIBIAL GROWTH PLATE INJURIES

Growth plate injuries in the proximal tibia are unusual because the major structural ligaments about the knee attach to the tibial metaphysis. When fractures do occur, a high incidence of vascular injury has been reported.[64] The fracture is adjacent to the popliteal artery as it divides into its three branches and to the anterior tibial artery as it crosses the top of the interosseous membrane to enter the anterior compartment.

FRACTURES OF THE PROXIMAL TIBIAL METAPHYSIS

As with proximal physeal injuries, metaphyseal fractures should be treated with respect because of the proximity of the blood vessels. Anterior compartment syndromes are not infrequent after surgery in this area or after injury. There is an innocent-appearing transverse fracture of the medial aspect of the proximal tibia that everyone should be aware of. Even when it is well reduced and maintained in long-leg plaster, this fracture may result in late valgus deformity of the leg, representing overgrowth of the adjacent physeal plate or local entrapment of soft tissues.

TIBIAL SHAFT FRACTURES

Tibial shaft fractures in children are relatively easy to manage; the majority of these children have only mild displacement and intact periosteal sleeves, which assist in maintaining reduction. Union can be expected in 6 to 8 weeks, whereas in teenagers this fracture might take 10 to 12 weeks to unite and in adults 16 to 20 weeks. The fibula is often intact but may be bent. Pathologic fractures are not infrequent in the tibial shaft, and congenital pseudarthrosis must be considered, especially when anterolateral bowing of the tibia, with the typical radiographic changes, suggests this diagnosis.

ANKLE FRACTURES

In children below the age of 14, while the physes are wide open, true ankle sprains are rare. Fractures about the ankle typically traverse one or the other of the physeal lines; and even during healing, the plain x-ray films may continue to appear normal. Local pain and swelling suggest injury, and stress radiographic studies are essential. Open reduction may be required to achieve anatomic alignment of the ankle joint in some distal tibial epiphyseal fractures. Premature closure of the physeal plate about the ankle is not unusual and may require intervention to prevent angulation.

Spinal injuries

Spinal injuries are relatively uncommon in children; the majority of the fractures take place in the upper cervical spine, and occasional fractures are seen in the thoracic or lumbar region. The few children who have neurologic deficit often develop subsequent spinal curvature and require spine fusion for stabilization.[78]

NEUROMUSCULAR DISEASE

The orthopedist is not uncommonly the first specialist to see a child with a peripheral neuropathy, a myopathy, or some other such disorder. Similarly, children with primarily neurologic disease are often brought to the primary care physician with what is apparently a skeletal complaint, such as lumbar lordosis, gait deviation, weakness, deformity, or failure of function of a specific part. An excellent example of this is toe walking, which is discussed later in this chapter.

Classically, the gradual development of pes cavus or a varus hindfoot may be the first sign of such mechanical problems with the spinal cord as diastematomyelia, tethering, or occult spinal dysraphism[22] (Fig. 23-18). A detailed workup, including muscle and nerve biopsy, electromyography, and conduction studies, combined with a history and physical examination should make the distinction from a simple local problem possible.

Treatment. Only when a definitive diagnosis is reached can one make an appropriate judgment as to how to treat the specific deformity, since a poor prognosis and/or extension of the condition to other adjacent muscles would alter any surgical plans. Peroneal nerve weakness as a result of a local disease process or trauma can be managed with tendon transfers to balance the strength of the foot. However, tendon transfers may not be appropriate in a progressive neuropathy in which the muscle groups considered for transfer may themselves become involved.

The general goal of the orthopedic management of children with neuromuscular conditions is to achieve a straight, stable spine over a level pelvis, aligned and mobile lower extremities, and plantigrade feet. Spinal curvature is not at all uncommon in many neuromuscular conditions and often progresses to severe deformity.[67] Scoliosis in neuromuscular disease does not respond well to bracing; but when the child is young, an orthosis may allow as much growth as possible before bracing fails and surgical stabilization is required. Scoliosis surgery for neurologic disease is compli-

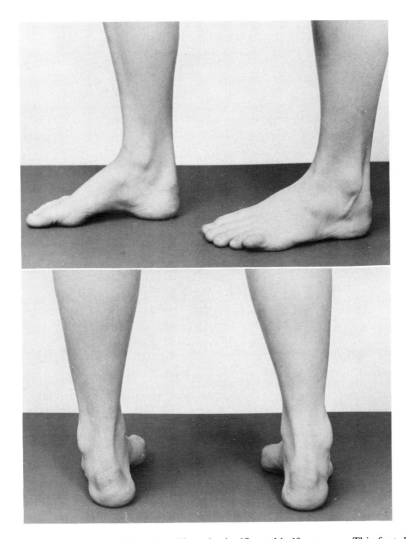

Fig. 23-18. Marked pes cavus deformity. There is significant hindfoot varus. This foot deformity may be the first sign of neuromuscular disease.

cated, requiring sophisticated support facilities in tertiary centers with extensive experience in spine reconstruction. Even orthopedic surgeons who manage large numbers of patients with idiopathic scoliosis may not have the necessary experience to manage children with neuromuscular scoliosis. Fusion often has to extend into the sacrum, and both anterior and posterior fusions may be required to achieve satisfactory fusion and long-term stability. A minimum pulmonary function of some 30% of predicted normal is necessary for such major procedures to succeed with acceptable mortality.

Children with neuromuscular scoliosis should be reviewed periodically in spinal treatment centers and major children's rehabilitation facilities, where experienced physical therapy, occupational therapy, and orthotic consultation are available to avail them of the most advanced orthotic techniques and wheelchairs (Fig. 23-19).

A level pelvis is necessary for a satisfactory gait, for brace fitting, and for good sitting posture; if there is sensory loss, a level pelvis is mandatory for distributing ischial pressure appropriately and preventing the development of decubitus ulcers. Pelvic obliquity may result from such suprapelvic causes as scoliosis and muscle contracture, from intrinsic pelvic distortion, or from such infrapelvic causes as muscle contractures about the hip.

Considerations for alignment of the remainder of the lower extremity are similar. A straight knee is required for walking; but for a person to arise from a chair without the use of the hands, at least one knee must flex beyond about 100 degrees; and for comfortable sitting, both knees should flex to close to 90 degrees. Below the knee, the goal is to obtain a plantigrade foot, that is, one in which the sole can be approximated to the floor, providing a firm base for gait. There are multiple and

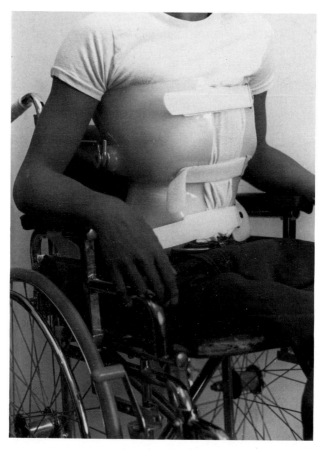

Fig. 23-19. Thoracic suspension orthosis. This specialized spinal support allows gravity to assist in maintaining spinal alignment and may assist in decreasing pressure on insensitive weight-bearing areas. Such advanced orthotic techniques as these are available only in comprehensive children's rehabilitation centers.

complex interrelated musculoskeletal imbalances and deformities that may develop over a period of time in the setting of neuromuscular disease. Even in progressive disorders, attention should be directed to these deformities, since they may significantly affect the function of a wheelchair-bound patient or even the care of a bedridden patient. Premature functional loss or severe, painful, or disfiguring deformities should not be allowed to develop in any neurologic condition.

Postoperative care. Postoperatively, external devices should be minimized to avoid the known loss of function that occurs with prolonged immobilization and/or bedrest in children with neuromuscular conditions. If sensation is absent, special considerations must be made for care of the underlying insensitive skin. Special children's orthopedic rehabilitation hospitals may provide the most appropriate setting for the recuperation involved.

Often the postoperative care is the most important determinant of the success of a surgical procedure, requiring intensive physical therapy with experienced pediatric therapists to achieve the functional goals. However, one of the major goals of the entire care program will be to minimize hospitalization and time spent in special facilities and to normalize the child's existence, making it possible for him to participate in local community activities and, perhaps, attend a regular school. An appropriate balance can usually be accomplished through good communication between the primary care physician and the specialty consultant.

Myelodysplasia

Early orthopedic surgical considerations combined with neurosurgical care and physical therapy and orthotic management will maximize function in children with myelodysplasia. As soon as rea-

Table 23-1. Functional levels in myelodysplasia

Neurosegmental level	Critical muscles	Deformity	Orthotic requirements	Mobility level
Sacral or S3-5	Intrinsics: feet	Variable Cavus Clawtoes	Shoe modification	Normal
S1-2	S-2 Gastrocnemius Lateral hamstrings Gluteus maximus Long toe flexors S-1 Peroneals Medial hamstrings Hip abductors	Calcaneovalgus	AFO (short leg brace)	Community Limited endurance May use crutch or cane as adult
L-5	Posterior tibial	Equinovarus	AFO > KAFO (long leg braces)	Child: community Adult: 50%+ household
L3-4	Anterior tibial Quadriceps	Hip Flexion External rotation Subluxation Dislocation Calcaneus	KAFO + pelvic band	Child: household Adult: 10% to 30% household
L1-2	Hip flexors Adductors	Hip Flexion Adduction Subluxation Dislocation	KAFO + thoracic extension	Child: household Adult: occasional household
Thoracic or T8-12	Abdominal	Postural: contracture Hip Flexion Abduction External rotation Scoliosis Kyphosis Lordosis	6 to 18 mo: standing brace 18 to 36 mo: walker, platform brace 36 mo+: triceps crutches, thoracic extension, KAFO	Child: pivot and drag to gait Adult: nonambulator

sonable neurologic assessment can be made, guidelines can be provided to the family for ultimate function, future surgical procedures, and the need for orthotic devices. Table 23-1 is one such compilation of guidelines and may be used as an initial approximation. There are, however, dangers in this form of categorization. It is extremely difficult to assess the functional musculature of a neonate, and often one overestimates paralysis. When children are assigned a "neurologic level," lifetime decisions are made on the basis of an initial exam; this early "tracking" may deprive a child of reaching his full potential. Neurologic level can be a guideline to ultimate function, but

it is significantly influenced by the presence of other congenital abnormalities, involvement of the upper extremities, hydrocephalus, intelligence, family setting, and many other factors. Furthermore, involvement of the lower extremities is often asymmetric.

When the lesion is in the thoracic region, the musculature of the lower extremities, including all the muscles about the hip, will generally be flaccid. Thus, the major problem of hip instability due to muscle imbalance does not occur. In lumbar-level lesions, the key cutoff appears to be L-3,[8] since very few individuals who do not have functional quadriceps muscles remain more than physiologic ambulators in their late teen or adult years. The standard classification below lists the levels of ambulation. In the midlumbar region, as can be seen from Table 23-1, there is muscle imbalance about the hips that may lead to hip dislocation. The ultimate functional level is not affected by the presence or absence of hip dislocation, and these hips are not painful.[36] Many children have been subjected to repeated surgical procedures and have had great periods of their childhood wasted in attempts to maintain reduction of their hips. On the other hand, contractures are usually lessened and brace fitting is generally easier when the hips are located. Particularly when one hip is dislocated, pelvic obliquity may well result, with all its attendant problems, in sitting balance, decubitus ulcers, and spinal deformity. It is our opinion that appropriate attempts can be made to maintain the hips located, particularly when the condition is unilateral. Alteration of orthoses may help, but often a surgical procedure is necessary. In these special instances, one attempt at maintaining hip reduction may be worthwhile.

Functional levels of ambulation

Nonambulator
    Wheelchair bound
    Able to transfer
Physiologic
    Nonfunctional, therapy in school or home
    Wheelchair for transportation
Household
    External support and apparatus
    Minimal assistance with bed-chair-standing
    Wheelchair for some indoor and all community activities
Community
    Indoor and outdoor
    May use braces and external support
    Wheelchair only for long trips

Categorizing neurologic defects in the lower segments is very difficult. Asymmetry is common, as are congenital abnormalities such as clubfoot. It is probably better for one to simply describe deformities and perform careful neurologic exams, listing the functioning muscles. Individual muscle testing not only serves as a guide to surgical intervention, but also provides an important record for possible later changes in neurologic status. One must always be alert for changing neurologic status and the need for current assessment of intraspinal abnormalities.

The management of clubfoot and congenital foot abnormalities in myelodysplastic children is the same as that in normal children, with the addition of concern for the insensitive skin.[50] Early intervention to correct fixed congenital abnormalities such as clubfoot is appropriate. Particularly because of the insensitive feet, plantigrade feet must be obtained in order to make weight bearing possible without recurrent ulceration. Foot deformities associated with myelodysplasia are among the most resistant to any form of treatment, and repeated surgical procedures are often necessary.

It can be seen from this brief discussion that we have a bias toward aggressive surgery and bracing. The goal is mobility. Almost all young children, regardless of neurologic level, can be made mobile in some form of orthotic device (Fig. 23-20). While this mobility may not persist into adulthood, it does provide significant benefit during childhood in the form of socialization, psychologic outlook, diminution of osteoporosis, improved urinary drainage, improved cardiovascular function,

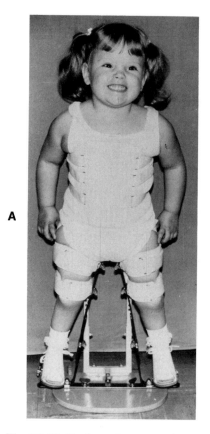

A

Fig. 23-20. For legend see opposite page.

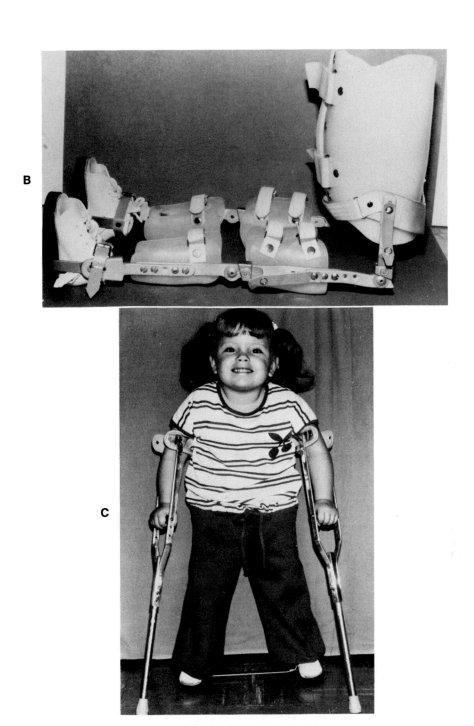

Fig. 23-20. Young girl with a thoracic-level myelomeningocele. There was complete flaccid paraplegia from T-10 down. This child had three ventriculoperitoneal shunt procedures. Early in life she became ambulatory in a platform standing orthosis (**A**). At about age 3 she was fitted with bilateral long leg braces with a single outside upright. Chest support was necessary. A similar device is seen in **B. C** Shows the child at age 4. At this time she was a community ambulator.

and a host of other secondary benefits. We are not discussing ambulation or "walking," but mobility in standing orthoses or braces at a young age and the use of a wheelchair when appropriate. It is possible to accomplish mobility without forgetting that the primary goals in the management of these children are psychologic, social, intellectual, educational, and, only very secondarily, physical.[107]

At least 50% to 80% of all children with myelomeningocele will develop significant spinal deformity.[129] Some 20% of these children have severe congenital abnormalities. The remaining group will develop spinal deformity with time. These deformities are made difficult by the problems of paralysis, gravity, and muscle imbalance. Extensive surgery is almost invariably required for spinal stabilization.

Postoperative complications in children with myelodysplasia are frequent. Because of urinary incontinence, poor skin, and problems with immobility, the wound infection rate is high (25% to 30%). Urinary tract infection and/or urinary stones are common and require great care to maintain hydration and urinary sterility. The long bones are often osteoporotic from disuse compounded by

postoperative immobilization and joint motion restriction. The most common postoperative complication is fracture during mobilization and the initiation of weight bearing.[89] Continued mobilization in braces can be utilized in any fracture in a myelodysplastic child, whether it is traumatic or postoperative. The exception to this rule is an epiphyseal fracture, in which traditional methods of external immobilization and limitation of weight bearing must be utilized to avoid nonunion and Charcot changes (Fig. 23-21).

Cerebral palsy

A precise definition of cerebral palsy is difficult because in reality it is a number of disorders. One approximation was put forth by Denhoff and Langdon[32]: ". . . a persistent, but not necessarily unchanging, abnormality of posture and movement due to (nonprogressive) damage to the central nervous system before its growth and development. . . ." While cerebral palsy is nonprogressive in terms of brain damage, its manifestations may seem to progress because of physical development and advancing social expectations for performance.

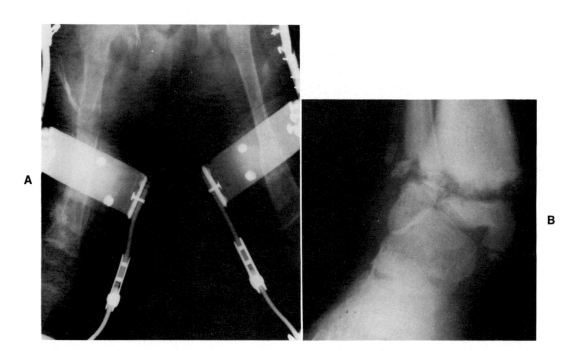

Fig. 23-21. Management of fractures in myelodysplasia. Many fractures may be managed by utilizing the child's braces for support and continuing mobilization (**A**). The exception is an epiphyseal fracture. If early weight bearing is allowed after an epiphyseal fracture, Charcot changes and nonunion may develop (**B**).

Understanding the orthopedic management of cerebral palsy is integrally bound to a complete understanding of its neurophysiology and pathology, as well as to an appreciation of the roles of the physiotherapist, occupational therapist, speech pathologist, and educational psychologist. The greatest problems in the surgical management of cerebral palsy are failure to set appropriate goals and errors in timing of surgical procedures. The procedures themselves are technically relatively simple.

Recent advances in gait analysis have helped in providing guidelines for surgical selection[125] but do not replace good judgment. Because muscle tone can be so severely affected by anxiety, strange circumstances, or fear, it is often difficult

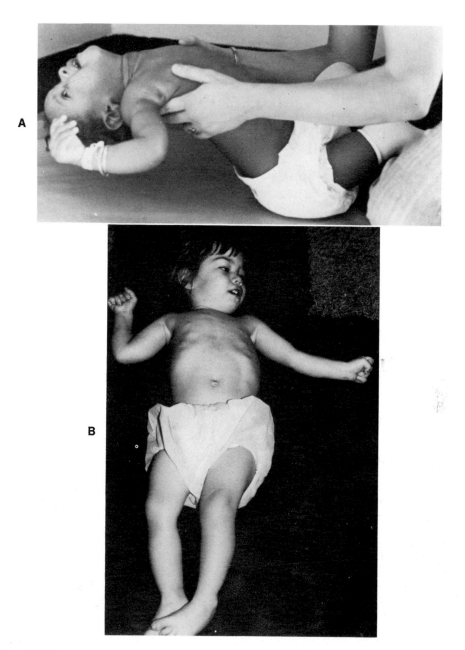

Fig. 23-22. A, The Moro response should not persist beyond age 6 months. **B,** Asymmetric tonic neck reflex. The persistence of such primitive motor patterns will significantly affect the child's ability to function when placed in certain positions.

to make treatment decisions based on a single evaluation. Only when the child has become accustomed to his surroundings will the examination accurately reflect daily function.

The lesion in cerebral palsy is in the central nervous system, and operating on the extremities will not alter spasticity, incoordination, and movement disorders. One can improve the gait by operating on the lower extremities and improve the function of the upper extremity, but the child will still have cerebral palsy.

The answer to the question "will this child walk?" depends on a number of factors, including overall involvement, strength, and balance and the persistence or absence of basic developmental reflexes and primitive motor patterns. Bleck[14] has categorized these persistent primitive reflexes (Fig. 23-22) and pathologic patterns (Fig. 23-23) and identified five important reflex patterns that are prognostic to the 90% confidence limit for ambulation as early as 1 to 2 years of age (see below).

The vast majority of children ambulate by age 7. Ambulation may require the assistance of orthoses but also implies a certain degree of independent functioning by the child.

Walking prognosis in cerebral palsy[14]

Score 1 if present
  Asymmetric tonic neck reflex
  Neck-righting reflex
  Moro reflex
  Symmetric tonic neck reflex
  Extensor thrust
Score 1 if absent
  Foot placement reaction
  Parachute reaction

2 or greater = Poor prognosis
1   = Guarded prognosis
0   = Good prognosis

When one speaks of surgery for cerebral palsy, often what comes to mind are heel cord lengthenings and perhaps adductor tenotomies; but there

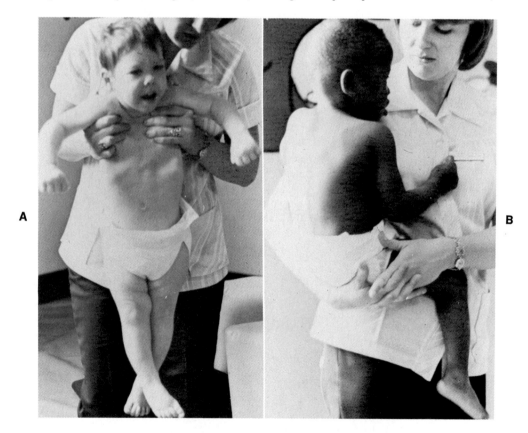

Fig. 23-23. A, When the child is improperly held, there is overflow of muscle tone with extensor thrust and scissoring. **B,** When the child is properly positioned, the abnormal tone is minimized. One of the important functions of physical therapy in cerebral palsy is to identify and reinforce positions and activities in which pathologic motor reflexes are minimized.

are a multitude of other surgical procedures that may be beneficial to individual children. Those interested in more detailed discussion of the orthopedic surgical management are referred to the excellent monographs by Samilson[140] and Bleck.[15]

Although most physicians recognize the importance, in cerebral palsy, of surgical procedures on the lower extremity, one question that often arises in a discussion of surgical indications is whether or not procedures on the upper extremity are ever useful. Some feel that since stereognosis is often deficient in the upper extremity, the hand will never be useful and, therefore, surgery may be little more than cosmetic. There is no reason, however, to withhold surgical procedures that will improve grasp and release, pinch, and ease of assistive movements simply because sensation is impaired.[49]

As with other neuromuscular disorders, the hospitalization surrounding the surgical procedure itself may be brief but prolonged hospitalization and/or physical therapy may be necessary in the postoperative period to obtain maximal benefit from the procedure.

Treatment of specific deformities

The general purpose of surgery in cerebral palsy is to release contracture and prevent deformity. The goal is to intervene at a time that does not interfere with the child's developmental progress, to make bracing possible, if desirable, or to allow the child to be brace free. The decisions regarding surgery should be delayed as long as possible because of the difficulties in goal setting and decision making; at the same time, however, surgery should be performed early enough that bony deformities do not develop and thereby necessitate surgery of even greater magnitude.

Numerous and varied surgical procedures have been utilized to correct specific deformities in cerebral palsy. Most are straightforward, requiring brief periods of hospitalization. Postoperatively, casting is usually required for several weeks and is followed by prolonged splinting, at least during sleep. The following is a brief discussion of the more common deformities and their surgical treatment.

EQUINUS

The most common deformity in cerebral palsy is equinus of the hindfoot (Fig. 23-24). Lengthening of the triceps surae muscle-tendon unit was one of the first surgical procedures to be performed in cerebral palsy over a hundred years ago. When proper indications are utilized, one anticipates a 90% incidence of good to excellent results from any of a variety of techniques, with most authors reporting a 10% incidence of recurrence of equinus.[9]

EQUINOVALGUS

Equinovalgus is a common deformity in spastic children that is often progressive and not well controlled by bracing. The Grice procedure commonly utilized to control progressive valgus[58,86] (Fig. 23-25), is an extra-articular arthrodesis of the subtalar joint, performed by inserting a bone block in the lateral talocalcaneal joint, and may be combined with a heel cord lengthening or with other transfers designed to balance the musculature about the foot.

KNEE FLEXION

Spastic hamstring muscles produce a flexed knee gait with short stride length, crouching, and

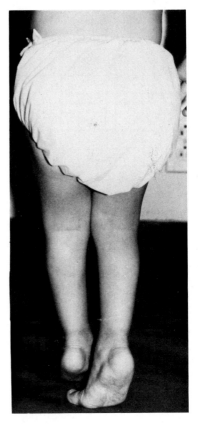

Fig. 23-24. The most common deformity in cerebral palsy is equinus of the hindfoot.

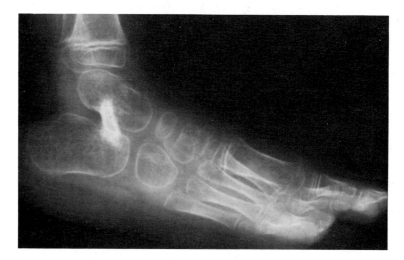

Fig. 23-25. The Grice procedure is a common method of correcting equinovalgus deformity. A bone block is placed to effect an extra-articular arthrodesis of the subtalar joint.

adduction and internal rotation of the hips. Often secondary deformities and contractures develop as a result of major hamstring surgery, and it has become increasingly evident that while hamstring surgery is useful, it should be done judiciously.[35] Usually fractional lengthening of the musculature without transfer will suffice. Often knee surgery is combined with other procedures on the hip, ankle, and foot.

HIP DEFORMITIES

Muscle imbalance and contracture make deformities of the hip common. Surgical procedures are usually designed to relieve these contractures, correct persistent anteversion, reduce the crouch gait, and prevent scissoring and progressive subluxation of the hip. Even in nonambulators, surgery may improve perineal hygiene and sitting balance and will, it is hoped, prevent pain from chronic dislocation of the hip. Most often these procedures are muscle releases of the flexors and adductors of the hip, with release of the iliopsoas from the lesser trochanter and transfer of the psoas tendon to the anterior capsule of the hip joint.[13] When the condition persists for a period of time, simple muscle release will not suffice, and a femoral derotation and varus osteotomy (p. 289) may become necessary.

Postoperative management from hip surgery will include either a body spica cast or at least bilateral long leg plasters fixed together with spreader bars. Since mobility is severely limited for several weeks, hospitalization in a rehabilita-

tion facility may be appropriate. On occasion, when all the contractures cannot be released without undue weakening, postoperative traction in the hospital may be useful (Fig. 23-26).

SPINAL DEFORMITIES

Significant spinal deformity may severely interfere with function, even in nonambulators. When one upper extremity must be utilized to maintain sitting, a significant portion of available function is lost. Standard scoliosis techniques may suffice, but anterior fusion and extension into the sacrum are often required.[18]

UPPER EXTREMITY DEFORMITIES

The typical spastic posture is adduction of the arm, elbow flexion, pronation of the forearm, flexion of the fingers, and thumb in palm. In general, surgical procedures on the upper extremity are designed to lengthen tight muscles and reinforce weak ones, and at the same time maintain mobility.[47]

• • •

Children with cerebral palsy often require many hospitalizations, have many surgical procedures, and deserve every effort to minimize their periods of immobilization and hospitalization. It is our feeling, based on long experience, that with careful preoperative assessment, multiple surgical procedures—such as on the hip, knee, and foot—can be performed at one sitting. Failure of surgical procedures in cerebral palsy comes not only from

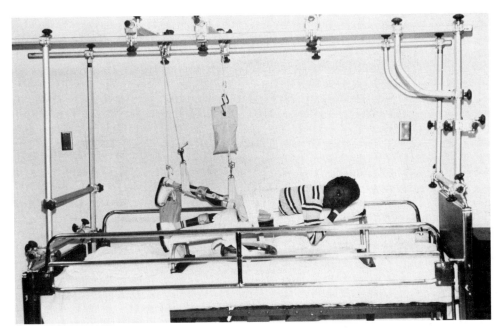

Fig. 23-26. Postoperative traction may be useful for continued correction of contracture.

preoperative misjudgment but also from underestimation of the extent of postoperative care that is necessary. Recurrence will all too often result when appropriate postoperative splinting and a careful program of postoperative physical therapy are not provided.

GENERALIZED CONNECTIVE TISSUE DISORDERS

Ehlers-Danlos syndrome and Marfan's syndrome are relatively rare, systemic, heritable diseases that have major manifestations in collagenous tissues and thus may require orthopedic attention because of the joint or skeletal abnormalities.

When hyperlaxity is a major feature of the condition, as it may be in some forms of Ehlers-Danlos syndrome, repeated dislocations are not uncommon.[104] Usually, these are easily reduced and do not require surgical procedures or corrections; subluxation and dislocation become less frequent with time and age. Reconstruction of the joint for repeated dislocation is difficult because of the inadequate collagenous tissues but occasionally must be undertaken when the dislocations are frequent and symptomatic.

An additional problem in Marfan's syndrome is scoliosis, which is often progressive and may be-

come quite severe.[132] Unlike idiopathic scoliosis, this lesion is more difficult to control with braces and more frequently requires surgery.

HEMOPHILIA

Although children with hemophilia should be followed at a tertiary care center where specialized hematologic coagulation laboratories are available for monitoring the nature and extent of their disease, the primary care physician must be fully informed as to the nature of the bleeding disorder, the status of the present level of bleeding factors, the presence or absence of inhibitors, and the patient's response to therapy in order to provide initial therapy for a bleeding episode. Prompt coagulation factor replacement may avoid many of the late complications of bleeding episodes.[73] No manipulation or invasive studies or therapeutic measures should be performed in children with bleeding disorders until after replacement therapy has been initiated, the therapeutic response to their infusion has been documented, and one is certain that inhibitors are not present.

Hemarthrosis

The most common problem that confronts the orthopedic surgeon in children with bleeding disorders is acute hemarthrosis.[127] All hemarthroses

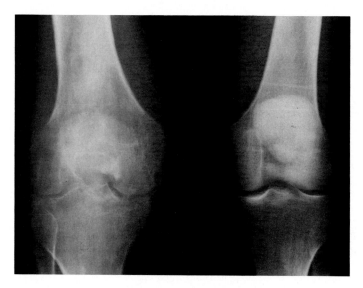

Fig. 23-27. Chronic hemophiliac arthropathy. There is widening of metaphyses and epiphyses, erosion of the intercondylar notch, loss of the articular space, and cyst formation and erosion of the subchondral bone.

do not require aspiration. Replacement should begin immediately, and aspiration should be reserved for joints that are taut and painful. All but the most minor hemarthroses should be briefly immobilized for patient comfort, reduction of pain, and control of muscle spasm and hemorrhage. As soon as the acute episode is under control, physical therapy should begin to restore range of motion and strength. Accepting a minor reduction in range of motion after hemarthrosis may not seem unreasonable at the time of a single episode, but the cumulative loss of motion with repeated episodes can be significant. Similarly, one must restore muscle power or be faced with a chronically weakened limb.

On certain occasions, despite the best measures, repeated hemorrhage into the joint results in chronic hypertrophic synovitis, which further contributes to the development of arthropathy, contracture, and repeated bleeding episodes. Intraarticular steroid injection may be beneficial, but careful consideration should be given to surgical synovectomy,[6] even though the cost for the replacement factor alone may be as high as $20,000 to $30,000. Reconstructive joint procedures, even total joint replacement, have been undertaken to correct the late results of repeated hemarthroses and chronic hemophiliac arthropathy (Fig. 23-27), but these very specialized surgical procedures should be undertaken only in highly specialized

centers with experience in surgery of children with bleeding disorders, and only after long consideration and trial of other therapeutic measures.

Bleeding into soft tissues

Spontaneous or posttraumatic hemorrhage into muscle bellies is not uncommon in children with bleeding disorders. A typical example is bleeding into the psoas muscle, which may present as a painful, apparently contracted hip held in flexion, abduction, and external rotation. It is important to distinguish a psoas hemorrhage from acute hemarthrosis of the hip. The treatment of both is rest, replacement, and immobilization; but because of the precarious blood supply of the hip in a child, attempts must be made to reduce the intra-articular pressure by aspiration of acute hemarthrosis. When the psoas is involved, gentle motion of the hip joint is not painful and the extremity is held in flexion and internal rotation. There may even be femoral nerve palsy as a result of local compression where the lumbosacral plexus passes through the origin of the iliopsoas muscle. There may be quadriceps paralysis and diminished sensation in the distribution of the saphenous nerve, which travels with the femoral nerve.

Where other muscle bellies, as in the forearm, are involved with hemorrhage, compartment syndromes may develop. Simple needle and catheter techniques are readily available for compart-

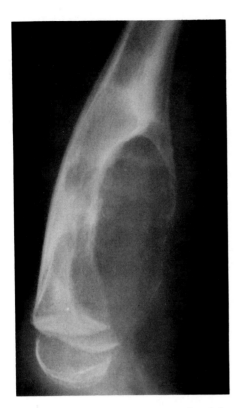

Fig. 23-28. A pseudotumor is an unusual and dramatic complication of hemophilia.

ment pressure assessment.[116,164] A progressive increase in pain, compartment tightness, inability to extend the fingers, pallor, loss of pulses, neurologic deficit, or elevated intracompartmental pressures are all indications for elective fasciotomy. The results of untreated compartment syndromes, Volkmann's ischemic contracture, are catastrophic.[48]

Pseudotumor

Massive soft tissue hemorrhage and organization of a hematoma may lead to a progressively enlarging mass known as a pseudotumor (Fig. 23-28), which is very difficult to manage. These have been successfully resected under coverage of appropriate replacement therapy[5]; but, as with other unusual situations in bleeding disorders, surgery should be undertaken only at very specialized tertiary care centers.

VASCULAR MALFORMATIONS

Vascular malformations of the extremities are hamartomatous, congenital malformations that may be composed of lymphatic, venous, or ar-

terial structures in varying combinations and may result in overgrowth and gigantism. They may be associated with more generalized conditions such as the Sturge-Weber syndrome or they may be associated with multiple enchondromas as in Maffucci's syndrome. Resection of the vascular malformation may be possible, depending on the extent and location of the lesion. Often the lesion is more extensive than is apparent, and an arteriogram and/or venogram is necessary to outline the three-dimensional anatomy of all but the smallest lesions. Extensive intramuscular extension is not uncommon, and massive bleeding can result when attempts are made to resect such lesions without due care. Steroids have been reported as being useful in controlling the venous aspect of massive or infiltrative lesions.[42]

ABNORMALITIES OF THE FEET
Minor abnormalities

The conditions described here can be considered minor only in a limited sense. They may represent the single largest group of foot problems that one sees in a primary care practice. Management should be simple; if one is not careful, however, the treatment may become worse than the disease.

Corns

A corn is always the response to a localized area of pressure,[101] most commonly resulting from ill-fitting shoes. The skin overlying a bony prominence responds to pressure by developing a hyperkeratotic area with a secondary deep, central nucleus that becomes exquisitely painful with persistent pressure or inflammation. If the corn is the result of a deformity of the foot or toe, this deformity should be corrected; more often, however, the solution lies in obtaining proper-fitting shoes. The corn itself is managed with salicylic acid plasters, which are commercially available. Surgical removal is rarely necessary.

Plantar warts

A plantar wart may occur on any part of the foot, not necessarily in a weight-bearing or pressure-sensitive area.[34] Like all other warts, these are papillomas resulting from viral infection; however, plantar warts are flattened with weight bearing and ultimately become embedded. Plantar warts are friable, bleed readily on irritation, and, when they are large or in a weight-bearing area, may be particularly tender.

Padding may be useful while one is awaiting spontaneous remission. Since surgery may lead to recurrence and/or a painful plantar scar, active treatment for plantar warts should be reserved for the particularly painful and persistent lesion.

Ingrown toenail

When the nail of the great toe is improperly trimmed, direct pressure at the corner of the nail may cause penetration of the nail into the adjacent soft tissues. With recurrent pressure and irritation, hypertrophy and inflammation result, followed by swelling, erythema, and tenderness. At this early stage of the ingrown toenail, the process may be aborted by soaks, elevation, and the insertion of

cotton beneath the edge of the toenail to allow it to grow free of the adjacent tissues. Recurrence can be prevented by proper transverse toenail clipping so that the nail corner extends beyond the soft tissues.[21]

If infection develops, drainage of the paronychia, soaks, and antibiotics will bring the infection under control and an attempt can be made to allow the nail to regrow properly. If the infection is chronic, with granulation and hypertrophy of the surrounding tissues, excision of a wedge of lateral tissue may be necessary, along with removal of a portion of the nail. When the nail has become deformed, resection of that segment of the nail and curettage of the nail bed to prevent regrowth will be definitive.

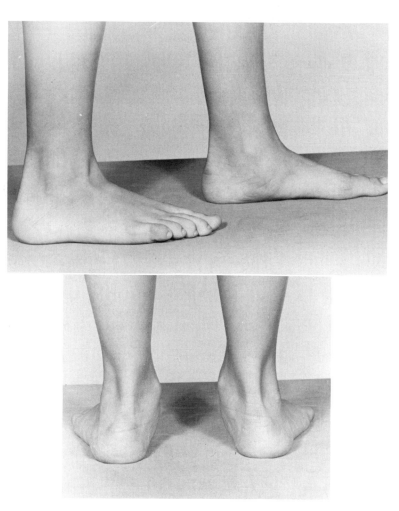

Fig. 23-29. Flexible flatfoot (pes planus). There is loss of the longitudinal arch, a pronated midfoot and forefoot, and a valgus position of the heels.

Flatfoot (pes planus)

Pes planus is an exceedingly frequent condition that is usually asymptomatic.[71,163] Only a very small percentage of children will ever experience significant or persistent pain because of this condition during their childhood.[31] All infants appear to have no longitudinal arch because of the fat overlying the abductor hallucis. Before the age of 2 years, most children have such hypermobile feet that the actual configuration of the longitudinal arch will be difficult to determine. Beyond age 2, a significant number of children will stand with pronated forefeet, valgus heels, and flattening of the longitudinal arch (Fig. 23-29). There is a prominence of the talus medially that is flexible, however, and subtalar motion is preserved. Gross motor and sensory function are normal, and in the relaxed, non-weight-bearing position the configuration of the foot is normal as well.

There appears to be a growing concensus among pediatric orthopedists that:

1. It is impossible to predict which children will become symptomatic, but their numbers are few.
2. It is probably impossible to prevent the development of symptoms if they are going to occur.
3. Most adults remain asymptomatic whether or not they had any form of orthotic management as children.
4. The orthoses, particularly some of the molded arch supports and molded plastic cups, may be useful in managing transient symptoms in childhood.
5. No orthosis affects the long-term configuration of the foot, and many adults discard their orthoses once they reach their majority and no longer have to satisfy their parents.

The child is usually seen at an early age, and the presenting complaint is almost invariably parental or grandparental concern. All that is usually required is reassurance to the parents. In the occasional child who does become symptomatic, heel cord stretching exercises and molded heel cups may be useful. Even more infrequently, surgical correction is indicated in children whose symptoms are persistent.

Surgical correction consists of reefing of the medial supporting structures of the longitudinal arch, advancement of the posterior tibial tendon, and tightening of the spring ligament.[111] Some authors have described various osteotomies of the metatarsocuneiform joint, the cuneiform bone, or the talus—all procedures designed to increase the arch and reduce the valgus of the hindfoot.[76] Generally satisfactory results have been reported, but whether this implies definitive correction of the problem or underselection and overtreatment is open to question. The hospitalization for flatfoot surgery will usually not extend beyond 5 to 7 days, but casting is required for 6 to 12 weeks and non–weight bearing for at least the initial several weeks of treatment.

Accessory tarsonavicular bone

Approximately 10% of all individuals will have an accessory ossicle at the medial end of the tarsonavicular bone early in childhood,[173] and this ossicle fails to unite with the main body of the navicular in 2% of the population. The ununited ossicle (Fig. 23-30) is referred to as a prehallux. The posterior tibial tendon, which is one of the main supporting structures of the longitudinal arch of the foot, has a major insertion into the tarsonavicular. Some authors believe that when an accessory or

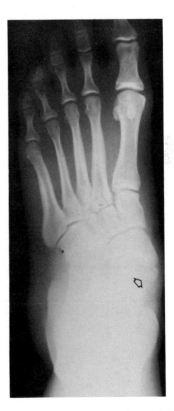

Fig. 23-30. Accessory tarsonavicular ossicle (arrow).

elongated navicular exists, the insertion of the posterior tibial tendon is more medial than normal and that loss of a portion of its plantar and lateral extension leads to collapse of the longitudinal arch.[151] There is no question that a significant number of individuals with an accessory navicular do have loss of the longitudinal arch, but the association may be coincidental rather than causative.

Whether or not a flatfoot deformity exists, some patients will develop activity-related localized pain and inflammation at the site of insertion of the posterior tibial tendon as well as a tenosynovitis of the tendon itself.

The symptoms of acute inflammation may be relieved by rest, anti-inflammatory agents, and, in some instances, the use of an ambulatory cast. Local injection of steroids should be avoided, since as much as 25% of the ultimate strength of a tendon or ligament may be lost as a result. Partial or complete rupture of the posterior tibial tendon might ensue, and such rupture has been cited as a cause of painful flatfeet. When pain persists, excision of the accessory navicular is indicated, with pain relief expected. If flatfoot is associated with the condition, formal reconstruction of the medial structures will be required in addition.

Rigid flatfoot

Rigid flatfoot, commonly called spasmodic or peroneal spastic flatfoot, is distinguished from the typical flexible flatfoot by the persistent loss of the longitudinal arch in non–weight bearing and by the absence or limitation of subtalar motion. Patients with this condition often have tenosynovitis and spasm of the peroneal tendons, the common toe extensors, and the anterior tibial tendon. Spasm is only an associated symptom; the underlying abnormality is coalition of two or more of the tarsal bones.[70] Tarsal coalition is an autosomal dominant trait, and a number of large families have been described.[172] Loss of the longitudinal arch does not always accompany a tarsal coalition, nor are patients with tarsal coalition always symptomatic.

The coalition may be fibrous, cartilaginous, or osseous and therefore may not be well visualized on routine radiographs (Fig. 23-31). The most common coalition is between the calcaneus and tarsal navicular, followed by talocalcaneal coalition.[97]

Symptoms appear during the teenage years, presumably as a result of increased activity, size, and solidification of the coalition. If the symptoms are mild and infrequent, rest and aspirin may be all that is necessary. In the more persistent cases, longitudinal arch supports or medial heel wedges may be effective. Surgical intervention is necessary for the recurrent or resistant case. When the bar is surgically accessible and degenerative arthritis has not yet occurred, resection with interposition of a local muscle flap is the procedure of choice. This procedure preserves motion, relieves

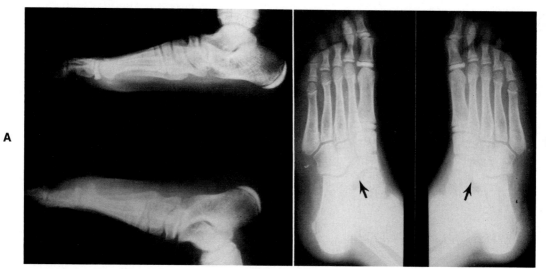

Fig. 23-31. A, Rigid flatfoot is almost invariably the result of tarsal coalition. **B,** These oblique x-ray films demonstrate the most common coalition, a calcaneonavicular bar.

pain, and should prevent long-term degenerative arthritis. If the bar is more extensive or if degenerative arthritis has already begun, surgical stabilization in the form of a triple arthrodesis is required.

Toe walking

Toe walking is a not uncommon reason for referral to a pediatric orthopedist. A partial list of the differential diagnosis is included in Table 23-2.

Table 23-2. Toe walking: differential diagnosis

Normal early walking	
Cerebral	Cerebral palsy (spastic)
	Behavioral
	Mental retardation
	Autism, schizophrenic
	Minimal brain dysfunction
Cerebellar	Cerebellar ataxia: olivoponto-cerebral atrophy
Myelopathy	Friedreich's
	Congenital
	Diastematomyelia
	Dysraphism
	Spastic
Familial spastic paraplegia	
Anterior horn cell	Spinal muscular atrophies
	Werdnig Hoffmann I
	Werdnig Hoffmann II
	Wohlfahrt-Kugelberg-Welander III
Peripheral nerve	Roussy-Levy
	Charcot-Marie-Tooth I, II
	Dejerine-Sottas
	Sciatic toxic neuropathy
Myoneural junction	Myasthenia
Muscle	Myositis
	Viral
	Collagen
	Vascular
	Muscular dystrophy
	Duchenne
	Becker
	Myopathy
	Glycogenosis
	Acid maltase deficiency
	Myotonic dystrophy
Joint	Clubfoot
	Hemophilia
	Short tendo calcaneus
	Idiopathic pes cavus and claw toes

This table was developed as a teaching outline for students and is not necessarily complete, but it does illustrate well the multitude of neuromuscular conditions that must be considered in evaluating a child who is a toe walker (Fig. 23-32). A careful physical examination, neurologic examination, and family history will usually exclude the majority of these disorders. The most common cause of toe walking in the toddler and young child is persistence of the normal infantile gait patterns, a temporary condition for which no intervention is necessary. Heel cord lengthening should be considered only after a prolonged period of observation to demonstrate that the condition is not going to improve spontaneously, and only after a thorough evaluation identifies, if possible, the primary cause. There are generalized neuromuscular conditions in which either the prognosis or the pattern of muscle weakness and mechanics of gait make heel cord lengthening unwise.

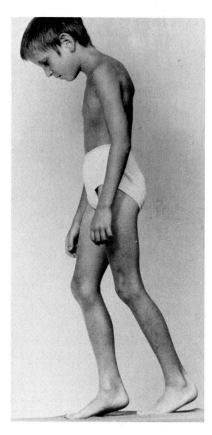

Fig. 23-32. This child developed toe walking, tight hamstrings, and a crouched gait. He was found to have a tethered spinal cord. This abnormal gait pattern resolved after surgical release.

AFFECTIONS OF THE HAND

In planning initial treatment and subsequent referral of hand problems, primary care physicians should keep in mind that because of the complexity of managing hand problems, an entire surgical subspecialty—hand surgery—has been developed in recent decades. Many general surgeons, plastic surgeons, and orthopedic surgeons will have adequate training and experience to manage some common hand problems, but complex nerve and tendon surgery or reconstruction of major congenital anomalies should not be undertaken by the average surgical practitioner. Because injuries to the hand occur so frequently, the primary care physician must have an appreciation of normal hand anatomy and function as well as common pathologic conditions so that the nature of any injury or underlying disease can be identified. An excellent introductory monograph has been prepared by the American Society for Surgery of the Hand[65] and is highly recommended for anyone dealing with extremity problems on a regular basis. It reviews the standard terminology for the structures of the hand as well as the basic anatomy, which is integral to the examination of the extremity.

Evaluation. The entire upper extremity must be examined as part of any hand examination. The usual cutaneous evaluation for swelling, edema, localized pain, tenderness, or warmth is performed. Individual anatomic structures must be tested, or significant injuries will be missed. The simple ability of the patient to make a fist and open the hand does not guarantee that major neurovascular structures or tendons have not been involved in an injury or disease process. Particularly with an uncooperative child, inspection of the hand posture at rest may reveal many clues to underlying injury without any physical manipulation.

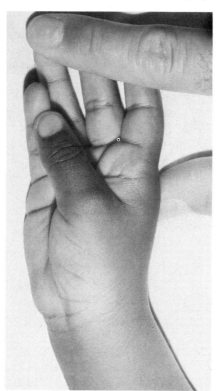

Fig. 23-33. During opposition the thumb is elevated, abducted, and rotated so that the pulp of the thumb approximates the pulp of the little finger.

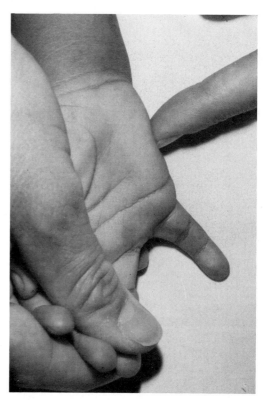

Fig. 23-34. The muscles of the hypothenar eminence are innervated by the ulnar nerve and can be tested by abduction of the fingers. Palpation of the muscle belly during the tested motion is an important part of the individual muscle examination.

It is most important for the primary care physician to recognize the potential seriousness of seemingly minor injuries and lesions of the hand and fingers. If he deals with such problems frequently, he should familiarize himself with hand anatomy and function; if he deals with them infrequently, he should readily avail himself of a competent consultant. Above all, he must maintain an attitude of suspicion toward every hand and finger injury, seeking assurance in each situation that no unrecognized injury is present. A missed lesion may result in severe loss of function that could have been avoided with early recognition and skilled therapy.

Innervation. The major cutaneous innervation of the hand is divided among three nerves. The median nerve enters the forearm proximally in the midline; it then travels from the volar surface of the forearm, passing through the carpal tunnel beneath the transverse flexor retinaculum, into the

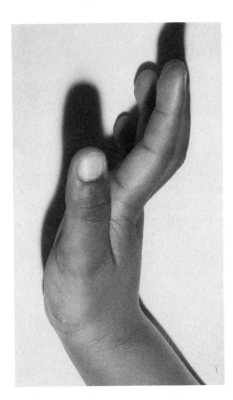

Fig. 23-35. The extrinsic extensors of the wrist and fingers are innervated by the radial nerve. The proximal interphalangeal (PIP) joints can be extended by the intrinsic muscles of the hand, and the extensor digitorum communis is tested by extension of the metacarpophalangeal joint.

hand, supplying the sensation on the volar aspect of the thumb, index, and long fingers as well as on half of the ring finger.

The dorsum of the distal portion of the same digits is also innervated by the median nerve. The ulnar nerve supplies the remainder of the volar surface of the hand as well as the dorsum of the lateral 1½ fingers through a separate dorsal branch. The radial side of the dorsum of the hand is supplied by the radial nerve through the superficial radial branch.

Sensation must be tested with care and, again, this evaluation may be difficult in an uncooperative child.[94] However, sweating and wrinkling of the skin after immersion in water are sympathetically innervated functions that do not require cooperation to evaluate. A dry area may therefore be an important diagnostic clue to an underlying nerve injury that can be confirmed by a formal "sweat test."[121] If the nerve injury has been present for any length of time, the fingerprint pattern may be lost. To test for wrinkling, the child's hand is immersed in water for a long-enough period of time to develop wrinkling.[122] Those areas that do not exhibit this phenomenon can be considered denervated.

Motor function. Motor function in the hand is provided by the intrinsic muscles—the small muscles about the hypothenar and thenar eminences as well as the interosseous and lumbrical muscles in the region of the palm—and the extrinsic muscles, whose muscle bellies lie in the forearm and whose innervation is proximal. The intrinsic muscles of the thenar eminence are primarily innervated by the median nerve, and a crude measure of median nerve function is thumb opposition (Fig. 23-33). The thumb should be elevated, abducted, and rotated so that the pulps of the fingers approximate and the nails are parallel. The thenar muscles must be palpated to be certain they are contracting and should be compared carefully with those of the opposite hand. Since the hand is a flexible and adaptable organ, other muscles can be substituted to accomplish apparent opposition. The ulnar innervated muscles are those of the midhand and hypothenar eminence, and these can be tested by having the child spread the fingers and bring them forcefully together (Fig. 23-34).

Some tests of hand functions are illustrated in Figs. 23-35, 23-36, and 23-37.

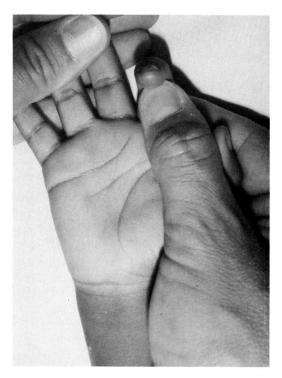

Fig. 23-36. The flexor digitorum profundus flexes the distal interphalangeal joint.

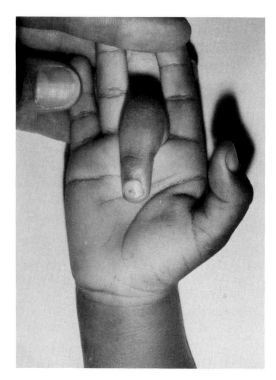

Fig. 23-37. The test for the flexor digitorum superficialis.

Trauma
Lacerations

One of the most important aspects of managing a laceration of the hand is to recognize whether or not a significant underlying structure has been injured (Fig. 23-38). The nerves, tendons, and blood vessels of the hand are all surprisingly close to the skin and may be involved in even the most insignificant-appearing injury.

Although the hand has an excellent blood supply and lacerations may bleed profusely, almost invariably the bleeding can be controlled with compression alone. Great care should be exercised in attempting to clamp bleeding vessels in the hand because there is danger of injuring an otherwise uninvolved vital structure. Since almost all lacerations of the hand will close satisfactorily by secondary intent or can be closed in the delayed primary manner, lacerations of the hand should be carefully debrided, irrigated, and dressed open unless one is certain of the cleanliness of the wound.

Radiograms of the hand are an important diagnostic adjunct, but remember that many common foreign bodies, such as glass and wood, may not be radiopaque. If a foreign body is suspected, how-ever, the radiographs are mandatory. Xeroradiograms may help.

Fractures and dislocations

Fractures and dislocations of the hand are little different from similar injuries that occur in other long bones. Injuries to the growth centers of the small bones of the hand can result in the same sorts of disabilities that occur when comparable structures are injured more proximally in the extremity.

Fractures of the hand are often underimmobilized. It is almost never satisfactory to immobilize a single finger. Even for minor injuries, the digit should be strapped to adjacent fingers to help prevent the development of malrotation, which will not remodel, even in a young child. One can use the plane of the fingernails as a guide for estimating normal rotation of the fingers, and comparison with the opposite extremity is helpful (Fig. 23-39). When a fracture is close to the joint, such as at the base of the proximal phalanx, the degree of angulation may not be appreciated because of the position of the other fingers on the x-ray film and because one of the fragments may be so short that one does not recognize the actual

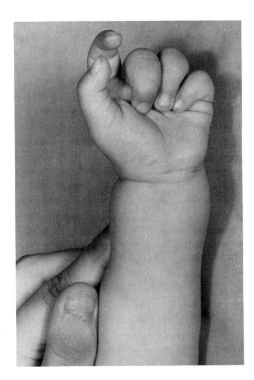

Fig. 23-38. The index finger remains extended when the remaining digits are flexed. This child had a laceration of the flexor digitorum superficialis.

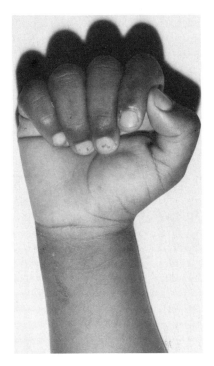

Fig. 23-39. The plane of the fingernails is a useful guide for estimating normal rotation of the fingers.

degree of angulation.[54] Unrecognized angulation may result in permanent interference with the delicate mechanical balance of the flexor and extensor mechanisms of the finger.

Another common error is failure to recognize that small avulsion chips seen on an x-ray film at the lateral border of the metaphysis may represent an avulsion of the collateral ligament. A chip at the base of the distal phalanx may signal an avulsion of the extensor mechanism—a mallet finger. When the fleck of bone is at the base of the volar side of the middle phalanx, it may represent a disruption of the volar plate, a strong fibrocartilaginous component of the proximal interphalangeal (PIP) joint. When the volar plate is disrupted, subluxation of the middle phalanx in relation to the proximal phalanx may occur and lead to significant long-term disability from posttraumatic arthrosis.

A fracture that involves the growth center of a bone must be reduced anatomically in order for normal growth and development to occur.[92] If the articular surface is disrupted, anatomic reduction accomplished by open surgical procedures may be necessary. Dislocations are common, and care must be exercised in their management; what ap-

pears to be a dislocation may in fact be an epiphyseal fracture. In a "complex dislocation," the volar fibrocartilaginous structures of the joint are entrapped within the joint and thereby prevent reduction. One clue will be dimpling of the skin, the dimple occurring in the thenar eminence of the thumb or at the level of the volar flexion crease in the other fingers. Radiographically, there may be significant widening of the joint space, which will suggest the interposed soft tissues. Sesamoid bones of the thumb become ossified after the age of 10 years and may be visible within the joint on radiographic evaluation. Complex dislocations require surgical reduction.

Fingertip injuries[39]

Subungual hematomas account for the severe pressure and pain that occur with the common crushing injuries of the fingertips. This pain can be relieved dramatically if the finger is treated early, before the blood begins to clot. Although the hematoma can be decompressed by drilling a hole in the nail overlying the blood with a sharp instrument or one of the commercially available drills that are designed for fingernails, burning a hole in the nail with a paper clip that has been heated over an alcohol lamp is probably just as effective; at any rate, the immediate relief of pain that comes with drilling or burning one or more holes into the hematoma can be dramatic. If a major laceration of the nail bed has occurred, it probably should be repaired in order to prevent late nail deformity. The question of whether or not to leave a loosened and obviously damaged nail in place often arises. An intact nail, even one that is going to be lost in the future, may well serve as a very satisfactory splint for any underlying soft tissue or bony injuries and will protect the extremely sensitive nail bed during the initial healing phase. If the nail is severely loosened or there is a question of infection, it can be discarded and the finger dressed until a new nail grows.

Amputation of the fingertip is a not uncommon sequel to a variety of sharp or crushing injuries. Even significant skin loss, however, will dramatically heal in time with simple dressing changes and soaking after initial cleansing and debridement of the wound. It is remarkable how much apparent deficit will fill in with epithelialization and contraction of the wound. On the other hand, a more significant amputation may require skin grafting. The tip of the finger should be saved, since it may serve either as a composite graft or as a source for split skin.

Replantation of severed digits or limbs

Recent advances in microsurgery have made replantation of severed digits (or even whole limbs) possible. Such procedures are regularly performed in several centers throughout the United States. The results of replantation in children are not quite as good as they are in adults—a fact that is not completely understood. Nevertheless, microsurgeons have managed such a high level of success that replantation should be considered whenever a part is amputated and retrievable. Since time is critical in such procedures, immediate referral and even air lift transportation to a center may be necessary to ensure the possible success of replantation. No attempts should be made to identify, cannulate, or manipulate the vessels in either the amputated part or the remaining stump. The amputated part should immediately be wrapped in moist sterile gauze and placed in Ringer's lactate solution. It is then cooled on ice and transported with the patient. The part should not come in direct contact with the ice, since freezing

may actually do further damage to the amputated tissues.[158]

Infection[29,41]

Infection in the hand can convert an innocuous laceration into a catastrophe. Infection in the hand presents with the same cardinal signs of inflammation seen in any portion of the body: redness, swelling, warmth, pain, and loss of function. A diffuse cellulitic process may be managed by elevation, soaks, or antibiotics; an abscess, on the other hand, requires drainage.

Paronychia

The most common infection in the hand, a paronychia, occurs in the soft tissues about the bed of the fingernail, usually the result of a staphylococcal infection in a "hangnail". Paronychias occur in children who pick at their nails or bite them; these often begin on one side of the nail and spread about the base of the nail in a horseshoe manner. Systemic antibiotics are rarely necessary, since a paronychia should respond to such local measures as drainage of the purulent material followed by soaks. Fig. 23-40 demonstrates the site of localization of a paronychia.

Drainage of the accumulation of pus can be accomplished by placing the tip of a No. 20 needle over the nail and beneath the epinychial soft tissue. If there is extreme pain, a local block of the finger will suffice for anesthesia. The common practice of making a radial incision at the base of the nail will drain the abscess, but only at the ex-

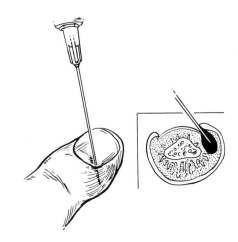

Fig. 23-40. Site of a paronychial infection and a simple method of drainage.

pense of making an incision through otherwise normal overlying tissues and is rarely necessary.

Felon

A felon is most commonly a staphylococcal abscess of the pulp space of the distal phalanx of the finger. It is caused by pressure, which results from constraint by radial fibrous bands existing in the finger pulp. A single lateral, hockey stick–type incision that divides the fibrous septi is often all that is required for drainage. Wide filleting of the finger in a fish mouth manner is not necessary. A neglected felon may proceed to osteomyelitis of the distal phalanx.

Tenosynovitis

Tenosynovitis involves the synovial sheaths of the flexor tendons of the fingers and may spread along this sheath proximally into the palm. Unlike a felon, tenosynovitis causes no well-localized changes in the pulp tip; rather, there is diffuse longitudinal swelling. The finger is held in a flexed attitude and is tender to palpation along the course of the flexor tendon; there is pain on extension of the digit. Untreated infection of the tendon sheath may result in significant long-term disability. If the diagnosis is uncertain, a period of 12 to 24 hours of observation is reasonable, during which time the hand is elevated in a compressive dressing and intravenous antibiotics are administered. However, surgical drainage should be instituted as soon as the diagnosis is confirmed and should always be performed in an operating room by a qualified hand surgeon.

Human bite infection

Most commonly, human bite infections occur after a tooth strikes a knuckle in a fight; but, obviously, they can also result from intentional bites. They often involve a joint, and the virulence of the aerobic and anaerobic flora of the mouth make them dangerous injuries with significant long-term morbidity. Human bite injuries often require hospital admission and surgical debridement in addition to appropriate antibiotic therapy and tetanus prophylaxis.

Tumors

Almost any bony or soft tissue tumor may present within the hand. Primary malignancies are rare but do occur and must always be considered. The most common bony tumor is an enchondroma;

this may occur either as an isolated lesion or as part of a syndrome of multiple enchondromas (Ollier's disease), which may be associated with multiple hemangiomas (Maffuci's syndrome).

The most common mass in the hand is a *ganglion cyst,* a well-defined round or ovoid mass that most commonly develops about the wrist but may present in a variety of locations. If the lesion appears cystic, is not pulsatile, does not have a bruit, transilluminates, and is not fixed to underlying structures, the diagnosis of a ganglion cyst is most reasonable. Occasionally, ganglions may develop within the deep structures of the hand and may present as a nerve compression syndrome with no palpable mass. One should be certain that the lesion is not attached to the underlying structures, since such other benign tumors as "giant cell tumors of the tendon sheath" and so-called fibro-histiocytoma are also common.

Treatment. Unless the cyst is compressing adjacent structures, the symptoms are usually mild and treatment is elective. Puncture alone will result in resolution of anywhere from 15% to 30% of all ganglion cysts.[119] Occasionally, injection of steroid material in and about the cyst mass is utilized. One should take care in injecting steroids in the subcutaneous region in black individuals: atrophy and hypopigmentation of the skin may produce an unsightly cosmetic defect that cannot be reversed. If the symptoms warrant it, and if the patient so desires, surgical excision can be accomplished. Tourniquet control, careful operating technique, and fine instruments should be utilized to avoid injury to an adjacent blood vessel, nerve, or tendon; but this does not preclude the use of local or regional block anesthesia and an ambulatory setting. Recurrence in anywhere from 10% to 20% of surgical cases and injury to adjacent structures are indirectly proportional to the skill and experience of the surgeon. The more careful and complete the dissection, the more likely it is that the lesion will not recur. Postoperative care and the period of recuperation should be limited.

COMMON DISEASES OF THE HIP JOINT

The diseases of the developing hip joint necessitate prompt diagnosis and early management so that disastrous complications can be obviated with successful treatment in the majority of cases. The most common entities include toxic synovitis of childhood, Legg-Calvé-Perthes disease, septic arthritis, and slipped capital femoral epiphysis.

A review of the examination of the hip is worthwhile here. After a careful history and a complete medical examination, the child should be undressed and observed while standing and walking. Any antalgic components of gait should be noted. Distinction should be made between pain and motor weakness about the hip joint. Inspection of the back, with the feet together, will help in establishing the presence of pelvic obliquity, spinal curvature, or leg length inequality.

The range of motion of both hips in flexion, extension, abduction, adduction, internal rotation, and external rotation is charted with the child supine on the examining table and any pain with motion noted. Simultaneous evaluation of both hips will detect subtle asymmetry in range of motion. A complete motor examination of both lower extremities is necessary. Thigh or calf atrophy can be detected with a tape measure and is often helpful in establishing the chronicity of a disease process. Both knees are examined for effusion, motion, and instability. In a similar fashion, the ankle joints, subtalar joints, and forefoot joints are examined. The involvement of other joints narrows the differential diagnosis of a hip lesion.

The initial laboratory evaluation might include a sedimentation rate, complete blood count, and urinalysis, as well as x-ray films: an AP and frog leg lateral view of the pelvis to include both hips and a true lateral view of the involved hip.

Transient synovitis

One of the more common causes of limping in a usually male child between the ages of 3 and 6 years is transient (toxic) synovitis, which may develop following an upper respiratory tract infection, trauma, or even an allergic episode.[81] A specific cause is yet to be determined.

Clinical presentation. The presenting complaint is an antalgic gait. Hip motion is limited in internal and external rotation, and abduction and a flexion contracture may be noted. A slight elevation in temperature may be found.

Evaluation. Laboratory examinations, including a white blood cell count and sedimentation rate, are normal. X-ray films of the pelvis may reveal evidence of an effusion with lateral displacement of the femoral head in the acetabulum. Bone changes are not present.

Differential diagnosis. The differential diagnosis includes juvenile rheumatoid arthritis, Legg-Calvé-Perthes disease, rheumatic fever, tubercu-

losis, and septic arthritis. Arthrocentesis of the hip joint is indicated, and all joint fluid studies will be normal except for a mild to moderate elevation of joint fluid white blood cell content, which makes the fluid appear turbid.

Treatment. Initial bedrest for relief of weight bearing is followed by progressive crutch ambulation as tolerated. Traction helps reduce pain and restore motion and should be continued for 2 to 3 days. Range of motion exercises may then begin; when motion is equal to the opposite hip and is painless, weight bearing may be allowed. A course of anti-inflammatory agents (salicylates) supplements the above.

Prognosis. Whether transient synovitis may lead to or be the prodrome of Legg-Calvé-Perthes disease is still conjectural.[147] Normally, one expects prompt and complete resolution of toxic synovitis with no lasting effects or disability. Repeated episodes do occur, but they are separated in time, and the symptoms should resolve each time in a few days or at most a few weeks. Any episode that lasts longer than 4 to 6 weeks is *not* transient synovitis, and another cause should be sought. Pauciarticular juvenile rheumatoid arthritis or the adolescent variation of ankylosing spondylitis may be the diagnosis in older children who do not have transient synovitis.

Legg-Calvé-Perthes disease

Legg-Calvé-Perthes disease occurs in approximately 1 out of 750 boys and 1 out of 3,700 girls (5:1) between the ages of 3 and 12 years, with the peak incidence being at about age 6 years. The disease occurs bilaterally in 10% to 15% of affected children and is rare in blacks.[37] A genetic predisposition is probable, but specific heritable factors have never been elucidated. Prenatal factors do not appear to play a significant role in the genesis of the disease. Bone age is retarded in 80% to 90% of affected children. Predisposing factors are previous nonspecific synovitis or trauma. In 25% of cases there is a history of trauma,[135] which is more frequent in boys, who historically have been more active than girls in contact sports and rough physical activity. The incrimination of synovitis is more tentative, but 6% to 10% of patients with "toxic synovitis of childhood" will progress into characteristic Legg-Calvé-Perthes disease.[147]

The clinical features are deceptively benign, and it is not uncommon for the child to have intermittent complaints for several months before medical attention is sought. A limp without pain is typical. If there is pain, it may be in the groin but is often localized to the thigh or knee. Physical abnormalities may vary, but the more common signs include an antalgic gait, a shortened extremity, limitation of internal rotation and abduction on the affected side, and atrophy of the thigh or calf. The child is afebrile, and the laboratory evaluation is within normal limits.

Legg-Calvé-Perthes is a self-limited disease of the secondary center of ossification of the proximal femur. The cause of this avascularity or hypovascularity of the capital femoral epiphysis is unknown. The living bony cells die, leaving intact the bony trabeculae composed of nonliving organic matrix, which is then reabsorbed and replaced by new, live bone.

The death and replacement process is classified radiographically and pathologically into four clinically indistinguishable stages.[145] The incipient, or initial, phase may occur weeks to months before the onset of symptoms. Radiographs characteristically demonstrate increased density of the femoral head and an occasional widening of the medial joint space, which produces an apparent lateral displacement of the femoral head. Small radiolucent metaphyseal defects or cysts may be seen. Pathologically, there is edema and hyperemia of the synovial membrane and capsule with excessive joint fluid and early abnormalities in the process of enchondral ossification as well as cartilage cell necrosis in the deeper zones of the epiphysis.

The second, or fragmentation, stage takes place during the 6 to 18 months that follow the onset of symptoms. Radiographs will reveal compression and fragmentation of the femoral head, usually in the anterolateral aspect of the epiphysis. Small bony islands will appear, representing osteolysis.

During this phase, vascular granulation tissue is invading the epiphysis. Dead bone is being removed while new precursor osteoid material is being deposited (creeping substitution). There is significant loss of structural stability during this phase, which, with diffuse, severe involvement, will result in fracture and collapse and permanent morphologic distortion.

The third stage, which usually occurs 1 to 3 years after the onset of the disease, is characterized by regeneration of bony tissue (Fig. 23-41). The deformity of the femoral head becomes apparent in this phase.

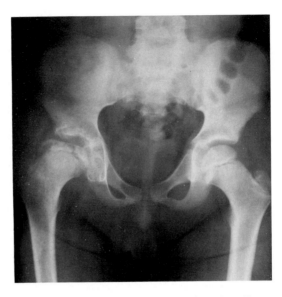

Fig. 23-41. Third stage of Legg-Calvé-Perthes disease. This stage occurs 1 to 3 years after the onset of the disease and is characterized by regeneration of bony tissue.

The final stage is often termed the healing and residual stage and evolves 2 to 5 years after the onset of symptoms. Any irregularity and deformity that have occurred during fragmentation and regeneration persist and may progress. Resulting deformities may include widening or flattening of the femoral head and widening of the femoral neck (Fig. 23-42). Concomitant dysplasia of the acetabulum may result.

Because Legg-Calvé-Perthes disease evolves over such a long period of time, identifying some indicator of eventual outcome has been the goal of many investigators. One of the more generally accepted prognostic classifications is that of Catterall.[27] Four groups, each describing a progressive radiographic involvement, are recognized. In group I only the anterior part of the epiphysis is affected, and no collapse is evident on x-ray films. Metaphyseal changes are minimal. Regeneration of the involved portion eventually ensues. In group II more of the anterior portion of the femoral head is involved, and sequestration is common. There is no collapse of the head, but cystic metaphyseal changes are more predominant. In group III nearly the entire proximal femoral epiphysis is sequestrated. The characteristic finding is a "head within the head," demonstrated by two distinctive areas within the epiphysis of different bony density. The head collapses, and there is often broadening of the femoral neck and generalized and extensive

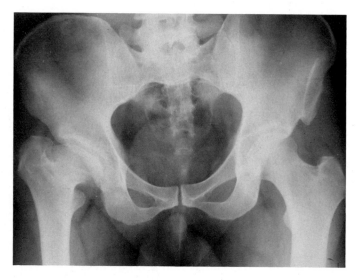

Fig. 23-42. Poor result several years after the onset of Legg-Calvé-Perthes disease. There is shortening and widening of the femoral neck, overgrowth of the greater trochanter, and flattening and enlargement of the femoral head.

metaphyseal changes. In group IV displacement of the epiphysis is common both anteriorly and posteriorly, total collapse of the epiphysis ensues, and metaphyseal changes are diffuse.

In group I over 95% of the patients studied had good results regardless of treatment. In each case with less than good results, the child was 8 years or older at the onset of the disease. In group II all patients 4 years of age or younger had good results without treatment or with nonoperative treatment, but 30% had only fair or poor results with or without treatment. In group III 70% to 90% of the patients had fair to poor results whether they were untreated or treated nonoperatively. Approximately 90% of the patients in group IV had fair or poor results. Age did not seem to be a factor in these groups.

Catterall has described an additional series of four radiographic signs that indicate a "head at risk." If these are found in any of the above-mentioned groups, the prognosis is less favorable. Basically, these signs describe significant alteration in the position of the femoral head from its normal position within the acetabulum. The potential for femoral head malformation is significantly increased and with it the possibility of degenerative joint disease in later years. If onset occurs at age 4 years or younger, the chances for a good result are extremely high. Girls tend to have worse results than boys.

One major difficulty with Catterall's classification is that it takes approximatley 6 months of observation before the final grade of involvement can be determined. For this reason, several other systems have been devised.[60]

Treatment. No uniformity of opinion exists regarding the treatment of Legg-Calvé-Perthes disease;[51,52,149] thus, there appears to be no clearly superior method. Nonsurgical methods range from bedrest and traction for early synovitis with loss of range of motion, to close observation to orthotic containment. Containment involves maintaining the femoral head reduced within the acetabulum in order to allow reciprocal spherical modeling and is the constant in most treatment protocols. Depending on the stage of femoral head involvement as well as the age of the child, containment can be affected nonsurgically by a weight-bearing brace or surgically by pelvic osteotomy or subtrochanteric femoral osteotomy (Fig. 23-43).

Many authors believe with Catterall that the age of onset is a major determinant of the ultimate results of Legg-Calvé-Perthes disease.[27,145] Others have reported some bad results even in the young patient. Close observation without active treatment is justified in patients under the age of 6 years whose disease remains limited in extent, but radiographic reevaluation should be performed at least every 3 months. Active treatment is indicated for all patients in the age group over 6 years and for

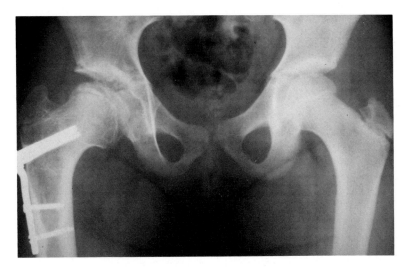

Fig. 23-43. One method of surgical containment is subtrochanteric varus derotation osteotomy of the proximal femur.

those of any age demonstrating full-head involvement or subluxation of the femoral head. Abduction bracing is also necessary in younger children who fail to maintain an adequate, painless range of motion despite 1 or 2 weeks of bed rest and traction. If there is any question about the severity of involvement, the safest course is to begin orthotic treatment; then, if after 6 months there has been no progression beyond stage I or II, the brace may be discontinued. Regardless of age or radiographic stage of involvement, bed rest, salicylates, and traction are appropriate for synovitis. A full, painless range of motion is the goal for all forms of treatment.

The treatment period ranges from 9 to 18 months.[62] Bracing is discontinued when radiography demonstrates regeneration of the femoral head.

Although subluxation of the femoral head is the major indication for surgery, an age of onset greater than 6 years, total head involvement (such as in Catterall's groups III and IV), the presence of the "head at risk" signs, and the inability to cooperate with abduction bracing are also considerations. Pelvic osteotomy affects containment by rotation of the acetabulum over the femoral head.[136] Coverage of the femoral head can be obtained just as easily with a femoral as with a pelvic osteotomy,[114] but a disadvantage is the shortening of the limb that results from femoral surgery. In certain unique instances, as in the older child with a complex problem, a combination of both procedures may be employed. Postoperatively, the child is placed in a spica cast for 6 weeks and is then begun on range of motion exercises and full weight bearing.

Pyarthrosis

The subject of pyarthrosis is dealt with earlier in this chapter, but a few of the admonitions regarding pyarthrosis or septic arthritis of the hip joint are worth repeating. Unlike the knee joint, where the capsule is attached to the epiphyseal portion of the bone, the metaphysis of the hip is intra-articular.

The continued buildup of bacteria and white blood cells in the joint fluid results in increased pressure and inhibition of normal vascular flow to the capital femoral epiphysis. In the short term, acute dislocation of the hip may result. As an intermediate response, avascular necrosis of the femoral head may appear; eventually, degenerative arthritis may ensue.

A white blood cell count of 50,000 to 100,000/ml^3 in the joint fluid is consistent with bacterial infection; the joint fluid in juvenile rheumatoid arthritis may be quite turbid, however, and the white blood cell count may exceed 50,000/ml^3. There is no time to await final culture results; it is far preferable to drain an occasional rheumatoid hip than to delay while the articular cartilage suffers under the influence of pus, bacteria, and their by-products.

There is no place for purely medical management of pyarthrosis of the hip. Incision and drainage must accompany antibiotics and immobilization.

Slipped capital femoral epiphysis

While a slipped capital femoral epiphysis may present below the age of 12 years, the peak incidence is in the adolescent and teenage years. The reader is referred to Chapter 28 in the section on the teenager for further discussion.

SPINAL DEFORMITIES

Classification. The spinal deformities of childhood are classified into three groups: scoliosis, lordosis, and kyphosis. Scoliosis refers to lateral curvature of the spine, lordosis (swayback) refers to a curvature in the sagittal plane directed anteriorly, and kyphosis (hunchback) refers to another curvature in the sagittal plane directed posteriorly. A normal lordosis occurs in the lumbar spine with a curve measuring between 30 and 50 degrees, and the thoracic spine has a normal kyphosis of 20 to 40 degrees. Pathologic curves may occur alone or in combination.

A scoliotic deformity can be considered either structural or nonstructural. The nonstructural curve is usually secondary to a postural problem, pain, pelvic obliquity, or leg length discrepancy; with resolution of the offending problem, the curve will normally resolve. Structural curves will not fully correct; they lack flexibility. Multiple subgroups of structural scoliosis exist. The idiopathic forms are characteristically grouped according to age. The infantile type occurs prior to the age of 3 years, the juvenile group is diagnosed between the ages of 3 and 10 years, and the adolescent group is noted between the age of 10 years and skeletal maturity.

Neuromuscular spinal curvature is classified into either neuropathic or myopathic subgroups. Neuropathic lesions include cerebral palsy, syringomyelia, poliomyelitis, and spinal muscular atrophy. The myopathic group includes such diseases as arthrogryposis or muscular dystrophy.

Scoliosis may be congenital, the result of vertebral body malformation. Scoliosis may also be seen in neurofibromatosis, rickets, and spinal tumors and after infection, trauma, or one of the osteochondrodystrophies.

Kyphosis may be secondary to many of the same processes that cause scoliosis. One of the more common types of kyphosis is Scheuermann's, an idiopathic condition defined as a roundback deformity with 5 degrees or more of wedging of at least three adjacent vertebrae at the apex of the curve.

Lordosis may result from a hip flexion contracture, as in arthrogryposis or cerebral palsy, but may also be postural or congenital.

Evaluation. The history of a young patient with a spinal deformity should include the age of onset or the time the spinal deformity was discovered and how it was determined that a deformity was present. It is also important to document the progression of the curve. The medical records should be obtained, as well as any previous spinal radiographs, and specific questions about previous treatment should be asked. Associated symptoms should be documented. Is there back pain or a radicular component? Idiopathic scoliosis is *not* painful. Are other systems involved? Has the child noted any weakness of an upper or lower extremity or bladder or bowel dysfunction? Did the child meet all the motor and mental milestones? Answers to these questions will help determine if neurologic compromise is present. It is worthwhile to inquire into the age of menarche in the girl or the onset of pubarche and voice change in the boy. These changes mark the beginning of the adolescent growth spurt and are helpful in planning specific treatment modalities.

Previous thoracotomy or radiation therapy predispose the patient to scoliosis,[142] and there is a definite increase in scoliosis in children with congenital heart disease.[11] The causative feature in thoracogenic scoliosis may be pleural scarring, and the curve always has its apex toward the contralateral side. Radiation-induced scoliosis is particularly common after treatment for Wilms' tumor.[131] Laminectomy when performed in the growing child often leads to progressive kyphosis.[96]

An in-depth family history is taken, with special attention given to spinal deformities. A general physical examination is performed with the child unclothed, and particular attention is paid to findings that may suggest a cause for the spinal deformity.

The skin is carefully examined for café au lait spots or skin lesions consistent with neurofibromatosis. One of the cardinal skeletal manifestations of neurofibromatosis is scoliosis. Hairy patches or dimples in the back may indicate underlying spinal dysraphism. The trunk and lower extremities should be carefully inspected for the presence of surgical scars. Secondary sex characteristics are recorded, including breast development and pubic hair development in the girl, or genital development and hair distribution in the boy. Obvious deformity of one extremity in comparison with the other is noted, as well as symmetry or asymmetry on the right and left. Tooth decay may well be a nidus of infection, with possible hematogenous spread to a vertebral body. A high-arched palate is found in Marfan's syndrome and in other syndromes. Scoliosis is often associated with Marfan's syndrome, and finding dilatation of the aortic root or mitral prolapse may help make the diagnosis. A thorough cardiac exam will indicate the presence or absence of cardiac abnormalities or arrhythmias.

The neurologic examination should be performed with great care. A spinal curvature may, in itself, compromise neurologic function, but usually only in severe cases. Congenital scoliosis is associated with a high incidence of diastematomyelia.[169] The first symptom of a spinal cord tumor may be scoliosis.

During the orthopedic examination for spinal curvature, a forward-bending test should be performed by having the child bend forward at the waist, leaving the arms dependent and free (Fig. 23-44). The patient is viewed from the back and the front. In this position the presence of a cervical, thoracic, or lumbar curve can be determined. Simple visualization is often all that is necessary. In the more obese patient, however, palpation of the spine is mandatory. A rib hump or paralumbar hump is almost always present to some degree in the more significant curves and is the result of vertebral body rotation, one of the cardinal features of structural scoliosis. The ribs are more prominent anteriorly on the side opposite the rib hump; the breast on this side will appear larger.

A plumb line is used to measure compensation or decompensation of the trunk as related to the fixed pelvis (Fig. 23-45). The plumb line is placed

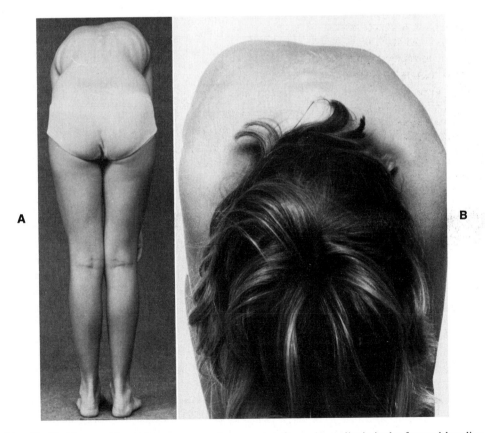

Fig. 23-44. The most important maneuver in screening for early scoliosis is the forward-bending test. The patient is viewed from both the back (**A**) and the front (**B**). A rib hump is usually visible before one can detect spinal deformity.

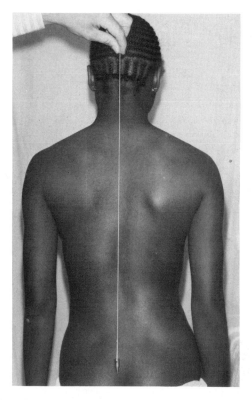

Fig. 23-45. Compensation is measured by dropping a plumb line from the occiput to the gluteal fold. Any deviation to the right or left is measured and recorded. Note, as well, the asymmetry of the waistline and the differing distances of the elbows from the trunk. This 16-year-old girl had thoracolumbar scoliosis and mild asymmetry of the shoulder.

proximally at the level of the seventh cervical spinous process and is allowed to hang free. Any deviation to the right or left of the midline immediately over the gluteal fold is measured and recorded. If a cervical curve is suspected, the measurement should be initiated from the occiput.

With the child standing and the feet together, the level of one shoulder is compared with that of the other. The higher shoulder will correspond to the convex side of the curve. The pelvis can be measured at this time for asymmetry or limb length inequality. The child is viewed from behind, the examining physician's hands are placed over the iliac crest, and any difference in height is recorded. If asymmetry is present, the exact difference may be measured by having the child stand on measured blocks.

The range of motion of all upper and lower extremity joints is recorded. Flexion contracture of the hip might explain hyperlordosis. The patient with tight hamstrings might have a spondylolisthesis. By this time one should have an excellent mental picture of any curve that is present.

Initial radiographic assessment. Radiographs will confirm the clinical impression and allow exact measurements. The initial radiographic assessment of the patient with a spinal deformity should include a standing AP and lateral view of the entire spine from occiput to sacrum. Further x-ray films at this point are probably not necessary, because referral to an experienced scoliosis center, where additional special views will be obtained, is recommended. Once a deformity is documented, referral to a physician experienced in the treatment of scoliosis is always indicated.

Scoliosis
Nonstructural scoliosis

Nonstructural scoliosis refers to a flexible curve that corrects on side bending toward the convex apical portion of the curve and is not associated with rotation of the vertebrae. Some common causes of nonstructural scoliosis are postural abnormalities, leg length discrepancy, hysteria, and inflammation.

The curve of *postural scoliosis* is quite long and may extend from the high thoracic region to the lower limits of the lumbar spine. There is no associated rib hump or elevation of one scapula. Correction of the curve is obvious when the child is prone, or when he is asked to stand with both feet together, both knees and hips in full extension, and both shoulders level. The diagnosis is confirmed by a standing AP x-ray film of the entire spine. Treatment consists of instruction on the proper postural attitudes and corrective exercises. These curves will not progress or become structural.

Leg length discrepancy likewise produces a nonstructural and nonprogressive curve involving both the thoracic and lumbar spine with the convex side directed toward the side of the short lower extremity. An appropriate-length shoe lift will correct the deformity.

Hysterical scoliosis is characteristically seen in an emotionally disturbed teenager. Although examination is often difficult because of the abnormal body contortions of the affected child, the curve will correct in the recumbent position and there is no associated rotation. Confirmatory x-ray films should be obtained with the child standing and recumbent. Emphasis is placed on psychiatric treatment rather than orthopedic care.

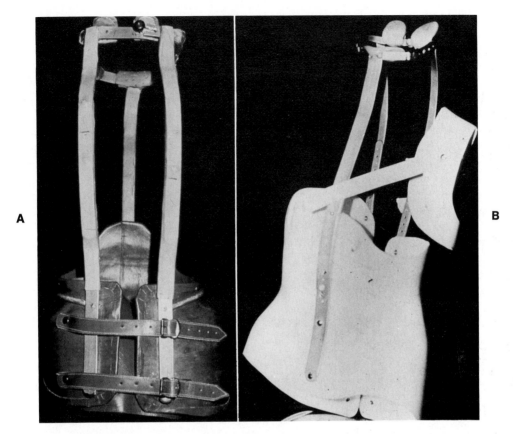

Fig. 23-46. A, One of the original Milwaukee braces, with a leather pelvic girdle and steel superstructure. Today, a variety of plastic molds are available for the pelvic girdle. Superstructures may be added to the pelvic module **(B).**

Nonstructural scoliosis secondary to inflammatory processes is less common. Typical sources include an intra-abdominal abscess, a ruptured appendix, or possibly irritation of a nerve root secondary to a herniated nucleus pulposus. Most often these flexible and nonprogressive curves are diagnosed incidentally during evaluation of the underlying disease. The curve will resolve without orthopedic intervention after treatment of the inflammatory process.

Structural scoliosis

The classification of structural scoliosis proposed by the Scoliosis Research Society includes no less than 14 major subclassifications with numerous individual causes within each major group. Only the more common entities are discussed here.

Idiopathic scoliosis represents the most common form of structural scoliosis. Three separate types according to age are recognized. Recent research has established a genetic predisposition, but the exact method of transmission has not been de-

fined.[171] Some investigators propose sex-linked transmission, whereas others believe that idiopathic scoliosis is an autosomal dominant trait or is multifactorial in origin. Overall, approximately 80% to 90% of all patients with scoliosis can be classified into the following three subgroups of idiopathic scoliosis.

Infantile scoliosis is a form of idiopathic scoliosis identified in the child from birth to the age of 3 years. It is rarely diagnosed in the United States; the majority of the work in this area is found in the European literature.[82] Infantile scoliosis occurs more often in boys than in girls and more commonly in the first year of life. Although the vast majority resolve spontaneously, the physician must determine whether this curve is progressive, static, or resolving. Some help can be obtained from specific measurements taken on a standing AP x-ray film of the spine.[105]

Curves greater than 30 to 40 degrees or those felt to be progressing should be treated by early bracing. Even a child less than 1 year of age can be fitted with a brace, although fitting an infant may require anesthesia. Except for short periods of bathing, the brace is worn around the clock, and treatment may be required for many years. If progression is noted within the brace, application of a body cast should be contemplated. Surgical intervention is necessary only when curves progress beyond 60 degrees despite conservative treatment.[77]

Juvenile idiopathic scoliosis is defined as idiopathic scoliosis occurring between the age of 4 years and the onset of puberty. The sex distribution is more even than in infantile scoliosis, and the average age at diagnosis is 6 years. Unlike the infantile curves, progression is the rule rather than the exception with the juvenile curve. Treatment consists of close follow-up alone for curves less than 20 degrees. Children with deformities greater than 20 degrees and those who have demonstrated progression are candidates for bracing[17] (Figs. 23-46 and 23-47).

Spinal fusion is indicated for all curves that are progressive despite attempts at conservative treatment and for curves greater than 50 to 60 degrees. Since spinal fusion is not encouraged in the young child because of cessation of growth of the spine and loss of trunk height, bracing may be continued even in a progressive curve until it reaches 60 degrees, after which the loss in stature from the curve will be greater than that from spinal fusion.[167]

Adolescent idiopathic scoliosis is a spinal curvature diagnosed between the age of puberty and skeletal maturity (Fig. 23-48). Obviously, there may be situations in which a juvenile or infantile curve will persist into adolescence. Girls are affected more than boys in a ratio greater than 2 to 1. The adolescent growth spurt is often a factor in the progression of the curves.

The specific treatment for structural scoliosis, orthotic or surgical, depends on the nature of the curve. Exercise alone is *never* adequate therapy for structural scoliosis. A general guideline is that

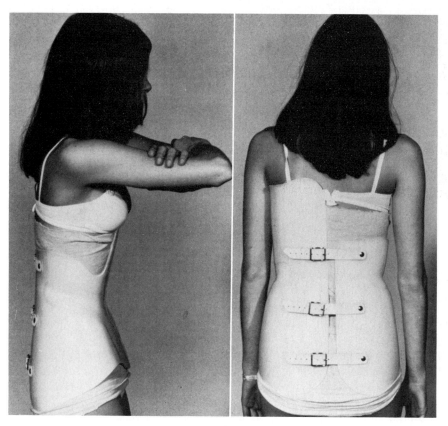

Fig. 23-47. In recent years, underarm orthoses have been devised that are effective in controlling some curves. One such device is pictured here. These braces are effective only in curvatures with an apex below T-8.

curves below 20 degrees do not require treatment unless they are thought to be progressive. Bracing is generally employed for curves between 20 and 40 degrees.[106] Spinal fusion, with or without Harrington rod instrumentation, is often required for progressive curves beyond 40 to 50 degrees.

It must be emphasized to both the patient and the parents that the objective of bracing is to stabilize and maintain the curve at its present level, not to correct the curve.[112] Generally, treatment initiated after the onset of puberty will be effective in maintaining the curve at the same degree that it was before treatment was started. True "correction" is achieved only when mild curves are treated in rather young patients.

Once bracing is started, the patient must wear the orthosis for 23 to 24 hours a day. Once skeletal maturity is complete, as demonstrated radiographically by such features as apophyseal fusion of the iliac crest and fusion of the ring epiphyses of the vertebral bodies, the child is weaned from the brace. The weaning must proceed slowly; the child should still be wearing the brace at night for some time after weaning is initiated.

A logical question that is commonly posed by parents is, "What will happen if the curve is allowed to progress?" Another is, "What is the natural history of the scoliotic curve in the untreated child?" Basically, curves below 60 degrees do not progress greatly after maturity and are not associated with significant cardiopulmonary compromise. However, if the curve progresses beyond 60 degrees, rotational deformities increase, as well as narrowing in the anteroposterior plane, resulting in decreased total lung volume and compression of the heart.[7] Decreased vital capacity, disturbed ventilation-profusion ratios, elevated $Paco_2$, atelectasis, emphysema, and cardiac failure have all been reported.

Some studies have addressed the subject of long-term follow-up of adults with untreated idiopathic scoliosis. In one study[28] the mortality was twice

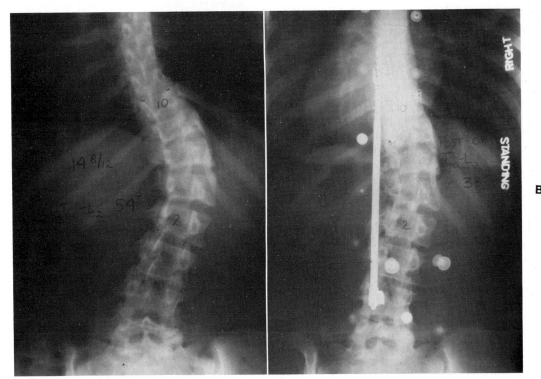

Fig. 23-48. Preoperative and postoperative x-ray films in idiopathic scoliosis. **A,** This curve was progressive, and the child had almost reached skeletal maturity (note the excursion of the iliac epiphyses). Because of her age, she was not a candidate for a brace program. **B,** A single Harrington distraction rod was selected to provide stabilization while the autogenous iliac crest bone graft was maturing. Complete correction of the curve is rarely achieved. The goal of surgery for scoliosis is stabilization and prevention of progression.

that of the normal population. Spinal deformities significantly compromised the activities of daily living. A significant number of these individuals had backaches, and over one fourth of them were disabled. Few, if any, were engaged in heavy labor. Other studies are not as pessimistic, but most authors would agree that severe scoliosis has significant social, emotional, and physical morbidity. Patients must be informed that spinal curvature and deformity are not necessarily arrested with cessation of skeletal growth. In fact, a significant number of patients with scoliosis will have progression of their curves during the adult years.

Kyphosis

Kyphosis is defined as a change in alignment in the sagittal plane that increases the posterior convex angulation. The thoracic spine has a normal kyphosis of 20 to 40 degrees.

Scheuermann's disease

One of the more common causes of increased thoracic kyphosis is juvenile kyphosis, or Scheuermann's disease. This is to be distinguished from the nonstructural entity called postural roundback, in which radiographs are normal. In Scheuermann's kyphosis, the child is unable to reverse the kyphosis voluntarily and radiographic examination demonstrates 5 degrees or more of vertebral body wedging in at least three of the apical vertebrae.[146] Schmorl's nodes and end-plate irregularity are seen (Fig. 23-49). The cause of Scheuermann's kyphosis is unknown.

Regardless of the cause, kyphosis may be the most malignant of spinal deformities and causes a significant risk of neurologic damage. Early diagnosis and experienced treatment are essential to avoid progression to a life-threatening deformity. Scheuermann's kyphosis has been documented in successive family generations, but there are many instances with a negative family history. Girls are affected more often than boys (2:1), and the diagnosis is usually made between the ages of 11 and 15.

The typical clinical complaint is slouching of the shoulder or roundback deformity associated with back pain. However, the deformity may be asymptomatic.

Physical examination reveals an increase in thoracic kyphosis with an associated hyperlordosis of the lumbosacral spine that is not fixed and cor-

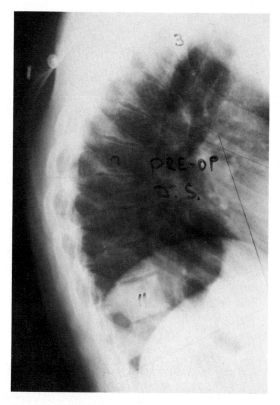

Fig. 23-49. Scheuermann's kyphosis is defined by the presence of at least three apical vertebrae with wedging of 5 degrees or more. Schmorl's nodes and vertebral end-plate irregularity are common.

rects on forward bending. (Thoracic kyphosis will not correct with posterior bending.) A mild degree of scoliosis is not uncommon in the thoracic spine. The neurologic examination is normal. Percussible tenderness may be elicited, especially over the apex of the kyphosis. Paravertebral muscle spasm may or may not be present.

The Milwaukee brace is particularly effective in Scheuermann's kyphosis.[20] Exercise should accompany the brace treatment but should never be instituted as a sole mode of treatment. Initially, the brace is worn for 23 hours each day. After 1 year and after maximum correction is obtained, weaning from the brace is attempted. For curves with severe wedging and structural abnormalities, immobilization must be continued until the completion of skeletal growth. Brace therapy for Scheuermann's kyphosis can be instituted at a much later age than is usually considered for idiopathic scoliosis, and definite clinical improvement can be obtained even during the late teen years. Surgical intervention is indicated only if chronic

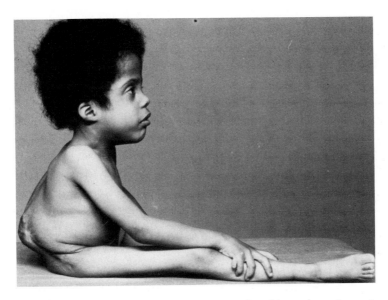

Fig. 23-50. Severe collapsing kyphosis in a child with myelomeningocele.

pain persists, the kyphosis exceeds 60 degrees, or neurologic compromise is present.[19]

Other types of kyphosis

Kyphosis can result from congenital malformations (Fig. 23-50) or follow laminectomy or spinal irradiation. Kyphosis may also occur following spinal trauma or as a manifestation of skeletal dysplasia.

Gravity would exaggerate the normal thoracic kyphosis if it were not for the compensatory forces of the posterior ligaments. If these ligaments are disrupted, relative weakness ensues that allows the anterior forces to predominate. This is essentially what occurs in the young child who has had posterior spinal surgery for a neoplasm or other pathologic process. Close follow-up is required by the orthopedist to document any changes in spinal morphology.[96]

More often than not, postlaminectomy spinal deformities are progressive and refractory to brace treatment. Brace treatment may still be instituted initially to impede progression and allow as much time as possible for spinal growth, but this therapy requires the guidance of the scoliosis specialist to ensure that the kyphosis does not progress significantly. Most patients require fusion. Anterior interbody fusion is indicated for the more severe curves, whereas posterior fusion may be employed for curves of lesser deformity.

POSTIRRADIATION KYPHOSIS

Wilms' tumor and neuroblastoma are the most common reasons for irradiation. Postirradiation kyphosis may be seen as an isolated entity or in association with scoliosis. The curve is caused by growth disturbance of the vertebral body endplate as well as by scarring and contracture of the spinal ligamentous complex. These children must routinely be referred for evaluation and follow-up until skeletal maturation decreases the likelihood of deformity.

Postirradiation kyphosis is treated with a combination of bracing and spinal fusion. The usual indication for fusion is a curve greater than 50 to 60 degrees.[131]

Lordosis

Lordosis is normally present in both the cervical and the lumbar spine. Normal lordotic curves range between 40 and 60 degrees. The Scoliosis Research Society recognizes several different types of lordosis: postural, congenital, neuromuscular, postlaminectomy, and that secondary to flexion contracture. Postural lordosis is nonstructural in nature and reversible at will (Fig. 23-51). Weakness of the abdominal musculature may be a causative factor. Congenital lordosis may be seen as an isolated entity or, more commonly, in association with scoliosis. Similarly, lordosis secondary to such neuromuscular disorders as cerebral

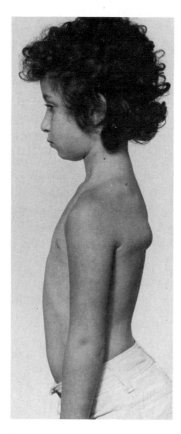

Fig. 23-51. Typical postural lordosis.

palsy, polio, spinal muscular atrophy, or myelomeningocele is commonly seen in association with scoliosis. As with progressive kyphosis in the thoracic spine resulting from a radical laminectomy, hyperlordosis may be seen after laminectomy in the lumbar spine or after the placement of a lumbo-peritoneal shunt. Flexion contractures of the hips produce hyperlordosis as a compensatory mechanism. Lordosis as a primary pathologic process is rarely encountered.[113]

Treatment is required only for progressive deformity or as a combined therapy for scoliosis. Postural hyperlordosis should respond to appropriate physical therapy. Emphasis is placed on pelvic tilt, strengthening of the abdominal musculature, and maintenance of a proper posture. Bracing is rarely indicated, but a ''low profile'' brace that forces a pelvic tilt can effectively reduce nonstructural lordosis. Surgery, either with instrumentation and/or fusion, is indicated for progressive deformity, cosmesis, and persistent pain.

If it is not treated, hyperlordosis may progress to compromise ambulation, may lead to a chronic low back syndrome, or may even alter the cardiopulmonary status of the patient by inducing compensatory thoracic kyphosis.

REFERENCES

1. Adams, J. B., and Fowler, P. D.: Wringer injuries of the upper extremity, South. Med. J. **52:**798, 1959.
2. Allen, B. L., Jr.: Segmental instrumentation for difficult spine deformities, Orthop. Trans. **3:**43, 1979.
3. Allen, B. L., and Lehmann, T. R.: Pelvic displacement osteotomy in young myelodysplastic patients with dislocated hips, South. Med. J. **171**(1):13, 1978.
4. Anderson, M. T., Green, W. T., and Messner, M. D.: Growth and predictions of growth in the lower extremities, J. Bone Joint. Surg. **45A:**1, 1963.
5. Arnold, N. D.: Pseudotumor of hemophilia, Prog. Pediatr. Hematol. Oncol. **1:**99, 1976.
6. Arnold, N. D., and Hilgartner, M. W.: Hemophilic arthropathy, J. Bone Joint Surg. **59A:**287, 1977.
7. Bake, B., and others: Regional pulmonary ventilation and perfusion distribution in patients with untreated idiopathic scoliosis, Thorax **27:**703, 1972.
8. Barden, G. A., Meyer, L. C., and Stelling, F. F., III: Myelodysplasia: fate of those followed for 20 years or more, J. Bone Joint Surg. **57A:**643, 1975.
9. Bassett, F. H., III, and Baker, L. D.: Equinus deformity in cerebral palsy. In Adams, J. P., editor: Current practice in orthopaedic surgery, St. Louis, 1966, The C. V. Mosby Co.
10. Bassett, F. H., III, and Goldner, L.: Fractures involving the distal femoral epiphyseal growth line, South. Med. J. **55:**545, 1962.
11. Beals, R. V., Kenney, K. H., and Lees, M. H.: Congenital heart disease and idiopathic scoliosis, Clin. Orthop. **89:**112, 1972.
12. Bell, J. S., and Thompson, W. A. L.: Modified spot scanography, A. J. R. **63:**915, 1950.
13. Bleck, E. E.: Hip deformities in cerebral palsy. In American Academy of Orthopaedic Surgeons: Instructional Course Lectures, vol. 20, St. Louis, 1971, The C. V. Mosby Co., p. 54.
14. Bleck, E. E.: Locomotor prognosis in cerebral palsy, Dev. Med. Child Neurol. **17:**18, 1975.
15. Bleck, E. E.: Orthopaedic management of cerebral palsy, Philadelphia, 1979, W. B. Saunders Co.
16. Bloch, E.: Personal communication, 1979.
17. Blount, W. P., and Moe, J. H.: The Milwaukee brace, Baltimore, 1973, The Williams & Wilkins Co.
18. Bonnett, C., and others: The evolution of treatment of paralytic scoliosis at Rancho Los Amigos Hospital, J. Bone Joint Surg. **57A:**206, 1975.
19. Bradford, D. S.: Scheuermann's kyphosis: results of surgical treatment by posterior spine arthrodesis in twenty-two patients, J. Bone Joint Surg. **57A:**439, 1975.
20. Bradford, D. S., and others: Scheuermann's kyphosis and roundback deformity, results of Milwaukee brace treatment, J. Bone Joint Surg. **56A:**749, 1974.
21. Brahms, M. A.: Common foot problems, J. Bone Joint Surg. **49A:**1653, 1967.
22. Brewerton, D. A., Sandifer, P. H., and Sweetmon, D. R.: ''Idiopathic'' pes cavus: an investigation of its etiology, Br. Med. J. **5358:**659, 1963.

23. Bright, R. W.: Surgical correction of partial epiphyseal plate closure in dogs by bone bridge resection and use of silicone rubber implants, J. Bone Joint Surg. **56A:**655, 1974.

24. Bryan, R. S., Lipscomb, P. R., and Chatterton, C. C.: Orthopedic aspect of congenital hypertrophy, Am. J. Surg. **96:**654, 1958.

25. Bryant, T.: The practice of surgery, vol. 2, London, 1876, J. & A. Churchill.

26. Cameron, J. M., and Rae, L. J.: Atlas of the battered child syndrome, London, 1975, Churchill Livingstone.

27. Catterall, A.: The natural history of Perthes disease, J. Bone Joint Surg. **53B:**37, 1971.

28. Collis, D. R., and Pouseti, I. V.: Long-term follow-up of patients with idiopathic scoliosis not treated surgically, J. Bone Joint Surg. **51A:**425, 1969.

29. Crandon, J. H.: Lesser infections of the hand. In Flynn, J. E., editor: Hand surgery, ed. 2, Baltimore, 1975, The Williams & Wilkins Co.

30. Crawford, A. H.: Neurofibromatosis in the pediatric patient, Orthop. Clin. North Am. **9**(1):11, 1978.

31. Crego, C. H., and Ford, L. T.: An end-result study of various operative procedures for correcting flatfeet in children, J. Bone Joint Surg. **34A:**183, 1952.

32. Denhoff, E., and Langdon, M.: Cerebral dysfunction: a treatment program for young children, Clin. Pediatr. **5:**332, 1966.

33. Dick, V. Q., Nelson, J. D., and Halatin, K. C.: Osteomyelitis in infants and children: a review of 163 cases, Am. J. Dis. Child. **129:**1273, 1975.

34. DuVries, H. L.: Disorders of skin and toenails. In Surgery of the foot, ed. 3, St. Louis, 1973, The C. V. Mosby Co.

35. Evans, E. B.: The knee in cerebral palsy. In Samilson, R., editor: Orthopaedic aspects of cerebral palsy, Philadelphia, 1975, J. B. Lippincott Co.

36. Feiwell, E., Sakai, D., and Blatt, T.: The effect of hip reduction on function in patients with myelomeningocele, J. Bone Joint Surg. **60A:**169, 1978.

37. Fisher, R. L.: An epidemiological study of Legg-Perthes disease, J. Bone Joint Surg. **54A:**769, 1972.

38. Fisk, J., Winter, R. B., and Moe, J. H.: Scoliosis, spondylosis and spondylolisthesis: their relationship as reviewed in 539 patients, Spine **3**(3):234, 1978.

39. Flatt, A. E.: The care of minor hand injuries, ed. 4, St. Louis, 1979, The C. V. Mosby Co.

40. Flynn, J. C., Matthews, J. G., and Benoit, R. L.: Blind pinning of displaced supracondylar fractures of the humerus in children, J. Bone Joint Surg. **56A:**263, 1974.

41. Flynn, J. E.: The grave infections of the hand. In Flynn, J. E., editor: Hand surgery, ed. 2, Baltimore, 1975, The Williams & Wilkins Co.

42. Fost, N. C., and Esterly, N. B.: Successful treatment of juvenile hemangiomas with prednisone, J. Pediatr. **72:**351, 1968.

43. Fries, I. B.: Growth following epiphyseal arrest, Clin. Orthop. **114:**315, 1976.

44. Gil, D.: Physical abuse of children: findings and implications of a nationwide survey, Pediatrics **44:**857, 1969.

45. Gilday, D. L., and others: Diagnosis of osteomyelitis in children by combined blood pool and bone imaging (radioactive bone scanning), Radiology **117:**331, 1975.

46. Goldner, J. L.: Volkmann's contracture, J. Bone Joint Surg. **37A:**621, 1958.

47. Goldner, J. L.: Upper extremity tendon transfers in cerebral palsy, Orthop. Clin. North Am. **5**(2):343, 1974.

48. Goldner, J. L.: Volkmann's ischemic contracture. In Flynn, J. E., editor: Hand surgery, Baltimore, 1975, The Williams & Wilkins Co.

49. Goldner, J. L., and Ferlic, D. C.: Sensory status of the hand as related to reconstructive surgery of the upper extremity in cerebral palsy, Clin. Orthop. **46:**87, 1966.

50. Goldner, J. L., Ruderman, R. J., and Somers, W.: Congenital equinovarus deformity in myelodysplasia, Z. Kinderchir., December 1980.

51. Gossling, H. R.: Legg-Perthes disease: analysis of poor results. In American Academy of Orthopaedic Surgeons: Instructional Course Lectures, vol. 22, St. Louis, 1973, The C. V. Mosby Co., p. 301.

52. Gossling, H. R.: Legg-Perthes disease: treatment by recumbency. In American Academy of Orthopaedic Surgeons: Instructional Course Lectures, vol. 22, St. Louis, 1973, The C. V. Mosby Co., p. 296.

53. Gowers, W. F.: Pseudohypertrophic muscular paralysis, London, 1879, J. & A. Churchill.

54. Green, D. P.: Hand injuries in children, Ped. Clin. North Am. **24**(4):903, 1977.

55. Green, D. P., and Terry, G. C.: Complex dislocation of the metacarpophalangeal joint: corrective pathological anatomy, J. Bone Joint Surg. **55A:**1480, 1973.

56. Green, W. T., Wyatt, G. M., and Anderson, M.: Orthoroentgenography as a method of measuring the bones of the lower extremities, J. Bone Joint Surg. **28:**60, 1946.

57. Greulich, W. W., and Pyle, S. I.: Radiographic atlas of skeletal development of the hand and wrist, ed. 2, Stanford, Calif., 1959, Stanford University Press.

58. Grice, D. S.: Extra-articular arthrodesis of the subastragalar joint for correction of paralytic flatfeet in children, J. Bone Joint Surg. **34A:**927, 1952.

59. Griffin, P. P., Anderson, M. A., and Green, W. T., Sr.: Fractures of the shaft of the femur in children, Orthop. Clin. North Am. **3:**213, 1972.

60. Griffin, P. P., Green, N. E., and Beauchamp, R. D.: Legg-Calvé-Perthes Disease: treatment and prognosis, Orthop. Clin. North Am. **11**(1):127, 1980.

61. Griffin, P. O., and Green, W. T., Sr.: Hip joint infections in infants and children, Orthop. Clin. North Am. **9**(1):123, 1978.

62. Gunther, S. F., and Gossling, H. R.: Legg-Perthes disease: treatment by aduction ambulation. In American Academy of Orthopaedic Surgeons: Instructional Course Lectures, vol. 22, St. Louis, 1973, The C. V. Mosby Co., p. 305.

63. Gutman, L. T., and others: H. influenza type B septic arthritis diagnosed by counterimmunoelectrophoresis; unpublished data, 1980.

64. Haas, L. M., and Staple, T. W.: Arterial injuries associated with fractures of the proximal tibia following blunt trauma, South. Med. J. **62:**1439, 1969.

65. The hand: examination and diagnosis, Aurora, Col., 1978, American Society for Surgery of the Hand.

66. Hardacre, J. A., and others: Fractures of the lateral condyle of the humerus in children, J. Bone Joint Surg. **53A:**1083, 1971.

67. Hardy, J. H.: Spinal deformity in neurological and muscular disorders, St. Louis, 1974, The C. V. Mosby Co.

68. Harrelson, J. M.: Infections and neoplasms of bone. In Sabiston, D. C., editor: Davis-Christopher textbook of surgery, ed. 11, Philadelphia, 1977, W. B. Saunders Co.

69. Harrington, P. R.: Treatment of scoliosis correction and internal fixation by spine instrumentation, J. Bone Joint Surg. **44A:**591, 1962.

70. Harris, R. I.: Retrospect: peroneal spastic flatfoot (rigid valgus foot), J. Bone Joint Surg. **47A:**1657, 1965.

71. Helfet, A.: A new way of treating flatfeet in children, Lancet **1:**260, 1956.

72. Herpe, L. B. V.: Fractures of the forearm and wrist, Orthop. Clin. North Am. **7**(3):543, 1976.

73. Hilgartner, M. W.: Hemophilic arthropathy, Adv. Pediatr. **21:**139, 1974.

74. Hilgartner, M. W., and McMillan, C. W.: Coagulation disorders. In Miller, D. R., and Pearson, H. A., editors: Smith's blood diseases of infancy and childhood, ed. 4, St. Louis, 1978, The C. V. Mosby Co.

75. Hodgson, A. R., Skinsnes, O. K., and Leong, C. Y.: The pathogenesis of Pott's paraplegia, J. Bone Joint Surg. **49A:**1147, 1967.

76. Hoke, M.: An operation for the correction of extremely relaxed flatfeet, J. Bone Joint Surg. **13:**773, 1931.

77. Hopper, W. C, and Lovell, W. W.: Progressive infantile idiopathic scoliosis, Clin. Orthop. **126:**26, 1977.

78. Hubbard, D. D.: Injuries of the spine in children and adolescents, Clin. Orthop. **100:**56, 1974.

79. Hunt, J. C., and Pugh, D. C.: Skeletal lesions in neurofibromatosis, Radiology **76:**1, 1961.

80. Irani, R. N., Nicholson, J. T., and Chung, S. M. K.: Treatment of femoral fractures in children by immediate spica immobilization, J. Bone Joint Surg. **52A:**1567, 1972.

81. Jacobs, B. N.: Synovitis of the hip in children and its significance, Pediatrics **47:**558, 1971.

82. James, J. I. P., Lloyd-Roberts, G. C., and Pilcher, M. F.: Infantile structural scoliosis, J. Bone Joint Surg. **41B:**719, 1959.

83. Jones, J. M., and Musgrave, J. E.: Effect of arteriovenous fistula on growth of bone, preliminary report, Proc. Mayo Clin. **24:**405, 1949.

84. Kahn, D. S., and Pritzker, K. P. H.: The pathophysiology of bone infection, Clin. Orthop. **96:**12, 1973.

85. Kawamura, B.: Limb lengthening, Orthop. Clin. North Am. **9**(1):155, 1978.

86. Keats, S.: Operative orthopaedics in cerebral palsy, Springfield, 1970, Charles C Thomas, Publisher.

87. Kempe, C. H., and Helfer, R. E.: Helping the battered child and his family, Philadelphia, 1972, J. B. Lippincott Co.

88. Klassen, R.: Pelvic fractures in children; presented at the Pediatric Orthopaedic Study Group, Montreal, May 1980.

89. Korhonen, B. J.: Fractures in myelodysplasia, Clin. Orthop. **79:**145, 1971.

90. Lam, S. F.: Treatment of fractures of the neck of the femur in children, Orthop. Clin. North Am. **7**(3):625, 1976.

91. Langenskjiold, A.: The possibilities of eliminating premature partial closure of an epiphyseal plate caused by trauma or disease, Acta Orthop. Scand. **38:**267, 1967.

92. Leonard, M. H., and Dubravcik, K. P.: Management of fractured fingers in the child, Clin. Orthop. **73:**160, 1970.

93. Limbird, T. J., and Ruderman, R. J.: Fat embolism in children, Clin. Orthop. **136:**267, 1978.

94. Lister, G.: The hand: diagnosis and indications, Edinburgh, 1977, Churchill Livingstone.

95. Lonstein, J. E.: Screening for spinal deformities in Minnesota schools, Clin. Orthop. **126:**43, 1977.

96. Lonstein, J. E., and others: Post laminectomy spine deformity, J. Bone Joint Surg. **58A:**727, 1976.

97. Lovell, W. W., Price, C. T., and Meehan, P. L.: The foot. In Lovell, W. W., and Winter, R. B., editors: Pediatric orthopaedics, Philadelphia, 1978, J. B. Lippincott Co.

98. Luke, M. D., and McDonnell, E. J.: Congenital heart disease and scoliosis, J. Pediatr. **73:**725, 1968.

99. MacEwen, G. D., Hardy, J. H., and Winter, R. B.: Evaluation of kidney anomalies in congenital scoliosis, J. Bone Joint Surg. **54A:**1451, 1972.

100. Mann, T. S.: Prognosis in supracondylar fractures, J. Bone Joint Surg. **45B:**516, 1963.

101. McElvenny, R. T.: Corns: their etiology and treatment, Am. J. Surg. **50:**761, 1940.

102. McGraw, M. B.: Neuromuscular development of the human infant as exemplified in the achievement of erect locomotion, J. Pediatr. **17:**747, 1940.

103. McGuire, T., and others: Osteomyelitis caused by B-hemolytic streptococcus Group B, J.A.M.A. **238**(19):1054, 1977.

104. McKusick, V. A.: The Ehlers-Danlos syndrome. In Heritable disorders of connective tissue, ed. 4, 1972, The C. V. Mosby Co.

105. Mehta, M. H.: The rib-vertebral angle in the early diagnosis between resolving and progressive infantile scoliosis, J. Bone Joint Surg. **54B:**230, 1972.

106. Mellencamp, D. D., Blount, W. P., and Anderson, A. J.: Milwaukee brace treatment of idiopathic scoliosis: late results, Clin. Orthop. **126:**47, 1977.

107. Menelaus, M. B.: Orthopaedic management of children with myelomeningocele: a plea for realistic goals, Dev. Med. Child Neurol. (Suppl.) **37:**3, 1976.

108. Merten, D. B., Kirks, D. R., and Ruderman, R. J.: Occult humeral epiphyseal fracture in battered infants, Pediatr. Radiol. **10:**151, 1981.

109. Meyers, M. H., and McKeever, F. M.: Fracture of the intercondylar eminence of the tibia, J. Bone Joint. Surg. **41A:**214, 1959.

110. Miller, H. H., and Welch, C. S.: Quantitative studies on the time factor in arterial injuries, Ann. Surg. **130:**428, 1949.

111. Miller, O. L.: A plastic flatfoot operation, J. Bone Joint Surg. **9:**84, 1927.

112. Moe, J. H., and Kettleson, D. N.: Analysis of curve pattern and preliminary results of Milwaukee brace treatment in 169 patients, J. Bone Joint Surg. **52A:**1509, 1970.

113. Moe, J. H., and others: Scoliosis and other spinal deformities, Philadelphia, 1978, W. B. Saunders Co.

114. Mose, K.: Legg-Calvé-Perthes disease: a comparison between three methods of conservative treatment, Oslo, Norway, 1964, Universitetsforlaget.

115. Moseley, C. F.: A straight-line graph for leg length discrepancies, J. Bone Joint Surg. **59A:**174, 1977.

116. Mubarak, S. J., and others: Acute compartment syndromes: diagnosis and treatment with the aid of the wick catheter, J. Bone Joint Surg. **60A:**1091, 1978.

117. Nasca, R. J., Stelling, F. H., and Steel, H. H.: Progression of congenital scoliosis due to hemivertebrae and hemivertebrae with bars, J. Bone Joint Surg. **57A:**456, 1975.

118. Neer, C. S., and Horwitz, B. S.: Fractures of the proximal humeral epiphysial plate, Clin. Orthop. **41:**24, 1965.

119. Nelson, C. L., Sawmiller, S., and Phalen, G. S.: Ganglions of the wrist and hand, J. Bone Joint Surg. **54A:**1459, 1972.

120. North Carolina Juvenile Code G.S. 7A-277 through G.S. 7A-289.

121. Omer, G. E., and Spinner, M.: Management of peripheral nerve problems, Philadelphia, 1980, W. B. Saunders Co.

122. O'Riain, S.: New and simple test of nerve function in the hand, Br. Med. J. **3:**615, 1973.

123. Orr, H. W.: Osteomyelitis and compound fractures, St. Louis, 1929, The C. V. Mosby Co.

124. Pennsylvania Orthopaedic Society: Traumatic dislocations of the hip in children, J. Bone Joint Surg. **50A:**79, 1968.

125. Perry, J., and others: Electromyography before and after surgery for hip deformity in children with cerebral palsy: a comparison of clinical and electromyographic findings, J. Bone Joint Surg. **58A:**201, 1976.

126. Ponseti, I. V., and Friedman, B.: Prognosis in idiopathic scoliosis, J. Bone Joint Surg. **32A:**381, 1950.

127. Qualls, D. M., Wolman, I. J., and Nicholson, J.: Management of musculoskeletal lesions in the hemophilia child, J. Bone Joint Surg. **41A:**1540, 1959.

128. Rang, M.: Children's fractures, Philadelphia, 1974, J. B. Lippincott Co.

129. Raycroft, J. F., and Curtis, B. H.: Spinal curvature in myelomeningocele: natural history and etiology; presented at the American Academy of Orthopaedic Surgeons Symposium on Myelomeningocele, St. Louis, 1972.

130. Reidy, J. A., and Van Gordon, G. W.: Treatment of displacement of the proximal radial epiphysis, J. Bone Joint Surg. **45A:**1355, 1963.

131. Riseborough, E. J., and others: Skeletal alterations following irradiation for Wilms' tumor, J. Bone Joint Surg. **58A:**526, 1976.

132. Robins, P. R., Moe, J. H., and Winter, R. B.: Scoliosis in Marfan's syndrome: its characteristics and results of treatment in 35 patients, J. Bone Joint Surg. **57A:**358, 1975.

133. Rosenfeld, A. A., and Newberger, E. H.: Compassion versus control: conceptual and practical pitfalls in the broadened definition of child abuse, J.A.M.A. **237**(19):2086, 1977.

134. Rowe, C. R., Pierce, D. S., and Clark, J. G.: Voluntary dislocation of the shoulder, J. Bone Joint Surg. **55A:**445, 1973.

135. Salter, R. B.: Experimental and clinical aspects of Perthes disease, J. Bone Joint Surg. **48B:**393, 1966.

136. Salter, R. B.: Legg-Perthes disease: treatment by innominate osteotomy. In American Academy of Orthopaedic Surgeons: Instructional Course Lectures, vol. 22, St. Louis, 1973, The C. V. Mosby Co., p. 309.

137. Salter, R. B., and Best, T.: The pathogenesis and prevention of valgus deformity following fractures of the proximal metaphyseal regions of the tibia in children, J. Bone Joint Surg. **55A:**1324, 1973.

138. Salter, R. B., and Harris, W. R.: Injuries involving the epiphyseal plate, J. Bone Joint Surg. **45A:**587, 1963.

139. Salter, R. B., and Zaltz, C.: Anatomic investigations of the mechanism of injury and pathologic anatomy of "pulled elbow" in children, Clin. Orthop. **77:**134, 1971.

140. Samilson, R. L.: Orthopaedic aspects of cerebral palsy, Philadelphia, 1975, Spastics International Medical Publications, J. B. Lippincott Co.

141. Schmid, F. R.: Principles of diagnosis and treatment of infectious arthritis. In Hollander, J. L., editor: Arthritis and allied conditions, Philadelphia, 1972, Lea & Febiger.

142. Scoles, P.: Scoliosis after thoracotomy, presented at the Pediatric Orthopaedic Study Group, Montreal, May 1980.

143. Scott, J. C.: Scoliosis and neurofibromatosis, J. Bone Joint Surg. **47B:**240, 1965.

144. Solomons, G.: Child abuse and developmental disabilities, Dev. Med. Child Neurol. **21:**101, 1979.

145. Somerville, E. W.: Perthes disease of the hip, J. Bone Joint Surg. **53B:**639, 1971.

146. Sorenson, K. H.: Scheuermann's juvenile kyphosis, Copenhagen, 1964, Munksgaard, International Booksellers & Publishers, Ltd.

147. Spock, A.: Transient synovitis of the hip joint in children, Pediatrics **24:**1042, 1959.

148. Statham, L., and Murray, M. P.: Early walking patterns of normal children, Clin. Orthop. **79:**8, 1971.

149. Stulberg, A. D.: Legg-Perthes disease: update, Proceedings of the Sixth Open Scientific Meeting of the Hip Society, 1978, p. 263.

150. Sutherland, D. H., and others: The development of mature gait, J. Bone Joint Surg. **62A:**336, 1980.

151. Tachdjian, M. O.: Pediatric orthopaedics, Philadelphia, 1972, W. B. Saunders Co.

152. Terminology Committee, Scoliosis Research Society: A glossary of scoliosis terms, Spine **1:**57, 1976.

153. Tetzlaff, T. R., and others: Antibiotic concentrations in pus and bone of children with osteomyelitis, J. Pediatr. **92:**135, 1978.

154. Thompson, S. A., and Mahoney, L. J.: Volkmann's ischemic contracture: relationship to fracture of the femur, J. Bone Joint Surg. **33B:**336, 1951.

155. Trveta, J.: The normal vascular anatomy at the femoral head, J. Bone Joint Surg. **39B:**358, 1947.

156. Trveta, J.: The three types of acute hematogenous osteomyelitis, J. Bone Joint Surg. **41B:**671, 1959.

157. Tupman, G. S.: Treatment of inequality of the lower limbs: the results of operations for stimulation of growth, J. Bone Joint Surg. **42B:**489, 1960.

158. Urbaniak, J. R.: Digit and hand replantation: current status, Neurosurgery **4**(9):51, 1979.

159. Vesely, D. G., and Mears, T. M.: Surgically induced arteriovenous fistula: its effect upon inequality of leg length, South. Med. J. **57:**129, 1964,

160. Wagner, H.: Operative beinverlarger-ung, Der. Chirurg. **42:**260, 1971.

161. Waldvogel, F. A., Medoff, G., and Swartz, M. N.: Osteomyelitis, Springfield, 1971, Charles C Thomas, Publisher.

162. Wall, J. J.: Acute hematogenous pyarthrosis caused by *Hemophilus influenzae,* J. Bone Joint Surg. **50A:**1657, 1968.

163. Wetzenstein, H.: The significance of congenital pes calcaneovalgus in the origin of pes plano-valgus in childhood, Acta Orthop. Scand. **30:**64, 1960.

164. Whitesides, T. E., and others: Tissue pressure measurements as a determinant for the need of fasciotomy, Clin. Orthop. **113:**43, 1975.

165. Wilensky, A. O.: Osteomyelitis: its pathogenesis, symptomatology and treatment, New York, 1934, MacMillan Publishing Co., Inc.

166. Wilson, P. D., and Thompson, T. C.: A clinical consideration of the methods of equalizing leg length, Ann. Surg. **110:**992, 1939.

167. Winter, R. B.: The effects of early fusion on spine growth. In Zorab, P. A., editor: Scoliosis and growth, Edinburgh, 1971, Churchill Livingstone.

168. Winter, R. B., and others: Congenital scoliosis, J. Bone Joint Surg. **50A:**1, 1968.

169. Winter, R. B., and others: Diastematomyelia and congenital spine deformities, J. Bone Joint Surg. **56A:**27, 1974.

170. Wynne-Davies, R.: Congenital vertebral anomalies: aetiology and relationship to spina bifida cystica, J. Med. Genet. **12:**180, 1975.

171. Wynne-Davies, R.: The inheritance of scoliosis. In James, J. I. P., editor: Scoliosis, Edinburgh, 1976, Churchill Livingstone.

172. Wynne-Davies, R.: Heritable disorders in orthopedics, Orthop. Clin. North Am. **9**(1):3, 1978.

173. Zadek, I., and Gold, A.: The accessory tarsal scaphoid, J. Bone Joint Surg. **30A:**957, 1948.

SECTION FIVE

The teenager

CHAPTER 24

General considerations

HOWARD C. FILSTON

Except for the ravages of major trauma, the teenage years are among the healthiest of one's life. There are few illnesses unique to this age group, most of those of infancy and childhood will already have made themselves known, and those diseases characteristic of adulthood rarely present in the teenage years. Thus, this age group, from the disease standpoint, is a relatively problem-free one. Major trauma casts a heavy shadow over this age group, however, as increasing independence and the use of motorized vehicles increase several fold the incidence of accidental injury to which these adolescents are exposed. The use of alcohol and drugs decreases their inhibitions and leads to risk taking with automobiles and motorcycles with resultant high mortality and morbidity. The considerations regarding major trauma in the childhood years are equally applicable to this age group.

CHAPTER 25

Specific problems

HOWARD C. FILSTON

INFLAMMATORY BOWEL LESIONS

Inflammatory lesions of the gastrointestinal tract are generally unusual in childhood. Perhaps the anxieties of increasing independence make these lesions somewhat more prevalent (though still uncommon) in the teenage years. Thus, peptic ulcer disease at the upper end of the gastrointestinal tract and Crohn's disease and ulcerative colitis at the lower end do begin to show themselves during this age.

Peptic ulcer disease

Peptic ulcer disease presents with the usual symptoms common to the adult, although acute onset with severe upper gastrointestinal hemorrhage as a complication may be slightly more common as a presentation in this age group than in adults. It is not unusual for a child to have severe upper gastrointestinal hemorrhage and yet have no significant previous history of epigastric pain or discomfort.

Evaluation of upper gastrointestinal hemorrhage in the child should utilize the advantages of modern endoscopy and radiographic techniques. In the acutely bleeding situation, a barium upper gastrointestinal study, once the mainstay of all bowel investigations, is all but contraindicated, for it leads to confusion and difficulty in subsequent endoscopy and angiography.[20] Endoscopy should be performed by an experienced endoscopist. This procedure will usually differentiate esophageal variceal hemorrhage from gastritis, diffuse ulceration, or an individual peptic ulcer. If endoscopy fails or is unavailable and acute hemorrhage is ensuing, arteriography is often helpful. This should be performed in a systematic fashion utiliz-

ing a nonselective aortogram initially, followed by selective major vessel evaluation, and then by highly selective individual vessel injection.[10]

When arteriography is utilized in diagnosis, consideration should be given to the indications for the use of vascular infusion therapy as a means of controlling the hemorrhage. Vasopressin injection through selective catheters is highly useful for diffuse gastric hemorrhage from gastritis, and infusion into the superior mesenteric artery has been a significant adjunct to the management of esophageal variceal hemorrhage.[1]

Initial therapy for upper gastrointestinal hemorrhage, however, should entail the passage of a nasogastric tube to confirm blood in the stomach, aspiration of the stomach, and irrigation with iced saline until the stomach is emptied and decompressed. Continued irrigation with iced saline until bleeding is well controlled is indicated and will usually suffice to control most cases of upper gastrointestinal hemorrhage. At the same time, a dependable intravenous line should be established and volume replacement initiated with balanced salt solution followed by type-specific blood. Once initial resuscitation is accomplished and the child is stable, the above-noted diagnostic maneuvers should be performed.

When the source of the bleeding is defined, the choice of therapy for bleeding unresponsive to iced saline lavage depends on the source of the hemorrhage. Vasopressin infusion through either a peripheral vein or, if arteriography has been used diagnostically, the superior mesenteric artery catheter is indicated for hemorrhage from variceal sources. Peripheral venous infusion has been shown to be as efficacious as superior mesenteric artery infusion for this lesion[8]; thus, peripheral venous infusion should be selected unless arteriography has already been utilized as a diagnostic method. On the other hand, bleeding from diffuse gastritis responds best to infusion therapy in the left gastric vessel, and bleeding from specific ulcers may respond to infusion therapy or may require embolization with autogenous clot or Gelfoam or other such material if the hemorrhage is from a single source of any magnitude.[10,15]

Finally, for variceal hemorrhage, the Sengstaken-Blakemore double-balloon catheter can be used to control hemorrhage by direct pressure on the varices by the inflated balloon. This instrument has a significant complication rate associated with it, however, and should be used only by experienced physicians in the setting of an intensive care nursing unit. Misplacement of the Sengstaken-Blakemore tube can lead to pressure expansion of the gastric balloon in the esophagus, resulting in severe disruption of the esophagus; and the complete occlusion of the esophagus achieved by inflation of the esophageal balloon can lead to aspiration of secretions above the inflated balloon if a second tube is not kept functioning to evacuate the secretions. Finally, the pressure that is required on the tube to pull the inflated gastric balloon up against the cardia may cause necrosis of the tissues of the nose if a proper traction setup is not utilized. If the balloons become deflated, the tube with one balloon inflated can be pulled into the hypopharynx, causing acute obstruction of the airway. Nevertheless, despite these disadvantages, the tube is a useful appliance when it is used in the proper setting by experienced personnel.

These nonsurgical means of control of upper gastrointestinal hemorrhage are highly successful; thus, surgery is rarely indicated for the acute hemorrhagic event in the child. If the bleeding is not controlled and surgery is required as a lifesaving endeavor, the surgeon must be one who realizes the acute nature of the lesion and also appreciates the ability of the child to tolerate hemorrhagic events if he is properly resuscitated and maintained. There is little place for radical surgical excision of organs, such as is often indicated for the control of hemorrhage in the aged patient who cannot sustain repeated hemorrhagic events without the risk of cerebral vascular accidents and myocardial infarcts. A child can tolerate repeated episodes of severe hemorrhage when these are properly corrected with vascular volume restoration. Thus, if surgery is required for control of hemorrhage in a child, the simplest procedure that will control the acute bleeding episode should be utilized. Oversewing of ulcers, highly selective vagotomies, and suture ligation of varices are indicated.[7,23] The latter procedure is only a temporizing one, and some form of shunt therapy would probably be necessary for any degree of permanent control of variceal hemorrhage.[6,22] Gastric resections are rarely indicated in the acute hemorrhagic situation in a child. For the child with chronic ulcer disease unresponsive to medical therapy, planned surgical procedures utilizing highly selective vagotomy and drainage procedures as the initial procedures of choice are indicated.

Crohn's disease and ulcerative colitis

For inflammatory lesions of the small and large intestine such as Crohn's disease and ulcerative colitis, surgical therapy is usually indicated in this age group only for complications of the disease.[9] Nevertheless, most patients eventually require surgery. Medical therapy includes attention to diet, the use of poorly absorbed sulfas (salicylazosulfapyridene), short-term steroid therapy, and azathioprine. When these fail, the use of moderate bowel rest for 4 to 6 weeks accompanied by total parenteral nutrition may allow healing of the inflammatory lesion and certainly is a useful adjunct in preparation for the patient who requires surgery.[9,14,16] Total parenteral nutrition prior to surgery will better prepare the patient to tolerate the surgical procedure, and in some instances the inflammatory process will subside to such a degree that the obstruction will ease.

Surgery is indicated in *Crohn's disease* for intestinal diversion proximal to significant fistulas or perforations, for persistent hemorrhage, and for obstructive intestinal lesions (Fig. 25-1). Surgical resection of diseased bowel has been followed by resumption of growth and maturation after developmental arrest.[5a] Resectional surgery for localized inflammatory lesions of Crohn's disease may be curative, but the recurrence —or perhaps better stated, persistence—rate of the disease is high. Ultimately, response to medical therapy is essential to prevent continual ravaging of the intestine by the disease process.[2,12,25]

For *ulcerative colitis,* the usual medical therapy is salicylazosulfapyridene and steroids. The short-term use of steroids is warranted to quiet down the acute inflammatory process, but long-term ste-

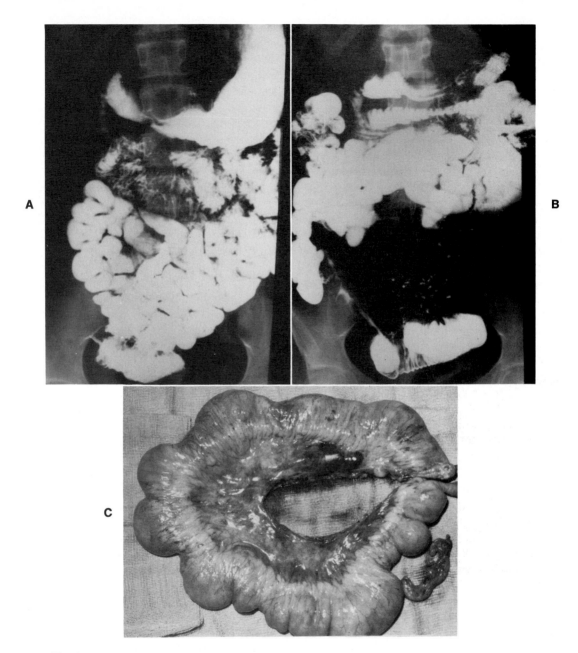

Fig. 25-1. A, This upper GI series with small bowel follow-through appeared normal until the very distal ileum began to fill and narrowing was encountered. **B,** Subsequent film showing a well-defined ''string sign'' with a fistula from the distal ileum to the cecum, demonstrating regional enteritis. **C,** Resected specimen of regional enteritis showing fat encroaching on the walls of the bowel.

roid management leads to numerous complications of chronic steroid therapy and does not prevent the prohibitive incidence of carcinoma of the colon that is known to occur when the disease persists for over 10 years.[19] Moreover, if significant inflammatory disease persists, ultimately colectomy will be required. Prolonged intensive steroid ther-

apy may increase the complication rate for the surgical procedure, and most surgeons would prefer that the patient not be pushed into a frankly cushingoid state before surgery is elected.

The tried and tested procedure for ulcerative colitis is total colectomy with ileostomy, although many subtotal colectomies with rectal-saving procedures have been utilized over the years. These leave the patient with the persistent high risk of developing carcinoma in the residual rectal segment. Recently an adaptation of the endorectal pull-through procedure utilized for Hirschsprung's disease has been gaining popularity among pediatric surgeons for ulcerative colitis. This actually brings the procedure full circle, since it was originally suggested and tried in the laboratory in 1946 by Ravitch and Sabiston[21] with the hope of utilizing it for patients requiring total colectomy and ileostomy for familial polyposis or ulcerative colitis. A modification of this procedure was adopted by Soave[26] for use in Hirschsprung's disease, and it was in this illness that the procedure gained its popularity. Martin, LeCoultre, and Schubert[18] have described the technical points essential for utilizing an endorectal pull-through procedure successfully for ulcerative colitis and have shown that the procedure is technically feasible. It nonetheless leaves the patient with a segment of ileum as the terminal intestinal segment, and considerable adaptation must take place before this ileal segment will function other than as a propelling conduit. Although the individual has frequent bowel movements, he is spared the encumbrance of an ileostomy appliance.

Finally, it must be emphasized that ulcerative colitis is a potentially fatal disease and that the toxic megacolon resulting from it can present as an extremely acute surgical emergency. The potential for the development of toxic megacolon in this disease must always be kept in mind by the physician applying medical therapy. Early surgical consultation for the patient who is acutely ill with this disease is certainly warranted.

BREAST LESIONS: MALE AND FEMALE

As the child passes on into adolescence, the development of secondary sex characteristics and the awakening of the functioning of the gonads may have effects on the breasts in either sex.

In the *male teenager* the end-organ may overrespond to transient hormonal imbalances, and this overresponse may lead to gynecomastia, a source of embarrassment to the male teenager. If no other sign of sexual abnormality is present, considerations regarding gynecomastia can be based essentially on the psychologic aspects of the lesion. Usually any significant degree of gynecomastia, especially if it is unilateral, will require excision of the breast. This requires a total excision of

mammary tissue, sparing the nipple, and is best done through an areolar incision, which will leave no obvious scar following healing. The advantage of this incision is that it leaves no scar for questioning that might serve to embarrass the child postoperatively as much as the gynecomastia itself. Thus, this technical point must be considered by the physician and the surgeon in planning the procedure for the child. When significant breast tissue is allowed to remain in the male, the possibility of developing carcinoma of the breast is present, just as it is in the female.

The *female teenager* may find herself confronted with various lesions related to the development of her breasts at puberty.[4,24,28] A frequent cause of concern is unilateral hypertrophy. This again is an end-organ response in which one breast responds earlier and more extensively to the developing sex hormones than does the other. This lesion is similar to that which occurs in childhood, where virginal hypertrophy of one or both breasts may develop as a result of end-organ response. Reassurance and the offer of careful follow-up are usually all that are needed in dealing with these problems, because in a short time the other breast will begin developing. Occasionally, the one breast will go on and hypertrophy to such an extent that surgical reduction becomes necessary, but this is the exception rather than the rule.

Subareolar breast buds typically develop at the onset of normal breast development. These may develop even in the very young child or infant as a result of transplacental hormones. Because of the wide concern for carcinoma of the breast in adult women, the population is imbued with the idea that masses in the breast are dangerous; and this idea is transmitted to the child. A great tragedy may ensue if the mother brings in the child with a breast bud development, especially if it is unilateral, and is referred to a surgeon whose knowledge of childhood breast development is lacking. Too often such surgeons have excised these so-called ''nodules'' only to find that the entire breast bud of the child has been removed. No breast will develop on the side of such a procedure. Thus, again it is incumbent on the primary care physician to ascertain the attitude, knowledge, and experience of the surgeons to whom he refers his pediatric patients.

With the onset of actual breast development in the growing teenager, several problems may develop. Most frequently seen are nodules developing in the breasts that may change size and become symptomatic coincident with the menstrual cycle. When these lesions are followed through several menstrual periods, they are found to enlarge and recede with each cycle. These are almost invariably fibrocystic changes, often related to anovulatory periods with excessive estrogen secretion. As the child's menstrual cycle regularizes and she becomes regularly ovulatory, this excessive stimulation recedes and the breast stabilizes. Most children can be reassured that this will be true, but occasionally the fibrocystic changes become so severe that some therapy is indicated. This therapy must be applied extremely judiciously, however, or the child's breast will be ravaged by surgical biopsy and partial excision before she reaches full adulthood.

Occasionally, these stimulatory cycles will result in the formation of a solid fibroadenoma. These lesions are discrete, firm, mobile masses that can enlarge to tremendous sizes. They do not recede with changes in the cycle and do require excision because of their size and the discomfort they frequently cause. These lesions are neither malignant nor premalignant and are excised simply because of their size and discomfort. They are the most common lesion resulting in breast surgery in this age group.[4,24,28] They can be excised through

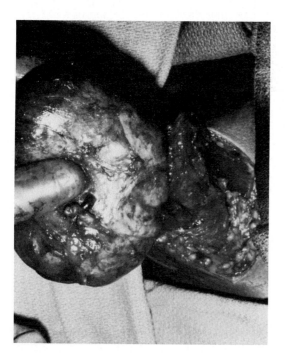

Fig. 25-2. Typical fibroadenoma being excised from the breast of a teenage girl.

an inframammary excision that lays the breast back and resects the fibroadenoma from behind the breast, leaving the breast normal in contour, to be resutured to the fascia of the chest wall (Fig. 25-2). Direct frontal attacks on these lesions often leave the breasts scarred and disfigured. Because of the exceedingly low malignant incidence in teenagers, cosmetic considerations can be foremost in the mind of the surgeon.

Occasionally, a mass thought to be a fibroadenoma will prove to be cystosarcoma phyllodes, usually a benign lesion.

The occasional development of an inflammatory lesion of the breast will be heralded by the usual signs of tenderness, redness, pain, and increased temperature and should be treated in the usual fashion for managing soft tissue infection. Cellulitis can be treated with antibiotics, but abscess formation will require incision and drainage.

GYNECOLOGIC PROBLEMS

The other area obviously unique to the teenage years is that of gynecologic problems. The incidence and differential complexity of these problems is increased by the precocious sexual activity of the present teenage population. Thus, consideration of pelvic inflammatory disease and ectopic pregnancy must enter into the differential diagnosis of abdominal pain in the young female teenager, and because of the hesitancy of the patient to admit to sexual activity, the history may fail to direct the physician's attention to the pertinent differential diagnosis. Once the teenager has reached the age of sexual activity, the acute abdomen must be looked on as something more than a clear-cut case of appendicitis. A careful, considerate history taken from the teenager in private may elicit answers that would not be available in the presence of the parents. If this history is elicited in such an atmosphere, that trust must not be broken by the physician without the permission of the teenager. Nevertheless, for the severely ill child who needs attention, careful guidance by the physician for both the patient and the family will help bridge the generation gap that has developed. A considerate but thorough and carefully performed pelvic examination must be part of any physical evaluation of the acute abdomen of a child who clearly has been sexually active. On the other hand, the child with a tight hymenal ring who seemingly has not engaged in sexual activity must be treated with the consideration and tenderness due the innocent child. Thus, the physician and the surgeon must individualize most carefully the questions and physical evaluations performed on each patient; yet thorough and accurate information must be obtained.

Some gynecologic lesions obviously do not require sexual activity for their development. These may present with acute abdominal pain and include such entities as tumors of the ovary,[5] torsion of ovarian cysts, ruptures of ovarian cysts, and the infrequently seen but dramatic imperforate hymen. Symptoms in the last-mentioned entity include severe monthly cramps and failure of menarche.[11] Pelvic examination may reveal the closed hymen and a midline pelvic mass. Occasionally, a severe urogenital sinus abnormality with hydrometrocolpos will fail to be diagnosed until cyclic monthly abdominal pain brings the child in for physical examination[31] (Fig. 25-3). Thus, although the child's innocence and dignity must be maintained, a thorough evaluation of the developing sexual organs, both external and internal, must be achieved or a significant pathologic condition may be missed to the detriment of the patient.

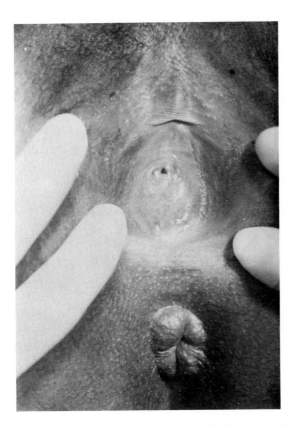

Fig. 25-3. Urogenital sinus deformity with distal vaginal atresia presenting in a teenager as primary amenorrhea and cyclic crampy pain.

To whom the primary care physician should refer a teenager with a potential gynecologic lesion may be a major consideration in itself. The child with a truly acute abdominal problem whose cause is not clearly gynecologic should probably be referred to a surgeon experienced in the care of abdominal lesions in childhood, but this individual must either have considerable experience with gynecologic lesions in this age group or be willing to consult quickly with a gynecologic colleague for help in dealing with any such problems that may arise. The child would benefit from both the conservatism of the pediatric-oriented surgeon and the experience and technical capability of the knowledgeable gynecologist. Ideally, a pediatric gynecologist would solve the problem, but few of these specialists are available. Thus, the adult-oriented general surgeon may fail to appreciate the gynecologic problems in the child, and the gynecologist inexperienced in dealing with lesions in children may be too radical in approaching the gynecologic lesion. For example, pyosalpinx due to gonococcus may require radical surgery for cure, but pyosalpinx can also result from systemic streptococcal infection in children and respond to intravenous antibiotic therapy with resolution of the process. Any of these lesions may present as an acute abdominal crisis with appendicitis or a perforated appendix as the major differential diagnosis. A perforated appendix with pelvic abscess may engulf both tubes and ovaries and present the adult gynecologist with a picture that usually leads him to recommend a radical pelvic clean-out. Nevertheless, these lesions may totally resolve with proper drainage and appendectomy and do not have the implications that venereal abscesses in the adult gynecologic patient have. That there is an increased incidence of ectopic pregnancy and infertility in patients whose tubes and ovaries have been involved in such appendiceal abscesses is true, but this incidence is nonetheless not an indication for such radical surgery.

It would seem, therefore, that it is incumbent on the primary care physician to maintain some control of the referral pattern for these children and to be in a position to call in additional consultants as needed.

MALE SEXUAL DEVELOPMENT PROBLEMS

The male teenager faces little in the way of sexual development problems that have surgical implications. One exception to this is epididymitis, which must be differentiated from torsion of the testicle. A child with an acutely swollen, tender testicle who has had no sexual activity must be considered to have torsion of the testicle until proved otherwise. However, the sexually active male teenager may well develop epididymitis, and a careful history and examination of any urethral discharge will help to differentiate epididymitis from torsion of the testicle. Nonetheless, if doubt exists in the mind of the experienced surgeon, either a pediatric surgeon or a pediatric urologist, exploration to rule out torsion of the testicle is certainly warranted.

LESIONS MISSED FROM EARLIER DAYS
Hirschsprung's disease

With few exceptions, most lesions common to the newborn and infancy periods of life will have long since been diagnosed and under therapy before the onset of adolescence. Probably the most

common exception to this, however, is that of Hirschsprung's disease. Children are still seen who go through infancy and childhood as chronic constipators and ultimately reach the teenage years and even adulthood with severe constipation even to the point of overflow soiling because of Hirschsprung's disease. Most of these individuals will have the onset of their disease in early childhood, and this fact should lead the physician to a direct workup for Hirschsprung's disease. As in other age groups, this evaluation should include a barium enema evaluation by a knowledgeable radiologist and, subsequently, rectal biopsy if indicated. Usually the barium enema is directly diagnostic and shows the classic pattern of Hirschsprung's disease (Fig. 25-4). Therapy for this lesion in this age group is similar to that in the infant and childhood age groups and should be accomplished expeditiously.

Important factors for the primary care physician to recognize is that Hirschsprung's disease can be associated with survival to teenage and adult years

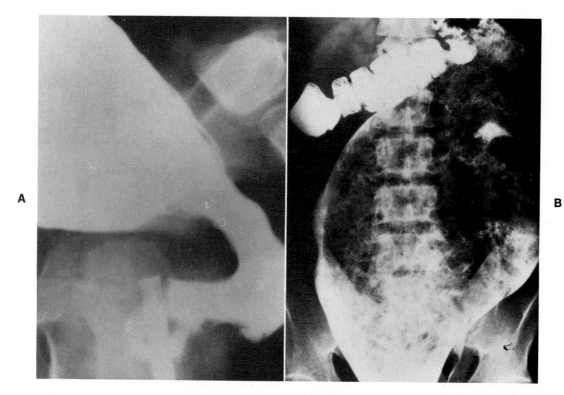

Fig. 25-4. A, Hirschsprung's disease in an older child with a long history of diarrhea. The radiograph shows the narrowed upper rectal segment, the transition zone, and the dilated distal sigmoid colon. **B,** Stool impacted in the sigmoid of a patient with long-standing Hirschsprung's disease. Note how the bowel tapers toward the upper rectum.

with a lifelong history of constipation but without the mortality that is the usual course of the disease. In addition, Hirschsprung's disease should be suspected in a child with irregular bowel habits or with diarrhea and soiling, because a lifelong chronic low-grade enterocolitis may hide the picture of constipation and of the underlying aganglionosis. We have seen such a child from whom we could elicit no history of constipation who at the age of 8 had colitis with rectal bleeding.

Imperforate anus

Another lesion that may go undetected is a mild degree of imperforate anus in which a stoma is present on the perineum but the anus is inadequate in either size, position, or elasticity. The stoma may be mistaken for a normal anus, but careful examination may reveal either a tight, strictured stoma or one that is so far anterior as to defeat the functioning of the puborectalis sling.[13,17] This may lead to problems with constipation or to soiling, and this possibility must be considered in

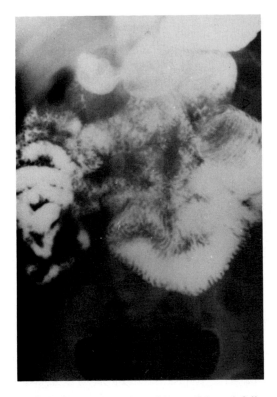

Fig. 25-5. Upper GI series with small bowel follow-through showing an intussuscepting hamartoma of the proximal jejunum (arrow).

any child seen with a long history of either problem.

Malrotation and intussusception

Other lesions that may be missed for long periods and present in late childhood or adolescence are malrotation and intussusception.

Malrotation rarely presents in later childhood with the acute life-threatening volvulus that is characteristic of this lesion in infancy. Rather, it presents with a history of chronic postprandial pain and occasionally vomiting. Often these children are considered to have psychosomatic gastrointestinal problems, and may even be referred for psychologic or psychiatric evaluation and therapy. The child with recurrent abdominal pain, particularly when it is postprandial and especially if it is associated with vomiting, should have an upper GI series performed by a radiologist experienced in looking for malrotation. The demonstration of a malpositioned ligament of Treitz with an accordionated duodenum, with or without evidence of duodenal obstruction and distention, should lead to the consideration that malrotation exists as an organic obstruction and is the cause of the child's symptoms.

Intussusceptions presenting in this age group usually are caused by some leading point such as an intussuscepted Meckel's diverticulum, a polyp, or a duplication. Occasionally, a lymphoma will present as an intussusception. Any child with chronic gastrointestinal problems such as abdominal pain, diarrhea, constipation, and particularly occult bleeding or anemia should be evaluated for such lesions.[3] When the intussuscepted lesion is in the small bowel, it may be demonstrated best by an upper GI series with small bowel follow-through (Fig. 25-5), rather than the traditional barium enema study used to demonstrate the typical idiopathic intussusception of infancy.

Cystic fibrosis

Infrequently, cystic fibrosis presents first in late childhood or the early teenage years with the complications of chronic liver disease. These are usually healthy children who have not had the pulmonary ravages of the disease and may have initial symptoms of acute upper gastrointestinal bleeding due to esophageal varices. Varices due to cavernous transformation of the portal vein usually make themselves known by upper gastrointestinal bleeding earlier in childhood; thus, such late onset of upper gastrointestinal hemorrhage, when demonstrated to be due to esophageal varices, should lead to an evaluation for cystic fibrosis.[27] These individuals often have an unusual form of the disease in which the liver sustains more of the damage than the lungs.

FOLLOW-UP OF EARLIER SURGICAL CONDITIONS

Once again it must be emphasized that any child who has had an intra-abdominal surgical procedure has a lifelong risk of adhesive bowel obstruction; thus, these children must be investigated for such a lesion earlier in the course of any abdominal illness characterized by crampy pain and vomiting. These children should be seen early, and an abdominal radiograph screening for signs of intestinal obstruction should be obtained. Careful follow-up must be provided until the child recovers from the illness or until a clear-cut obstruction is identified. The use of barium instilled into the stomach and followed through with plain x-ray films at intervals is a useful maneuver to rule out obstruction when it is not clearly present on plain abdominal films.

Intestinal atresias

Children who have had atresias of the intestine with reconstruction, particularly when there has been great disparity in size between the dilated proximal segment and the narrowed unused distal segment, may experience late complications. These are due to distention of the proximal segment, which leads to stretching and elongation and ultimately to the positioning of the stoma to the side of the original proximal segment. This may eventually lead to the development of a blind loop syndrome with stasis of intestinal contents, change in bacterial flora, and a change in the bile-salt, bile-acid ratio that may interfere with distal ileal absorption of specific nutriments and to a catharsis-like effect on the colon, leading to salt and water loss. Any child with failure to thrive or a spruelike malnutrition syndrome who has such surgery in his history should be investigated for such a development.

Portal hypertension

The child with portal hypertension due to cavernomatous transformation of the portal vein will usually have had bleeding episodes from early childhood and will have been followed at regular intervals. It should be recognized, however, that in late childhood or in the early teenage period, the incidence of bleeding episodes may increase. Along with the increased incidence there is increased severity and markedly increased difficulty in stopping the bleeding. The child who for years responded to simple bowel rest, nasogastric intubation, and ice saline lavage, perhaps requiring a 1-unit transfusion or even none at all, may now require a Sengtaken-Blakemore tube and vasopressin (Pitressin) infusion with each bleeding episode. The blood loss may be more massive, requiring more extensive volume transfusion. Nonetheless, if the episodes can be controlled, conservative therapy is still warranted, both because increasing collateral vessels may form with the passage of time, decreasing the frequency of the bleeding episodes, and because the complications of shunt therapy in teenagers may be considerable.[29]

Recent interest in the Warren distal splenorenal shunt with partial gastric devascularization has led to the hope that this procedure will be associated with fewer complications in the form of hepatic encephalopathy.[22,30] This entity has been recognized in recent years in many children who have had successful shunt therapy for cavernomatous transformation of the portal vein. Until the Warren shunt is shown to control hemorrhage reliably and to lessen the incidence of ammonia-related encephalopathy, conservative therapy remains the cornerstone of treatment so long as the child's life is not unduly threatened. Obviously, there comes a time when either the frequency and severity of the bleeding episodes are so great that they encumber the child's life and daily activities, or one episode of bleeding is uncontrollable and surgical intervention is clearly indicated. In these individuals, it must be hoped that a Warren shunt will be successful and that the encephalopathic complications will prove to be minimal.

REFERENCES

1. Athanasoulis, C. A., and others: Angiography: its contribution to the emergency management of gastrointestinal hemorrhage, Radiol. Clin. North Am. **14:**265, 1976.
2. Benner, J., and others: Crohn's disease in children and adolescents: is inadequate weight gain a valid indication for surgery? J. Pediatr. Surg. **14:**325, 1979.
3. Blackburn, W. W., and Filston, H. C.: Common symptoms in children: routine illness or abdominal lymphoma, Am. J. Surg. **130:**539, 1975.

4. Bower, R., Bell, M. J., and Ternberg, J. L.: Management of breast lesions in children and adolescents, J. Pediatr. Surg. **11:**337, 1976.
5. Bronsther, B., and Abrams, M. W.: Ovarian tumors in childhood. In Bronsther, B., editor: Sex related surgical problems, part 1, Pediatr. Ann. **4:**565, October 1975.
5a. Castile, R. G., and others: Crohn's disease in children: assessment of the progression of disease, growth, and prognosis, J. Pediatr. Surg. **15:**462, 1979.
6. Clatworthy, H. W., Jr.: Extrahepatic portal hypertension. In Childs, C. G., III, editor: Portal hypertension, Philadelphia, 1974, W. B. Saunders Co.
7. Curci, M. R., and others: Peptic ulcer disease in childhood reexamined, J. Pediatr. Surg. **11:**329, 1976.
8. Davis, G. B., Bookstein, J., and Hagan, P. L.: The relative effects of selective intra-arterial and intravenous vasopressin infusion, Radiology **120:**537, 1976.
9. Drucker, W. R.: Regional enteritis (Crohn's disease). In Sabiston, D. C., Jr., editor: Davis Christopher textbook of surgery, Philadelphia, 1977, W. B. Saunders Co., pp. 1011-1023.
10. Filston, H. C., Jackson, D. C., and Johnsrude, I. S.: Arteriographic embolization for control of recurrent severe gastric hemorrhage in a 10-year-old boy, J. Pediatr. Surg. **14:**276, 1979.
11. Gerbie, A. B.: Congenital anomalies of the female genital tract, Pediatr. Ann. **3:**20, December 1974.
12. Harris, B. H., Hollabaugh, R. S., and Clatworthy, H. W., Jr.: Surgery for developmental and growth failure in childhood granulomatous enteritis, J. Pediatr. Surg. **9:**301, 1974.
13. Hendren, W. H.: Constipation caused by anterior location of the anus and its surgical correction, J. Pediatr. Surg. **13:**505, 1978.
14. Homer, D. R., Grand, R. J., and Colodny, A. H.: Growth, course and progress after surgery for Crohn's disease in children and adolescents, Pediatrics **59:**717, 1977.
15. Johnsrude, I. S., and Jackson, D. C.: A practical approach to angiography, Boston, 1979, Little, Brown & Co.
16. Layden, T., and others: Reversal of growth arrest in adolescents with Crohn's disease after parenteral alimentation, Gastroenterology **70:**1017, 1976.
17. Leape, L. L., and Ramenofsky, M. L.: Anterior ectopic anus: a common cause of constipation in children, J. Pediatr. Surg. **13:**627, 1978.
18. Martin, L. W., LeCoultre, C., and Schubert, W. K.: Total colectomy and mucosal proctectomy with preservation of continence in ulcerative colitis, Ann. Surg. **186:**477, 1977.
19. Moody, F. G.: Ulcerative colitis. In Sabiston, D. C., Jr., editor: Davis Christopher textbook of surgery, Philadelphia, 1977, W. B. Saunders Co., p. 1120.
20. Oddson, T. A., and others: Acute gastrointestinal hemorrhage: the changing role of barium examinations, Radiol. Clin. North Am. **16:**123, 1978.
21. Ravitch, M. M., and Sabiston, D. C., Jr.: Anal ileostomy with preservation of the sphincter: a proposed operation in patients requiring total colectomy for benign lesions, Surg. Gynecol. Obstet. **84:**1095, 1947.
22. Rodgers, B. M., and Talbert, J. L.: Distal spleno-renal shunt for portal decompression in childhood, J. Pediatr. Surg. **14:**33, 1979.
23. Schuster, S. R., and Gross, R. E.: Peptic ulcer disease in childhood, Am. J. Surg. **105:**324, 1963.
24. Seashore, J. H.: Breast enlargements in infants and children, Pediatr. Ann. **4:**542, 1975.
25. Sherman, N. J., and others: Regional enteritis in childhood, J. Pediatr. Surg. **7:**585, 1972.
26. Soave, F.: Hirschsprung's disease: a new surgical technique, Arch. Dis. Child. **39:**116, 1964.
27. Stern, R. C., and others: Symptomatic hepatic disease in cystic fibrosis: incidence, course, and outcome of portal systemic shunting, Gastroenterology **70:**645, 1976.
28. Turbey, W. J., Buntain, W. L., and Dudgeon, D. L.: The surgical management of pediatric breast masses, Pediatrics **56:**736, 1975.
29. Voorhees, A. B., Jr., and others: Portal-systemic encephalopathy in the noncirrhotic patient: effect of portal systemic shunting, Arch. Surg. **107:**659, 1973.
30. Warren, W. D., and others: Selective distal splenorenal shunt: technique and results of operation, Arch. Surg. **108:**306, 1974.
31. Williams, D. I., and Bloomberg, S.: Urogenital sinus in the female child, J. Pediatr. Surg. **11:**51, 1976.

CHAPTER 26

Urologic considerations

JOHN W. DUCKETT and HOWARD C. FILSTON

GENERAL CONSIDERATIONS

Most of the problems associated with the urogenital system of a developmental nature will present themselves by the time the child reaches puberty. There are few entities unique to the teenage years in the urologic system; but, of course, any of the anomalies that have been previously mentioned may have been missed throughout childhood. In addition, all of the problems of venereal infection that plague the adult may be found in the sexually active teenager.

Because trauma from automobile accidents, falls, or sports is the most common cause of death in late childhood and the teenage years, trauma as it affects the urologic system is discussed in this chapter.

TRAUMA
Renal injuries

Trauma to the kidney is frequently part of a generalized picture of blunt trauma in which other organ systems are involved. Renal trauma is recognizable by the presence of hematuria, but this is not always present. Evaluation of the urinary tract, particularly the kidneys, should be part of any workup for generalized blunt trauma. The intravenous pyelogram may show frank extravasation but more often merely shows some deficiency of function in comparison with that of the opposite, uninjured side. A renal scan may be confirmatory in doubtful cases. Arteriography is rarely necessary in blunt trauma unless complete avulsion of the vascular pedicle is suspected by the fact that there is no function whatsoever on the intravenous pyelogram (IVP). In the shattered kidney, arteriography is helpful to determine viable segments.

Nonsurgical treatment consists of maintaining a good urine output and providing coverage with antibiotics. Careful daily observation may avert an unnecessary exploration. Delayed surgical treatment is often more appropriate. Drainage of urinary extravasation is not usually necessary. More renal substance can be spared during secondary procedures than could be spared during the acute hemorrhage of the initial injury. The long-term prognosis for salvaging significant functioning renal tissue is generally good, although careful observation for late development of hypertension is needed.

When renal injury is discovered after seemingly minimal trauma, an underlying congenital anomaly or tumor is present in about 15% to 20% of cases.[1,2]

Ureteral injuries

The ureters are relatively immune to injury from blunt trauma because of their well-protected retroperitoneal location. They are frequently injured in gunshot wounds, however, and hematuria may not be present as a sign of such injury. Consequently, the ureters must be thought of along with other intra-abdominal and retroperitoneal structures when a gunshot wound to the abdomen is being evaluated.

Urethral injuries

With demonstration of a pelvic fracture, one should immediately suspect a ruptured urethra in the male patient. A catheter should not be passed until a urethrogram is performed and, if possible, a cystogram obtained. The passage of a catheter can then be accomplished by someone aware of the potential problems of catheterizing a patient with a urethral injury. A suprapubic catheter is the safest and most effective way to manage a urethral injury initially.

Rupture of the bladder will be detected by a cystogram, especially with a postemptying film. Transperitoneal rupture will require surgical closure, whereas retroperitoneal tears will heal with urethral catheter drainage.

REFERENCES

1. Miller, R. C.: The incidental discovery of occult abdominal tumors in children following blunt abdominal trauma, J. Trauma **6**:99, 1966.
2. Persky, L., and Forsythe, W. E.: Renal tumors in childhood, J.A.M.A. **182**:709, 1962.

CHAPTER 27

Neurosurgical considerations

W. JERRY OAKES and ROBERT H. WILKINS

GENERAL CONSIDERATIONS

The format of this text attempts to group symptoms into those age ranges in which they are most commonly seen. This is done with a clear understanding that no age group is immune from any particular disease process. Included in this chapter on teenage neurologic problems are brief comments on vascular and neoplastic diseases that occur predominantly in younger patients. This was done to enhance the continuity of the presentation of the particular type of disease rather than present a fragmentary comment under the appropriate age heading.

VASCULAR DISORDERS

Disease processes of children that affect the blood vessels of the brain and spinal cord are uncommon. In the past, interest in these disorders was primarily academic, for little more than symptomatic treatment could be offered except for the simplest of aneurysms and arteriovenous malformations. Today, recent advances in neuroradiology have greatly increased diagnostic accuracy. Angiography and computerized tomographic (CT) brain scanning can now define aneurysms and arteriovenous malformations in more detail than was previously thought possible. Accompanying the improvement in diagnosis has been an improvement of the anesthetic and preoperative management of patients with these lesions. Controlled hypotension can reduce blood loss, an intraoperative risk associated with these lesions. With the use of the surgical microscope and bipolar coagulation, neurosurgical removal of large vascular lesions is now not only possible but routine. As experience is gained, lesions that lie deep in the brain

and are surrounded by functioning cortical tissue can be considered surgically accessible. Frequently these lesions can be excised precisely, with little to no functional damage to the surrounding structures. In addition to the excision of vascular anomalies, adequate blood flow may be restored by microvascular anastomosis.

Possible findings. The clinical presentation of vascular disorders is largely dependent on the age at presentation. Nontraumatic intracranial bleeding in the premature or low–birth weight neonate characteristically begins in the subependymal germinal matrix and is frequently followed by rupture into the ventricular system. These neonates almost always have significant respiratory embarrassment that is associated with their intraventricular hemorrhage. The respiratory distress syndrome, with hyaline membrane formation, pneumonia, or other respiratory difficulties, is almost always present in these neonates. Once intracranial bleeding has occurred, the neonate may develop generalized seizure activity, increased muscular tone, and tremulousness. Evidence of increased intracranial pressure with bulging of the anterior fontanelle and increase of the head circumference may occur. The patient is listless, apathetic, febrile, feeds poorly, and frequently needs increased respiratory assistance to maintain ventilation. If significant bleeding has taken place, there may be a moderate, unexplained decrease in the hematocrit value.

A small but interesting group of patients develop congestive heart failure within the first few days of birth. Cardiac catheterization will be seen to be normal; however, oxygen saturation of the venous blood in the superior vena cava or in the internal jugular vein will be high. The cardiac failure is secondary to high output; as much as 80% of the cardiac output is directed through a cerebral arteriovenous malformation.[56] The most common malformation presenting in this manner is composed of small- to medium-size intracranial arteries anastomosing directly into a dilated venous outflow channel. This usually occurs deep in the substance of the brain with dilatation of the vein of Galen (Fig. 27-1). Although a misnomer, these lesions are termed aneurysms of the vein of Galen because of the massive dilatation of that structure. Large arteriovenous malformations within the cerebral hemisphere that may or may not empty by the deep venous system have also been reported

to present in this fashion.[34,47] The cardiac failure will frequently be refractory to medical management and demand surgical therapy within the first few days of life to decrease the arteriovenous shunt. If the cardiac failure is not sufficient to arouse clinical suspicion, the infant may escape detection until late infancy, when he may be found to have macrocrania. This entity usually occurs when the vascular malformation is large and is located adjacent to a narrow point of the cerebral spinal fluid (CSF) pathway, usually the aqueduct of Sylvius, and internal hydrocephalus develops. In both of these presentations, a cranial bruit may be prominent, the anterior fontanelle will be full,

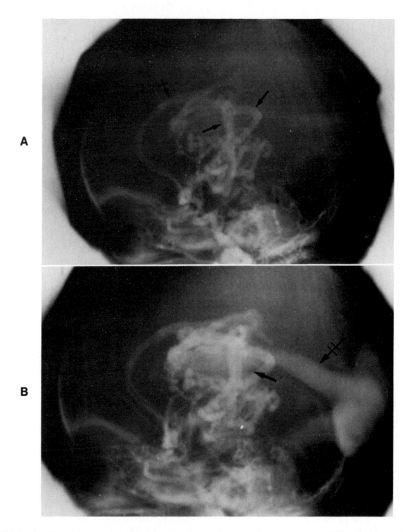

Fig. 27-1. A, Fistulous communication between the anterior ($\rightarrowtail$) and middle ($\rightarrow$) cerebral arteries and the vein of Galen (vein of Galen aneurysm) in a neonate. All involved vessels are grossly dilated. **B,** The vein of Galen ($\rightarrow$) and straight sinus ($\nrightarrow$) are enlarged to accommodate the outflow from the malformation. The neonate developed uncontrollable cardiac failure within the first 24 hours of life.

and the cardiac examination will demonstrate high-output cardiac failure.

In childhood, vascular lesions frequently present because of hemorrhage. The hemorrhage characteristically is located either in the subarachnoid space or within the substance of the surrounding neural tissue. Spontaneous subarachnoid hemorrhage is characterized by the sudden onset of lethargy and severe headache. Depending on the location of the malformation, focal neurologic findings will frequently not be present. Altered mental status, meningismus, and photophobia are the clinical hallmarks of subarachnoid hemorrhage. Some lesions may produce hemorrhage not only in the subarachnoid space but also within the surrounding brain. These patients will frequently manifest focal neurologic deficits. Lesions near the precentral gyrus may present with the sudden onset of hemiparesis. Those located within the posterior fossa usually cause cranial nerve deficits, and lesions in the occipital lobe will cause homonymous hemianopsia. In some patients the blood will dissect through the parenchyma of the brain, rupture the ependymal lining of the ventricular system, and cause intraventricular hemorrhage. As the blood dissects through the foramen of Monro and occludes the aqueduct of Sylvius, acute hydrocephalus develops and frequently will result in acute raised intracranial pressure and death within hours. Rarely, a lesion will be found that bleeds into the subdural space and presents as an acute subdural hematoma without predisposing trauma.

Although the majority of patients with vascular disorders are seen by the clinician because of a bleeding episode, approximately 20% of patients with arteriovenous malformations will initially have seizure activity.[40,56] Such activity may be relatively easily controlled with anticonvulsants or occasionally will be seen to be refractory to medical therapy. The presence of an intracranial bruit or minor alteration of the neurologic examination may be the only clue that the underlying cause of the seizure disorder is a vascular malformation. A small group of malformations will present with a gradually increasing focal neurologic deficit that is thought to be secondary to a steal of arterial blood from the surrounding functional brain to the malformation. CT scans of arteriovenous malformations have shown peripheral infarction of the brain, which may account for this gradual progression.[2,55,83] Headaches may also be the primary symptom bringing the patient to the physician. The headache may be episodic and take on a migraine-like character. Again, the presence of a bruit or mild focality to the neurologic examination may be the only clue to the underlying malformation. Strategically located aneurysms of the posterior communicating artery may present with ophthalmoplegia with pain located behind the involved eye, associated with ptosis, pupillary dilatation, and altered extraocular muscle function.

When the sudden onset of focal neurologic deficit occurs without alteration of mental status, the cause may be arterial occlusive disease of childhood.[15,78] This entity may be seen with primary thrombosis of an intracranial artery or may be secondary to an embolic phenomenon. As opposed to occlusive disease in adult life, which primarily affects the large extracranial vessels, occlusive disease in childhood primarily affects the intracranial vessels. Cerebral arteritis, collagen vascular disease, and granulomatous disorders, among others, may cause spontaneous thrombosis of intracranial arteries. Following the arterial occlusion, hemorrhage may occur into the ischemic and softened brain, converting a thrombotic (white) infarction into a hemorrhagic (red) infarction with subsequent mass effect and alteration of the mental status. This situation is seen most commonly following embolic infarction where the embolus breaks up, allowing blood to flow into the area of infarction.

The intracranial venous system also may become occluded. Infection surrounding the venous drainage of the brain will frequently be associated with venous stasis and infarction,[76] which can occur at multiple levels of the venous system, from cortical veins that thrombose secondary to meningitis to dural sinuses that thrombose because of adjacent otitis. Occasionally, direct neoplastic infiltration of a dural sinus will cause thrombosis. Other factors that predispose the patient to venous infarction include dehydration of the neonate and hematologic disorders associated with polycythemia; both cause a hyperviscosity syndrome.

A recently recognized syndrome of undetermined cause is characterized by progressive vascular occlusions involving the large arteries at the base of the brain. This condition was first recognized in Japan, where the term *moyamoya disease* was first applied.[13,63,81] These children have multiple ischemic infarctions in the distribution of the involved vessels. In response to occlusion of the

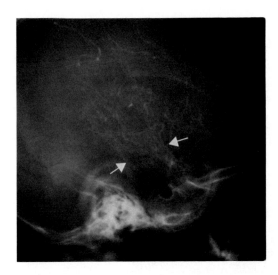

Fig. 27-2. Lateral projection of a carotid angiogram—late arterial phase showing a diffuse network of small vessels at the base of the brain (arrows) attempting to bypass a middle cerebral artery occlusion. The patient came to medical attention with a history of focal neurologic deficits caused by arterial occlusion.

intracranial vessels, a large network of anastomotic channels develops. At the time of angiography, the large number of these small vessels give the appearance of a puff of smoke (moyamoya) (Fig. 27-2).

Common occurrences. The cause of a subarachnoid hemorrhage not secondary to trauma is relatively evenly divided between arteriovenous malformations and intracranial aneurysms, each making up between 35% and 40% of the patients seen. The remainder are caused by an assortment of conditions, including hematologic disorders with a bleeding diathesis, intracranial tumors, and hemorrhagic encephalitis secondary to herpes simplex. There is also a small group of patients in whom the cause of the subarachnoid hemorrhage is never found.

Arteriovenous malformations are congenital lesions that frequently do not become manifest clinically until the second or third decade of life. Lesions that do present in children do so most commonly in the teenage years. The majority of lesions present with hemorrhage into either the subarachnoid space or the parenchyma of the brain. Most lesions are located in the cerebral cortex, most frequently in the distribution of the middle cerebral artery followed by lesions in the

anterior and finally the posterior cerebral arterial distribution. Another group are located deep within the substance of the supratentorial compartment along the corpus callosum or in the deep gray matter. These locations make up greater than 90% of the lesions seen. Additional locations where malformations may be encountered include the brain stem, cerebellum, and spinal cord. The sizes of the lesions vary considerably. Small cryptic malformations imbedded in the cerebral hemisphere are thought to be responsible for many atraumatic intraparenchymal hemorrhages for which a cause cannot be found.[50]

Patients are characteristically neurologically normal until the hemorrhage occurs. Depending on the location of the malformation, a focal neurologic deficit may result. Lesions in the distribution of the middle cerebral artery will frequently cause hemiparesis and cortical hemisensory loss. Those in the posterior fossa will more often cause cranial nerve abnormalities. Lesions within the cerebellum present with ataxia, whereas malformations within the spinal cord may cause paraplegia. Some 20% of malformations will present primarily with seizure activity. These lesions are located in the cerebral hemispheres. Older children may have a migrainelike history, whereas infants may develop congestive heart failure, cardiomegaly, or hydrocephalus as a result of their malformation.

In childhood, *intracranial aneurysms* come to clinical attention much less frequently than arteriovenous malformations. However, they become clinically apparent much more readily because of their increased tendency to bleed. These lesions are thought to be congenital in origin with the exception of the rare traumatic aneurysm and lesions associated with infectious arterial emboli from subacute bacterial endocarditis, pulmonary infection, and cyanotic heart disease with a right-to-left shunt. Aneurysms that result from septic emboli are termed mycotic aneurysms. They frequently develop in the distribution of the middle cerebral artery distal to the usual location of congenital aneurysms. Congenital aneurysms have an increased incidence in patients with coarctation of the aorta, polycystic kidney disease, or essential hypertension of childhood. Their incidence of clinical presentation seems to have a bimodal distribution, with lesions presenting in infancy and again in teenage years. Lesions that become manifest within the first few months of life are usually

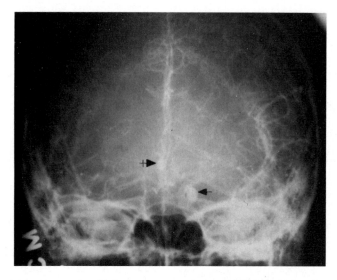

Fig. 27-3. Carotid angiogram in which an aneurysm (→) can be seen arising from the junction of the internal carotid artery and the posterior communicating artery. A second aneurysm is suspected in the anterior communicating complex (↠).

found beyond the circle of Willis and are frequently much larger than those encountered in adult life.[3] Greater than 40% of the aneurysms in infancy are considered to be giant (greater than 2½ cm in diameter). In addition, in comparison with those in adults, a higher percentage of aneurysms in infants present predominantly with the mass effect of the aneurysm rather than with subarachnoid hemorrhage. A recent study emphasized that antecedent head injury in a child may so prejudice the initial clinical impression that aneurysm may be overlooked diagnostically.[3] Some 35% of aneurysms found in teenagers occur at the bifurcation of the internal carotid artery.[66] In adult life, aneurysms at this location make up only 4% of lesions.[46] The other, more common locations in adults—at the anterior communicating artery complex (Fig. 27-3) and at the junction of the internal carotid and posterior communicating arteries—are also relatively common sites in teenagers.

Evaluation. In the child with a suspected vascular lesion of the brain, plain x-ray films of the skull are routinely normal. Occasionally, calcification within an aneurysmal dilatation of the vein of Galen or within an arteriovenous malformation may be seen (Fig. 27-4). The electroencephalogram (EEG) may be of help in demonstrating a focal abnormality with or without evidence of epileptic activity. This information is especially useful when one is planning angiography. As with many other lesions, however, computerized

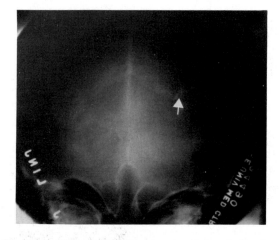

Fig. 27-4. Frontal skull film showing light calcification within the arteriovenous malformation (arrow) in an 11-year-old patient with mental retardation and seizures. Early in life the child had been known to have well-compensated congestive heart failure.

tomography has become the mainstay in diagnosing intracranial hemorrhage from vascular malformations. By CT scan, the location and extent of the hemorrhage, as well as the size and position of the ventricular system, can be determined easily. With enhancement, large aneurysms or arteriovenous malformations may become evident. It should be emphasized, however, that the CT scan is an unreliable tool in excluding the presence of a vascular anomaly.[56] Aneurysms smaller than 1 cm and smaller arteriovenous malformations may

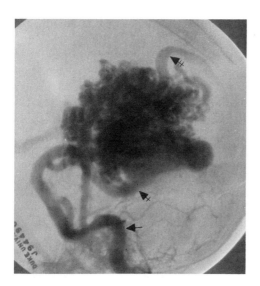

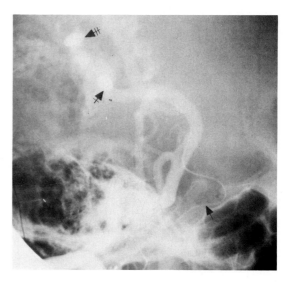

Fig. 27-5. Lateral vertebral angiogram in which the vertebral artery is massively enlarged (→), as are the posterior cerebral arteries (↛). The malformation is located adjacent to the vein of Galen. An early draining vein is visible at the superior aspect of the malformation (↠). A lateral carotid angiogram demonstrated a significant contribution from the anterior and middle cerebral arteries as well.

Fig. 27-6. Lateral vertebral angiogram during gluing of arteriovenous malformation in the patient seen in Fig. 27-4. A large catheter has been introduced into the internal carotid artery. Through the parent catheter a small double-lumen inner catheter (→) has followed the stream of flow up the carotid artery through the posterior communicating artery to the posterior cerebral artery, which is a dominant feeding vessel of the malformation. The inner catheter has a balloon blown up at its tip (→). Through the other lumen of the inner catheter, a rapidly hardening glue is injected into the malformation (↛). The inner catheter is then quickly withdrawn following the release of the glue to prevent it from being glued in place. Gluing is still primarily used as an adjunct to surgical removal. (Courtesy E. Ralph Heinz, M.D., Durham, N.C.)

be undetected by this technique. Cerebral angiography is essential in defining the vascular lesion and planning subsequent therapy (Fig. 27-5). With arteriovenous malformations that are large or deeply seated, angiography of all the major intracranial vessels is essential, since the malformation can recruit feeding vessels from any vascular distributions found within the brain or dura. Although the incidence of multiple aneurysms is not as high in children as it is in adults, complete angiography is important in evaluating intracranial aneurysms before planning therapy.

Referral. Children with suspected intracranial hemorrhage of acute onset are obviously candidates for immediate referral to an appropriate neurosurgical center. Children without evidence of altered mental status but with the sudden onset of severe headache associated with photophobia and meningismus are also at significant risk of renewed bleeding within the first few weeks following the initial episode. Because of this, their referral should also be urgent. In addition, infants with unexplained congestive heart failure and cranial bruits demand immediate neurosurgical evaluation. Patients who present with episodic headaches that are thought to be possibly sec-

ondary to an intracranial malformation and patients whose initial symptoms are seizure activity can be evaluated on a more elective basis.

Medical versus surgical treatment. In the relatively recent past, even the most aggressive of neurosurgeons would frequently recommend conservative therapy for many intracranial aneurysms and arteriovenous malformations.[52,86] This was because the operative risk was high and the natural history of these disease processes was not known. In the past several years, however, operative mortality associated with surgery for intracranial vascular anomalies has decreased significantly.[68,88-90] This is a result of the ability of the neuroradiologist to identify the major feeding vessels involved accurately and precisely. Arteriovenous malformations that have large feeding vessels and high flow that then narrow into a plexiform configuration within the parenchyma of the cerebral hemispheres are sometimes considered for embolization, either as a preoperative adjunct to resection or as an alternative to surgical resection (Fig. 27-6). Embolization has been attempted with plastic spheres of various sizes, as well as with gelatin sponge and tissue adhesives. These techniques, while helpful, frequently lack the specificity of careful surgical dissection. Patients with lesions that are not considered resectable, however, may benefit from this type of therapy.[20,48]

Many factors are involved in making the decision regarding resectability of an arteriovenous malformation. These include the location and size of the malformation and its proximity to vital neural structures. Lesions located in the dominant hemisphere and involving the speech centers are viewed differently from lesions in relatively silent areas of the brain. The extent and accessibility of feeding vessels are also important. The goals of surgery for arteriovenous malformations are to prevent subsequent bleeding episodes, to evacuate localized intracranial hemorrhage, to relieve congestive heart failure, and rarely, to help in the therapy of refractory seizures. An additional indication for surgical resection is the halting of a progressive neurologic deficit thought to be associated with arterial steal secondary to the malformation. Experience is still being gained with resection of arteriovenous malformations. The brain within the malformation is gliotic and nonfunctional. Therefore, if the resection is restricted to the border of the malformation, little or no increased neurologic deficit should be caused by the resection. Even deep-seated malformations are now being resected with minimal morbidity and mortality.[22,89,90]

The indications for surgical elimination of intracranial aneurysms in childhood are more clearly established than those for resection of arteriovenous malformations. Aneurysms that present either as mass lesions compromising surrounding neural structures or as the source of intracranial bleeding should be strongly considered for operation. Many of these lesions can now be corrected safely with little risk of increasing the preoperative neurologic deficit. Deep-seated giant lesions with broad bases and fusiform dilatations of intracranial arteries are exceptions, however.

Surgical options. The goal of surgery with arteriovenous malformations and intracranial aneurysms is to eliminate the abnormal vessel or vessels from the circulation. This is done by exci-

sion of the malformation and exclusion of the aneurysm from the circulation. Arteriovenous malformations that are not completely excised tend to recur and grow, recruiting additional blood supply from neighboring vessels. As previously mentioned, embolization to decrease the vascular input into a lesion prior to surgical excision is frequently helpful. Control of blood pressure with hypotension during surgical exposure of both arteriovenous malformations and aneurysms has greatly reduced blood loss and aided visualization of these lesions. Following the cortical exposure of the lesion, the main arterial feeders are occluded before any venous outflow is interrupted. This prevents the surgeon from increasing the resistance of the venous outflow and risking major intraoperative hemorrhage. Following resection of the lesion, intraoperative angiography will confirm the absence of further malformation.

Aneurysms are now routinely approached through a small osteoplastic craniotomy. The use of glucocorticoids, hyperosmotic agents, and spinal drainage to slacken the tension of the brain has facilitated exposure. The operating microscope has reduced the amount of retraction necessary to visualize many of these lesions, which lie at the base of the brain in relation to the circle of Willis. Careful dissection and preservation of small perforating arteries adjacent to the aneurysm have greatly improved the morbidity and mortality of this procedure.

Postoperative course. Frequently following surgery, these children will resume their preoperative condition within a few days. Because of the small degree of brain retraction necessary to visualize many of these lesions, cerebral swelling is less than was previously the case. Seizure activity in the postoperative period remains a possibility; thus, prophylactic anticonvulsants are routinely administered with resection of arteriovenous malformations. Hematoma formation within the operative site, which used to be a feared complication, is now rarely seen because of improved surgical technique. Postoperative in-hospital recuperation usually takes 7 to 10 days, at which time the patient is ready for discharge. Postoperative angiography to ensure the complete removal of arteriovenous malformations and the elimination of aneurysms is performed routinely. If residual malformation or aneurysm is seen, secondary resection is considered. If a secondary procedure is performed, it is advisable to do it within 2 weeks of the primary procedure to minimize the amount of postoperative scarring present in the operative site and decrease the amount of further dissection necessary.

Prognosis. Current operative mortality for most arteriovenous malformations and aneurysms is less than 5% when the patient is in experienced hands. Certain exceptions to this rule include aneurysms of the vein of Galen that present within the first few days of life with severe congestive heart failure. These lesions continue to be a major challenge to neurosurgery and have a current operative mortality greater than 75%. It should be realized, however, that without surgery virtually all of these patients will die from intractable congestive heart failure. Additional morbidity associated with surgical resection of vascular anomalies is low; it occurs in less than 10% of cases. Although the exact natural history of these lesions is not known, it is realized that recurrent hemorrhage that is life threatening continues to be a possibility until the lesion has been eliminated. Because of the long life expectancy in children, there is more reason to resect a malformation in a child than in an older patient. In addition, vascular surgery appears to be particularly well tolerated by children, with the morbidity and mortality statistics lower in this group than in comparable adult patients.

Important aspects of follow-up. Children who are left with focal neurologic deficits that include hemiparesis and speech disturbance will benefit from aggressive speech therapy and physical therapy. Maximum rehabilitative efforts should be directed at the young child to enable him to function as normally as possible during his lifetime.

Complications. Many patients whose initial symptoms included seizure activity will continue to manifest this tendency and will need postoperative anticonvulsants. In addition, some 20% of patients who did not have seizures prior to intracranial surgery will develop seizure activity at some point in the postoperative course.[27] Because of this, prophylactic anticonvulsants are administered routinely in some centers for 6 to 9 months following craniotomy. Should seizures recur following the slow withdrawal of anticonvulsants, the medication should be reinstituted. Patients who originally show evidence of either subarachnoid or intracerebral bleeding may develop communicating hydrocephalus. This occurs in 10% to 20% of patients.[11,56] A CT brain scan following craniotomy will quickly evaluate the size of the ventricular system and the need for ventriculoperitoneal or ventriculoatrial shunting (Fig. 27-7). Subsequent episodes of bleeding may be associated with partially resected arteriovenous mal-

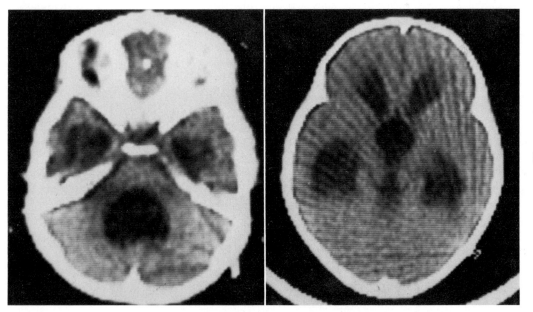

Fig. 27-7. An infant who survived neonatal subarachnoid and intraventricular hemorrhage developed macrocrania and accelerated head growth. **A,** CT brain scan demonstrating moderate to severe enlargement of the fourth ventricle and both temporal horns. **B,** Higher section showing enlargement of the third ventricle and both frontal horns. (The streak artifact is from a recently placed right parietal shunt valve.)

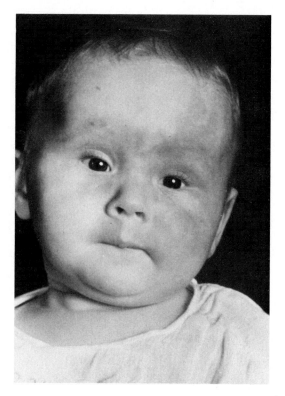

Fig. 27-8. Child with the typical port wine stain over the left side of the face indicative of Sturge-Weber syndrome. The child initially came to medical attention because of a generalized seizure disorder. The child developed a progressive loss of intellectual function and was institutionalized.

formations or inadequately clipped aneurysms. An alternative explanation is the presence of a second lesion that had been unrecognized previously. Although the incidence of multiple aneurysms is said to be lower in children, they occur in 15% to 20% of adult patients. For this reason, subsequent bleeding episodes should be evaluated carefully for the source of the hemorrhage.

Other less common lesions. Arteriovenous malformations that occur in or around the spinal cord are rare. They may present with the acute onset of paraplegia or they may cause unexplained subarachnoid hemorrhage when vascular studies of the brain are unremarkable. In addition, they may present with a slowly progressive paraplegia that is thought to be secondary to either the mass effect of the malformation compressing the spinal cord or the spinal equivalent of the cerebral arterial steal phenomenon. These lesions can now be demonstrated by spinal angiography; and with the use of bipolar coagulation and the operating microscope, they can be resected. This approach is indicated in patients with progressive neurologic deterioration and evidence of spinal subarachnoid hemorrhage.[56]

The Sturge-Weber syndrome is one of the phacomatoses that has as one of its component signs a capillary facial nevus in the distribution of the trigeminal nerve (usually the ophthalmic division) (Fig. 27-8). Children with this rare condi-

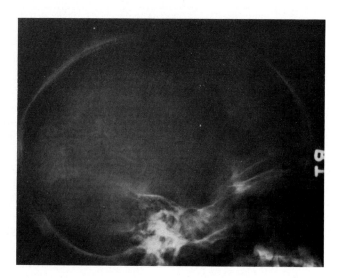

Fig. 27-9. Lateral skull film of a patient with the Sturge-Weber syndrome. Characteristic parietal occipital calcification is seen to occur within the cortex and is described as a "railroad track."

tion have seizure disorders, mental retardation, and delay in motor development. Plain x-ray films of the skull will frequently show the pathognomonic calcification of the cerebral cortex (Fig. 27-9). These patients come to surgical attention because of intractable seizures. Resection of the involved cortex or undercutting of the cortical connections are alternatives that should be used only when medical therapy for the seizures has failed.

The surgical role in occlusive arterial disease in childhood is small. Occasionally, consideration can be given to revascularization of the ischemic brain by use of extracranial-intracranial microvascular anastomosis. The role of this procedure in childhood is currently not well defined but is under study.

TRAUMA

Injuries are the most common cause of death in children and young adults. After the first few months of life, accidents account for more deaths below the age of 14 than the next nine causes combined.[87] At least 25% of such deaths are a direct result of head injury.[25] In addition to the children who actually die as a result of their injury, many who survive are left with a permanent neurologic deficit. The causes of head injury in children and adolescents include automobile accidents (more frequently as a pedestrian than as a passenger), falls, play injuries, and parental abuse.[32,37] The scope of this last category has only recently been recognized and guidelines for diagnosis and follow-up established.[8,41] Although fatal head injuries are common, many more children will suffer an injury that will require medical attention but will be associated with recovery. It is estimated that 10% of children will experience head trauma sometime during childhood that is associated with loss of consciousness,[53] but the vast majority will show complete and full recovery of neurologic function.

Injury to the brain, spinal cord, and peripheral nerves are also important causes of death and disability associated with birth trauma. One third of all neonates dying within 2 weeks of birth do so as a direct result of trauma associated with delivery.[26]

The problem facing the clinician dealing acutely with the traumatized child is to differentiate serious injuries needing immediate referral from those that are trivial and associated with spontaneous and rapid recovery. Such differentiation is particularly important to the clinician who does not have immediate access to neurosurgical support.

Possible findings. Birth trauma of the head is common. Autopsies of full-term stillborns demonstrate that as many as 40% had macroscopic intracranial hemorrhage.[26] This figure is higher in infants born by breech delivery and in premature neonates. Blood or xanthochromia in the CSF is so common as to be considered a normal finding in the newborn.

The scalp is the most commonly affected tissue of the head to be involved with birth trauma. It may demonstrate hemorrhage or swelling as fluid accumulates in various compartments of the scalp. In the usual vertex presentation, the portion of the scalp first seen through the cervical os will become edematous and swollen as the contracting uterus forces this portion of the head through the constricted opening. If the face is the presenting part, it too will demonstrate extravasation of fluid into the soft tissues and become edematous and discolored. This swelling of the newborn scalp is termed caput succedaneum and is not confined by the cranial sutures as a boundary of extension. The swelling is present immediately at the time of delivery and will become less prominent over the following period of hours. Caput succedaneum is commonly seen with vaginal deliveries, particularly in firstborn infants. Pathologically, it represents an accumulation of blood and serum into the scalp. No treatment is required, and no further diagnostic procedures are necessary.

In approximately 1.5% of newborns, scalp swelling will be seen to become more pronounced following the delivery.[91] In addition, this swelling is limited in its extension by the adjacent cranial sutures. This type of scalp mass or swelling is secondary to hemorrhage beneath the pericranium of the skull and cannot extend beyond the suture lines, because the pericranium is firmly attached to the skull at these points. This type of swelling is termed a cephalohematoma. An underlying linear skull fracture will be seen in 5% to 25% of these patients.[91] A cephalohematoma may be responsible for a significant loss of blood and may result in hypotensive shock, anemia, and hyperbilirubinemia. Therapy with fluid and blood replacement may be necessary if the lesion is large. Aspiration of a cephalohematoma, even under relatively sterile conditions, is ill advised for fear of infecting the area. If septicemia is superimposed on a neonate with a cephalohematoma, the avascular hematoma may become secondarily infected with the formation of an abscess. In such cases, culture of the infected hematoma, as well as incision and drainage, continues to be the therapy that will result in the most rapid and predictable improvement. Ordinarily, uncomplicated cephalohematomas require no specific therapy and will resolve in a period of weeks. They may, however, be responsible for skull asymmetry that persists beyond the neonatal period. If radiographs of the skull are obtained after the neonatal period, they may demonstrate calcification of both the inner and outer layers of the hematoma, with asymmetry of the skull (Fig. 27-10). As the outer layer progressively calcifies, the hematoma will eventually be reabsorbed. If the asymmetry is striking, there is some justification for excising the enclosed hematoma cavity for cosmetic purposes. This procedure is suggested only in cases that have persisted for months and show little spontaneous resolution.

In the newborn, massive scalp hemorrhage may also rarely occur in the subgaleal space and is usually associated with a coagulation defect. This also requires prompt therapy to avoid anemia and shock. Hyperbilirubinemia frequently results and may require exchange transfusion.

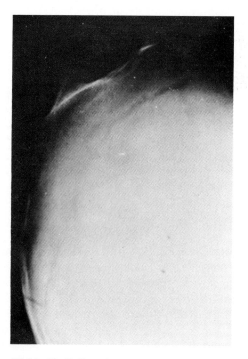

Fig. 27-10. Skull film of a patient with calcified cephalohematoma. Calcification is occurring along the outer aspect of the hematoma while bone is being reabsorbed along the inner aspect.

Hemorrhage within or under the scalp after the first few months of life can almost never be the cause of shock from blood loss. If shock occurs in the setting of a head injury in childhood or adolescence, an alternative cause must be sought (ruptured spleen, hemothorax, retroperitoneal hematoma, etc.). Lacerations of the scalp, on the other hand, can result in significant loss of blood externally and not be appreciated by the physician caring for the patient away from the scene of the accident. Scalp lacerations can also be associated with a depressed skull fracture and laceration of the dura and brain. At the time of suturing of even small scalp or facial lacerations, the integrity of the underlying bone and soft tissue must be evaluated. This is true whether or not x-ray films of the skull have demonstrated a fracture.

The patient's clinical condition—rather than the presence or absence of a skull fracture—remains the best indicator of the degree and severity of the underlying injury. Skull fractures take on importance only as they show the mechanism of injury or as they are a sign of the degree of brain or dural injury. They imply that the force of the blow was sufficient to interrupt the integrity of the bony covering of the brain but do not necessarily imply significant underlying brain injury. Linear skull fractures are associated with some adjacent hemorrhage and tenderness of the surrounding pericranium. If a linear fracture is located across the course of a major dural sinus or extends in the occipital bone to the foramen magnum, it takes on added significance with regard to the possible coexisting accumulation of an extradural or subdural hematoma. Linear skull fractures that occur in the temporal bone and pass through the foramen spinosum or across the course of the middle meningeal artery can be associated with the rapid accumulation of an arterial epidural hematoma. Linear temporal skull fractures may also represent the lateral extent of a more extensive basilar skull fracture.

In general, fractures of the base of the skull result from more severe head trauma than do fractures of the cranial vault. They are usually diagnosed by their associated clinical findings, including hemotympanum, CSF rhinorrhea or otorrhea, subcutaneous ecchymoses about the eyes or over the mastoid, and scleral hemorrhage. Such physical findings are important in establishing the diagnosis because the direct visualization of the fracture on routine x-ray films is frequently not possible.[9]

Hemotympanum may be unilateral or bilateral and is diagnosed simply by visualizing blood behind the tympanic membrane. Blood that is found in the external auditory canal and is not the result of a facial or scalp laceration also implies a basilar skull fracture with a tear of the epithelial lining of the canal. Acutely, the hemotympanum and underlying basilar skull fracture may be associated with decreased hearing, altered equilibrium, and peripheral facial weakness. Detailed examination, including audiometry following recovery from the accident, is essential to assess return of normal cochlear and vestibular function. If disruption of the ossicular chain is the cause of diminished hearing on the follow-up audiogram, referral to an otologist for appropriate therapy will frequently allow restoration of significant function.

CSF otorrhea is suspected if watery fluid is noted to be draining from the ear. *CSF rhinorrhea* is suspected if a similar clear, watery fluid is seen to come from the nose or pharynx with changes of position or with the Valsalva maneuver.

Subcutaneous ecchymoses that occur over the mastoid tip (Battle's sign) or around the eye limited sharply by the palpebral fascia (raccoon sign) imply the presence of a basilar skull fracture. Neither type of ecchymosis is due to soft tissue injury from a direct blow to the area. They result from the dissection of blood into the soft tissues from an underlying fracture of either the mastoid tip and petrous bone or orbit and floor of the anterior fossa. Associated with the raccoon sign may be a *scleral hemorrhage* that originates from the posterior aspect of the globe and dissects forward. Its posterior extent cannot be seen by the examiner; it may thus be differentiated from scleral hemorrhage due to direct trauma to the globe, where the posterior limit of the scleral hemorrhage can usually be appreciated. These subcutaneous ecchymoses usually develop hours after the trauma and are usually not present during the initial clinical evaluation. The presence of either Battle's sign or periorbital ecchymosis strongly suggests an underlying fracture, even if the fracture is not evident on standard radiographs. Epistaxis without nasal or facial trauma can also be a symptom of basilar skull fracture.

Depressed skull fractures that are seen in the neonate's and infant's skull are frequently referred to as "ping-pong" fractures. Clinically, a depression of the surface of the cranial vault can be seen and felt over the fracture site (Fig. 27-11). The depression may disappear when swelling and superficial hemorrhage accumulate over the site itself. Easily confused with the findings of a depressed skull fracture in a neonate or infant, however, is a subperiosteal hematoma. This lesion can mimic the clinical findings of a depressed skull fracture and be difficult to differentiate. Because of this, radiographic confirmation of all depressed skull fractures is necessary. In the more mature and rigid skull of the older child and adolescent, depressed fractures are frequently comminuted and may be associated with underlying dural and cortical lacerations. If a scalp laceration is seen in addition, a traumatized cortex may present on the skin surface when the child is first examined. This type of lesion with a small compound comminuted skull fracture may result from the edge of a swing, or a golf club, hammer, or other object striking the frontal or parietal areas of the skull. Areas of the skull that are particularly vulnerable to penetrating low-velocity wounds include the temporal area just above and in front of the ear and the orbital roof (floor of the anterior cranial fossa), with the point of skin penetration being the upper eyelid or nasal cavity. Sticks and other sharp wooden objects may penetrate these areas, leaving little superficial evidence of trauma.

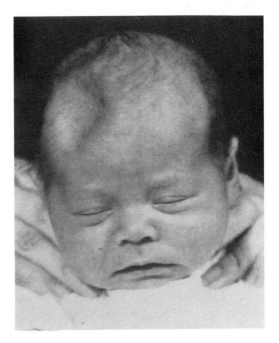

Fig. 27-11. Neonate with "ping-pong" depressed skull fracture in the right frontal area. (From Matson, D. D.: Neurosurgery of infancy and childhood, ed. 2, 1969. Courtesy Charles C Thomas, Publisher, Springfield, Ill.)

Gunshot wounds of the head are relatively common in this country and are a major cause of death and disability in children and adolescents. Depending on the area of the brain involved and the velocity and mass of the missile, clinical findings secondary to tissue destruction will be prominent or absent. Through-and-through gunshot wounds to the head usually cause marked tissue destruction along and adjacent to the path of the bullet. The volume of tissue destroyed is directly related to the mass of the missile and to the square of its velocity. Missiles that enter the skull and do not exit but have their entire course within the substance of the brain may ricochet within the skull and result in massive cerebral destruction. High-velocity bullets that do not penetrate the skull but are simply reflected off the outer table may still cause significant brain destruction under the point of impact. Low-velocity weapons such as pellet guns and BB guns do not usually cause extensive tissue destruction.

Blunt injury of the brain is most frequently mild and associated with minor symptoms. Typically, the patient with minor head injury initially appears stunned or dazed, becomes confused, and then complains of being tired and wants to sleep. He may become nauseated and refuse to eat or actually vomit. Occasionally, there may be a short, generalized seizure, after which the patient will remain postictal for several minutes to hours. If the occipital lobes have received the brunt of the injury, there may be little alteration of the state of consciousness; however, the child may develop cortical blindness: the pupils remain reactive to light but the child is functionally blind. Cortical blindness may persist for several hours and then usually resolves spontaneously.[28] It rarely persists as a permanent sequela of blunt trauma to the head. The patient's lethargy and malaise may persist for several hours or days. During this period he will continue to refuse food, although he may be able to drink and avoid vomiting. The lethargy will slowly improve, and improvement of the appetite will follow. Headaches, dizziness, and inability to concentrate and read may persist for days, weeks, or even months, depending on the severity of the injury. Amnesia for the events associated with the accident (and for the period of time immediately before and for some time after the accident) may also be evident. With time, the amount of memory loss will decrease.

With more severe injuries, the child will be unconscious from the time of the injury. He will not respond to verbal commands and will not talk or open his eyes.[82] Spontaneous decerebrate or decorticate posturing may occur. These responses can also be seen in response to painful stimulation. Decerebrate rigidity is characterized by extension of the arms and legs with internal rotation of the upper extremities. Decorticate rigidity involves extension of the lower extremities but flexion of the upper extremities at the elbows. Respiration may become irregular when the child assumes either of these postures. Various respiratory patterns can be seen, depending on the level of brain stem dysfunction.[69] In the presence of progressive deterioration, the unattended child with increased intracranial pressure may demonstrate transtentorial herniation. In addition to the alteration of consciousness and the development of either decerebrate or decorticate posturing, the child will be seen to develop progressive dilatation of the pupil and paralysis of the extraocular muscles innervated by the third cranial nerve. The eye will assume a position of abduction and slight inferior displacement with preservation of the function of the fourth and sixth cranial nerves. In addition, there will be ptosis. These eye findings may be seen unilaterally or bilaterally. With transtentorial herniation, they will occur first on the side of the mass lesion. Before death the child will lose his decerebrate rigidity and become flaccid as the level of dysfunction extends below the pons.[69] Severe respiratory irregularities develop, and death becomes imminent. Severe elevation of the intracranial pressure may also cause the sudden onset of pulmonary edema.[23] Increased intracranial pressure may be secondary to an extracerebral collection of blood (subdural or epidural hematoma), an intraparenchymal hematoma, or massive cerebral contusion and edema unassociated with significant focal hemorrhage. Following trauma to the head or neck, the carotid artery may thrombose, resulting in infarction in the distribution of the occluded vessel.

Injury to the spinal cord is uncommon in childhood in comparison with head injury. In addition to being infrequent, the diagnosis in infancy and childhood may be made more difficult by the minimal radiographic evidence. At the time of delivery, excessive traction may be transmitted to the cervical spine, either in an attempt to deliver the infant's shoulder or in an attempt to deliver the aftercoming head of a breech presentation. The ligamentous connections and disc bonds of the cervical spine may be stretched beyond their elastic limit, and the cervical or upper thoracic spinal cord may actually be severed or torn. Neonates who suffer from spinal cord injury are seldom diagnosed correctly during their initial evaluation.[33] Spinal reflexes can easily be mistaken for spontaneous movement. In addition to the obvious presentation of the paraplegic or quadriplegic newborn with spinal reflexes only, multiple other presentations can be seen. A neonate with respiratory distress syndrome may, on close examination, be found to have respiratory distress not from hyaline membrane disease but from a lack of contraction of the intercostal muscles, resulting in diaphragmatic breathing. An alternative presentation is that with fever of unknown origin. These neonates are frequently evaluated extensively before it is found that the infant has actually lost central control of temperature regulation. Spinal reflex activity in the newborn will initially confuse all but the most astute clinician.

In older children and teenagers spinal cord injury occurs in association with automobile accidents, diving accidents, and falls. The older the child, the less laxity there is to the spinal ligaments and the more likely there is to be radiographic evidence of bony trauma to the spine. Occasionally in the young child with a spinal injury, the entire radiographic diagnosis will depend on indirect evidence of spinal trauma, including development of a paraspinal mass with loss of definition of structures that are normally seen around the spine, including the normal psoas muscle shadow and the fat stripe anterior to the cervical spine. Physical examination will almost always reveal pain at the point of spinal damage, forcing the child to guard and protect the involved area. An important exception to this rule is the child who is unconscious and has a spinal injury. These patients cannot protect themselves against spinal manipulation, which may result in further neurologic damage. For this reason, all posttraumatic comatose patients should be regarded as having a spinal injury until it is proved otherwise. Transportation and care of these children should reflect the possibility of this association. The injury to the spine most frequently results in myelopathy from injury to the spinal cord. Frequently, there is evidence of weakness of the legs and/or arms, a sensory level roughly corresponding to the level of motor dysfunction, and a decrease in or absence of anal tone and voluntary control of the bladder. Sacral sensation may be spared with intramedullary lesions (hematomas) and should always be evaluated in cases of spinal cord disease. An alternative presentation of spinal trauma is with radiculopathy from injury to the nerve roots as they exit the spine. In this case, pain may be radicular, radiating down the involved extremity in a specific nerve root distribution. In addition, decreased strength and sensation in the same nerve root distribution may be demonstrated.

Peripheral nerve defects in the neonate and young child are more easily diagnosed than spinal cord or brain injury because of the total lack of movement in the involved muscles secondary to interruption of the final common pathway. Birth injuries can occasionally affect the brachial plexus or facial nerve. These lesions are becoming increasingly uncommon because of improved obstetric care. Brachial plexus lesions may involve the upper plexus (Erb's palsy) or the lower plexus (Klumpke's palsy). Erb's palsy results from a traction injury to the upper aspect of the brachial plexus, usually involving the C-5 and C-6 innervated muscles. With this type of lesion, the neonate's arm will lie limply by his side. Weakness will easily be demonstrated in the deltoid, biceps, and supinator muscles. Movement of the hand and flexors of the wrist will usually continue to be active. The arm will be held in an adducted and internally rotated position. With stimulation, Moro's reflex will be strikingly asymmetric with little to no movement about the involved shoulder and elbow but with preservation of vigorous movement about the wrist and hand on the involved side. This type of traction lesion is much more common than involvement of the lower aspect of the brachial plexus. Klumpke's palsy is characterized by involvement of the C-8 and T-1 innervated muscles; there is profound weakness of the small muscles of the hand and development of ipsilateral Horner's syndrome.

Beyond the newborn period, peripheral nerve injuries occur secondary to lacerations, injections, and fractures. The weakness and sensory loss is in the distribution of the involved nerve. It is important to assess the initial extent of the injury accurately so that subsequent change can be evaluated properly.

Common occurrences. Cerebral concussion is by far the most common form of head injury. The blow to the head may be associated with a brief period of loss of consciousness, followed by rapid and complete recovery. Following recovery of consciousness, the patient is frequently bothered by headache, lethargy, malaise, nausea, anorexia, and dizziness. The infant or young child will be irritable and easily upset. The resolution of these nonspecific complaints is usually complete in a period of hours to days.

Cerebral contusion also results from blunt head injury and occurs at a point where the brain contacts the inner table of the skull or the free edge of the tentorium. Areas of frequent injury include the undersurface of the frontal lobes and the frontal, temporal, and occipital tips. In addition, the brain may become contused directly under the site of trauma to the skull, as in a depressed skull fracture. Contusion may involve extensive areas of the brain and is frequently associated with cerebral edema. Focal neurologic dysfunction will occur if the contusion involves a critical area of brain function. Unconsciousness is usually more prolonged with cerebral contusion, and the degree of cerebral swelling is greater. The cerebral edema may be so extensive that transtentorial herniation results. Contusions that occur directly under the point of impact are referred to as *coup* injuries, whereas those that occur away from the direct area of the injury are referred to as *contrecoup* lesions.

Brain stem contusion is seen relatively frequently in childhood.[17] In addition to unconsciousness, these children may exhibit dysfunction of multiple cranial nerves. Evidence of brain stem compromise in adults carries a grave prognosis. In children, however, injuries to this sensitive structure may be associated with complete recovery. This may occur after a prolonged period of unconsciousness lasting several weeks. Residual cranial nerve dysfuncion may persist despite the recovery of consciousness and motor function of the extremities.

Accumulation of blood within the subdural space commonly occurs as the result of trauma in the anteroposterior (AP) plane. The large cortical veins that drain the cerebral hemispheres attach to the sagittal sinus, which is fixed and held in place by the fibrous and inelastic dura. With sudden and excessive movement, these bridging veins tear near their point of entrance into the sagittal sinus as the brain moves in relationship to the dura. Venous blood will then accumulate in the subdural space. If large quantities of blood are accumu-

lated quickly, or if the injury is associated with significant cerebral contusion with swelling of the underlying cerebral hemisphere, the child may have acute symptoms of an altered mental status, seizures, hemiparesis, and finally transtentorial herniation. Lesions that present for clinical evaluation less than 24 hours after the injury are termed *acute subdural hematomas*. They are usually associated with severe brain injury, for which the overall mortality is high (greater than 50%). This is not because of the difficulty of treating the extracerebral blood collection but because of the frequently associated severe brain contusion or laceration that accompanies lesions presenting acutely. This type of lesion may be encountered in the neonate in association with birth trauma, in the child as a result of being hit by an automobile, or in the teenager as the driver or passenger involved in an automobile accident. This lesion can also be seen in association with fractures of the long bones and ribs and with retinal hemorrhages. The fractures can often be dated prior to the time of the head injury and are strong evidence of child abuse.

Subacute subdural hematomas come to clinical attention between 1 and 14 days following injury. The consistency of the hemorrhage in this case, which can be likened to currant jelly, may make evacuation by needle or through a burr hole or limited craniectomy difficult. The degree of associated brain injury is less than that associated with the acute presentation of a subdural hematoma.

Chronic subdural hematomas of infancy are discussed in Chapter 12 in the section on the infant and toddler. If these lesions are seen in a child or teenager, however, they do not present with macrocrania but with evidence of compromise of the supratentorial compartment. Clinically, this compromise may become manifest by the onset of seizures, hemiparesis, headache, or lethargy. In response to the accumulation of blood in the subdural space, membranes are formed around the hematoma. Classically, the inner membrane is adjacent to the arachnoid and is thin and transparent. The outer membrane is much thicker and will contain multiple delicate and friable blood vessels. Chronic subdural hematomas may be associated with repeated episodes of hemorrhage. In this case, hematomas of different ages will be seen in the subdural space. These compartments will frequently not communicate one with the other, and at the time of surgical removal significant variation in the thickness of the outer membrane of each of the compartments may be seen. The fluid within a chronic subdural hematoma can be likened to crankcase oil. Following the evacuation of the chronic subdural hematoma, the brain may not immediately expand to refill the subdural space. (Acute subdural hematomas, on the other hand, are associated with a rapid and alarmingly quick reexpansion by the underlying edematous brain.)

The accumulation of blood within the subdural space may also be seen outside the setting of trauma and result from coagulation disturbances or as a result of rapid decompression of a dilated ventricular system secondary to a shunting procedure. Blood may also accumulate in the subdural space over the cerebellum. This is most frequently encountered with fractures overlying the dural sinuses, with bleeding occurring in the subdural space from the lacerated sinus. As the mass accumulates, the child becomes increasingly somnolent and develops hypotonia ipsilateral to the lesion. Respiratory irregularities are also common. If prompt action is not taken to evacuate the posterior fossa subdural hematoma, the child will rapidly deteriorate over a period of hours and die.

Intracranial hemorrhage that accumulates in the epidural space in the adult and in the older child is frequently associated with bleeding from a laceration of the middle meningeal artery.[56,64] This may or may not be seen in conjunction with a fracture of the squamous portion of the temporal bone. Clinically, the adolescent or older child will receive a blow to the head that may result in unconsciousness lasting for several minutes. Following this, there may be a spontaneous recovery, as is seen with most cerebral concussions. Over the ensuing several hours, the patient will progressively complain of headache, anorexia, and lethargy and begin to vomit. This lucid interval corresponds to the time necessary for the accumulation of blood in the epidural space from the lacerated middle meningeal artery. Finally, a critical mass of blood is reached and the patient will lose consciousness. Quickly following the onset of unconsciousness, the pupil ipsilateral to the epidural hematoma will dilate and become nonreactive to light. Increased tone and a positive Babinski response may be seen contralateral to the dilated pupil. If the lesion continues to be unrecognized and untreated, the contralateral pupil will become dilated and fixed. The spastic weakness will then involve all four extremities and quickly be seen to progress into decorticate or decerebrate posturing. Blood pressure elevation, bradycardia, and finally respiratory irregularities will follow, resulting in the patient's death.

Because the hematoma is a consequence of arterial bleeding, the time between the onset of unconsciousness and irreversible brain stem hemorrhage or death may be short (minutes to hours). In more than half of the children, however, epidural hematomas may accumulate over days before they reach a size that may cause clinical symptoms. Such bleeding is frequently venous in origin.[52,56] Fractures across suture lines, over the posterior fossa, or separation of a suture (e.g., lambdoid) should bring this diagnosis to mind. Here again, however, once a critical mass of blood is reached and the patient develops clinical symptoms, further decompensation may be quite rapid. Epidural hematomas are usually unilateral and occur much less frequently than subdural hematomas (a ratio of 1 to 10). Because the degree of underlying brain damage is usually relatively small with an epidural hematoma in comparison with that of an acute subdural hematoma, complete recovery of neurologic function is usually seen if appropriate therapy is accomplished prior to the development of irreversible changes. Clinical recognition of an epidural hematoma is unparalleled in its importance in the treatment of traumatic injuries of the head.

Subarachnoid hemorrhage is most commonly seen secondary to head trauma. This can be seen with varying degrees of head injury and can be recognized clinically by the development of meningismus, photophobia, and hyperthermia. Blood in the subarachnoid space is associated with xanthochromic discoloration of the spinal fluid. Bloody spinal fluid as a result of a subarachnoid hemorrhage may be differentiated from a traumatic lumbar puncture by the presence of xanthochromia in the supernatant following centrifugation. No active therapy is necessary for the treatment of posttraumatic subarachnoid hemorrhage. The normal resorptive pathway for the CSF may be temporarily occluded by the subarachnoid blood. If this persists, communicating hydrocephalus may develop, which will require the insertion of a shunting device. This is an unusual but well-recognized complication of head injury.

Blood may also accumulate within the substance of the brain at the site of a cerebral laceration or contusion. The hemorrhage may be large and associated with major shifts of the ventricular system away from the hemorrhage, or the hemorrhages may be multiple, scattered, and small. Intraparenchymal brain hemorrhage commonly occurs in areas of the brain that are predisposed to cerebral contusion and are usually associated with large areas of cerebral edema. If the intraparenchymal hemorrhage is large and responsible for clinical symptoms of increased intracranial pressure or focal neurologic deficit, the patient may improve by the evacuation of the hematoma. Smaller hemorrhages associated with large amounts of cerebral edema are not generally considered for surgical evacuation. Hemorrhage may also be seen within the brain stem secondary to transtentorial herniation. In this location it is thought to be associated with irreversible clinical changes and a frequent cause of permanent unconsciousness.

Evaluation. The most important aspect of the initial evaluation is a detailed neurologic and general physical examination. The extent of the examination is dictated by the patient's clinical condition. Patients with normal vital signs who are alert and awake, or who are easily arousable, may be examined in a deliberate and complete fashion, whereas patients with airway obstruction, shock, or other life-threatening signs are best served by immediate attention to the maintenance of ventilation and perfusion.

As mentioned previously, patients with a history of head injury associated with an initial cerebral concussion followed by rapid return of neurologic function to normal should be monitored carefully for further neurologic deterioration. This may occur minutes, hours, or even days following the initial trauma. The rapidity with which the secondary deterioration occurs dictates the evaluation that is indicated. A most important aspect of the patient's care is to determine the tempo of neurologic change. If the patient is initially evaluated in the emergency room following an automobile accident, for example, and is seen to be conscious, cooperative, and without focal neurologic signs and in a period of minutes becomes comatose with evidence of a third-nerve palsy and contralateral hemiparesis, further evaluation is contraindicated. The patient is assumed to have an expanding extracerebral hematoma, which should be evacuated immediately without further diagnostic procedures. If the patient is brought to the operating room and no extracerebral hematoma is found, he

should then be returned for further evaluation. This tactic is necessary to prevent irreversible changes in the brain stem as a result of a rapidly expanding supratentorial mass. Although some patients with generalized cerebral edema may be unnecessarily subjected to burr holes during a search for extracerebral hematomas, the reward is in finding patients who have deteriorated rapidly and who do, in fact, have an epidural hematoma as a result of the rapid accumulation of arterial blood from a torn middle meningeal artery. The additional time required preoperatively to prove the existence of an epidural hematoma will frequently be associated with permanent neurologic damage that could have been avoided by the rapid evacuation of the suspected lesion. This approach has limited applicability, and the vast majority of patients with stable examinations can be evaluated carefully by physical examination and radiographic means prior to the consideration of surgery.

In the unconscious patient as well as in the conscious patient, trauma to other organ systems must be evaluated carefully. After the first few months of life, shock cannot be accounted for by blood loss under the scalp or within the cranial vault. An alternative site of blood loss must then be sought. Cervical spinal injuries should also be assumed to be present in all posttraumatic unconscious patients until spinal x-ray films show no evidence of spinal trauma or instability.

Following the initial history and physical examination, the patient should be considered for x-ray examination of the cervical spine and skull. In the patient who has never lost consciousness or was only momentarily dazed or frightened and who has minimal complaints of head or neck pain in addition to a normal neurologic examination, the necessity and usefulness of these examinations can be questioned.[7,30] Much has been written about the necessity to study radiographically every patient who has sustained even the slightest head injury. Guidelines should therefore be set up to aid the emergency room physician in determining which patients should and should not receive x-ray films of the skull and cervical spine. In general, infants and young children who cannot localize pain well should receive x-ray evaluation of the head and cervical spine. The ability to perform a critical evaluation of the nervous system in these patients is frequently compromised because of their lack of cooperation. In addition, patients who are unconscious or who demonstrate evidence

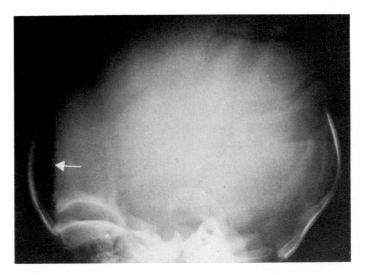

Fig. 27-12. Communicated and widely diastatic skull fracture and frontal pneumocephalus in a young child. The radiograph was taken with the child in the supine position, allowing for an air fluid level (arrow). The injury occurred as a result of child abuse and resulted in the child's death soon after this radiograph was taken.

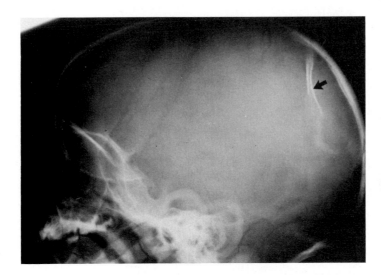

Fig. 27-13. Depressed parietal skull fracture associated with a dural laceration.

of a focal neurologic deficit should also have the advantage of films of the skull and cervical spine. These may demonstrate evidence of pneumocephalus (Fig. 27-12) (air within the skull that implies a fracture of the skull base involving the paranasal sinuses or mastoid air cells). The extent and location of fractures may also be appreciated. Fractures that cross dural sinuses (Fig. 27-13) and those over the posterior fossa with extension to the foramen magnum bear close clinical evaluation.[56] Patients with evidence of focal trauma consistent

with the possibility of a depressed skull fracture should also have radiographs made. In addition to routine views, tangential views of the involved area may demonstrate the extent of the depression more clearly. Children suspected of having penetrating wounds of the head are also candidates for skull films. Of importance in evaluating linear skull fractures is the degree of diastasis. If the lines of the fracture are separated by more than 3 mm, there is a strong likelihood that a dural laceration is also present at that point. Linear fractures with

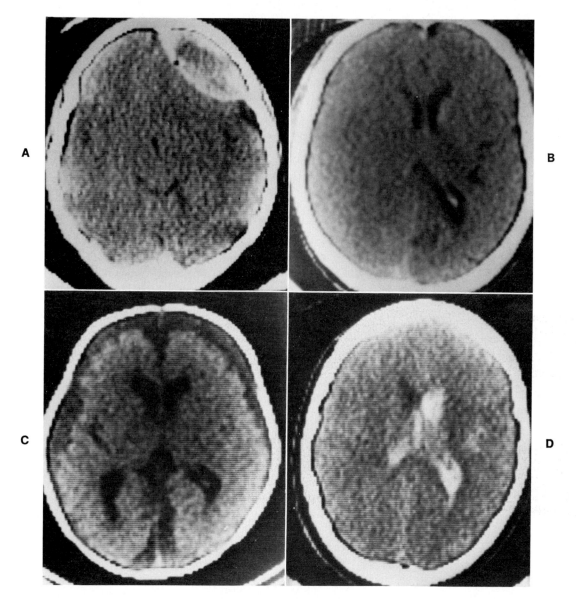

Fig. 27-14. A, Unenhanced CT brain scan of a patient with an acute epidural hematoma in the right frontal area. The lesion's high attenuation in comparison with that of brain and its biconcave appearance are both indicative of an acute epidural hematoma. **B,** Subacute subdural hematoma over the left convexity. The exact size of the lesion is much more difficult to outline because of its isoattenuation with the surrounding brain. This problem is encountered more frequently with lesions that are 7 to 15 days old. When bilateral symmetric lesions are present, the diagnostic difficulty is compounded, since no midline shift may be present. **C,** Chronic subdural hematomas are easily recognized by their low attenuation. **D,** Posttraumatic intraventricular hemorrhage is an unusual occurrence but is easily diagnosed by CT scanning wherein the hemorrhage conforms to the position and shape of the ventricular system.

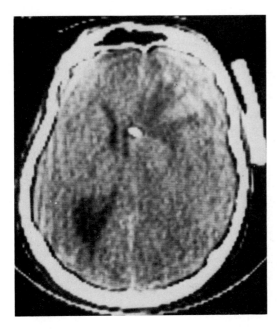

Fig. 27-15. CT brain scan of a patient with scattered intracerebral right frontal hemorrhage and contusion. The shift away from the area of damage is apparent. The dense white dot in the right frontal horn is an intraventricular catheter used to monitor intracranial pressure and periodically remove CSF to decrease the intracranial tension. The patient recovered uneventfully after several days of coma and elevated intracranial pressure.

this degree of diastasis are then considered for exploration and repair of the lacerated dura in an attempt to prevent the formation of a leptomeningeal cyst.

Although they are of significant help in the evaluation of patients sustaining head injury, x-ray films of the skull by no means give the detailed information that can be obtained from a CT scan of the brain. Trauma has been one of the areas in which CT scanning has proved most helpful.[54] Evidence of extracerebral or intracerebral blood collections can easily be recognized with the aid of this diagnostic modality (Fig. 27-14). In addition, the degree of cerebral swelling and shift of the ventricular system can easily be seen (Fig. 27-15). CT scanning has now almost totally replaced cerebral angiography as the diagnostic procedure of choice in the evaluation of acute head trauma. The EEG is helpful in the diagnosis of episodic disorders of the cerebral cortex (seizures) but is unreliable and frequently misleading in the evaluation of surgically correctable posttraumatic intracranial hematomas. Lumbar puncture in the setting of

acute head trauma has little value and can be dangerous if it precipitates transtentorial herniation. The information that can be obtained in the immediate posttraumatic period almost never justifies the risk involved in performing a lumbar puncture in the presence of increased intracranial pressure from either an intracranial hematoma or acute brain swelling.

Children who come to medical attention with evidence of head trauma and retinal hemorrhage are likely victims of child abuse.[24] Infants and children sustaining head injury under ill-defined or mysterious circumstances can be evaluated by a radiographic skeletal survey looking for healing fractures of various ages. In addition, a detailed social history taken by a knowledgeable and compassionate social worker will be of significant help. Burns of the fingers and palms are also indicative of this problem, which is now being recognized as having an alarming frequency.[41]

Children with suspected spinal lesions are carefully immobilized and then studied radiographically. Frequently, infants and young children with spinal injuries will have relatively normal plain x-ray films (Fig. 27-16, *A*). Subtle changes such as those of paraspinal hemorrhage may be the only indication of recent trauma. In patients with strong indications of spinal injury, tomography and myelography may be of benefit in confirming abnormalities that may correspond to the clinical level of neurologic dysfunction (Fig. 27-16, *B*). If the patient is ambulatory, complaining of pain only, further information can sometimes be gained by asking the child to carry the painful area of the spine through the extremes of flexion and extension while being radiographed to see if instability is, in fact, present. An additional helpful diagnostic tool that will confirm the level of trauma is the radionuclide bone scan of the spine. Areas of recent trauma will show increased activity, which can then add additional weight to the findings present on routine x-ray studies (Fig. 27-17).

Peripheral nerve trauma can largely be diagnosed by the clinical examination. An electromyogram performed in the recovery phase of the illness may help to localize the lesion and give early evidence of regeneration in incomplete lesions.

Referral. All patients with serious head injuries, suspected spinal cord injuries, and peripheral nerve lacerations should be evaluated on an emergency basis. Children who sustain minor head injuries without loss of consciousness and are sim-

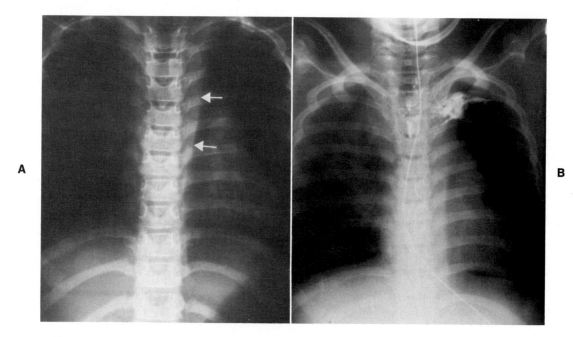

Fig. 27-16. A, AP spinal film of a 6-year-old child hit by an automobile. The child was paraplegic with a sensory level at T-4. The bony elements of the spine were thought to be normal. Detailed tomography of the area of clinical suspicion failed to reveal any significant bony injury. The strongest evidence of spinal trauma on the plain spinal films is the paraspinal swelling on the patient's left (arrows). **B,** The myelogram, in contrast to the plain films, is grossly abnormal, with contrast leaving the spinal canal and entering the left chest. The spinal cord and dura are disrupted between T-2 and T-3. The film also shows evidence of bilateral pneumothoraces.

ply dazed or stunned may be safely evaluated by the primary care physician and then observed for the next several hours. If the child returns to normal and remains without complaint, serious sequelae from the head injury are unlikely. All patients who were unconscious even for a relatively brief time should be observed for at least 12 hours in a facility capable of evacuating an extracerebral hematoma on an emergency basis. Commonly, these children are observed overnight, either in the emergency room or on the hospital ward. Their condition is evaluated on an hourly basis, and any fluctuation in the level of consciousness or responsiveness should be reported quickly to the neurosurgical staff caring for the patient. Ambulatory patients with persistent symptoms of headache, neck pain, altered vision, weakness, or seizure activity should also be evaluated by a neurosurgeon. This can usually be done on an outpatient basis with x-ray films of the skull and/or spine and a CT brain scan.

Medical versus surgical treatment. The vast majority of children with cerebral concussions need neither medical nor surgical therapy and will recover completely without evidence of residual neurologic dysfunction. Many patients with cerebral contusions will also recover without specific therapy. In the setting of increased intracranial pressure with alteration of the mental status and without CT evidence of either an extracerebral or intraparenchymal hematoma, medical therapy directed toward decreasing cerebral swelling will frequently benefit the patient. Such therapy includes elevation of the head to enhance venous drainage; administration of dehydration agents (e.g., mannitol, urea, or glycerol) or diuretics (e.g., furosemide); intubation and mechanical hyperventilation, paralyzing the patient if necessary to maintain the Pco_2 in the range of 25 to 30 torr; removal of intraventricular fluid;[49,59] and administration of barbiturates (e.g. thiopental, phenobarbital).[51] Using one or more of these techniques, intracranial hypertension can be controlled in the majority of children, even those with massive cerebral contusions and increased intracranial pressure. Patients with evidence of increased intracranial pressure and accumulation of either extracerebral or intraparenchymal hemorrhage should

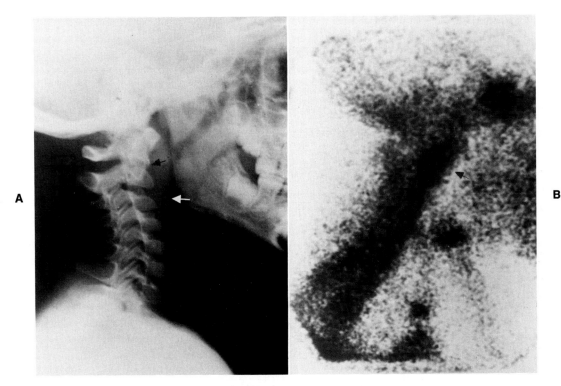

Fig. 27-17. A, Lateral cervical spine film of a patient who fell while playing and refused to move his neck voluntarily. The lower spine is normal. The paraspinal soft tissue anterior to the spine is thickened (white arrow), and the junction of the odontoid and the body of C-2 appears irregular (black arrow). An open-mouth view of the base of the odontoid appeared relatively normal. **B,** A regional bone scan shows the area in question at the junction of the odontoid and the body of C-2 to have unquestionable increased activity (arrow), implying recent trauma.

have consideration given to removal of the hemorrhage.

Patients with evidence of penetrating wounds of the head must have the entry site debrided of bony spicules and debris. Penetration of the skull by a piece of wood is particularly apt to produce a brain abscess. Every effort should be made to recognize such penetration and to remove the foreign body prior to the development of a serious infection.[58] Low-velocity missiles should be removed along with fragments of bone that have been driven into the brain. High-velocity missiles are considered sterile, and removal is unnecessary; however, bony spicules and debris should be removed, as in any other lesion.

Linear skull fractures in general require no therapy. Those that are widely diastatic and have suspected underlying dural lacerations should be surgically explored and the lacerated dura repaired. A significantly depressed skull fracture (>5 mm) should be elevated. Again, the dura should be inspected for laceration and repaired if necessary.

Basilar skull fractures rarely need surgical attention except when they are associated with persistent CSF rhinorrhea or otorrhea.

Typical spinal injuries in children may be managed conservatively with immobilization to allow for healing of the ligamentous and soft tissues that have been disrupted. Penetrating wounds of the spine, like those of the head, must be debrided to the point of their maximum penetration. It is important to perform this debridement acutely, before infection can take place. The indications for surgical exploration of nonpenetrating spinal injuries include progressive neurologic deterioration despite immobilization, all injuries associated with lesions of the conus medullaris or cauda equina with a neurologic deficit, and patients with a complete myelographic block and a neurologic deficit compatible with a spinal cord lesion at that point. The myelographic block may be secondary to a traumatically herniated nucleus pulposus, to an extradural or intramedullary hematoma, or, more commonly, simply to swelling of the traumatized spinal cord. If bony spicules can be seen to penetrate the spinal canal and impinge on the spinal cord, these should be removed. In the patient with an unstable thoracic or thoracolumbar fracture, even in the face of complete neurologic dysfunction, an argument can be made for early surgical exploration of the spinal lesion and stabilization with Harrington rod instrumentation and posterior fusion to allow for early mobilization and rehabilitation. Quadriplegic patients may benefit from surgical exploration of a cervical fracture site if signs of an incomplete lesion in an important cervical root are present. It is important here, however, to emphasize some conditions that contraindicate surgical exploration. Patients with evidence of a central cord syndrome[75] (with weakness of the arms out of proportion to weakness of the legs), patients with stable spinal fractures and no evidence of myelographic block, and patients with unstable fractures that are associated with a high rate of spontaneous fusion if they are simply immobilized (e.g., hangman's fracture) are usually not surgical candidates.

Peripheral nerve injuries associated with either stretch or compression of the nerve are treated conservatively and watched for 4 to 6 weeks. If evidence of regeneration exists, a further period of conversative therapy is indicated. If no clinical or electrical evidence of regeneration has occurred, the patient should be considered for surgical exploration of the involved nerve or plexus. Peripheral nerves that have been cleanly lacerated by either a knife, razor, or other sharp object may be considered for immediate reanastomosis if the wound is considered to be relatively clean. If a question exists as to the viability of the cut ends of the peripheral nerve, primary repair should be delayed for 4 to 6 weeks, at which time the devitalized area of the peripheral nerve will be well demarcated and can be amputated.[71] Birth injuries of the brachial plexus are frequently followed conservatively for at least 6 months before surgical exploration is considered.

Surgical options. Trauma to the scalp without interruption of the integrity of the skin is frequently associated with the formation of a subgaleal or subperiosteal hematoma. Blood collecting in either of these spaces needs no surgical evacuation or needling. In fact, such aspiration or surgical drainage introduces the risk of infection. Over a period of days to weeks, the hematoma will usually resolve spontaneously. In neonates cephalohematomas associated with birth may occasionally calcify. If the cephalohematoma is large and has not shown a tendency to resolve by 6 months of age, consideration should be given to the surgical excision of the calcified cephalohematoma. This is a cosmetic procedure that carries low risk but is only rarely indicated. Recently formed cephalohematomas may become secondarily infected as a result of septicemia. In this case, the hematoma itself will become tender and warm and will be associated with systemic evidence of infection, including hyperpyrexia, an elevated white blood cell

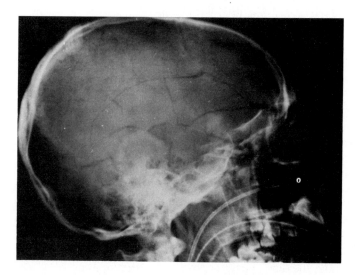

Fig. 27-18. Severely comminuted skull fracture from a motorcycle accident.

count, and malaise. The infected hematoma should be incised and allowed to drain, and appropriate antibiotic therapy begun.

Scalp lacerations are sutured after the hair-containing skin around the laceration is shaved. The eyebrow is an exception to this general rule and is never shaved because of its slow rate of regrowth and resultant cosmetic defect.[39] The laceration is then vigorously irrigated to clean it of debris and foreign material, and the underlying skull is carefully inspected for evidence of fracture. Devitalized pericranium or galea is excised, and the laceration is reapproximated with a single layer of monofilament suture. If areas of the scalp have been avulsed, the hair is shaved from the adjacent skin and a rotation flap is designed to cover the exposed skull. In some patients it may be necessary to place a split-thickness skin graft over the exposed intact pericranium from which the rotation flap has been moved. When large areas of the scalp have been devascularized and avulsed, microvascular reanastomosis has been shown to be of value.[14]

Most skull fractures are linear and nondisplaced and require no specific therapy. As mentioned previously, fractures that cross the course of the middle meningeal artery, the dural sinuses, or the paranasal sinuses or that extend to the foramen magnum require careful and close follow-up for fear of the development of an extracerebral hematoma or CSF leakage. Linear skull fractures in children associated with separation of the lambdoid suture are not infrequently associated with accumulation of an epidural hematoma, and these also require special attention. Basilar skull fractures, like linear skull fractures of the vault, usually require no specific therapy for the fracture itself. If persistent CSF rhinorrhea or otorrhea develops, surgical repair of the dural laceration may be indicated. It should be emphasized that basilar skull fractures may be associated with traumatic subarachnoid hemorrhage. They are, however, rarely associated with extracerebral hematomas of clinical significance. Linear skull fractures that are widely diastatic are frequently associated with a dural laceration, particularly if the radiographic measurement of the diastasis is greater than 4 mm. In these cases, repair of the suspected dural laceration should be performed to prevent the formation of a leptomeningeal cyst.[84]

Grossly comminuted skull fractures are almost always associated with very significant cerebral contusion (Fig. 27-18). No specific therapy for the skull fracture is indicated; however, much effort will be necessary to control the intracranial pressure associated with the contusion. Depressed skull fractures should be elevated if the amount of depression is greater than 5 mm. In infancy the "ping-pong" fracture occurs; and although a small number will elevate spontaneously, most will require surgical therapy to hasten this process. This can be done simply by placing a small linear incision adjacent to the depressed fracture. A limited craniectomy is performed, and a periosteal elevator is inserted under the depressed fracture, manipulating it into a normal position (Fig. 27-19). This procedure is preferred to continuing clinical observation while hoping for spontaneous resolution as the brain applies sufficient pressure to the depressed fracture to correct the deformity. Severely depressed fractures are frequently associated with interruption of the overlying skin and contamination of the brain. It is important in such cases to

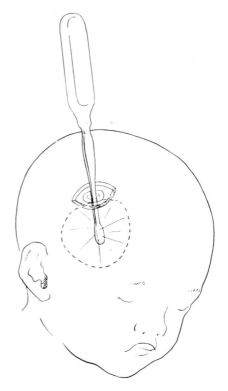

Fig. 27-19. Technique of elevating a "ping-pong" depressed skull fracture through a limited scalp and bony opening. (From Matson, D. D.: Neurosurgery of infancy and childhood, ed. 2, 1969. Courtesy Charles C Thomas, Publisher, Springfield, Ill.)

explore the wound, debride it of foreign material (including devitalized and necrotic brain), and restore an intact dural layer to prevent further brain herniation (cerebral fungus). If the wound is grossly contaminated, it is best to remove the fracture fragments and return the child for an elective cranioplasty at a future time. If the bone fragments are easily cleaned, they may be replaced and cranioplasty avoided. Any dural laceration must be sutured.

Penetrating wounds of the brain, like compound depressed fractures, must be debrided of contaminated material. High-velocity gunshot wounds will be associated with multiple small bony spicules driven into the adjacent brain. These must all be located at the time of surgical exploration and removed.[29] The high-velocity missile itself may be left in place. Penetrating wounds from sticks or branches will be associated with a particularly high rate of infection unless the foreign material is totally removed. Again, the dura is reapproximated, cranioplasty is not performed, and the scalp is sutured in a single layer after the devitalized tissue has been debrided.

Epidural hematomas that present with acute deterioration of neurologic function may be primarily evacuated through a twist drill or burr hole in the emergency room. The patient should then be brought quickly to the operating room; the head is shaved, and a small linear incision is made in a coronal plane anterior and superior to the external auditory canal. The overlying temporal muscle is split, and a limited craniectomy is performed. The source of bleeding is identified and coagulated, usually through a craniectomy with a hole the size of a silver dollar. It may be necessary to find the foramen spinosum and occlude the middle meningeal artery at its point of intracranial penetration. The wound is then irrigated to ensure that all bleeding has stopped, and the soft tissues are reapproximated. A more deliberate procedure can be carried out in the patient with chronic presentation of an epidural hematoma that has been outlined by a CT scan. Again, a limited craniectomy is performed directly over the clot and the source of bleeding is identified and stopped.

In the emergency situation it may be difficult to differentiate an acute subdural hematoma from an epidural hematoma clinically. Both lesions may present with an acute deterioration of neurologic function. In general, however, epidural hematomas are much less common and are associated

with less underlying cerebral contusion. If the child is thought to be a surgical emergency and is taken directly to the operating room without diagnostic studies, it may be necessary to place multiple burr holes on both sides of the head to search for the suspected hematoma. The position of these holes is such that they can be used to fashion a craniotomy flap should this be desired (Fig. 27-20). If clotted blood is present that can be only subtotally removed, a craniotomy will be necessary to evacuate the hematoma completely. In the presence of transtentorial herniation, consideration may be given to amputation of the anterior portion of the temporal lobe to relieve brain stem compression and restore third-nerve function. In general, however, removal of traumatized brain should be avoided except as a lifesaving measure. Occasionally, in the setting of transtentorial herniation and ocular motor palsy, the patient may develop hemiparesis ipsilateral to the dilated pupil. This hemiparesis is thought to be secondary to compression of the contralateral cerebral peduncle against the free edge of the tentorium as the brain stem is pushed to the opposite side of the skull (Kernohan's notch). This situation occurs uncommonly but it emphasizes the fact that ocular motor dysfunction is a more reliable sign as to which side of the brain is being maximally compressed and is associated with an extracerebral hematoma. In addition to burr holes placed over the temporal

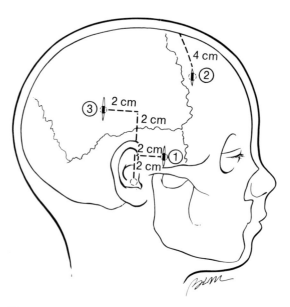

Fig. 27-20. Position and sequence of exploratory burr holes following severe head injury.

area, a burr hole will be placed anterior and lateral to the anterior fontanelle and above and behind the top of the ear (Fig. 27-20). If all three burr holes reveal no extracerebral hematoma in either the epidural or subdural space, the opposite side is then explored in a similar fashion.

If the tempo of the patient's illness has allowed a CT scan to be performed and either a subdural or epidural hematoma is diagnosed, exploratory burr holes are unnecessary. Burr holes are then made directly over the lesion, and the hematoma is evacuated. If the consistency of the clotted blood does not allow adequate evacuation through a small burr hole, a craniotomy may be necessary to evacuate the clot completely. In addition, the cortex can be inspected and any bleeding points on the cortex coagulated. In this case, the dura is grafted to accommodate cerebral swelling. The bone flap is not replaced. If the patient recovers, the bone flap can be replaced once the intracranial pressure has normalized.

Posterior fossa epidural hematomas in general are treated in a similar manner, with a burr hole over the hematoma, control of the bleeding points, and complete evacuation of the clotted blood. As previously mentioned, however, posterior fossa epidural hematomas in childhood, as well as posterior fossa subdural hematomas, commonly occur as a result of dural sinus lacerations. Provisions should then be made for immediate transfusion and repair of the lacerated sinus.

The treatment of chronic subdural hematomas in infancy is covered in Chapter 17. In brief, these lesions are treated by repeated subdural taps for 10 to 14 days. If this fails to alleviate the problem, burr holes are placed and a drain is left in the subdural space for 24 to 48 hours. This combination of procedures will be effective in the vast majority of young children and infants with chronic subdural hematomas. Because subdural taps cannot easily be performed in the older child or adolescent, burr holes are placed over the hematoma cavity and tubes are placed in the subdural space to allow drainage. This is the initial therapy and treatment of choice for chronic subdural hematomas in older children and teenagers.

Severe cerebral contusion with increased intracranial pressure is best dealt with by medical means, as outlined previously. In unusual circumstances, this will be inadequate to control intracranial pressure and consideration must be given to surgical forms of therapy. In the setting of trans-

tentorial herniation from diffuse cerebral swelling, anterior temporal lobectomy is resisted until all other avenues of therapy have failed. Large decompressive craniectomies are also of questionable value except in very selected patients.

Large intracerebral hematomas that are acting as mass lesions producing clinical symptoms and that are unresponsive to medical therapy can be evacuated. Deeply situated hematomas are generally not considered for surgical evacuation. At the time of surgery, a limited craniectomy is placed over the point at which the hematoma is most superficial. The dura is opened, the cortex is incised, and the hematoma is evacuated. Care is taken not to remove adjacent edematous brain. Adequate differentiation of viable edematous brain from nonviable cerebral cortex cannot be made in the acute setting. For this reason, limited cerebral tissue is evacuated.

Epineural repair continues to be the accepted form of therapy for lacerated nerves. Frequently the operating microscope is helpful in the anastomosis of the nerve. If significant retraction of the nerve ends has occurred during the period of waiting for demarcation, the nerve may need extensive mobilization to ensure a tension-free anastomosis. In this way, additional length may be gained. If necessary, the bony length of the extremity can be shortened to allow for adequate primary epineural anastomosis. If the nerve is believed to be contused or stretched, it is important to postpone repair until the extent of the neural damage can be visually appreciated. This usually requires 4 to 6 weeks. If no clinical or electrical evidence of recovery exists at that time, the nerve should be explored. Neuromas in continuity can be excised if there is no electrical evidence of function in the nerve beyond the neuroma. If possible, primary reanastomosis is then accomplished. If primary anastomosis cannot be accomplished, the alternative of an interposition sural nerve graft should be considered.[73]

Postoperative course. Simple scalp lacerations not associated with loss of consciousness are sutured in the emergency room, and the patient is discharged home. Stitches are removed on the tenth day following suturing, and the wound is inspected for infection. Patients with scalp avulsions, with or without rotation flaps, require hospital admission. These patients will routinely stay in the hospital until suture removal is possible at 7 to 10 days. Patients with diastatic or depressed skull fractures with few symptoms of cerebral contusion can be discharged after they have been watched in the hosptial for 3 to 4 days. Wounds with a high probability of becoming infected may need prolonged in-hospital observation. If the patient is discharged, he should also be watched for the same possibility, with frequent outpatient visits.

The timely evacuation of an epidural hematoma is usually associated with a gratifying and rapid recovery of neurologic function. These children, however, are routinely kept in the hospital for the period of time necessary for suture removal and the institution of rehabilitative efforts that may be necessary. Patients with acute subdural hematomas associated with severe cerebral contusion will need prolonged hospital admission. Medical control of increased intracranial pressure following the evacuation of an acute subdural hematoma will be most difficult in the first week following the injury. Intracranial pressure monitoring and attention to respiratory function and nutrition are important in the immediate postinjury or postoperative period. During prolonged unconsciousness, the ability to clear the patient's airway and avoid pneumonia will be enhanced by the placement of a nasotracheal tube. Tracheostomy may be required if intubation is necessary for more than 7 days, because prolonged intubation can be associated with the development of subglottic stenosis. This problem can be avoided by early tracheostomy or by carefully managed, appropriately sized endotracheal tubes. If no abdominal trauma is present and the patinet has normal bowel sounds, a nasogastric tube is passed, both for the administration of medicines and for nutrition. This aspect of care is frequently neglected. Growing children will quickly exhaust their supply of available nutrition and will develop a negative nitrogen balance after several days of receiving no calories. This development may prolong their postoperative recovery and can easily be avoided by providing the patient with feedings through a nasogastric tube. Patients with combined cranial and abdominal trauma should be considered for hyperalimentation.

Medically, penetrating wounds of the brain are dealt with in a manner similar to that for severe cerebral contusion. However, in addition to controlling the intracranial pressure, antibiotics are administered in an attempt to prevent infection from occurring and prophylactic anticonvulsants are begun.

After laminectomy for traumatic lesions of the spine, the patient is monitored carefully for the return of neurologic function. If the patient is paraparetic with no urinary function, intermittent catheterization is performed every 4 to 6 hours, and physical therapy with strengthening exercises to weakened muscles and stretching of involved tendons is performed on a routine basis. In cases where the child is paraplegic, frequent turning is necessary in order to avoid the formation of decubitis ulcers. Patients with cervical spine trauma with instability are managed preoperatively and postoperatively in a halo jacket. This device provides significant stabilization of the cervical spine and can be kept in place for several months while fractures heal or fusion takes place. Patients with thoracic spine trauma and instability who are stabilized with Harrington instrumentation can be transferred to a rehabilitation unit after 2 to 3 weeks of acute in-hospital therapy. During this period of time, active physical therapy to strengthen the remaining muscle groups is helpful in allowing the patient to utilize maximally what muscle power remains following his injury.

Patients with simple peripheral nerve lacerations that are reapproximated acutely under no tension should have range of motion exercises to the involved joints to avoid contractures and enhance recovery of motor function. Frequently, the physical therapy can be administered on an outpatient basis following immediate recovery from the surgery. Patients with delayed primary reanastomosis of lacerated or contused peripheral nerves are followed postoperatively in a similar way. It is emphasized to the patient preoperatively as well as postoperatively that recovery of peripheral nerve function is a slow process, usually requiring months of continued physical therapy to prevent contracture formation while the peripheral nerve is regenerating. The regenerating nerve will regrow at the rate of approximately 1 inch per month. When short distances are involved, recovery is relatively quick. When longer distances are involved, incomplete recovery commonly occurs.

Prognosis. Patients with simple scalp lacerations, scalp avulsions, and cerebral concussions, as would be expected, have a rapid and complete recovery of function. The eventual prognosis for patients with cerebral contusions is a function of the severity of the injury and its location.[31,61] Children who show rapid improvement of their level of consciousness and other parameters of clinical function usually experience complete recovery. Children may regain consciousness after even weeks of unconsciousness. In general, the younger the child, the greater the expectation of eventual recovery. Children possess a remarkable ability to recover from prolonged unconsciousness and severe neurologic deficits. It is often very difficult to predict within the first few days which children will eventually recover consciousness and significant neurologic function and which children will be left in a vegetative state. The recovery of function, particularly of intellectual function, may continue for years following the injury.[43] Long-term follow-up of children sustaining severe brain injury shows only half recovering sufficiently to perform "fairly normally" in school.[31]

Patients sustaining an extradural hematoma can frequently be returned to normal by prompt evacuation of the extracerebral mass. Following development of signs of brain stem compression, however, irreversible changes may have taken place; and despite the evacuation of the epidural hematoma at that point, recovery is not possible. It is seen, then, that epidural hematomas will fall into one of two categories, those that are recognized and treated quickly (associated with gratifying recovery) and those where prolonged brain stem compression results in permanent and severe neurologic compromise or death.

As previously mentioned, acute subdural hematomas are almost always associated with severe cerebral contusion; and for this reason, rapid recovery is unusual. The mortality from an acute subdural hematoma associated with cerebral contusion continues to be greater than 50%. The best therapy in this situation is the avoidance of the injury. Children who do survive acute subdural hematomas recover function slowly and usually incompletely. Permanent intellectual deficits, hemiparesis, and visual defects are common.

The prognosis for children with depressed fractures, cerebral lacerations, and penetrating wounds of the brain is a function of the portion of the brain that is injured. If the depressed fracture occurs over the primary motor area and is associated with either severe cerebral contusion or cerebral laceration, it is likely that the child will have permanent spastic hemiparesis. If the depressed fracture or cerebral laceration is limited to one frontal lobe, the residual neurologic deficit may be undetectable.

Children who are seen to have no evidence of function in the spinal cord for greater than 24 hours can be assumed to be permanently paraplegic. Children with lesions that are incomplete and who show rapid improvement over several hours to days may have significant return of function to allow for ambulation. Spinal cord injury as opposed to brain injury in childhood is not associated with continued significant recovery weeks to months after the accident.

Peripheral nerve and plexus injuries are generally associated with evidence of permanent neurologic injury. Birth injuries that affect the upper brachial plexus show much better return of function than those involving the lower portion of the plexus because the regenerating nerves from the lower plexus must travel a greater distance before they can attach to the target muscles. In addition, the muscles innervated by the lower brachial plexus are responsible for intricate and complicated movements of the fingers. The muscles supplied by the upper brachial plexus are involved with grosser motion about the shoulder. An additional consideration in the prognosis of recovery of peripheral nerve function is the composition of the nerve. Nerves that are predominantly motor (e.g., radial) will have their regenerating axon travel down the residual neurilemmal sheaths with little possibility of going astray. In contrast, mixed nerves (e.g., median) will have a greater proportion of the regenerating axons enter inappropriate neurilemmal sheaths and thereby not contribute to the regeneration process. Clinical evidence supports this view; recovery of radial nerve function is much more complete than recovery of median nerve function, with lacerations doing better than stretch or contusion injuries. In summary, the prognosis following a peripheral nerve injury is a function of (1) the length between the site of nerve injury and the target muscle, (2) the type of muscle to be reinnervated, (3) the mix of the affected nerve (pure motor versus mixed motor-sensory), and (4) the type of lesion (laceration, contusion, or stretch).

Important aspects of follow-up. Following scalp lacerations or scalp avulsions, the patient is monitored for the continued integrity of the scalp. After several days the wound will gradually lose its tenderness and edema. The area around the wound may demonstrate some sensory loss, particularly if the laceration has included a major nerve (occipital or supraorbital).

Following the common condition of cerebral

concussion, the patient should be reevaluated 4 to 6 weeks following the trauma. At this examination the detailed neurologic examination is repeated. Specifically tested for is function of the child's first cranial nerve. This is somewhat difficult to test for in young children; in older children and teenagers, however, the olfactory nerves may be seen to be damaged and this is an indication of the severity of the injury. Motor function and fine coordination should be normal. Following severe contusion, the follow-up should be more detailed and extensive. Outpatient physical and speech therapy may be of benefit in the appropriate patient. Frequently, the parents can be taught to help the child with specific exercises, and returning to the hospital on a daily basis is not necessary. The child may not be able to return to a normal classroom for several months, if at all. During this period of time, special instruction at home or in a class of very limited size will be of significant benefit. Endocrine disturbances with diabetes insipidus or panhypopituitarism may also be seen occasionally following severe head injury.[18,67]

Patients who were prophylactically placed on anticonvulsants because of cerebral laceration or a penetrating wound of the brain should have this decision reevaluated 6 months following the trauma if the patient has remained seizure free. The EEG is repeated, and if no evidence of active epileptic discharges is present, the anticonvulsants are slowly tapered off over a period of weeks. It should be remembered, however, that epilepsy may become clinically evident early (within the first weeks after injury) or late. Early posttraumatic epilepsy is relatively common, occurring in 5% of patients with head injuries who are admitted to the hospital. Depressed skull fractures, intracerebral hematomas, and more than 24 hours of posttraumatic amnesia increase the likelihood of early posttraumatic epilepsy.[38] Children under 5 years of age are also at greater risk of developing epilepsy even after trivial injuries. Posttraumatic status epilepticus of childhood is not associated with as grave a prognosis as that following head injury in adults. Late posttraumatic epilepsy also occurs in approximately 5% of patients with head injuries who are admitted to the hospital.[38] Half the patients will have their first seizure more than a year after the trauma. Depressed fracture, dural laceration, and early posttraumatic seizures add to the risk of the development of late posttraumatic epilepsy.[38]

Older children and adolescents who sustain depressed or diastatic skull fractures without scalp laceration and undergo craniectomy may be considered for cranioplasty following recovery from the injury. Patients with compound wounds should have cranioplasty deferred for 1 year following the trauma. If no evidence of infection is present at that time, cranioplasty can be considered. Infants and young children may spontaneously regenerate bone and fill in small cranial defects, making cranioplasty unnecessary. Older children and teenagers do not possess the capability of regenerating large areas of bone. Therefore, cranioplasty frequently will be needed to protect the underlying brain from trauma and improve the cosmetic appearance. Cranioplasty is a relatively uncomplicated procedure that can be accomplished extradurally with the insertion of an acrylic plate fashioned at the operating table.

Patients with epidural hematomas and acute subdural hematomas frequently need prolonged physical therapy and speech therapy to help them recover from deficits inflicted by the trauma. When extended recuperation is anticipated, the rehabilitation wing of a hospital or other facility designed to aid in the recuperation and prolonged therapy of injured or damaged children will be a source of great help. In such situations, children can continue their schoolwork along with active physical and speech therapy, frequently returning home on weekends.

Following severe spinal injuries, a similar unit can be of great help. Control of the neurogenic bladder is a critical part of the continued care of any paraplegic or quadriplegic patient, and special attention to this aspect of the patient's care is necessary. Following some spinal injuries and frequently following peripheral nerve injuries, orthopedic procedures to strengthen the weakened extremity by transferring tendons or other maneuvers should be considered. Any decision regarding this type of procedure should be delayed until maximum recovery of motor function (which may take months) has been allowed to occur. During that period of time, contractures can be avoided by frequent range of motion exercises of the involved joints. If contractures have developed, as for instance at the heel cord or hamstring, tendon-lengthening exercises may be of help in restoring a full range of motion.

Complications. The most serious complication following simple scalp laceration or even scalp avulsion involves local infection and cellulitis. This rarely can be associated with propagation of the infection through a venous channel, resulting in a subdural empyema or brain abscess. Osteomyelitis from compound depressed skull fractures occasionally occurs from inadequately debrided wounds. In these children the area of trauma continues to be tender and edematous days or weeks after the trauma. There are frequently systemic signs of infection accompanying the acute infection, although radiographic changes will lag weeks behind.

Following diastatic fractures or depressed fractures that may not have been treated surgically, the development of a leptomeningeal cyst should always be considered.[42,74] This lesion occurs predominantly in children less than 3 years of age as a gradually enlarging CSF-containing cyst that presents through the disrupted dura and bone as a subcutaneous mass. Serial x-ray films of the skull will show progressive widening of the fracture site, hence the synonym "growing fracture." Occasionally, the brain will also be seen to herniate out through the dural tear, and hemiparesis may develop. Leptomeningeal cysts occur weeks to months after the trauma and if left unattended will result in progressive neurologic compromise. The presence of a leptomeningeal cyst can be easily confirmed by comparing current skull x-ray films with those that were obtained at the time of initial trauma. These lesions should be repaired surgically with grafting of the lacerated dura and cranioplasty.

CSF rhinorrhea or otorrhea that develops as a consequence of basilar skull fracture will frequently resolve spontaneously with time. With rhinorrhea, clear fluid can be seen to drain from the nose, depending on the patient's position. If a question arises as to whether or not the fluid draining from the nose is CSF or watery mucus, the presence of glucose in the fluid will confirm it as being CSF. Tomograms through the area of the cribriform plate and sphenoid may disclose the area of trauma. On tomography, if buckling of the floor of the anterior fossa is seen with bony spicules penetrating the intracranial cavity, there is little reason to contemplate conservative therapy. These lesions will rarely close on their own, and surgery is indicated to restore the integrity of the dura. Without such unusual circumstances, CSF rhinorrhea is treated conservatively for a period of 7 to 10 days. During that time the CSF pressure is lowered by intermittent or continuous drainage of spinal fluid through lumbar punctures or a lumbar subarachnoid drain. In addition, penicillin G is given in an attempt to prevent more fulminant forms of meningitis (e.g., streptococcus pneumoniae). For the occasional patient who persists with CSF rhinorrhea despite lumbar drainage, consideration of craniotomy and repair of the dural leak should be given. This is done to prevent repeated bouts of meningitis, which will develop if a persistent subarachnoid nasal fistula exists. Usual sites of dural tears are in the area of the cribriform plate or sphenoid sinus. Isotope cisternography may be of value in determining the site of CSF leakage.

Posttraumatic otorrhea with accumulation of fluid in the middle ear is also initially treated conservatively. Fortunately, the vast majority of these patients spontaneously seal their leak as well. Surgical repair of this lesion is technically more challenging than the repair of CSF rhinorrhea. Neurosurgeons will frequently allow a 3-week period of conservative therapy before further investigation and consideration of surgical repair of persistent CSF otorrhea.

If neither CSF rhinorrhea nor otorrhea is discovered in the immediate posttraumatic period, the patient may develop these symptoms months or years later. This possibility should be kept in mind, particularly in patients having repeated bouts of meningitis cause by respiratory flora. These organisms include *Streptococcus pneumoniae* and *Hemophilus influenzae*. An indirect sign of disruption of the dura over the paranasal sinuses or mastoid air cells is the development of pneumocephalus. This usually can be appreciated readily on x-ray films of the skull. The air can be seen to accumulate in the extradural, subdural, subarachnoid, or cerebral intraventricular compartment. When the amount of air progressively increases or is unchanged for days, a wide dural tear is implied and is a relative indication for early surgical repair.

Following a head injury, epidural or subdural hematomas may accumulate in a relatively gradual fashion and may not be recognized within the first 24 to 48 hours after the injury. In any patient who fails to improve progressively following head trauma and in whom the initial CT brain scan shows evidence of contusion only, a repeat scan several days following the initial study may be of help. Chronic subdural hematomas may become manifest clinically weeks or even months following a head injury. Communicating hydrocephalus as a result of traumatic subarachnoid hemorrhage can also be seen as a late complication of head trauma. This possibility can also be assessed easily by a CT brain scan. Follow-up examinations of patients with basilar skull fractures should include an audiogram if any symptoms or findings indicate hearing difficulties. Disruption of the ossicular chain can then be detected and repaired.

Children who sustain head injuries and develop the postconcussion syndrome may develop symptoms quite different from adults.[21] The vast majority of affected children will develop an alteration of personality, becoming more aggressive and antisocial. Sleep disturbances and enuresis may be seen. Adolescents may develop the more easily recognized headache, dizziness, irritability, and difficulty with concentrating. Symptoms may persist for weeks or months after the injury and are best treated with reassurance and symptomatic therapy of the specific complaints. Heavy sedation should be avoided. Early return to regular school activities during the recovery phase may be frustrating to the patient and may prolong his convalescence.

With compound and penetrating wounds of the head, the possibility of brain abscess formation should also be considered. It is clear that the child with progressive neurologic dysfunction following a head injury may have multiple causes for his problem. An additional source of further neurologic compromise, however, is repeat injury. This, unfortunately, is common in the child who is the victim of parental abuse. Characteristically, multiple lesions are present with fractures of the long bones and ribs, as well as retinal and subdural hemorrhages. Infants and children who come to medical attention because of subdural hematomas, either chronic or acute, should have their fundi searched carefully for the presence of retinal hemorrhages. A bone survey as well as a chest x-ray film for rib detail may give further evidence in support of abuse. Careful follow-up of these patients by the primary care physician and local health authorities is essential to prevent further injury to the child.

Further neurologic complications from spinal injuries are uncommon. Occasionally, spinal instability will not be recognized at the time of the initial evaluation, and with ambulation or further movement the neurologic compromise can be accentuated. However, children will usually complain of pain and be extremely reluctant to become active in the presence of a spinal injury. This should be a strong sign to those taking care of the child to consider spinal instability as a cause of the patient's discomfort. An unusual complication following spinal cord injury is the development of a posttraumatic syrinx.[6] This may occur months to years following spinal cord injury and will present as a progressive intramedullary neurologic dysfunction. The diagnosis may be confirmed by myelography if the lesion is large. Therapy centers around drainage of the syrinx cavity into the subarachnoid space. In general, however, the long-term complications from spinal injuries are not neurologic; rather, they are urologic and orthopedic.

Long-term complications from peripheral nerve injuries are unusual. In adults peripheral nerve and plexus injuries may be associated with the development of causalgia, dysesthesia, or other chronic pain syndromes. The discomfort may become overwhelming and inhibit rehabilitation. Fortunately, chronic pain syndromes are unusual in childhood.

Other, less common lesions. Intervertebral disc herniation is uncommon in childhood. The occasional older child or adolescent may come to medical attention with back pain and limited mobility of the lumbar spine. There may be no objective evidence of neurologic compromise. The findings are frequently limited to loss of the lordotic curve, limited straight-leg raising, and forward bending with typical back pain radiating in a sciatic distribution down the posterior lateral aspect of the leg. The two most common levels of disc herniation are the L4-5 and L5-S1 levels. With a disc herniation at L4-5 and an L-5 radiculopathy, the patient may have no alteration of the reflexes. Pain and occasionally paresthesia will radiate into the great toe. If weakness develops, it involves the extensor hallucis longus and anterior tibial muscles. With involvement of the S-1 nerve root from the L5-S1 disc space, the patient will have pain and paresthesia radiating into the lateral aspect of his foot, primarily the little toe. The ankle jerk will be lost or diminished, and in advanced cases weakness will be present in the gastrocnemius muscle. As with disc disease in adult patients, the first course of action is to pursue conservative therapy, including a prolonged trial of bed rest, usually 10 to 14 days. If clear weakness is present, however, and conservative therapy has failed, consideration of myelography and spinal surgery is appropriate. At the time of operation, free disc fragments are rarely encountered. The bulging annulus and herniated nucleus will be densely adherent to the cartilaginous end-plate, and diskectomy is performed with some difficulty. Results of appropriately selected cases show excellent relief of symptoms. The fact that weakness that is profound prior to surgery will frequently not return supports a policy of early surgery if weakness is present.

SUPRATENTORIAL TUMORS

In the pediatric age group, more solid neoplasms occur in the brain than in any other location.[87] Brain tumors account for more childhood deaths than any other form of cancer except leukemia. The frequency of involvement of the various intracranial locations varies with the age of the patient. As a group, children tend to have a greater percentage of neoplasms occur below the tentorium. This is particularly true when one looks specifically at the group of children between 3 and 11 years of age, where greater than 70% of the intracranial neoplasms occur in this location.[44] Before age 3, however, the incidence of infratentorial tumors is roughly equivalent to the incidence of supratentorial tumors. After 11 years of age, the ratio of supratentorial tumors to infratentorial tumors gradually increases until adult life, when 70% of recognized intracranial tumors occur above the tentorium.

Some significant differences exist between the supratentorial tumors found in children and those found in adults. Meningioma and pituitary adenoma, which occur relatively frequently in adults, are both rarely seen in children. Metastatic tumors, which are common in adults, are also rarely seen in children; when they do occur, however, the primary tumor from which the metastasis originated is most likely to be a neuroblastoma, rhabdomyosarcoma, or Wilms' tumor.[85] Between 70% and 80% of the tumors that do occur in the supratentorial compartment in childhood are gliomas. Within this group glioblastoma multiforme occurs less frequently in childhood than in adult life. Not uncommonly, the microscopic examination of a childhood supratentorial tumor will reveal bizarre and unusual histologic features that may defy classification.

Tumors that occur above the tentorium are more easily understood and analyzed when they are considered by location and histologic type. The supra-

tentorial tumor sites to be considered in this discussion include the cerebral hemispheres, the sellar and suprasellar regions, the pineal region, and the ventricles.

Possible findings. The clinical presentation of supratentorial tumors varies significantly, depending on the location of the neoplasm. Some features, however, may be seen with tumors in any location. Neoplasms that occur adjacent to normal constrictions in the CSF pathway will frequently become clinically apparent initially with internal or noncommunicating hydrocephalus, which will occur early in the course of the illness. Increased intracranial pressure can also be seen without obstruction to the flow of CSF as a direct result of the mass created by the growth of the neoplasm. Rarely, excessive CSF production from a choroid plexus papilloma will lead to the development of communicating or external hydrocephalus.[56] Increased intracranial pressure in infants can be readily recognized by palpation of the anterior fontanelle with an estimation of the intracranial tension and by serial head circumference measurements to document accelerated head growth. Infants frequently will not demonstrate obvious lateralizing neurologic signs, even in the presence of a large hemispheric tumor. Minor degrees of motor asymmetry that may be present can be extremely difficult to detect in the uncooperative and irritable infant or young child. Not infrequently, the first clinically detectable signs of abnormality will be delay in the development of motor skills. As the child becomes older, subjective complaints become more specific. Before 5 years of age, children with increased intracranial pressure usually develop irritability, malaise, and anorexia without complaints of localized pain such as headache. The older child develops the classic triad of headache, nausea and vomiting, and papilledema. This triad is somewhat less frequent in patients with supratentorial tumors than in the initial clinical presentation of lesions occurring within the posterior fossa.

Lesions that begin within the cerebral hemispheres not uncommonly present with seizure activity as their initial manifestation. This is seen in approximately one third of patients with supratentorial tumors.[52] The seizure activity may be of a variety of types, including brief bouts of akinetic activity or lapses of awareness of the environment.[65] A sensory or visual aura is rarely described by younger children. Occasionally, lesions located within the medial aspect of the temporal lobe may present with uncinate seizures. These are characterized by the initial detection of a nonexistent unpleasant odor followed by a generalized seizure. Older children may be able to remember the aura when questioned specifically. Adversive seizures that are thought to originate in the area of the frontal eye field are characterized by tonic deviation of the head and eyes away from the involved hemisphere and are also a helpful localizing sign.[8] During the immediate postictal period, significant information can be gained by examining the patient for the presence of asymmetric weakness (Todd's postictal paralysis). Persistent focal weakness may be the only indication that the observed seizure activity may be secondary to a structural lesion of the brain. Similarly, seizures that have an obvious focal onset must be considered to be the initial manifestation of a structural lesion until it is proved otherwise.

Frequently, the initial complaints of children with neoplasms of the cerebral hemispheres are vague and nonspecific. Irritability, inability to con-

centrate, change of personality, and a decrease in school performance may be the earliest symptoms of tumors in this location. The child will tire easily and lose the ability to compete physically with his peers at play. Eventually, signs and symptoms of increased intracranial pressure will develop, with papilledema being present in greater than 60% of children at the time of initial diagnosis.[52] Alteration of muscular tone and strength is commonly present. Disturbances of gait with ''stiffness'' of the involved leg, as well as difficulty with fine-coordinated activities, occur commonly. Occasionally, confusion can occur when ataxia is found to be secondary to a frontal lobe lesion rather than a posterior fossa mass. With evidence of increased intracranial pressure and spastic hemiparesis without seizure activity, the possibility of a thalamic neoplasm should be considered. Visual field deficits and cortical sensory alterations can be difficult to determine in younger children. The use of opticokinetic nystagmus to detect parietal lobe lesions may be of some assistance. As the tape or drum is moved horizontally, the fast component of the

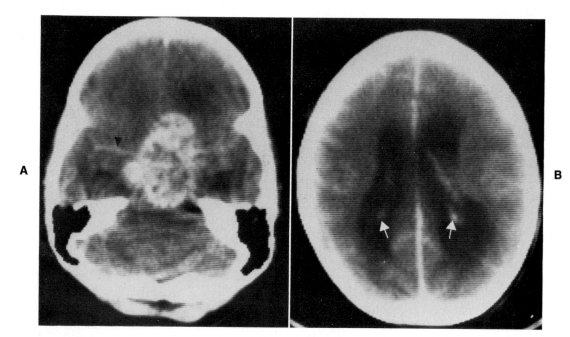

Fig. 27-21. A, Enhanced CT brain scan of a patient with visual and growth failure and recent onset of headaches. The lesion was seen to be calcified on plain films and the unenhanced scan. The left middle cerebral artery (arrow) seems to emerge from the lesion. **B,** Bodies of the lateral ventricles are moderately dilated from the obstruction to CSF flow at the foramen of Monro. The choroid plexus and glomus can be seen in the atrium of the ventricles (arrows). The lesion was histologically confirmed to be a craniopharyngioma and was macroscopically totally removed without major complication.

nystagmus will be lost as the targets move toward the side of the lesion. The loss of opticokinetic nystagmus can be seen with parietal lobe lesions but is not specific for that location.

Dysfunction of the hypothalamic-pituitary axis and visual apparatus occurs with tumors in the sellar and parasellar locations. As lesions become large and compress the anterior third ventricle, hydrocephalus can occur as a result of the obstruction of CSF flow at the foramina of Monro (Fig. 27-21). These patients frequently develop the classic symptoms of headache, nausea and vomiting, and papilledema as evidenced on funduscopic examination. Disturbances of pituitary function often occur with tumors in this location. With pressure on the infundibulum and pituitary gland itself, younger children will demonstrate growth failure secondary to deficiency in the secretion of somatotrophin, usually the earliest of the hypothalamic pituitary functions to be disturbed. In the older child or adolescent, delay or lack of development of secondary sexual characteristics is also common. Thyrotrophin abnormalities may result in the development of pale, thin, hairless skin. Occasionally, the patient will demonstrate panhypopituitarism. The least likely pituitary function to be deficient is secretion of corticotrophin. Diabetes insipidus is uncommon with the majority of tumors that occur in this area. When diabetes insipidus does occur, particularly as an initial manifestation of the patient's illness, the presence of a suprasellar germinoma should be strongly considered. Under these circumstances, diabetes insipidus may precede visual or other endocrine disturbances by several months or years. Rarely, precocious puberty is a presenting sign of tumors of the posterior hypothalamus. These children develop secondary sexual characteristics before 10 years of age in the boy and before 8 years of age in the girl. This is considered to be an irritative phenomenon, since precocious puberty is not seen following trauma or other destructive processes that involve the hypothalamus. Children who develop precocious puberty will usually have no other disturbance of the endocrine system. They will not have evidence of diabetes insipidus or alteration of somatotrophin, thyrotrophin, or corticotrophin function. With invasion and destruction of the anterior hypothalamus, patients will fail to thrive, will fail to gain both height and weight, and will lose subcutaneous fat despite adequate caloric intake. Most patients who develop this syndrome are evaluated for gastrointestinal disease and metabolic disturbances before a central nervous system origin for their difficulty is considered. Headaches, seizures, and visual changes with direct hypothalamic involvement are usually lacking. Autonomic seizures with wide fluctuations of the pulse, blood pressure, and flushing of the skin are occasionally seen with hypothalamic tumors.

With tumors that originate within the orbital portion of the optic nerve, proptosis is the most common initial complaint. The proptosis that occurs is directed forward initially. However, after the tumor has obtained significant size, the eye will deviate inferiorly and laterally (Fig. 27-22). The extraocular movements are characteristically preserved with tumors of the optic nerve. This will help to differentiate this tumor from other neoplasms that occur within the orbit. Visual acuity is frequently affected. On funduscopic examination the tumor may actually be seen as it presents through the optic nerve head and fungates into the vitreous chamber. Intracranial neoplasms that originate in the anterior visual apparatus are brought to clinical attention initially because of decreased visual acuity or decreased visual fields. This disturbance may occur unilaterally or bilaterally. As the tumor grows, disturbances of hypothalamic function commonly occur.

Tumors that originate within the ventricular system occur uncommonly. As previously discussed, choroid plexus papillomas that present in

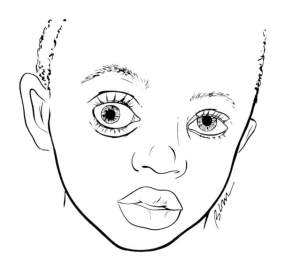

Fig. 27-22. Child with right optic nerve glioma. The globe is proptotic and displaced inferiorly and laterally.

childhood tend to occur in the trigone of the lateral ventricle. The signs and symptoms are usually those of hydrocephalus. Uncommonly, the tumor will come to clinical attention as a result of subarachnoid hemorrhage. The hydrocephalus that is produced by this tumor has been proved in a few selected patients to be due to the overproduction of CSF.[57] Diminished CSF resorption may also play a role in the production of the hydrocephalus that is commonly found with this tumor. If the intraventricular mass is located near a narrowing of the ventricular system, the resultant hydrocephalus may be secondary to obstruction to the intraventricular flow of CSF. In this case, internal or noncommunicating hydrocephalus develops. Ependymomas that originate near the ventricular lining and enlarge into the ventricular system are characteristically associated with elevations of the CSF protein content. Hydrocephalus may also result from this tumor as it enlarges and obstructs the CSF pathway.

Tumors that originate in the area of the pineal gland also commonly present with evidence of hydrocephalus and raised intracranial pressure. The position of the pineal immediately above the aqueduct of Sylvius explains the internal hydrocephalus that is commonly seen with tumors in this location. In addition, however, because of the compression of the quadrigeminal plate and the fibers coursing down from the cerebral cortex to the area of the superior colliculus, patients frequently develop paralysis of upward gaze, mild ptosis, and pupillary asymmetry. Nystagmus retractorius with synchronous retraction of the globe on attempted upward gaze may also be seen. This constellation of symptoms in association with hydrocephalus is strongly suggestive of a neoplasm in the area of the pineal. Rarely, precocious puberty may be seen with tumors that occur in this location in boys.

Children with clinical evidence of neurofibromatosis or tuberous sclerosis should have special attention directed to the nervous system during routine evaluations. It is well recognized that neurofibromatosis carries with it an increased risk of the development of gliomas of the cerebral hemispheres, hypothalamus, optic nerves, and chiasm, as well as other central nervous system tumors. Children with tuberous sclerosis may develop neoplasms in the subependymal area that protrude into the ventricular system. Their ventricular lining may appear studded with multiple small neoplasms

that take on the configuration of "candle guttering." Occasionally, a subependymal tumor may grow to a large size and occlude CSF circulation.

Arachnoid cysts occurring above the tentorium present with symptoms of a focally expanding mass. It may not be possible clinically to separate the presentation of these cysts from other mass lesions. Occasionally, patients will come to clinical attention acutely following head trauma with hemorrhage into the cystic cavity. In this case, the patient's clinical condition will appear more severe than would be expected from the history of the accident.[1,72]

Common occurrences. Most neoplasms that occur within the cerebral hemispheres are gliomas. Histologically, this group is made up of glioblastoma multiforme, both benign and malignant astrocytomas, ependymoma, ganglioglioma, and occasionally oligodendroglioma or the unusual primary intracerebral neuroblastoma.

Glioblastoma multiforme, which appears so commonly in adult life, is unusual in childhood. Many tumors, however, may be identified as being glial and yet the specific cell of origin or histologic classification may be difficult to establish. The primitive nature of the elements of many tumors may predominate and make their exact classification difficult. Numerous series of patients with cerebral hemisphere gliomas have been published in the literature with varying frequencies of the various tumor types.[4,19,44,52] This inconsistency most probably does not represent a variation in tumor population; rather, it may be a variation in the histologic classification.

The *astrocytoma* is thought to be the most common cerebral neoplasm in childhood. It may arise in any area of brain, including the cerebral hemispheres, and will grow by infiltration of the adjacent brain tissue. The dura is an effective barrier in preventing direct extension of the tumor. Calcification, which can be detected radiographically, occurs infrequently. Metastases, either within the central nervous system via the CSF or outside the central nervous system, occur rarely. As previously mentioned, the clinical presentation of most astrocytomas of the cerebral hemispheres involves headache and emotional or personality change followed by the development of motor weakness. Nausea, vomiting, and anorexia, which are so common with posterior fossa tumors, appear to be less frequent with tumors of the cerebral hemispheres. Approximately 67% of patients with tumors of the cerebral hemispheres have papilledema at the time of their initial clinical presentation.[52] Seizures may also herald the occurrence of this tumor. Of particular importance are seizures that are focal in onset. Occasionally, a cerebral glioma will be found in a patient with a long-standing seizure disorder. It behooves all clinicians following patients with childhood epilepsy to be aware of this fact and maintain a close vigil of the patient's neurologic examination for signs of a progressive neurologic deficit.

Cerebral astrocytomas may be solid (Fig. 27-23) or, less commonly, cystic (Fig. 27-24). Fluid within the cystic cavity will appear light yellow and contain little cellular debris. Hemorrhage within the tumor or the accompanying cyst occurs infrequently. Glioblastoma multiforme, which may originate in an area of astrocytoma, is commonly associated with hemorrhage and necrosis within the tumor. Both of these tumors will show no distinct point of cleavage between tumor and adjacent brain.

Ependymomas of the cerebral hemispheres occur much less commonly than astrocytomas. This tumor is thought to rise adjacent to the ventricular system and extend either into the ventricle or into the substance of the brain. A favorite location is in the area of the trigone of the lateral ventricle. As the tumor grows into the ventricle, it frequently takes on a papillary configuration and may be confused with the choroid plexus papilloma. Ependymomas are noted for their vascularity and frequent calcification in comparison with astrocytomas. This tumor also may occur as a solid mass or be associated with single or multiple cysts of varying sizes. Fluid within the cyst differs from that commonly seen with astrocytomas because of its darker color; it frequently appears deep amber and is occasionally hemorrhagic. Characteristically, the entire cyst wall is lined by neoplasm. Because of their occurrence near the ventricular system, ependymomas may spread within the central nervous system through the CSF pathways. Occasionally, metastases will cause the initial clinical manifestation. Despite their apparent separation from normal brain structures, histologically ependymomas will be found to be infiltrative. Cure of a supratentorial ependymoma is unusual.[16,45]

Pure *oligodendrogliomas* are rare in childhood. Not uncommonly, however, mixed gliomas can be found to have areas most consistent with an oligodendroglioma.[52] Of the supratentorial gliomas, this tumor calcifies most frequently.

Neoplastic lesions that characteristically occur in the area of the sella turcica in childhood include craniopharyngioma, glioma of the hypothalamus, glioma of the optic nerve or chiasm, and suprasellar germinoma. The frequency of their occurrence is as listed, with craniopharyngioma being seen most often. Together these lesions make up some 10% to 15% of intracranial neoplasms seen in childhood.

The *craniopharyngioma* has been reported to occur as a congenital tumor presenting within the first few days of life. The peak incidence, however, is in the second half of the first decade. This tumor is a benign growth of tissue of ectodermal origin that is thought to represent a remnant of Rathke's pouch. The tumor may be solid or cystic containing a thick brownish yellow fluid (Fig. 27-25), which is extremely irritating if it is allowed to enter the subarachnoid space. A pathognomonic characteristic of the fluid is the presence of cholesterol crystals, which can be appreciated using polarized light. Some tumors are mainly solid and are composed primarily of squamous epithe-

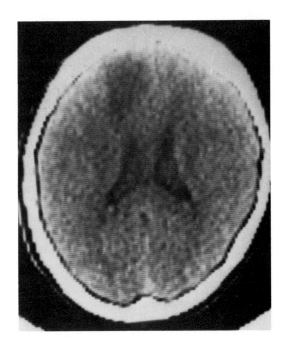

Fig. 27-23. Unenhanced CT brain scan showing low attenuation in the left frontal lobe of a patient who developed an adversive seizure disorder (head and eyes turned toward the right). The lesion proved to be a solid anaplastic astrocytoma.

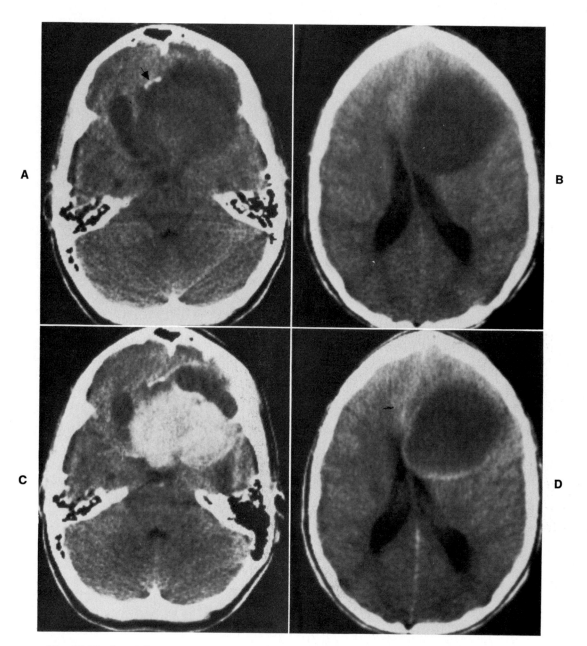

Fig. 27-24. A and **B,** Unenhanced CT brain scan showing a large right frontal lobe mass in an 11-year-old child whose initial symptoms were right-sided visual failure and headache. A small area of calcification is seen near the tip of the right frontal pole (arrow). **C,** Following contrast enhancement, the inferior portion of the lesion enhances diffusely and represents the solid portion of the tumor. **D,** The superior aspect of the mass enhances at the periphery only. The central area of the upper portions of the mass proved to be a large cyst containing proteinaceous fluid. (Courtesy A. A. Zeal, M.D., Jacksonville, Fla.)

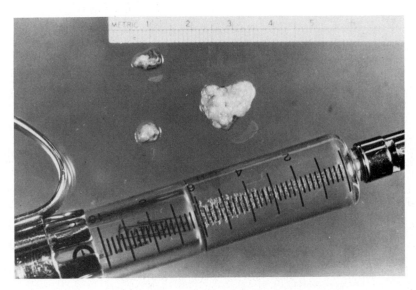

Fig. 27-25. Specimen of excised craniopharyngioma and cyst fluid. The solid portion of the neoplasm is lightly calcified. The fluid within the cyst contains cholesterol crystals, which are characteristic for this tumor. (Courtesy G. L. Odom, M.D., Durham, N.C.)

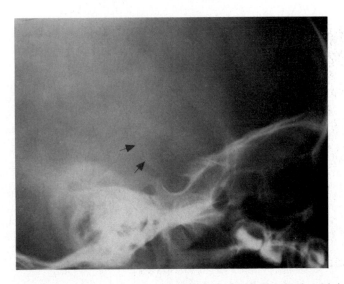

Fig. 27-26. Lateral skull radiograph of a 2-year-old child who suffered a head injury. The curvilinear calcification of a craniopharyngioma (arrows) can be seen above and behind the sella turcica. The tumor was completely excised to macroscopic inspection.

lium and associated cell debris. Surrounding the tumor is an inflammatory reaction that may reach a thickness of 5 mm. This lining is composed of fibroblasts and reactive astrocytes. Calcification occurs within the wall of the tumor and can be seen on routine radiographs in greater than 90% of patients (Fig. 27-26). Additional symptoms that may be present relate to increased intracranial pressure and internal hydrocephalus secondary to obstruction of the foramen of Monro on one or both sides. Visual field defects, decreased visual acuity, and small stature are also common findings. The extent of pituitary and hypothalamic dysfunction depends on the degree of encroachment of the tumor on these structures. Rarely, the tumor will spontaneously leak irritating cholesterol-laden

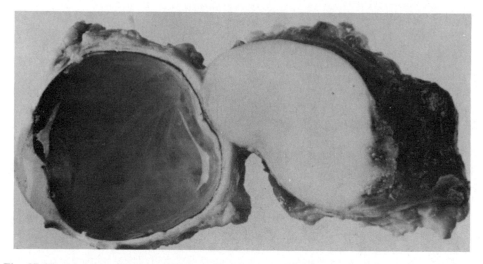

Fig. 27-27. Specimen of an excised optic nerve glioma demonstrating the marked expansion of the nerve by the infiltrative neoplasm. (From Vogel, F. S.: Special aspects of neoplasms: the nervous system. In Brunson, J. G., and Gall, E. P., editors: Concepts of disease: a textbook of human pathology. Copyright © 1971 by McMillan Publishing Co., Inc.)

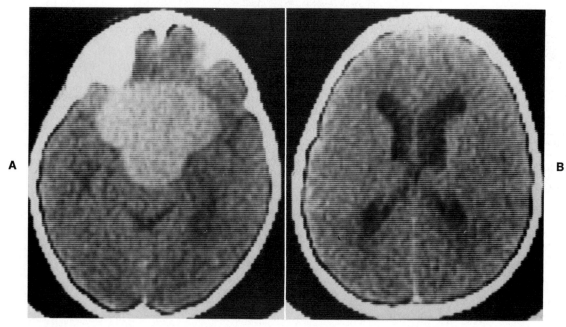

Fig. 27-28. CT brain scan of a 2-year-old child seen because of a bobbing motion of the right eye present since birth. The child was blind in the right eye and had mild macrocrania and increased intracranial pressure. **A,** The tumor enhanced homogeneously and is quite large when appreciated in the light of the child's minimal symptoms. **B,** The lateral ventricles are dilated secondary to compression of the foramina of Monro. The tumor was histologically confirmed to be an optic chiasm astrocytoma.

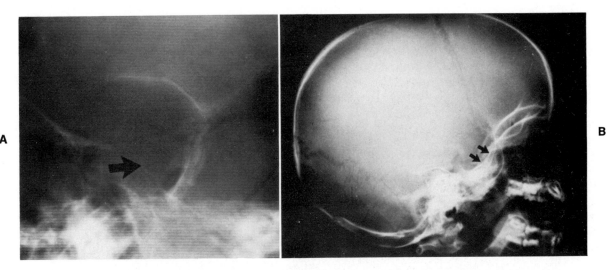

Fig. 27-29. A, Optic foramen view of a skull radiograph. The grossly enlarged optic foramen (arrow) is indicative of an optic nerve tumor. **B,** Lateral skull radiograph of another patient with erosion of the tuberculum sella (arrows) and amputation of the dorsum sella from a large optic chiasm glioma.

fluid into either the ventricular system or the subarachnoid space, resulting in the abrupt onset of sterile meningitis. Careful examination of the CSF will document the presence of cholesterol crystals and secure the diagnosis.

Gliomas occurring in the structures around the sella turcica may come to clinical attention in a variety of ways. Tumors confined to the intraorbital portion of the optic nerve will characteristically present with proptosis and decreased vision in the involved eye. It is currently believed that these tumors have a rather benign course with little evidence of progression when they are followed over many years.[35] There is an increased incidence of these tumors in the presence of neurofibromatosis. Histologically, the tumor is composed of benign-appearing astrocytes that infiltrate between the fibers of the optic nerve and expand it (Fig. 27-27). The exophthalmus associated with these tumors is characteristically nonpulsatile, and the globe is usually displaced slightly laterally and inferiorly. Extraocular movements are characteristically preserved. The optic disc is almost always abnormal with evidence of either papilledema or optic atrophy. Occasionally, the tumor itself may be seen as it penetrates the optic disc.

If the tumor is located more posteriorly and primarily involves the optic chiasm, the clinical presentation and implications for the patient are quite different. Since children will infrequently com-

plain of decreased visual acuity, these tumors may attain a large size and present primarily with evidence of increased intracranial pressure by obstruction of CSF flow at the foramen of Monro (Fig. 27-28). Visual loss will be apparent on careful testing and will frequently involve both eyes, although asymmetrically. If the portion of the optic nerve within the optic canal is involved, there may be enlargement of this structure when appropriate x-ray films are taken (Fig. 27-29, *A*). Enlargement of the optic foramen or the presence of an abnormal sella turcica is seen in greater than 90% of the gliomas that involve the optic chiasm (Fig. 27-29, *B*).

Tumors that primarily involve the hypothalamus present with one of two clinical pictures. In the first few years of life, the presentation is that of the diencephalic syndrome of Russell. This syndrome is characterized by marked emaciation with loss of subcutaneous fat, cachexia, and failure to thrive despite adequate caloric intake. As the tumor enlarges, it will eventually occlude the foramen of Monro and cause increased intracranial pressure. In addition, infiltration of the optic tract and chiasm may cause alteration of the visual fields and visual acuity. Pathologically, the tumors vary from a hamartomatous malformation with little neoplastic growth potential to a highly malignant astrocytoma with rapid growth characteristics. Typically, an extensive gastrointestinal evaluation

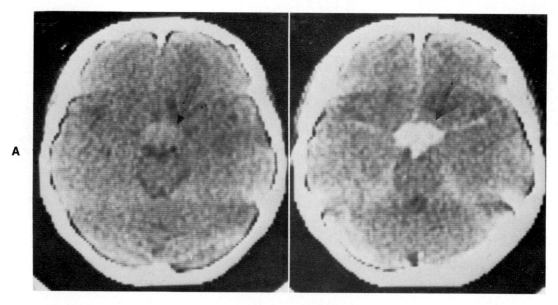

Fig. 27-30. CT brain scan of a patient with a long history of diabetes insipidus and recent development of visual failure. **A,** The unenhanced CT brain scan demonstrates a mass in the suprasellar cistern that is of slightly higher attenuation than brain. No calcification can be appreciated. **B,** With enhancement the lesion developed a homogeneous white appearance. The lesion was histologically confirmed to be a germinoma.

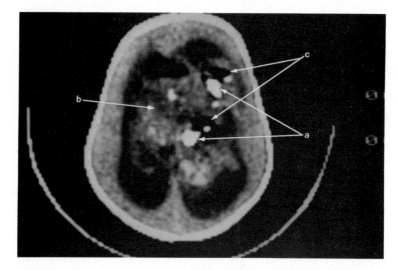

Fig. 27-31. CT brain scan of a 6-week-old infant with macrocrania and increased intracranial pressure. Within the dilated ventricular system is a large neoplasm composed of high-attenuation bone *(a)*, isoattenuation soft tissue *(b)*, and low-attenuation fat *(c)*. The tumor was histologically confirmed as an intraventricular teratoma. (Courtesy Norman Grant, Hospital for Sick Children, London, Eng.)

is carried out in these children before it is realized that the primary problem lies within the central nervous system. If the tumor presents in the older child or adolescent, precocious puberty can be the clinical presentation. Development of secondary sexual characteristics in the boy less than 10 years old or the girl less than 8 years old is considered abnormal. Associated findings may include marked obesity; periods of excessive sweating, flushing, or tachycardia; chorioathetoid movements; and occasionally diabetes insipidus. The tendency to develop evidence of increased intracranial pressure is much greater in the older child.

Germinomas that occur above the sella turcica (ectopic pinealoma, suprasellar atypical teratoma) may appear well encapsulated or may infiltrate the hypothalamus. Greater than 90% of patients will have evidence of diabetes insipidus prior to surgery.[12] Other common complaints include visual loss and growth failure or other signs of pituitary insufficiency. Calcification occurs uncommonly, but CT brain scanning will usually demonstrate the tumor well (Fig. 27-30). Cytologic examination of the CSF may reveal histologically specific cells.

Neoplasms that occur in the area of the pineal gland include gliomas of the posterior third ventricle that extend into this area, as well as primary neoplasms of the posterior fossa that secondarily invade the pineal region. The germinoma (atypical teratoma) that originates in the pineal gland occurs infrequently in the United States and Europe. Its incidence is somewhat higher in Japan, where it makes up more than 4% of intracranial tumors seen in childhood. This tumor is also known to affect males predominantly, usually in adolescence or early adult life. Because of the location of the tumor lying directly above the quadrigeminal plate, small tumors will frequently become manifest early in their clinical course with evidence of increased intracranial pressure by compression of the aqueduct of Sylvius. In addition to having headache and vomiting, the patient may be ataxic secondary to compression of the superior cerebellar peduncle. As mentioned previously, ocular mobility is frequently affected. Paralysis of upward gaze, sluggish reaction of the pupils to light, and nystagmus retractorius, help to localize the area of involvement accurately to the dorsal midbrain adjacent to the pineal gland. Occasionally, tumors present with precocious puberty or mild spastic quadriparesis with extensor plantar responses. The

germinoma that occurs in this location most commonly is composed of two cell types: small, round, lymphocytic-appearing cells scattered among large epithelial cells. This same pattern can be appreciated by cytologic examination of the CSF. Other tumors that are occasionally encountered in this area include teratomas, dermoids, pineocytomas, pineoblastomas, gliomas, and cysts.

Aside from the occasional supratentorial ependymoma that will secondarily extend into the ventricular system, choroid plexus papillomas make up the majority of tumors seen in this location. The characteristic presentation of this tumor is within the first 3 years of life and includes evidence of increased intracranial pressure secondary to the overproduction of CSF. The characteristic location is in the area of the trigone, and CSF cytology taken at the time of lumbar puncture or at the time of surgery will frequently show cells that are diagnostic of the tumor. Total resection of the tumor is usually possible. Rarely, secondary implants will occur within the central nervous system, or malignant degeneration of the tumor may be seen. Occasionally, teratomas will be found within the midline ventricular system, presenting with hydrocephalus (Fig. 27-31).

Supratentorial arachnoid cysts occur in characteristic locations (sylvian fissure, cortex, and between the hemispheres). Most commonly, cysts occur in the sylvian fissure (Fig. 27-32). The presentation of these cysts is indistinguishable from that of other focal supratentorial masses. Headache, vomiting, and seizures commonly occur in older children and adolescents. With compression of the primary motor area, hemiparesis develops. With cysts occurring in the middle fossa, a prominent temporal bulge is frequently appreciated on inspection of the head. The intracranial structures surrounding the cyst will be displaced away from it by the mass effect of the lesion (Fig. 27-32). This helps to differentiate a symptomatic arachnoid cyst from a porencephalic cyst. A porencephalic cyst that occurs as a result of cerebral damage and tissue loss does not act as a mass; rather, it may have the surrounding structures shifted toward it (Fig. 27-33). Occasionally, a porencephalic cyst will loculate and no longer freely communicate with the CSF pathways. In this special circumstance, it may then begin to act as a mass and require treatment.

Evaluation. Although x-ray films of the skull may be abnormal with supratentorial tumors, par-

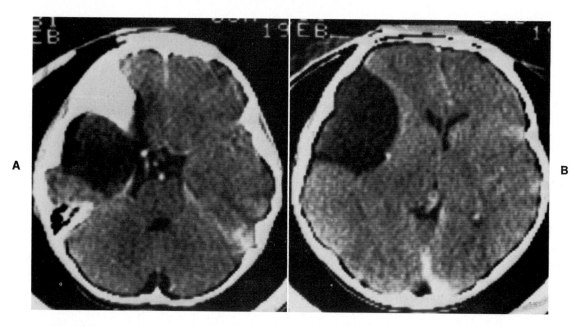

Fig. 27-32. CT brain scan of a 9-year-old child who came to medical attention with progressive left-sided weakness and headaches. On examination the patient was seen to have a left temporal bulge. **A,** The enhanced CT brain scan demonstrates a CSF-attenuation lesion in the left middle fossa (sylvian fissure). **B,** The higher section again demonstrates the cyst and the internal carotid artery viewed end-on immediately before its bifurcation. A shift of the midline structures away from the cyst is apparent. (Courtesy G. L. Odom, M.D., Durham, N.C.)

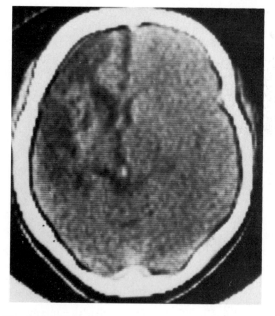

Fig. 27-33. CT brain scan of a teenager with sickle cell anemia and multiple left cerebral infarctions. The scan demonstrates a shift of the midline structures toward the infarcted hemisphere, as well as compensatory enlargement of the ipsilateral ventricle. The tissue loss has been long-standing and resulted in thickening of the vault on the involved side. (Courtesy Thomas Kinney, M.D., Durham, N.C.)

ticularly with craniopharyngiomas, the CT scan has greatly simplified the screening of many patients whose clinical presentation could be secondary to an intracranial supratentorial tumor. Abnormalities that can be seen on x-ray examination of the skull include intracranial calcification, which may be seen in as many as 25% of cerebral gliomas in children.[52] Our ability to detect intracranial calcification has been greatly enhanced by the use of the CT brain scan. Radiographs of the skull may show evidence of increased intracranial pressure. Suture separation can be appreciated best by looking at the coronal or sagittal sutures (Fig. 27-34). This finding is present in almost two thirds of patients with gliomas of the cerebral hemispheres at the time of clinical presentation.[52] In addition to suture separation and erosion of the dorsum of the sella, increased intracranial pressure may cause exaggeration of the digital impressions on the inner aspect of the skull (beaten silver appearance). The sella turcica and optic foramina are frequently found to be abnormal in the presence of sellar and parasellar tumors. Enlargement of the optic foramen, which can be demonstrated with special views of the skull, is highly suggestive of a tumor involving the portion of the optic nerve that passes through the optic canal. If the optic chiasm is in-

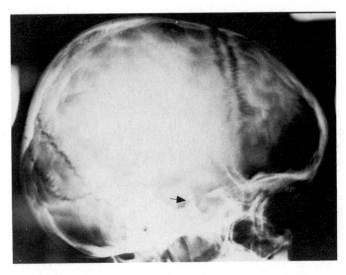

Fig. 27-34. Lateral skull film of a patient with increased intracranial pressure and separation of both coronal sutures. The pattern of interdigitation of the coronal sutures is exaggerated and the posterior clinoids (arrow) are blunted.

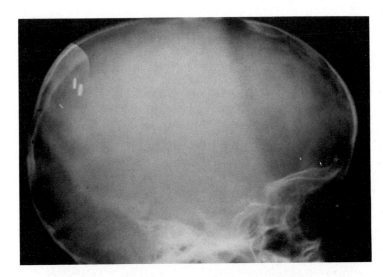

Fig. 27-35. Radiograph of a 4-year-old child seen because of irritability and vomiting. Examination disclosed evidence of increased intracranial pressure. The coronal and lambdoid sutures are separated, supporting a diagnosis of increased intracranial pressure. The sella turcica is of normal size and position; however, calcification within only one anterior clinoid can be seen. Bony destruction was secondary to a middle fossa meningioma. (The surgical clips in the posterior parietal area are from the evacuation of an epidural hematoma at 1 year of age, from which the child had recovered fully.)

volved, the sella turcica may take the appearance of the letter *J*. This finding, however, is not specific for this tumor, and normal children may have a J-shaped sella turcica. Gliomas of the hypothalamus rarely calcify and are frequently associated with a normal x-ray film of the skull. Craniopharyngiomas, on the other hand, will cause radiographic abnormalities of the skull in greater than 90% of affected patients.[5] These abnormalities include calcification within the tumor in 80% of patients. In addition, the dorsum sellae may be eroded or shortened, the sella turcica enlarged, or one or both of the anterior clinoids amputated (Fig. 27-35). Suprasellar germinomas are characteristi-

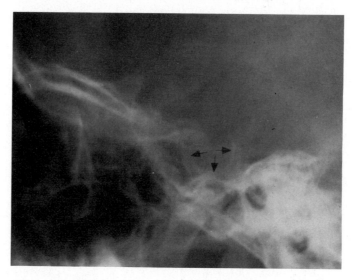

Fig. 27-36. Cone-down lateral skull film of a 12-year-old child evaluated because of severe obesity. The child was seen to have hypertension, hirsutism, diffuse muscular weakness, impaired linear growth, and purplish striae. The skull film demonstrates an enlarged and ballooned sella turcica from a cortisol-producing adenoma (Cushing's syndrome). Arrows outline the expanded bony aspect of the sella turcica. The double floor of the sella turcica can also be appreciated.

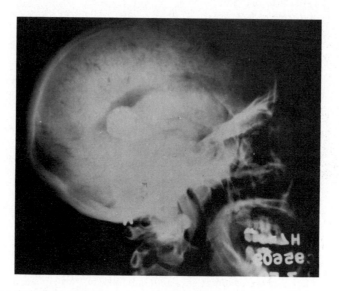

Fig. 27-37. Lateral skull film during a pneumoencephalogram showing a densely calcified pineal neoplasm measuring more than 1 cm in greatest diameter.

cally associated with normal radiographs of the skull, which will help differentiate them from craniopharyngiomas. The rare pituitary adenoma may primarily expand the sella turcica, usually without calcification within the tumor (Fig. 27-36).

Germinomas (atypical teratomas) in the pineal area may be associated with premature calcification of the pineal gland. This finding is abnormal and demands further evaluation when it is found on x-ray films of the skull in a patient below the age of 10 years or on CT scans in a patient less than 2 years of age.[30] In any age group, calcifica-

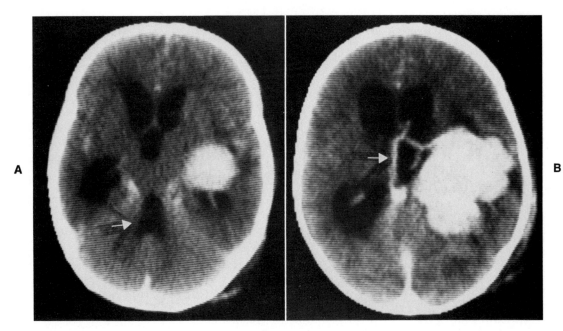

Fig. 27-38. CT brain scan of a 10-month-old infant evaluated because of irritability and macrocrania. The examination was unremarkable save for macrocrania and evidence of increased intracranial pressure. **A,** The enhanced CT scan demonstrates significant enlargement of the entire ventricular system, including the fourth ventricle (arrow). The hydrocephalus was thought to be secondary to a combination of CSF overproduction from a choroid plexus tumor in addition to communicating hydrocephalus from a subarachnoid hemorrhage from the tumor. The lesion was shown to be a choroid plexus carcinoma originating from the atrium of the lateral ventricle. **B,** The higher section shows more of the extent of the tumor, as well as the dilated venous outflow (arrow).

tion of the pineal greater than 1 cm in its greatest diameter when viewed sagittally is also suggestive of neoplastic growth and is an indication for further evaluation[30] (Fig. 27-37).

The CT brain scan is now accepted as the screening procedure of choice for supratentorial neoplasms and cysts, particularly in the presence of infiltrating gliomas of the cerebral hemispheres, in which case angiography may be normal. Pneumoencephalography would show displacement of the ventricular system and subarachnoid spaces; however, frequently more information is obtained by CT scanning (Fig. 27-38). CT scanning combined with the injection of contrast medium into the ventricular system or subarachnoid space may elucidate which cysts communicate with the ventricular system or subarachnoid space and which do not. The cyst that is loculated is much more likely to act as a mass lesion (Fig. 27-39). Cysts associated with neoplasms can easily be demonstrated. In addition, the relative position of the cyst in relation to the neoplasm can be appreciated.

Intraventricular tumors and neoplasms in the region of the pineal gland may also be readily appreciated by CT scanning. Less diagnostic accuracy, however, is present when the suprasellar areas are being evaluated. Neoplasms in this location may have attenuation coefficients that are similar to those of brain. The diagnosis is then contingent on visualization of the suprasellar cistern and soft tissue encroachment into it. These findings are frequently subtle, and further studies are required. Pneumoencephalography is still employed to outline the structures in the suprasellar areas, as well as the anterior third ventricle. The role of angiography is to assess tumor vascularity and outline vascular displacements secondary to the mass lesion, both of which are important in planning the surgical approach.

The EEG may demonstrate epileptiform activity or focal slowing in patients with supratentorial tumors and cysts. The EEG should not be used as a screening device for the presence of a structural lesion of the brain. Lumbar puncture is not

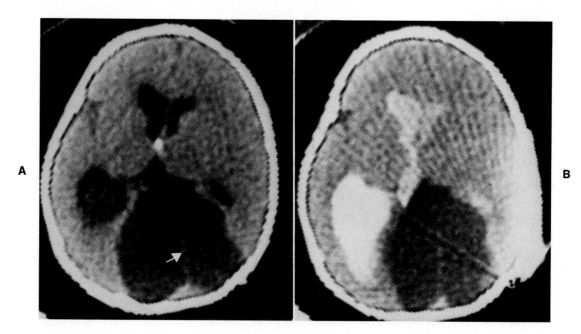

Fig. 27-39. A, Unenhanced CT brain scan of a child with hydrocephalus following shunting of the ventricular system. (The tip of the ventricular catheter can be seen as the white dot in the midline.) A large right occipital CSF attenuation mass can easily be seen displacing the surrounding structures. Within the mass is the suggestion of a septum (arrow). **B,** Following the injection of metrizamide into the ventricular system, the cyst is seen to have no contrast within it. This finding implies that the cyst is not in communication with the shunted ventricular system. Since the cyst was acting as a mass, a separate proximal catheter was used to connect the cyst with the previously placed shunt.

routinely employed in evaluating intracranial tumors unless it is thought that CSF cytology would be helpful and no evidence of increased intracranial pressure is present.

Referral. Children with the atraumatic onset of seizure activity unassociated with a fever should be screened for the presence of an intracranial mass. Even following a negative preliminary evaluation, a change in the patient's seizure pattern or breakthrough of seizure activity once control has been established on a specified dose of medication should raise the suspicion of a structural lesion of the brain. This may occur months or years following the onset of the seizure activity.[52] Seizures that are focal in onset or are associated with focal postictal paralysis or a focal EEG abnormality suggest the presence of a structural lesion of the brain. In addition to seizure activity, unexplained visual loss in any patient needs immediate and careful evaluation. The child may come to clinical attention by asking to be moved to the front of the class in school or by one of the routine visual screening programs now available. Children, particularly those who are mentally retarded, may have unrecognized loss of vision for some time before clinical detection. In general, the younger the child, the worse the visual loss prior to detection. Patients with proptosis, visual field defects, optic nerve atrophy, or papilledema all require further evaluation to identify the cause of their problem. Headache associated with nausea or vomiting, or that which is nocturnal or present in the early morning on arising, may indicate the presence of increased intracranial pressure. Additional signs on the physical examination can then be sought, including the presence of papilledema or focal neurologic deficit; and if these are present, immediate referral is indicated.

There are many causes for alteration in the endocrine system, only one of which is compression or invasion of the pituitary gland or hypothalamus. Neoplasms and cysts of the suprasellar and sellar area should be considered when other causes have been excluded. The endocrinologic abnormality may predate neuroradiologic alterations by several years, even when the most sophisticated equipment is used to detect abnormalities. Therefore, if no apparent cause of the endocrinopathy is found initially, continued surveillance is necessary; reevaluation is indicated particularly if visual complaints develop.

Medical versus surgical treatment. In general, the demonstration of an intracranial supratentorial neoplasm should be followed by histologic confirmation and attempted removal. The goal of surgery is to excise totally encapsulated or well-demarcated neoplasms, such as craniopharyngiomas or intraventricular choroid plexus papillomas. Gliomas that are diffusely infiltrative should be treated by generous internal decompression, removing as much gross tumor as possible without endangering vital brain structures and increasing the preoperative neurologic deficit. Frequently, tumors located in the temporal or frontal lobe, especially those presenting with seizure activity early in their course, can be treated by total macroscopic surgical removal. This plan is advocated in all cerebral neoplasms located in surgically accessible areas. The number of patients with surgically inaccessible lesions is decreasing. Technical advances now allow visualization of areas of the brain that previously could be approached only with acceptance of high operative risk. The pineal region is such an area. Currently, this area can be visualized with the use of the operating microscope and microinstrumentation with little increase in risk as compared with other procedures performed to visualize and remove intracranial tumors.

Even with tumors that are considered surgically inaccessible utilizing standard techniques, stereotactic biopsy guided by the CT scanner can now be considered. Lesions of the basal ganglia and thalamus fall into this category. The "blind" treatment of suspected supratentorial tumors with radiation therapy or chemotherapy without histologic confirmation and attempted surgical removal is becoming unnecessary. Neoplasms of the parasellar area present a special problem in management. The preservation of function despite the infiltrative nature of gliomas of the hypothalamus and optic chiasm makes attempted removal ill advised. In these patients biopsy and consideration of adjunctive therapy is recommended. Optic nerve gliomas confined to the orbit are followed with CT scanning. When all useful vision is lost or the eye becomes significantly proptotic, surgical resection of the tumor should be considered. The growth potential of gliomas that lie in the orbit is limited, justifying this conservative therapeutic approach.[35] Radiotherapy in this group of patients is of questionable value.

Supratentorial arachnoid cysts presenting clinically with a mass effect require surgical therapy. As previously mentioned, a porencephalic cyst that freely communicates with the CSF pathway does not require therapy, because it will not act as a mass lesion. Those that do become loculated and expand should be treated in a manner similar to that for expanding arachnoid cysts.

Surgical options. Tumors located within the substance of the cerebral hemispheres are routinely approached through an osteoplastic craniotomy. The overlying gyri may be widened and pale, as well as edematous and soft. A cortical incision is made through a gyrus thought to be maximally involved with tumor and yet not in a vital area. Within the cortical incision, the neoplasm is identified by its altered texture, consistency, and color. Once the neoplasm is located, an attempt is made to stay within the tumor during the resection. The alternative to this debulking approach to supratentorial gliomas is to assume from the preoperative radiographic studies that the neoplasm is confined to an anatomically defined lobe of the brain such as the temporal lobe or the occipital or frontal pole. An attempt is then made to excise the involved lobe, leaving a portion of uninvolved brain along the surgical margins. This approach is justified only when the neoplasm is thought to be relatively confined anatomically and when surgical cure is possible by a more radical procedure. Even though total macroscopic tumor removal may be possible, microscopic infiltration of the surrounding cortex is commonly present.

Tumors that lie in the suprasellar area are usually approached through a right frontotemporal osteoplastic craniotomy using lumbar drainage and osmotic diuretics to shrink the brain and minimize the retraction necessary to visualize the optic nerve, optic chiasm, sella turcica, and large vessels at the base of the brain. If the tumor is large and extends superiorly and posteriorly with compression of the anterior third ventricle, a combined subfrontal and transventricular approach may be helpful. In this way, both the dome of the tumor and that portion of the tumor intimately involved with the delicate vascular and neural structures at the base of the brain may be seen and freed from surrounding tissue prior to removal. If the tumor expands posteriorly from the sella and lies in the interpeduncular cistern, it may be advantageous to lift the temporal lobe and split the tentorium to allow maximal visualization. It is emphasized here that in treating a craniopharyngioma, which is a histologically benign neoplasm, every effort should be made during the initial resection to remove the tumor totally. Secondary and tertiary attempts at tumor removal are notoriously difficult, carrying with them a high morbidity and mortality. Partial resection followed by radiation therapy is associated with a significant rate of recurrence of the tumor and should not be employed unless total removal is not possible. If the suprasellar area is explored and an intrinsic glial tumor of the hypothalamus or optic chiasm is found, simple biopsy in a clinically silent area or of an exophytic mass is the procedure of choice. Optic nerve gliomas lying in the orbit may be exposed through a frontal craniotomy. The bony roof of the orbit is removed, and the optic nerve with its tumor is resected. The globe is routinely left to act as a prosthesis.

Recent experience with successful surgical approaches to the pineal region have encouraged surgeons to explore neoplasms that were previously not confirmed histologically but treated presumptively with radiation therapy and shunting procedures for hydrocephalus.[36,79,80] An advantage to surgical exploration is finding the occasional patient with a totally benign congenital tumor (dermoid, teratoma), which would have been ineffectively controlled by radiotherapy. Surgical resection of these benign tumors is the procedure of choice and may result in cure.

Intraventricular tumors are approached through the corpus callosum or through a cortical incision over the tumor. The goal of surgery is to locate the vascular pedicle and ligate the feeding vessels prior to resection of the tumor. With the use of this technique, blood loss can be minimized. Tumors that have caused hydrocephalus, particularly in the pineal and suprasellar areas, will benefit from normalization of the intracranial pressure prior to removal of the tumor. This is routinely done by inserting a ventriculoperitoneal shunt 7 to 10 days prior to the tumor resection.

Supratentorial cysts are most easily treated by diverting their contents to a compartment where resorption may take place. Craniotomy with excision of the cyst wall and communication of the cyst with the subarachnoid space will frequently be associated with recurrence of symptoms.[10] A simpler approach is to shunt the cyst primarily, either to the peritoneal cavity or to the cervical subarachnoid space, depending on whether or not communicating hydrocephalus is thought to be present.

Postoperative course. Following craniotomy for a supratentorial neoplasm, the patient needs careful physiologic monitoring of multiple functions. Such monitoring is most easily done in a neurosurgical intensive care unit in which the personnel are familiar with the care of children. Adequate renal output is maintained by intravenous fluid infusion; total fluid intake is minimized, however, to limit cerebral edema. High-dose corticosteroids are given to control cerebral edema. The head is elevated to 30 degrees above the horizontal to enhance venous drainage of the brain. The tendency to develop inappropriate secretion of antidiuretic hormone (ADH) both preoperatively and postoperatively is carefully monitored. Hyponatremia, which is most commonly caused by inappropriate ADH secretion in the postoperative period, is routinely treated by fluid restriction and the occasional use of intravenous infusion of hypertonic saline when the patient develops seizures from the hyponatremia. Procedures that have involved the sellar and suprasellar structures with either manipulation or trauma to hypothalamic or pituitary tissue may be followed by either transient or permanent diabetes insipidus and/or panhypopituitarism. Corticosteroids are routinely given both preoperatively and postoperatively to these patients until their physiologic pituitary function can be assessed, usually several months following the craniotomy. During this time maintenance corticosteroids are given, but thyroid replacement is not. Diabetes insipidus may become manifest within the first few hours following surgery or may be delayed in onset and not be seen until several days after the craniotomy.

In the stuporous or comatose patient, urinary output must be very carefully monitored by hourly recording of the volume and specific gravity, as well as by frequent estimation of the serum electrolytes and osmolarity. As long as urinary output remains at a reasonable level that can easily be replaced either orally or intravenously, little difficulty arises. However, when the output becomes excessive, particularly in the patient with a depressed mental status and inability to verbalize thirst due to hyperosmolarity, it has been our practice to administer aqueous vasopressin (Pitressin) to control the urinary output. Once the child is urinating more than 150 to 200 ml an hour of very dilute urine (specific gravity less than 1.002), the ability of the nursing staff to replace this fluid intravenously becomes strained. It is then safer to control the urinary output by the administration of aqueous vasopressin and wait for the patient's mental status to improve so that the thirst mechanism may help establish a homeostatic balance. Once the patient is fully conscious and able to drink, he is allowed to drink freely. During the nighttime, to ensure adequate rest, vasopressin is again administered to prevent the patient from having to awaken every hour to void and then drink. Longer-acting antidiuretic drugs such as vasopressin tannate in oil (Pitressin Tannate) are avoided in the immediate postoperative period. The diabetes insipidus may frequently resolve over a period of days, and this can be more easily recognized when the short-acting antidiuretic compounds are used.

The presence of postoperative hemorrhage and wound infection are always kept in mind as possible complications following craniotomy. Again, the CT scan has greatly facilitated evaluation of the presence of postoperative hemorrhage. Unexplained fever is routinely evaluated by lumbar puncture and wound examination to ensure that meningitis and wound infection are not present.

When cortical contusion has occurred, postoperative seizures can be seen. These are not treated prophylactically with anticonvulsants because of their low incidence. However, patients who have seizure activity prior to surgery and are receiving one or more anticonvulsants have their medication continued at the same dosage schedule in the postoperative period. Even if a portion of the epileptic focus has been excised, rapid withdrawal of anticonvulsants may promote seizure activity from the area surrounding the cortical excision. EEGs are used to help the physician determine if the anticonvulsants may be gradually tapered over several weeks or months following the surgical procedure. It should be emphasized that cerebral neoplasms associated with seizure activity will continue to demonstrate this activity despite removal of the inciting neoplasm. Surgery to remove these intrinsic gliomas or compressive neoplasms of the brain will frequently not remove the seizure focus. This is because the brain that surrounds the neoplasm and that is either partially infiltrated with tumor or simply compressed by the tumor will continue to demonstrate seizure activity after the tumor resection. There is no justification for removing this surrounding cortex at the time of the tumor resection, since functional neural tissue will be mixed with the epileptic focus. Therefore, the tendency to have seizure activity will continue in most patients following resection of the tumor. Seizure control may be somewhat simpler postoperatively, but anticonvulsants are usually still necessary.

If radiation therapy is not necessary, the routine hospital stay following a supratentorial craniotomy for tumor is 7 to 14 days.

Prognosis. The eventual outcome of patients with supratentorial neoplasms is influenced by many factors. The most important of these are the histologic nature of the tumor and its location. Histologically benign choroid plexus papillomas that are totally removed can be considered to be cured. The hydrocephalus that routinely accompanies this tumor may continue to require a shunt. However, in approximately 50% of patients, the hydrocephalus resolves with resection of the tumor.

Patients with gliomas of the cerebral hemispheres may survive for many years following their resection. Histologically aggressive tumors will usually show clinical recurrence within a few months to years of the initial resection. Patients with benign astrocytomas treated with surgical resection and postoperative radiation frequently survive for several years prior to clinical recurrence. Occasional long-term survivors without clinical or radiographic evidence of recurrence will be seen, particularly when the tumor has been located in a clinically silent area of the brain, allowing radical removal. Ependymomas above the tentorium have a particularly unfavorable outcome despite surgery and radiation.[60,77] Radiation therapy is frequently given to patients with known partial resection of histologically benign cerebral gliomas, although the advantage is marginal.

Tumors that occur in the area of the pineal gland to a large extent have their outcome predicted by their histology. The atypical teratoma or germinoma is radiosensitive. Craniospinal radiation is given following surgical exploration and attempted resection. Chemotherapy may be of significant benefit in isolated cases.[62] The 5-year-survival rate for patients with this tumor is greater than 50%. With a more aggressive surgical approach prior to adjunctive therapy, this figure may improve.

Gliomas that involve the hypothalamus are associated with a generally poor prognosis, with the majority of the patients dying within 5 years of

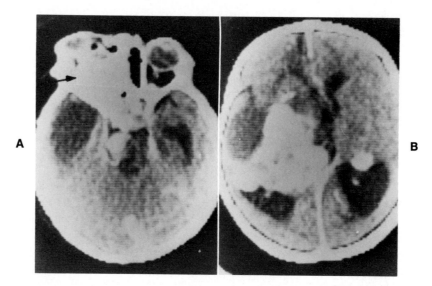

Fig. 27-40. Enhanced CT brain scan of a child who had left-sided visual loss. Evaluation disclosed a markedly enlarged left optic foramen. A mass was present within the chiasm and presumed to be a glioma. The child received radiation therapy. **A,** Four years after the initial therapy, the CT scan demonstrates massive enlargement of the tumor within the orbit (arrow) and intradurally. The brain stem is compressed from the front and the left. **B,** The higher section shows more of the extent of the tumor with a significant shift of the midline structures to the right. The study demonstrates the progressive nature of some anterior visual pathway gliomas.

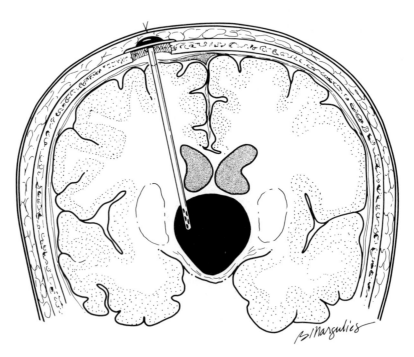

Fig. 27-41. Coronal section of a patient with cystic craniopharyngioma. The cystic portion of the tumor is cannulated with Silastic tubing and attached to a subcutaneous reservoir for periodic aspiration.

diagnosis despite radiation therapy. Gliomas that are confined to the anterior aspect of the optic nerve usually follow a benign course, either remaining static or growing slowly over a period of years. Tumors of the optic chiasm may follow a similar benign course for many years; however, the growth potential of this tumor is significantly greater than that of gliomas confined to the optic nerve. Many tumors that originate in the optic chiasm are seen to enlarge rather rapidly and threaten life (Fig. 27-40).

Patients with craniopharyngiomas approached aggressively during the initial resection may survive for extended periods of time, with more than half presumed to be cured.[52] However, the morbidity of an aggressive surgical approach is significant and includes diabetes insipidus, panhypopituitarism, and increased visual loss. If only partial excision is possible, radiation therapy is given; however, long-term cure of these patients is unlikely. Secondary tumor resections carry increased risks of intraoperative damage and should be performed selectively. Occasionally, patients with large cystic components to their tumors will benefit from periodic aspiration of the cyst (Fig. 27-41). Most patients with arachnoid cysts enjoy an excellent outcome. However, continued surveillance of the patient for adequate shunt function is necessary.

Important aspects of follow-up. After craniotomy and resection of supratentorial neoplasms or shunting of cysts, patients can now be followed easily for recurrence by repeat CT brain scans. Not only can the size of the tumor or cyst be estimated, but also the ventricular size is easily seen and the necessity for either shunt placement or shunt revision can be made. A most important aspect of follow-up relates to tumors in the area of the hypothalamic-pituitary axis. Very frequently these patients receive total endocrine replacement. Patients with total dependence on exogenous corticosteroids and thyroid replacement must be made aware that if they encounter additional physical stress, including virtually any systemic illness, they must increase their steroid dosage. This fact needs continual reinforcement from the patient's primary care physician. On occasion, death has occurred following successful resection of a benign tumor of the suprasellar area because inadequate steroid replacement was maintained during a subsequent stressful situation.

Diabetes insipidus is currently managed by the nasal installation of the antidiuretic compound desmopressin acetate (DDAVP) or by the injection of the relatively long-acting vasopressin tannate in oil. Should the patient lose consciousness for any reason, the tendency toward diabetes insipidus should always be remembered. This is particularly true if repeated seizure activity occurs and adequate fluid replacement is not maintained. The patient will rapidly develop a hyperosmolar syndrome and compound his tendency for seizure activity.

Complications. As previously stated, tumor recurrence and the presence of hydrocephalus can be evaluated easily in most patients by CT brain scans. Epilepsy is a well-recognized complication of any neoplasm occurring in the supratentorial compartment or from a craniotomy with manipulation of the cortex. Seizures can usually be controlled quite adequately with anticonvulsants. Progressive focal neurologic deficits may be due to recurrent tumor growth or can occasionally be seen with cyst formation at the site of the cortical resection. Again, CT scanning will frequently differentiate amenable causes from those that could not be helped by further surgery. As tumors in the hypothalamus and anterior visual pathway slowly enlarge, further visual compromise will take place. Careful attention to repeated visual field examinations and assessment of visual acuity are important to help document the rate of this progression. In addition, the function of the hypothalamic-pituitary axis should be remembered.

Other, less common lesions. There are many additional types of tumors that are occasionally encountered in the supratentorial compartment. Among these are the congenital developmental tumors, including the dermoid, epidermoid, and teratoma. When one of these tumors is suspected, it should be approached with the preoperative plan of total excision.

Rarely, primary tumors of neurons occur above the tentorium and are classified as ganglioneuromas and gangliogliomas. Characteristically, these tumors occur in the third ventricle, hypothalamus, and temporal lobe; they frequently present with seizure activity and are noted for their propensity to calcify. These tumors are slow growing and usually have a long clinical history. The supporting glial elements have been seen to undergo malignant degeneration in some patients.

Meningiomas, pituitary adenomas, and metastatic tumors of the brain are rarely encountered

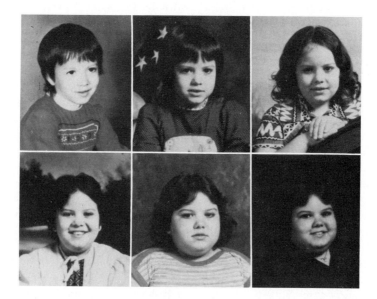

A

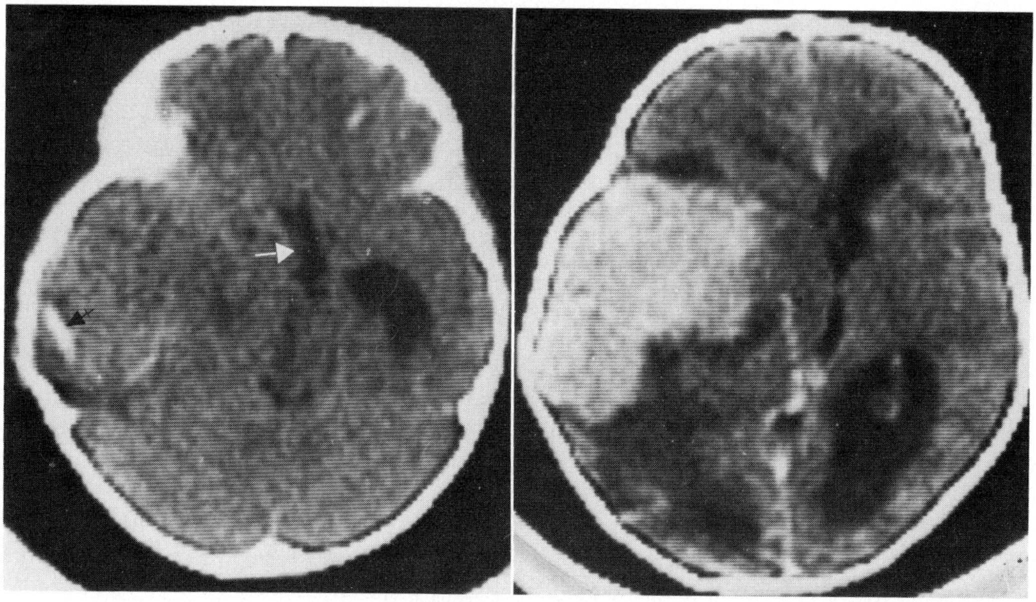

B

Fig. 27-42. A, Unenhanced CT brain scan of the patient seen in Fig. 27-35 demonstrates displacement of third-ventricle (→) dilatation of the right temporal horn, expansion of the left middle fossa, and pathologic calcification within the tumor (↦). **B,** Following contrast administration, the tumor enhances homogeneously. Surrounding the tumor are areas of low attenuation compatible with edema of the surrounding brain. The lesion was histologically confirmed to be a meningioma originating in the area of Meckel's cave (dural covering of the gasserian ganglion).

Fig. 27-43. Serial photographs demonstrating the facial changes of a child with Cushing's syndrome (same patient as seen in Fig. 27-36). The tumor is clinically evident in the last four pictures.

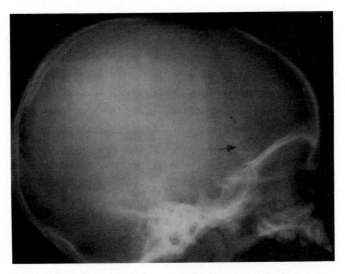

Fig. 27-44. Lateral skull film of a child with an epidermoid tumor in the inferior frontal bone. The lesion appears "punched out" and is completely surrounded by a sclerotic border. The lesion is encapsulated and should be excised when diagnosed to prevent compression of the intracranial contents.

in children as compared with adults, in whom these tumors make up a very significant portion of the neoplasms seen. The meningiomas that do occur do so with an increased propensity for the intraventricular and posterior fossa locations. The diagnosis is simplified by contrast-enhanced CT scanning (Fig. 27-42).

Pituitary tumors are being recognized with increased frequency in childhood because of raised clinical suspicion and improved methods of detection.[70] The most common presenting complaint is that of failure of sexual maturation. However, 80% of patients will demonstrate evidence of pituitary hypersecretion (Cushing's syndrome [Fig. 27-43], gigantism, acromegaly, or the amenorrhea-galactorrhea syndrome). X-ray films of the sella turcica are abnormal in the majority of patients when hypocycloidal polytomography is used. Fractional pneumoencephalography will help differentiate pituitary adenomas from other tumors that occur in this area (e.g., craniopharyngioma). Recommended therapy consists of transsphenoidal or transcranial resection followed by radiation therapy when only incomplete resection is possible.

TUMORS OF THE SKULL AND SCALP

Primary tumors of the skull and scalp are occasionally encountered throughout the pediatric age range. Commonly seen are epidermoids and dermoids. *Epidermoids* in the skull tend to occur off the midline and are surrounded by a sclerotic border that is easily appreciated on skull films (Fig. 27-44). These lesions come to clinical attention as a result of swelling and tenderness over the lesion or as a result of routine radiographs taken following head trauma. Only rarely will laterally placed epidermoids be associated with significant intracranial extension. Therapy consists of removal of the encapsulated mass. *Dermoids* tend to occur in the midline, primarily over the occiput. The subcutaneous tumor will frequently be associated with a dermal sinus tract leading to the skin. Occasionally, these lesions will extend intracranially and be associated with recurrent bouts of bacterial meningitis or an intracranial mass (Fig. 27-45). Skull x-ray films will demonstrate a bony defect under the mass when intracranial extension exists. The dermal sinus tract through the skull may become sclerotic. Therapy consists of excision of the tumor. Delay in excision is unjustified when extension of a dermal sinus tract to the skin is found. Mobile subgaleal masses over the anterior fontanelle are most frequently found to be inclusion dermoid tumors. Lesions in this location rarely demonstrate intracranial extension and can easily be excised without elaborate preoperative evaluation.

Eosinophilic granulomas may be solitary or multiple and frequently involve the skull. Patients come to clinical attention with immobile scalp swelling that may be somewhat tender. Radio-

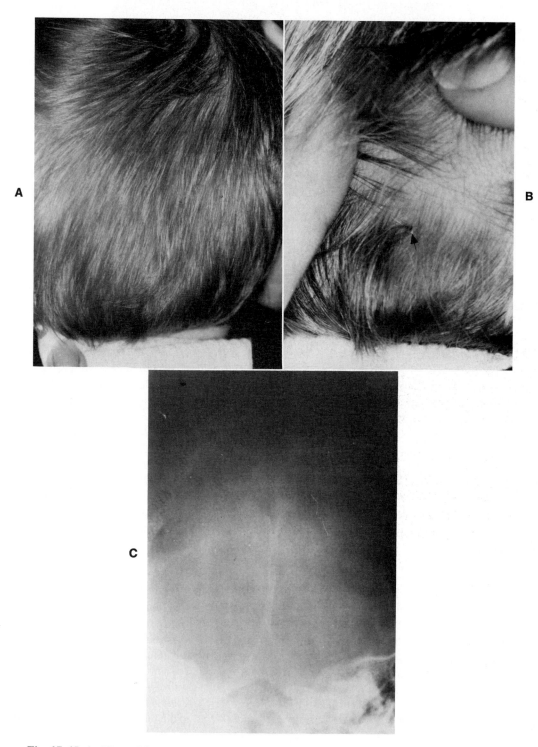

Fig. 27-45. A, View of the occipital area of a child with no obvious abnormality. **B,** Careful inspection reveals a dermal sinus tract (arrow) that had been responsible for a previous bout of staphylococcal meningitis. **C,** Skull film demonstrating a vertically oriented sclerotic tract within the occipital bone, implying intracranial extension.

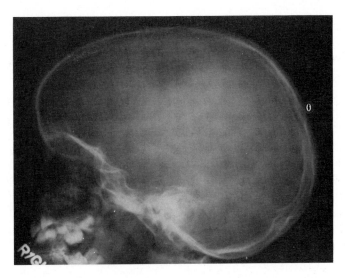

Fig. 27-46. Lateral skull film of a patient with an eosinophilic granuloma. The lesion is near the coronal suture in the parietal bone. The lesion is characterized by an area of irregular bony destruction without a surrounding sclerotic border.

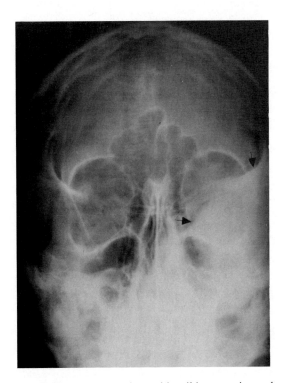

Fig. 27-47. Teenage patient with mild proptosis on the left and left-sided orbital pain and headache. The greater and lesser wings of the sphenoid bone (arrows) are densely sclerotic from fibrous dysplasia.

graphs of the skull demonstrate a well-defined "punched out" area without a sclerotic border (Fig. 27-46). The radiographic appearance is not diagnostic, and these lesions should be removed to confirm their histology. If multiple areas of the skull are involved, biopsy of a single lesion for histologic confirmation combined with low-dose radiation therapy is the therapy of choice.

Fibrous dysplasia is thought to be a mesenchymal developmental anomaly that frequently affects the bone about the orbit. Involved areas may demonstrate bony prominence without evidence of pain. The disease generally comes to clinical attention in late childhood and early adolescence. The diagnosis can be strongly suspected from the radiographic appearance (Fig. 27-47). Therapy consists of removal of the excessive bony growth that compromises neurologic function (e.g., optic nerve) or leads to progressive proptosis.

REFERENCES

1. Aicardi, J., and Bauman, F.: Supratentorial extracerebral cysts in infants and children, J. Neurol. Neurosurg. Psychiatry **38**:57, 1975.
2. Amacher, A. L., Allcock, J. M., and Drake, C. G.: Cerebral angiomas: the sequelae of surgical treatment, J. Neurosurg. **37**:571, 1972.
3. Amacher, A. L., and Drake, C. G.: Cerebral artery aneurysms in infancy, childhood, and adolescence, Child's Brain **1**:72, 1975.
4. Bailey, P., Buchanan, D. N., and Bucy, P. C.: Intracranial tumors of infancy and childhood, Chicago, 1939, University of Chicago Press.

5. Banna, M.: Craniopharyngioma: based on 160 cases, Br. J. Radiol. **49:**206, 1976.

6. Barnett, H. J. M., Foster, J. B., and Hudgson, P.: Syringomyelia, London, 1973, W. B. Saunders Co., Ltd.

7. Bell, R. S., and Loop, J. W.: The utility and futility of radiographic skull examinations for trauma, N. Engl. J. Med. **284:**236, 1971.

8. Bell, W. E., and McCormick, W. F.: Increased intracranial pressure in children: diagnosis and treatment, ed. 2, Philadelphia, 1978, W. B. Saunders Co.

9. Bergeron, R. T., and Rumbaugh, C. L.: Skull trauma. In Newton, T. H., and Potts, D. G., editors: Radiology of the skull and brain. Vol. 1. The skull, St. Louis, 1971, The C. V. Mosby Co.

10. Bhandari, Y. S.: Non-communicating supratentorial subarachnoid cysts, J. Neurol. Neurosurg. Psychiatry **35:**763, 1972.

11. Brackett, C. E.: Special problems associated with subarachnoid hemorrhage. In Youmans, J. R., editor: Neurological surgery, Philadelphia, 1973, W. B. Saunders Co.

12. Camins, M. B., and Mount, L. A.: Primary suprasellar atypical teratoma, Brain **97:**447, 1974.

13. Carlson, C. B., Harvey, F. H., and Loop, J.: Progressive alternating hemiplegia in early childhood with basal arterial stenosis and telangiectasis (moyamoya syndrome), Neurology **23:**734, 1974.

14. Chater, N. L., Buncke, H., and Brownstein, M.: Revascularization of the scalp by microsurgical techniques after complete avulsion, Neurosurgery **2:**269, 1978.

15. Chiofalo, N., and others: Occlusive arterial disease of the child and young adult, Child's Brain **4:**1, 1978.

16. Coulon, R. A., and Till, K.: Intracranial ependymomas in children, Child's Brain **3:**154, 1977.

17. Crompton, M. R.: Brainstem lesions due to closed head injury, Lancet **1:**669, 1971.

18. Crompton, M. R.: Hypothalamic lesions following closed head injury, Brain **94:**165, 1971.

19. Cuneo, H. M., and Rand, C. W.: Brain tumors of childhood, Springfield, Ill., 1952, Charles C Thomas, Publisher.

20. Debrun, G.: Treatment of certain intracerebral vascular lesions with releasable balloon catheter. In Schmidek, H. H., and Sweet, W. H., editors: Current techniques in operative neurosurgery, New York, 1977, Grune & Stratton, Inc.

21. Dillon, H., and Leopold, R. L.: Children and the postconcussion syndrome, J.A.M.A. **175:**110, 1961.

22. Drake, C. G.: Cerebral arteriovenous malformations: considerations for and experience with surgical treatment in 166 cases, Clin. Neurosurg. **26:**145, 1979.

23. Ducker, T. B.: Increased intracranial pressure and pulmonary edema, J. Neurosurg. **28:**112, 1968.

24. Eisenbrey, A. B.: Retinal hemorrhage in the battered child, Child's Brain **5:**40, 1979.

25. Elliott, H.: Deaths from skull fracture and other head injuries in Canada. In DeVet, A. C., editor: Proceedings of the Third International Congress of Neurological Surgery of the World Federation of Neurosurgical Society, Copenhagen, August 23-27, 1965, Amsterdam, 1966, Excerpta Medica Foundation.

26. Ford, F. R.: Diseases of the nervous system in infancy, childhood, and adolescence, ed. 6, Springfield, Ill., 1973, Charles C Thomas, Publisher.

27. Forster, D. M.C., Steiner, L., and Hakanson, S.: Arteriovenous malformations of the brain: a long-term clinical study, J. Neurosurg. **37:**562, 1972.

28. Griffith, J. F., and Dodge, P. R.: Transient blindness following head injury in children, N. Engl. J. Med. **278:**648, 1968.

29. Hammon, W. H.: Retained intracranial bone fragments: analysis of 42 patients, J. Neurosurg. **34:**142, 1971.

30. Harwood-Nash, D. C., and Fitz, C. R.: Neuroradiology in infants and children, St. Louis, 1976, The C. V. Mosby Co.

31. Heiskanen, O., and Kaste, M.: Late prognosis of severe brain injury in children, Dev. Med. Child Neurol. **16:**11, 1974.

32. Hendrick, E. B., Harwood-Nash, D. C., and Hudson, A. R.: Head injuries in children: a survey of 4465 consecutive cases at the Hospital For Sick Children, Toronto, Canada, Clin. Neurosurg. **11:**46, 1964.

33. Hoffman, H. J., Hendrick, E. B., and Humphreys, R. P.: Spinal cord injuries. In Care for the injured child, Baltimore, 1975, The Williams & Wilkins Co.

34. Holden, A. M., and others: Congestive heart failure from intracranial arteriovenous fistula in infancy, Pediatrics **49:**30, 1972.

35. Hoyt, W. F., and Baghdassarian, S. A.: Optic gliomas of childhood: natural history and rationale for conservative management, Br. J. Ophthalmol. **53:**793, 1969.

36. Jamieson, K. G.: Excision of pineal tumors, J. Neurosurg. **35:**550, 1971.

37. Jennett, B.: Head injuries in children, Dev. Med. Child Neurol. **14:**137, 1972.

38. Jennett, B.: Trauma as a cause of epilepsy in childhood, Dev. Med. Child Neurol. **15:**56, 1973.

39. Johnson, E.: Cycles and patterns of hair growth. In Jarrett, A., editor: The physiology and pathophysiology of the skin, New York, 1977, Academic Press, Inc.

40. Kelly, J. J., Mellinger, J. F., and Sundt, T. M.: Intracranial arteriovenous malformations in childhood, Ann. Neurol. **3:**338, 1978.

41. Kempe, C. H.: Pediatric implications of the battered baby syndrome, Arch. Dis. Child. **46:**28, 1971.

42. Kingsley, D., Till, K., and Hoare, R.: Growing fractures of the skull, J. Neurol. Neurosurg. Psychiatry **41:**312, 1978.

43. Klonoff, H., Low, M. D., and Clark, C.: Head injuries in children: a prospective five year follow-up, J. Neurol. Neurosurg. Psychiatry **40:**1211, 1977.

44. Koos, W. T., and Miller, M. H.: Intracranial tumors of infants and children, St. Louis, 1971, The C. V. Mosby Co.

45. Liu, H. M., Boggs, J., and Kidd, J.: Ependymomas of childhood, Child's Brain **2:**92, 1976.

46. Locksley, H. B.: Report on the cooperative study of intracranial aneurysms and subarachnoid hemorrhage. Sect. 5, part 1. Natural history of subarachnoid hemorrhage, intracranial aneurysms, and arteriovenous malformations, J. Neurosurg. **25:**219, 1966.

47. Long, D. M., and others: Giant arteriovenous malformations of infancy and childhood, J. Neurosurg. **40:**304, 1974.

48. Luessenhop, A. J., and Presper, J. H.: Surgical embolization of cerebral arteriovenous malformations through internal carotid and vertebral arteries: long-term results, J. Neurosurg. **42:**443, 1975.

49. Lundberg, N., and others: Non-operative management of intracranial hypertension, Adv. Tech. Stud. Neurosurg. **1:**3, 1974.

50. Margolis, G., Odom, G. L., and Woodhall, B.: Further experiences with small vascular malformations as a cause of massive intracerebral bleeding, J. Neuropathol. Exp. Neurol. **20:**161, 1961.

51. Marshall, L. F., Smith, R. W., and Shapiro, H. M.: The outcome with aggressive treatment in severe head injuries, J. Neurosurg. **50:**26, 1979.

52. Matson, D. D.: Neurosurgery of infancy and childhood, Springfield, Ill., 1969, Charles C Thomas, Publisher.

53. Melchior, J. C.: The incidence of head injuries in children, Acta Paediatr. **50:**47, 1961.

54. Merino-DeVillasante, J., and Taveras, J. M.: Computerized tomography (CT) in acute head trauma, A.J.R. **126:** 765, 1976.

55. Michelsen, W. J.: Natural history and pathophysiology of arteriovenous malformations, Clin. Neurosurg. **23:**307, 1979.

56. Milhorat, T. H.: Pediatric neurosurgery, Philadelphia, 1978, F. A. Davis Co.

57. Milhorat, T. H., and others: Choroid plexus papilloma: proof of cerebrospinal fluid over-production, Child's Brain **2:**273, 1976.

58. Miller, C. F., Brodkey, J. S., and Colombi, F. J.: The danger of intracranial wood, Surg. Neurol. **7:**95, 1977.

59. Miller, D., and Adams, H.: Physiopathology and management of increased intracranial pressure. In Critchley, M., O'Leary, J. L., and Jennett, B., editors: Scientific foundations of neurology, London, 1972, William Heinemann Medical Books, Ltd.

60. Mork, S. J., and Loken, A. C.: Ependymoma: a follow-up study of 101 cases, Cancer **40:**907, 1977.

61. Natelson, S. E., and Sayers, M. P.: The fate of children sustaining severe head trauma during birth, Pediatrics **51:**169, 1973.

62. Neuwelt, E. A., and others: Malignant pineal region tumors: a clinico-pathological study, J. Neurosurg. **51:** 597, 1979.

63. Nishimoto, A., and Takeuchi, S.: Abnormal cerebrovascular network related to the internal carotid arteries, J. Neurosurg. **29:**255, 1968.

64. Northfield, D. W. C.: The surgery of the central nervous system, Oxford, 1973, Blackwell Scientific Publications, Ltd.

65. Page, L. K., Lombroso, C. T., and Matson, D. D.: Childhood epilepsy with late detection of cerebral glioma, J. Neurosurg. **31:**253, 1969.

66. Patel, A. N., and Richardson, A. E.: Ruptured intracranial aneurysms in the first two decades of life, J. Neurosurg. **35:**571, 1971.

67. Paxson, C. L., and Brown, D. R.: Post-traumatic anterior hypopituitarism, Pediatrics **57:**893, 1976.

68. Peerless, S. J., and Drake, C. G.: Surgical treatment of aneurysm of the posterior fossa. In Ransohoff, J., editor: Modern techniques in surgery, Mount Kisco, N.Y., 1979, Futura Publishing Co., Inc.

69. Plum, F., and Posner, J. B.: The diagnosis of stupor and coma, ed. 3, Philadelphia, 1980, F. A. Davis Co.

70. Richmond, I. L., and Wilson, C. B.: Pituitary adenomas in childhood and adolescence, J. Neurosurg. **49:**163, 1978.

71. Rizzoli, H. V.: Treatment of peripheral nerve injuries. In Meirowsky, A. M., editor: Neurological surgery of trauma, Washington, D.C., 1975, Office of the Surgeon General, Department of the Army.

72. Robinson, R. G.: Congenital cysts of the brain: arachnoid malformations, Prog. Neurol. Surg. **4:**133, 1971.

73. Samii, M.: Modern aspects of peripheral and cranial nerve surgery, Adv. Tech. Stud. Neurosurg. **2:**33, 1975.

74. Sato, O., Tsugane, R., and Kageyama, N.: Cerebrospinal fluid pulsatile force and focal ventricular dilatation in cases of growing skull fracture, Neurochirurgia. **17:**1, 1974.

75. Schneider, R. C.: Trauma to the spine and spinal cord. In Kahn, E. A., and others, editors: Correlative neurosurgery, ed. 2, Springfield, Ill., 1969, Charles C Thomas, Publisher.

76. Scotti, L. N., and others, editors: Venous thrombosis in infants and children, Radiology **112:**393, 1974.

77. Shuman, R. M., Alvrod, E. C., and Leech, R. W.: The biology of childhood ependymomas, Arch. Neurol. **32:** 731, 1975.

78. Solomon, G. E., and others: Natural history of acute hemiplegia of childhood, Brain **93:**107, 1970.

79. Stein, B. M.: The infratentorial supracerebellar approach to pineal lesions, J. Neurosurg. **35:**197, 1971.

80. Suzuki, J., and Iwabuchi, T.: Surgical removal of pineal tumors (pinealomas and teratomas), J. Neurosurg. **23:** 565, 1965.

81. Taveras, J. M.: Multiple progressive arterial occlusion: a syndrome of children and young adults, A.J.R. **106:**235, 1969.

82. Teasdale, G., and Jennett, B.: Assessment of coma and impaired consciousness, Lancet **2:**81, 1974.

83. Terbrugge, K., and others: Computed tomography in intracranial arteriovenous malformations, Radiology **122:**703, 1977.

84. Thompson, J. B., and others: Surgical management of diastatic linear skull fractures in infants, J. Neurosurg. **39:**493, 1973.

85. Vannucci, R. C., and Baten, M.: Cerebral metastatic disease in childhood, Neurology **24:**981, 1974.

86. Ver Brugghen, A.: Neurosurgery in general practice, Springfield, Ill., 1952, Charles C Thomas, Publisher.

87. Vital statistics of the United States, 1977, Rockville, Md., U.S. Department of Health, Education, and Welfare, Public Health Service.

88. Yarsargil, M. G., and Fox, J. L.: The microsurgical approach to intracranial aneurysms, Surg. Neurol. **3:**7, 1975.

89. Yarsargil, M. G., and others: Arteriovenous malformations of the anterior and the middle portions of the corpus callosum: microsurgical treatment, Surg. Neurol. **5:**67, 1976.

90. Yarsargil, M. G., and others: Arteriovenous malformations of vein of Galen: microsurgical treatment, Surg. Neurol. **6:**195, 1976.

91. Zelson, C., Lee, S. J., and Pearl, M.: The incidence of skull fractures underlying cephalohematomas in newborn infants, J. Pediatr. **85:**371, 1974.

CHAPTER 28

Orthopedic considerations

ROBERT J. RUDERMAN and PETER W. WHITFIELD

KNEE PROBLEMS

The knee is the largest joint in the body. Because of its anatomic location between two weight-bearing long bones, and because of its relatively unprotected location, the knee is particularly susceptible to significant stresses, trauma, and alterations in metabolism.

Examination of the knee: general considerations

Almost all aspects of the orthopedic examination are discussed in one or another of the preceding chapters on orthopedic considerations. There are no major changes during the teenage years that alter the basic elements of that examination. However, during the teenage years, injuries and afflictions of the knee become increasingly frequent clinical occurrences. For that reason, it is appropriate to review the examination of the knee in some detail.[38]

The examination of the knee is performed with both lower extremities exposed from at least mid-thigh distally. A quick component on one lower extremity during the swing phase of gait may indicate pain. Because a painful knee may well indicate primary disease in the hip joint, examination of the hip and spine should accompany any evaluation of the knee. With the patient standing and the knee viewed from the side, an imaginary line drawn from the anterior superior iliac spine bisects the lateral aspect of the knee joint. If the tibia is posterior to the femur, as a result of internal derangement of the knee, recurvatum is obvious. Flexion of the knee might indicate a leg length discrepancy, with the flexed knee compensating for a shorter contralateral extremity. If the knee cannot be straightened on command, the knee may

have an effusion or it may be locked, indicating, perhaps, a loose body or a torn meniscus.

Two of the most common knee deformities in the adolescent are genu varum (bowleg) and genu valgum (knock-knee). Genu varum is documented by determining the distance between the medial knee joints, and genu valgum by measuring the distance between the medial malleoli at the ankle. Swelling in the popliteal space might represent a Baker's cyst.

With the patient sitting on the examining table with the knees overhanging the table edge, the patellas should be at the same level and facing forward. Prominence of the tibial tubercle may indicate Osgood-Schlatter disease.

Prior to manual examination, the active range of motion should be demonstrated. Zero degrees begins with the knee in full extension. Extension above zero would indicate genu recurvatum. Flexion is usually possible through approximately 135 degrees.

Measurement of thigh and calf circumference is important because atrophy may indicate disuse secondary to pain or internal derangement, or possibly congenital or acquired dysplasia. The knee is then examined for an effusion. One hand is placed above the kneecap over the suprapatellar pouch. With firm pressure, any fluid accumulation will be forced toward the joint. Pressure on one side of the knee may produce a fluid wave on the opposite side. Ballottement of the patella will be present if there is significant fluid within the joint, and the patient may lack full extension of the knee joint. With the examiner's hand on the patella during active range of motion, subpatellar grating or pain may indicate irregularity of the articular cartilage (chondromalacia patella), a common

546

finding in the adolescent patient. With the knee in 30 degrees of flexion, there should be little if any movement of the patella medially or laterally. If movement is present, subluxing patella must be a diagnostic consideration.

With the patient lying supine, pain with full extension often indicates a traumatic or degenerative tear of a meniscus. If the knee cannot be fully extended, locking may be present.

With the patient's hips flexed at 45 degrees, the knee flexed at 90 degrees, and the foot flat on the table, palpation of the medial and lateral joint lines is performed. Pain along the medial joint line may be associated with a tear of the medial meniscus, strain or tear of the medial collateral ligament, or possibly pes anserinus bursitis. The pes anserinus is a confluence of tendinous insertions of the sartorius, gracilis, and semitendinosus muscles. In a similar fashion, palpation of the lateral joint is performed for evidence of lateral collateral or lateral meniscus tears. Palpation of the patellar ligament is performed. Tenderness in this area may be associated with jumper's knee or possibly Osgood-Schlatter disease.

To test the medial collateral ligament, a valgus stress is applied with the knee in approximately 20 to 30 degrees of flexion. The ankle is secured with one hand, and the opposite hand is placed proximal to the knee joint. If opening of the knee joint occurs without a corresponding gap on testing of the opposite extremity, evidence exists to suggest medial collateral ligament instability. If the joint remains closed but pain is present, a sprain or strain of the collateral ligament exists. To test for lateral collateral ligament stability, a varus stress is applied to the knee in a similar fashion.

Anterior or posterior cruciate ligament instability is indicated by forward or backward displacement of the tibia on the femur. Obviously, the results of these tests must be compared with those of tests on the opposite extremity. The tests become somewhat complicated when one attempts to distinguish between cruciate instability and medial or lateral ligamentous and/or capsular instability.[30,50] Abnormalities warrent orthopedic consultation for a more detailed evaluation of the knee.

Osgood-Schlatter disease

The etiology of Osgood-Schlatter disease is unclear, but some evidence suggests that the disease is actually a traumatic patellar tendinitis.[39] Heterotopic bone results in elevation of the tibial tubercle associated with pain and often, localized edema. Another theory holds that fragmentation of the tibial tubercle results from necrosis of the epiphysis.[1]

The usual patient is male, between the ages of 11 and 16, active in sports, and perhaps obese. Commonly, the problem is bilateral. The chief complaint is localized pain and swelling, which is exaggerated by exertion, particularly running and jumping. Examination of the knee joint is normal.

Radiographs demonstrate localized soft tissue edema, thickening of the patellar tendon, and free fragments felt to be ectopic bone formations rather than fragments from the tibial tubercle.

Osgood-Schlatter disease is self-limiting and requires only ice and aspirin for pain relief. Fusion of the tibial tubercle occurs with maturation of the skeleton and usually ends the symptomatic period. Activity need not be restricted unless symptoms are severe enough to compromise the patient's activities, in which case cylinder cast immobilization for 6 to 8 weeks may be useful.

Late complications associated with Osgood-Schlatter disease that may persist after skeletal maturation include elevation and prominence of the tibial tubercle, bursitis, chronic pain with kneeling, and painful small fragments of heterotopic bone.[85] The most important part of treatment is educating the parents that this condition is *painful* but not *harmful*.

Abnormalities of the patella

The bipartite patella has no clinical significance and is asymptomatic, but it must be distinguished from a fracture of the patella at the time of injury. Radiographs of both knees should be obtained, since the variant is usually found bilaterally. A bipartite patella is usually noted to be fragmented in the upper pole and has characteristic smooth, round edges.

Subluxation of the patella

Recurrent dislocation or subluxation of the patella is a common problem among adolescents that often requires surgical treatment.[17] The causes of the subluxation, or frank dislocation, are multiple and include lax joints, abnormalities in the medial supporting structures that allow lateral deviation of the patella, and contracture of the iliotibial band and lateral retinaculum, which creates greater lateral stress. Patella alta, genu valgum,

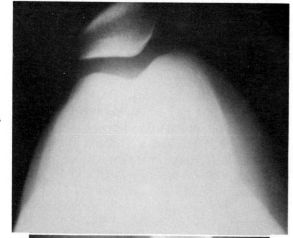

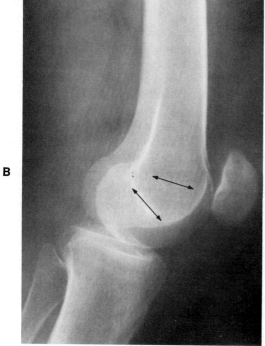

Fig. 28-1. X-ray findings in chronic subluxation of the patella. **A,** Tangential view of the patella demonstrating lateral tilt and some hypoplasia of the lateral femoral condyle. **B,** Lateral view demonstrating patella alta. The patellar tendon (measured from the inferior pole of the patella to the tibial tubercle) should be approximately the same length as the patella. Here it is much longer. In a lateral view taken in mild flexion, the patella should fall between two lines (arrows) that correspond to the old physeal plate and the intercondylar notch. In this view the superior pole of the patella is well above the upper line. Note, as well, the irregularity and sclerosis of the subchondral bone beneath the articular surface of the patella.

and external tibial torsion all predispose the patient to subluxation.

Subluxation of the patella may begin early in childhood, but the symptoms usually do not become manifest until adolescence or even early adulthood, when the child may experience a sensation of the knee giving way.[48] Although the child may be brought to the emergency room with a complete lateral dislocation of the patella, usually there is lateral subluxation of the patella on flexion of the knee and spontaneous reduction with extension. With recurrent episodes, pain and occasionally an effusion occur.

Examination may reveal one of the predisposing conditions; occasionally, however, only a painful knee joint with the discomfort poorly localized to the subpatellar region is found. Subtle changes in patellar morphology may be demonstrated, as well as abnormal tracking of the patella with flexion and extension.

Although routine x-ray views of the knee should be taken in the anteroposterior (AP) lateral, oblique, and intercondylar projections, these will usually be normal. If this is the case, special patellar views should be obtained, including tangential views of the patella with the knee flexed between 20 and 30 degrees (Fig. 28-1).

Treatment. Initial conservative treatment includes physical therapy to strengthen the quadriceps mechanism, specifically the vastus medialis muscle, aspirin for relief of the pain of chondromalacia (which may accompany subluxation), and immobilization in a cylinder cast for 4 to 6 weeks. If conservative treatment is not successful, one may try one of the numerous surgical approaches described that combine procedures on both the patellar tendon and the retinaculum surrounding the knee joint and patella.[13] Medial transfer of the tibial tubercle by a bone block (Hauser) was popular in the past, but today it is usually avoided because of an unacceptable incidence of growth disturbance and compartment syndromes. Immobilization after surgery will last anywhere from 3 to 6 weeks and is followed by a period of crutch ambulation and physical therapy. All procedures performed for subluxation carry a 5% to 10% recurrence and complication risk.

Chondromalacia patella

Chondromalacia patella refers to softening of the cartilage beneath the patella, but it may also involve the patellofemoral groove and synovitis.[28]

Chondromalacia patella typically becomes symptomatic between the ages of 11 and 14. Girls are more frequently affected than boys. Some adolescents develop symptoms of retropatellar pain and effusion after direct trauma to the patella; others relate the onset of pain to episodes of patellar subluxation or dislocation. Another group develops progressive pain after repeated athletic activities, ultimately with only mild activity. In addition to pain in the retropatellar region, the child may experience locking, which represents either a synovitis, an effusion, an osteochondral fracture, or muscle spasm.[80] It has been suggested that the source of the pain is a separation of the cartilage from the subchondral bone, which is richly supplied with nerves and believed to be the site of the pain.[72]

The differential diagnosis should include suprapatellar plica, meniscal lesions, synovitis, loose body, osteochondral fracture, and even Osgood-Schlatter disease. If clinical suspicion warrants further investigation for chondromalacia, arthroscopy can be considered.[10] However, the early lesion may not be noted at arthroscopy, because the surface cartilage may not be sufficiently involved.

Treatment. Since osteoarthritis does not follow chondromalacia, except in instances where surgical intervention has occurred, every effort should be made to treat the lesion by conservative means. Nonsurgical measures should include aspirin, which has a specific action in preventing cartilage degeneration, and isometric and isotonic quadriceps exercises, especially emphasizing the last 30 degrees of extension. Steroid injections are condemned. When exercise, rest, and salicylates do not relieve the symptoms, a cylinder cast may be applied for approximately 4 weeks, followed by a course of physical therapy.

Surgery should be considered only if activities of daily living are significantly compromised after an adequate course of conservative therapy. The procedure selected depends on the cause of the chondromalacia patella but might involve correction of a subluxing patella, arthroscopic shaving, arthrotomy for drilling and shaving, or elevation of the tibial tubercle (Macquet procedure) to diminish stress on the patellofemoral joint. Patellectomy, although a satisfactory procedure, is performed only after everything else fails.

Osteochondritis dissecans

Osteochondritis dissecans is thought by some to be a form of epiphyseal ischemic necrosis similar to Osgood-Schlatter disease; it commonly involves the distal femoral epiphysis, specifically the subchondral bone and articular surface. Because of inadequate collateral circulation from the metaphysis, a localized area of bone necrosis occurs shortly after the time of epiphyseal closure. Others believe that the area in question is actually a tertiary ossification center that is initially vascularized but that loosens after trauma and becomes a free fragment.[73]

Probably because of the size and location of the joint, the medial side of the lateral femoral condyle is the most likely site for this lesion to appear. Other bones commonly involved include the talus, the capitellum of the distal humerus, the patella, and the proximal humerus. Osteochondritis dissecans may be asymptomatic and noted on x-ray films of the knee taken for another problem, but more commonly there is localized pain or the sen-

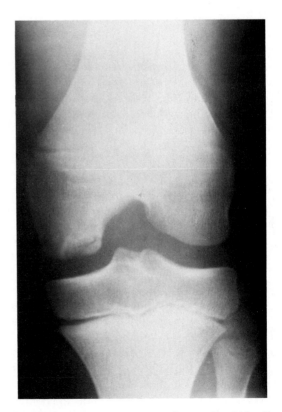

Fig. 28-2. X-ray appearance of osteochondritis dissecans. This lesion is typically located on the lateral aspect of the medial femoral condyle.

sation of something floating within the knee. Other associated findings include thigh atrophy, effusion, and even true locking.[32]

The early lesion may appear as a radiolucent area on the articular surface associated with a small fleck of bone (Fig. 28-2). In more mature lesions an obvious section of bone is separated from the major bony condyle by a radiolucent line.

Treatment. When there is good evidence for a loose body, an arthrogram or arthroscopy will delineate the loose fragment, which is then removed at arthrotomy, and the base of the osteochondral defect is drilled. In cases not involving a loose body, cast immobilization is usually successful for early lesions and should be tried for periods of up to 6 months. If 3 to 6 months of conservative therapy fail, a surgical technique may be tried that involves pinning the lesion in position to avoid complete separation and to allow healing or coalescence within the subchondral bone.[53] Others have suggested removing the fragment and drilling the subchondral surface in hopes that the defect will fill in with fibrocartilage.

Discoid meniscus

Discoid meniscus is an acquired morphologic alteration in the meniscus from its characteristic semilunar shape to a discoid shape. Recurrent trauma to an already altered meniscus is thought to deform the cartilage, making it prone to degeneration and cyst formation.[45] The lateral meniscus is involved more commonly than the medial meniscus.

The patient will usually have a history of snapping or clicking associated with pain along the joint line. There may be a sensation of the knee giving way or true locking and a small palpable mass in the area of the joint line that changes with activity.

On physical examination, the presence of snapping or clicking associated with a lateral joint cyst is highly suggestive of a discoid meniscus, but the diagnosis should be confirmed by arthrography and/or arthroscopy. A discoid meniscus that causes locking and effusion or that is associated with a cyst should be excised.[72] Postoperative care will consist of a short period of immobilization to allow soft tissue healing, followed by a course of physical therapy and weight bearing to tolerance.

Popliteal cysts

The popliteal or Baker's cyst is typically asymptomatic and is located on the medial aspect of the popliteal area. Joint symptoms are not commonly related to the cyst, but the cyst may arise as a result of synovitis secondary to internal derangement of the knee. Neoplasm should also be included in the differential diagnosis. Unless there is suspicion that internal derangement is the cause or the mass is thought to be a neoplasm, treatment is probably not necessary. If the cyst causes discomfort or limits motion because of its size, surgical excision can be performed.

The plica syndrome

The plica syndrome refers to a thin, filmy band or fold of synovial tissue that represents the remnants of the three embryologic compartments of the knee.[31] As a result of blunt trauma or repeated stress, the synovial fold becomes inflamed, edematous, and thickened.[7] Trauma, loose bodies, meniscus tears, and chondromalacia patella can all be confused with plica syndrome and all may be present in addition to a symptomatic plica.

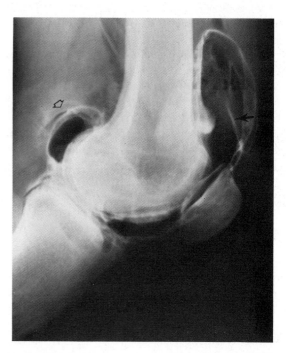

Fig. 28-3. Double-contrast pneumoarthrogram illustrating a small popliteal cyst (open arrow) and a suprapatellar plica (closed arrow). The plica is only mildly thickened and straightened and may not have been the source of the knee pain.

Usually the patient has a history of blunt trauma to the knee or a recent increase in such physical activity as running, jogging, or repetitive exercise. Similar to the discomfort of chondromalacia patella, the pain of a symptomatic plica may be intermittent and dull, worse with climbing stairs or with sitting with the knee flexed for long periods of time. On examination of the knee, the findings characteristic of chondromalacia patella or internal derangement may be demonstrated. However, in addition, an audible and palpable snap or click with associated localized pain is demonstrated. The clinical suspicion of plica syndrome can be confirmed by knee arthrography (Fig. 28-3) or arthroscopy.

The majority of patients will respond to non-surgical treatment consisting of rest, aspirin, heat, and hamstring-stretching exercises.[34] If the symptoms recur or persist with conservative treatment, excision of the plica is indicated, possibly using the operative arthroscope.

FOOT PROBLEMS

Since most major foot abnormalities have been identified before the teenage years, relatively little attention is directed to the teenager's foot. However, several important conditions become prominent during the teenage years.

Adolescent bunion

Bunions can develop during adolescence and can become an important cause of foot pain. The underlying abnormality is a medial deviation of the first ray (metatarsus primus varus), a genetic condition that is autosomal dominant with incomplete penetrance.[46] There are rotary abnormalities in the midfoot and forefoot as well, the end result of all being lateral deviation of the great toe in relation to the metatarsal shaft. Bunions are anatomic-mechanical abnormalities and are seen even in populations that do not wear shoes, but ill-fitting shoes contribute to the disability. One or both ends of the shoe are bound not to fit a child with a relatively narrow hindfoot and a splayed and widened forefoot, and the result will be painful calluses, corns, or pressure areas. The secondary changes are less frequent in the adolescent than in the adult (Fig. 28-4).

Treatment. It is possible to obtain shoes with wide forefeet and narrow heels, but these are generally special-order items that are expensive and difficult to find. Therefore, the usual treatment of adolescent bunion is surgical. The first ray (either at its base or more distally) is redirected so that it becomes approximately parallel to the other metatarsals.[29,77] Resection of the medial osteophyte and plication of the medial first metatarsophalangeal joint capsule are performed to realign the great toe, and tendon lengthenings or transfers balance the bony correction.

Correction of an adolescent bunion is a major surgical procedure requiring several days of hospitalization, a postoperative period of non–weight bearing of several weeks, and cast immobilization for 6 to 8 weeks.

Most often, complications are avoided and a gratifying result with long-term pain relief and the ability to wear regular shoes is achieved.

Clawtoe

The true clawtoe hyperextends at the metatarsophalangeal joint and flexes at both the proximal

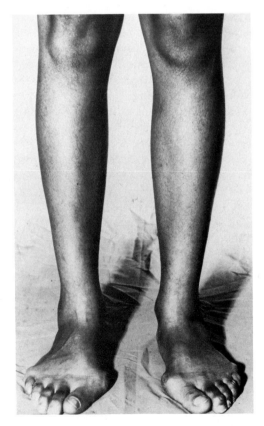

Fig. 28-4. Severe splay foot with hallux valgus and bunion formation in a 14-year-old.

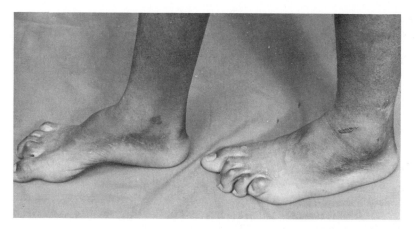

Fig. 28-5. Cavovarus feet and clawtoes in a 15-year-old. The clawing is bilateral, and all the lesser toes are affected. The metatarsophalangeal joint is hyperextended, and the proximal and distal interphalangeal (PIP) joints are flexed. Note the callous and corn formation on the dorsum of the PIP joints.

and distal interphalangeal joints (Fig. 28-5). Almost invariably, clawing is bilateral, affects all the lesser toes, and is commonly associated with cavus feet. The great toe may be clawed as well. While these deformities may be isolated abnormalities, a diligent search for an underlying neurologic disorder is mandatory whenever clawtoes present in an adolescent. The workup should include electromyography and motor and sensory nerve conduction studies.

Whatever the etiology, the clinical course is constant: progressive depression of the metatarsal heads with metatarsalgia, shortening of the extrinsic extensor and flexor tendons, joint contracture with fixation of the deformity, and painful dorsal callosities and corns. Some form of surgical correction is usually required.[65] The hospitalization for clawtoe correction is short, but immobilization in casts will be required for several weeks.

Hammertoe

Hammertoe is often confused with clawtoe, but initially hyperextension deformities at the metatarsophalangeal joints are absent.[76] With the subsequent development of metatarsalgia and hyperextension at the basilar joint, the toe assumes the appearance of the clawtoe, including painful callosities beneath the metatarsal heads, over the tips of the toes, and on the dorsum of the proximal interphalangeal joint. The second toe is the most commonly affected, particularly when there is an element of hallux valgus. There is a strong familial incidence of hammertoes, but an underlying neurologic deficit is unlikely.

In the adolescent, surgical correction is probably preferable to shaving callosities, wearing corn pads, or padding.

Mallet toe

Mallet toe is characterized by a flexion deformity at only the distal interphalangeal joint and may be limited to a single toe.[76] A painful corn develops over the tip of the toe and can be alleviated by releasing the long toe flexor or fusing the distal interphalangeal joint, a surgical procedure so simple that surgery seems the most efficacious course.

HIP PROBLEMS
Avascular necrosis of the femoral head

There is a variant of Legg-Calvé-Perthes disease that presents during adolescence, has a poor prognosis, and is difficult to manage. Joint replacement may become necessary in young adulthood.

A similar poor course is seen in the avascular necrosis of the femoral head that occurs in certain chronic diseases (Fig. 28-6); the best studied is that following renal transplantation.[18] Steroids have often been implicated as the primary offender in avascular necrosis, but recent studies have failed to show a direct correlation with steroid dose.[67] The degree of necrosis seems to be more related to the degree of pretransplant renal osteodystrophy, and this observation is consistent with the finding of aseptic necrosis in children who are un-

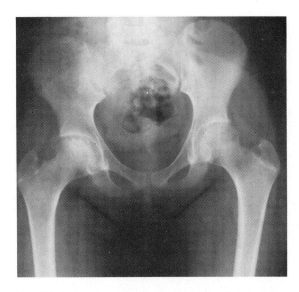

Fig. 28-6. Aseptic necrosis of the proximal right femur in a 15-year-old girl with lupus erythematosis. The patient had undergone steroid treatment for several months.

dergoing renal dialysis and have never had courses of steroids.[6]

A parallel clinical problem is present in sickle cell disease and other hemoglobinopathies.[62] Clinically apparent aseptic necrosis appears to be the cumulative result of repeated intravascular sludging. When the radiographic changes are minimal and the contour of the head is preserved, rest, crutches, and limitation of activity will allow reconstitution of the head to occur. Unfortunately, collapse of a large segment is more typical, and total joint replacement becomes necessary.

Slipped capital femoral epiphysis

Slipped capital femoral epiphysis occurs during the rapid growth phase between the ages of 10 and 16; it affects boys much more frequently than girls. There is a cephalad and anterior displacement of the femoral neck in relation to the capital femoral epiphysis, which, in turn, displaces posteriorly and inferiorly.[49]

The etiology of slipped capital femoral epiphysis is unknown. Two types of children are typically affected. The first type is an obese and knock-kneed adolescent boy who has underdeveloped genitalia—the adiposogenital habitus, or Fröhlich's syndrome. The second type is a tall, thin ectomorph who recently had a rapid growth spurt. In each case, the predominant influence may be

growth hormone,[37] which weakens the physeal plate, decreases sheer strength, and makes the child susceptible to trauma. Another theory proposes that although in childhood the periosteum surrounding the physeal plate is quite thick and strong, during adolescence this periosteal layer thins, making the child more prone to slipping of the epiphysis during the period of rapid growth.[33] The plane of the physeal plate may also play an integral part in the predisposition to a slip; a more vertically placed physeal plate will withstand less stress. Slipped capital femoral epiphysis has also been associated with parathyroid adenomas,[12] acquired hypothyroidism,[60] and renal osteodystrophy.[11]

Displacement of the proximal or capital femoral epiphysis occurs gradually through the physeal cartilage, and the periosteum remains intact. If slipping is severe, a bony prominence of the femoral neck will develop and may impinge against the acetabulum and limit abduction, internal rotation, and complete flexion. Avascular necrosis rarely results from the slip but may be iatrogenically induced during an attempt to manipulate the slipped head into a more anatomic position. Deformity, incongruity, and loss of articular cartilage all predispose the child to early degenerative disease.

The child may come to medical attention with insidious onset of hip or possibly knee pain, an antalgic gait, a hip limp, an externally rotated lower extremity, and little history of antecedent trauma. Localized tenderness over the joint may be present. The range of motion of the hip will be limited and often associated with pain. Characteristically, the hip will rotate externally as flexion is increased.

The diagnosis is confirmed by radiographic examination. An AP and frog lateral view of the pelvis affords the opportunity for comparison as well as an excellent view of the proximal femur. In the preslipping stage, widening and irregularity of the physeal plate are apparent. In true slipping, there is a posterior and medial displacement of the epiphysis. Slips of lesser degree may be difficult to diagnose (Fig. 28-7). In 15% to 25% of patients, some degree of slippage may be present on the contralateral side.[47]

Treatment. The goal of surgery is immobilization to prevent further slipping and arrest of physeal growth. This is achieved by bone graft or by passing pins across the physis.[61,75] Reduction depends on numerous factors, including the sur-

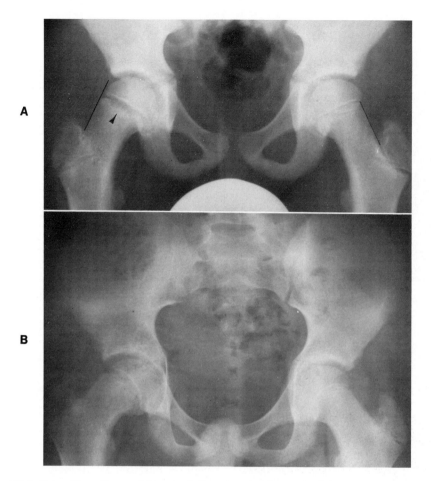

Fig. 28-7. X-ray films of two mild cases of slipped capital femoral epiphysis. **A,** A line drawn along the superior neck of the right femur does not pass through the capital femoral epiphysis. There is widening and irregularity of the physeal plate (arrow). **B,** In this slightly more advanced case, the rounding and prominence of the right superior femoral neck is indicative of the chronicity of the problem.

geon's experience, the chronicity of the slip, and the degree of slippage. Acute slipping can be reduced manually or by traction, but chronic slips are usually fused in situ, since late manipulation increases the risks of avascular necrosis. Ossification of the physeal plate usually occurs within several months following surgery, at which time weight bearing can be initiated. Follow-up examination should continue until skeletal maturity and beyond.

TUMORS OF SKELETAL STRUCTURES

Tumors are infrequent but not rare skeletal lesions, most of which are benign and easy to diagnose; occasionally, the critical distinction from malignancy is difficult.[19] Even if the diagnosis is apparent, the rapidly changing technology of tumor management makes referral to a tertiary care center appropriate in many instances. There, a "tumor team" consisting of an orthopedist, a skeletal radiologist, an oncologist, an orthopedic pathologist, a radiation therapist, and specialized nursing personnel provides complete care for the patient.

Of paramount importance is the need to establish a diagnosis early; however, if one is not prepared to treat the lesion in question, it is probably not appropriate even to initiate the diagnostic workup. An inadequate or improperly placed biopsy not only may delay and confuse the diagnosis but may actually adversely affect the treatment, prognosis, and survival.

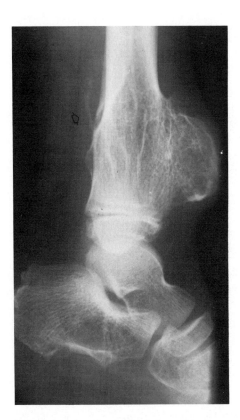

Fig. 28-8. Lateral radiograph of the ankle in a patient with multiple osteochondromas (osteocartilaginous exostoses). There is a large sessile lesion anteriorly. The cortical margins at the base of the lesion are contiguous with the cortex of the bone. There is a small pedunculated lesion posteriorly (arrow). Pedunculated osteochondromas always lie in the long axis of the bone and point away from the epiphysis.

Osteochondroma

An osteochondroma, the most common benign primary bone "tumor,"[25] is probably not a neoplasm but the reflection of disordered growth at the periphery of the physeal plate. It appears at or near the physis in bones formed by enchondral ossification and grows away from the epiphysis, at right angles to the long axis of the bone or toward the midshaft of the bone (Fig. 28-8). The advancing cartilaginous cells protrude into adjacent soft tissue, while those behind undergo enchondral ossification and form a bony base that is contiguous with the cortex of the bone, either as a wide base or as a long, narrow stalk.

The osteochondroma normally will cease growth as the physeal plate closes; however, the cartilaginous cap persists into maturity. An autosomal

dominant pattern is seen in families affected by multiple exostoses.[74]

Osteochondromas become symptomatic only when their growth reaches a point at which a nerve or a tendon is impinged on or when the bursa that develops over the tip of the cartilaginous cap becomes inflamed. Large or multiple lesions may distort normal longitudinal growth, producing dwarfing, bowing, and angulation in severely affected individuals. Malignant degeneration occurs in less than 1% of single osteochondromas; lesions of the flat bones or axial skeleton are more likely to undergo malignant degeneration than lesions of the appendicular skeleton.[20] In the multiple form, the rate may be higher. Malignant degeneration is suggested when a lesion that has been quiescent for some time becomes symptomatic, particularly in the skeletally mature patient. If malignant degeneration should occur, the transformation is usually into chondrosarcoma. Fibrosarcoma or osteosarcoma also develop.[4]

Excision is indicated when the lesion becomes symptomatic or compromises function, and prophylactic excision of lesions of the axial skeleton is warranted. Depending on the location of the lesion, cast immobilization may or may not be necessary. The closer to a joint or the larger the size of the lesion, the more immobilization is apt to be required after excision.

Enchondroma

An enchondroma is a benign, cartilaginous tumor that is believed to originate from portions of the physeal plate that failed to undergo the characteristic transformation into bone.[57] These cartilaginous rests then continue their growth within the shaft of long bones but may expand to erode (but not violate) the cortex. They develop, most often, in the bones of the feet and hands but may be found throughout the skeleton.

Enchondromas are extremely slow growing and asymptomatic until early adult life, with the child noticing only a painless swelling of a digit in the hand or foot (Fig. 28-9). Malignant degeneration is extremely rare in the adolescent. Multiple enchondromas (Ollier's disease) are usually discovered as a result of growth disturbance. In Maffucci's syndrome, there is associated hemangiomatosis.

In the small tubular bones of the hand or foot, total excision or curettage may be possible with or without insertion of a bone graft. If the enchon-

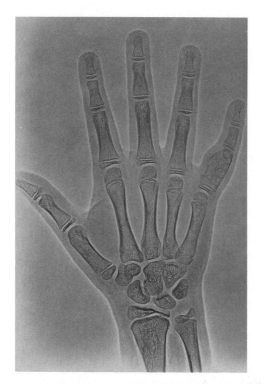

Fig. 28-9. Xeroradiogram of an enchondroma of the proximal phalanx of the little finger. The child's only symptom was painless swelling of the digit.

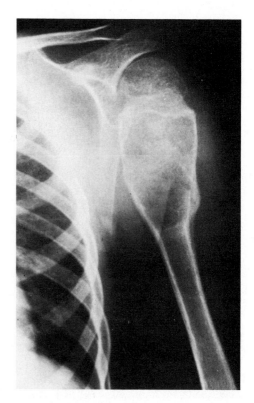

Fig. 28-10. Typical appearance of a unicameral bone cyst of the proximal humerus.

droma is first noted as a cause of pathologic fracture, treatment must be individualized according to the location. Treatment of major long bone enchondromas may well necessitate internal fixation.

Chondroblastoma

Chondroblastoma (Codman's tumor) is a tumor of cartilaginous origin that is almost invariably located within the epiphysis, usually about the knee or proximal humerus.[14] Radiologically, it appears as a radiolucent area measuring anywhere from 1 to 5 cm in diameter.

Chondroblastomas become manifest during the second decade of life with pain being the characteristic presenting complaint. Tenderness is elicited over the epiphyseal portion of the involved long bone. Joint effusion may be present.

Definitive treatment is total local excision or curettage.[57] Recurrence is possible; malignant degeneration is rare but does occur.

Unicameral bone cyst

The unicameral bone cyst is a fluid-filled cavity with a thin membranous lining, located beneath the physeal plate in the metaphyseal region of the long

bone[15] (Fig. 28-10). The origin is unknown.[43] The cyst fluid may be clear, yellowish, or frankly hemorrhagic, indicating bleeding after a pathologic fracture through the cyst. It may expand the width of the medullary cavity, increasing the diameter of the bone and thinning the cortex, predisposing it to fracture.

The proximal humerus is the site of the lesion in well over 50% of cases. The proximal femur is the second most common area. The cysts occur in children between the ages of 6 and 16 and are usually asymptomatic unless expansion has caused compression of a nerve or interferes with tendon excursion. Pain after trauma usually indicates a pathologic fracture. In other cases, the lesion is diagnosed on routine chest radiographs. A fracture through a unicameral bone cyst will heal with immobilization. Growth retardation or angular deformity may result as a consequence of epiphyseal plate involvement.

Treatment. The mere presence of the cyst is not an indication for treatment unless the lesion progressively enlarges to include a major portion of the diaphysis or involves weight-bearing bones. If a lesion has sustained a pathologic fracture on

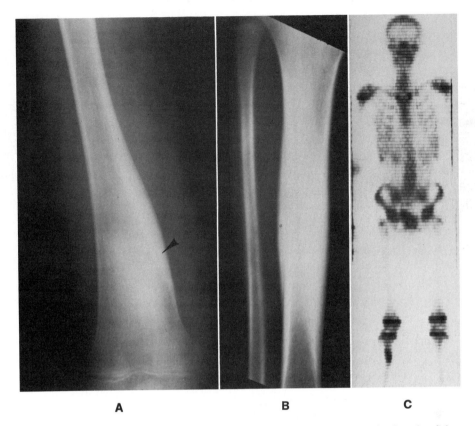

A   **B**   **C**

Fig. 28-11. A, Osteoid osteoma of the distal femur. There is thickening and sclerosis of the surrounding cortex and metaphyseal bone. The arrow indicates the small, circular, lucent nidus. One can just detect a central fleck of calcification within the nidus. **B** and **C,** Osteoid osteoma of the midshaft of the tibia. The dense reactive new bone obscures the nidus. The lesion is displayed prominently on the technetium 99 polyphosphate bone scan.

two occasions, treatment is necessary. Classically, curettage or excision of the lesion *en bloc* is supplemented with autogenous bone grafting. The recurrence rate is quite significant, especially in girls and in cysts close to the physis, perhaps reflecting the surgeon's ability to excise the lesion widely without fear of injury to the physeal plate.[25] Recently there have been encouraging reports of successful obliteration of unicameral bone cysts following aspiration and steroid injection.[16]

The hospitalization for surgery may be only 3 to 5 days. Following surgery, the extremity must be immobilized several weeks to months and crutches will be necessary for a weight-bearing extremity.

Osteoid osteoma

It is not clear whether osteoid osteoma is a neoplasm, an inflammatory process, or a vascular malformation, but it is benign and is usually diagnosed during the second decade of life.[41] Any bone may be affected, but the femur and tibia are most frequent sites. Microscopically, an osteoid osteoma has a small central nidus of vascular fibrous tissue filled with a delicate network of trabeculae of osteoid surrounded by reactive new bone.

Perhaps half the patients will describe the "classic" history of localized pain, which is worse at night and specifically relieved by aspirin. Radiographically, a small, circular, lucent area surrounded by dense hyperostosis (Fig. 28-11, *A*) is diagnostic, but the reactive bone may be so dense as to obscure the nidus. On the other hand, if the osteoid osteoma is located in trabecular bone, sclerosis may be minimal, making diagnosis difficult.[71] A bone scan and/or arteriograms may illuminate the lesion (Fig. 28-11, *B* and *C*) because of the extreme vascularity of the nidus.[52]

Immediate and complete relief of pain is ex-

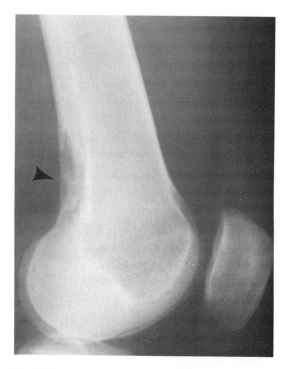

Fig. 28-12. A fibrous cortical defect has the same histology as a nonossifying fibroma. This small lesion (arrow) in the distal femur is slightly larger than many fibrous cortical defects and shows the eccentric, bubbly, scalloped appearance of the nonossifying fibroma (fibroxanthoma).

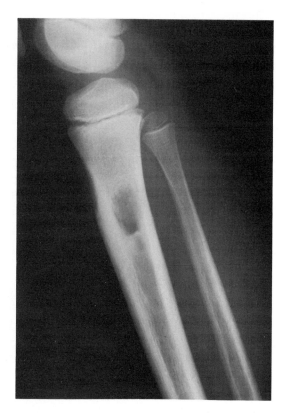

Fig. 28-13. Eosinophilic granuloma of the proximal tibia. The x-ray appearance is usually that of a "punched out" lytic lesion; but this appearance is highly variable, and a definitive diagnosis requires a biopsy.

pected after removal of the nidus. Recurrences probably represent incomplete resection.

Nonossifying fibroma

There is no mistaking the bubbly, scalloped, eccentric, metaphyseal x-ray appearance of this common lesion (Fig. 28-12). Histologically, one sees a swirling fibrous background with lipid-laden histiocytes (xanthoma cells);[20,70] biopsy is not necessary, however, since these lesions are invariably benign and asymptomatic unless the lesion enlarges significantly, resulting in a pathologic fracture.[24] Curettage and bone grafting should result in cure.

Eosinophilic granuloma

Eosinophilic granuloma, either solitary or multiple, is composed of a mass of histiocytes or other reticuloendothelial elements interspersed with varying numbers of eosinophilic leukocytes. It is not known whether this is a neoplastic or inflammatory process. The lesion represents one end of

the spectrum of disorders grouped as histiocytosis X, which includes Letterer-Siwe disease and Hand-Schüller-Christian disease.

Radiographically, a "punched out" lytic lesion is typical, but a definitive diagnosis rests on biopsy (Fig. 28-13). Eosinophilic granuloma is the most common cause of complete vertebral collapse in the child (vertebral plana or Calvé's disease). Curettage, with or without bone grafting, is the treatment of choice, but the lesion is exquisitely sensitive to radiation therapy.

Fibrous dysplasia

This lesion is probably a disorder of the normal metaphyseal process of bone formation and may involve one (monostotic) or more bones (polyostotic). In the polyostotic form, there is a tendency for the lesion to cluster in one extremity or on one side of the body. When polyostotic fibrous dysplasia is coupled with precocious puberty (invariably in a girl) and café au lait spots, it is called Albright's disease.[2]

The central canal of the bone is filled with cellular fibrous tissue with multiple small trabeculae of metaplastic bone (''alphabet soup'' appearance) interspersed. Radiographically, a central lytic lesion with scalloped edges and a ''ground glass'' appearance expands and thins the bony cortex. If the lesion is strategically placed, growth disturbance or pathologic fracture may occur.[36]

In the polyostotic form of fibrous dysplasia, the adverse effects of the multiple lesions are additive, and deformity and growth retardation are more frequent. When the lesions are in the proximal femur, coxa vara, the so-called shepherd's crook deformity, develops. When the bones of the skull are involved, as they frequently are, there may be severe facial deformity, visual disturbance from narrowing of the foramen for the optic nerve, or endocrinopathy as a result of involvement of the sella turcica.

The frequency of endocrine changes makes integrated medical-surgical management essential. Malignant degeneration is rare, unless the lesion is radiated (it shouldn't be!).[69] Pain and deformity are indications for curettage, bone grafting, and, possibly, internal fixation.

Giant cell tumor of bone

Giant cell tumors of bone never appear until after closure of the physes; therefore, they are rare in childhood, only occasionally presenting in the late teenage years. The patient usually comes to medical attention with a painful swelling or mass at the end of the long bone, but not uncommonly with a pathologic fracture. The distal femur, the proximal tibia, and the distal radius are three of the more common areas of tumor location. Typically, the lesion is eccentrically located in the metaphysis and epiphysis and is one of the few tumors that involves both of these areas. In some cases, the tumor will expand the cortex and initiate periosteal reaction and new bone formation. The differential diagnosis should include aneurysmal bone cyst as well as brown tumor of hyperparathyroidism.

The distinction between a benign and malignant lesion depends on histologic evaluation and grading.[44] Metastases are usually pulmonary.

Even benign giant cell tumors are locally aggressive and have a high rate of recurrence. Wide, en bloc resection is recommended. Malignant degeneration may follow repeated excision. Radiation is reserved for lesions that are surgically in-

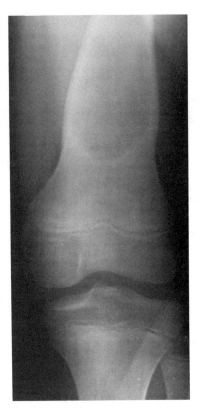

Fig. 28-14. The aneurysmal bone cyst can be differentiated from a giant cell tumor on this radiograph because the lesion is central, metaphyseal-diaphyseal, and the physeal plate is still open. Cortical expansion can be more extensive, and some aneurysmal bone cysts have a bubbly appearance.

accessible. Cryotherapy has been reported as being as successful as surgery, but it must still be considered investigational.[56]

Aneurysmal bone cyst

The aneurysmal bone cyst is so named because of its clinical and radiographic similarity to a vascular aneurysm.[23] Some authors believe that hemorrhage within the bone from trauma matures and organizes, resulting in fibrous-walled septae filled with old blood. Others have suggested a confluence of congenital hemangiomas or arteriovenous malformations, or degeneration and involution of some other primary lesion.[42]

Approximately 60% to 70% of aneurysmal bone cysts are found in the second decade of life. There appears to be no sex predilection, and any bone may be affected.

The most common presenting complaints are localized pain and swelling. Associated muscle weakness, nerve root or peripheral nerve irritation, limited joint motion, and evidence of vascular compromise depend on the anatomic location and the size of the lesion. Radiographically, the lesion is radiolucent and located in either the diaphysis or metaphysis. The cyst may expand beyond the normal anatomic bony boundaries or thin the cortex to an egglike shell. Pathologic fracture is not uncommon (Fig. 28-14).

The differential diagnosis should include osteosarcoma and giant cell tumor.[21]

Localized lesions within the diaphysis or metaphysis of long bones can easily be treated by simple curettage. Aneurysmal bone cysts located in the spine, which are inaccessible or difficult to eradicate completely by curettage, may be treated by supplemental irradiation. Malignant degeneration of the cyst is thought to be rare, and lesions that "transform" into a malignant state may well have been low-grade malignant tumors from the outset.

Malignant tumors of bone
Osteosarcoma

Osteosarcoma is a rather general term for a group of malignant tumors originating from differentiated mesenchymal cells that have the potential for osteoid (uncalcified bone matrix) production.[20] These tumors were previously called osteogenic sarcoma, an even more general term encompassing such tumors as chondrosarcoma and fibrosarcoma. Primary osteosarcomas are more common than such secondary osteosarcomas as those arising from Paget's disease, chronic osteomyelitis, and other osteosarcoma variants.[58]

The incidence of osteosarcoma peaks in the second and third decades; 75% to 80% are found between the ages of 10 to 25 years. The tumor may arise anywhere in the skeleton but is found most frequently in the distal femur, proximal tibia, and proximal humerus. Often, insignificant trauma may induce symptoms, thus prompting medical attention. Pain, edema, erythema, and in-

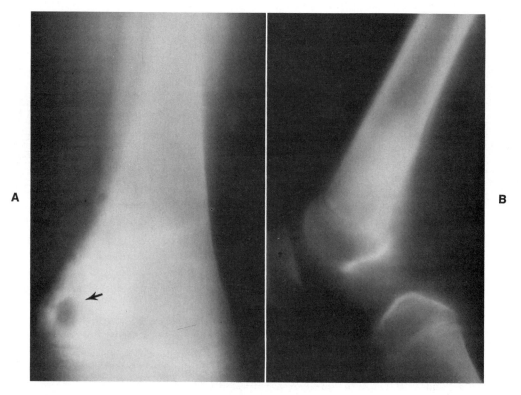

Fig. 28-15. AP **(A)** and lateral **(B)** tomograms of an osteogenic sarcoma of the distal femur. The arrow indicates a biopsy site. This x-ray is typical, and the diagnosis can be made without a biopsy, although pathologic confirmation is desirable.

creased warmth may be localized or diffuse within the extremity. A mass may be palpable, and fever, chills, malaise, and weight loss may be present.

The diagnosis of osteosarcoma can be made from the typical radiographic features: cortical destruction, periosteal reaction with new bone formation, tumor expanding outside the confines of the cortical margins, and either sclerotic or lytic areas within the medullary canal (Fig. 28-15). Bone scanning is often employed to confirm the full extent of skeletal involvement. Skip lesions,[26] areas of tumor extension within the same bone, or metastatic areas of the tumor to other bones are characteristic of osteosarcoma.

Treatment. Treatment regimens consisting of combinations of chemotherapy, irradiation, and surgical ablation are complex and constantly changing and should be planned at a tertiary care facility.[66] Results are currently being reassessed, but survival has clearly been prolonged as a result of contemporary treatment. A minimum 5-year disease-free rate of 40% is expected.

Metastasis to the lungs, if not already present at the time of initial diagnosis, typically occurs within 6 to 12 months of diagnosis. With aggressive surgical intervention and chemotherapy, the prognosis has improved even for these patients, and pulmonary resection of multiple lesions is now commonplace.[55] Periosteal and parosteal osteosarcoma generally have a more favorable prognosis that the classic type of osteogenic sarcoma, but telangiectatic osteosarcomas have a more virulent course. These three lesions are significantly less common than the classic type.

The initial hospitalization for children with osteogenic sarcoma may be prolonged, with visits from multiple physicians and nursing personnel involved in both direct care and consultations. After initial evaluation which may include arteriograms and tomograms or computerized tomographic (CT) scans of the lungs, a diagnostic biopsy will be necessary. If surgical ablation is entertained, the prosthesis will probably not be fitted until after proper wound healing, but immediate fitting may be possible. Adjuvant chemotherapy, prosthesis fitting, and gait training may necessitate repeated hospitalizations and evaluation over an 18- to 24-month period. Subsequent treatment will be based on any evidence of recurrence or metastasis.

Ewing's sarcoma

Ewing's sarcoma is a primary malignancy of bone that is believed to arise from the endothelial cells of the bone marrow.[64] Light microscopy demonstrates closely packed masses of round tumor cells that may be difficult to distinguish from other round cell sarcomas and metastatic neuroblastoma. Ewing's sarcoma is a neoplasm of childhood without predilection for either sex; 70% of all tumors are diagnosed before the age of 20. Between 50% and 60% of cases are found in the long bones. The tumor commonly arises within the marrow or medullary cavity of the metaphysis and may also be found within the shaft, but rarely in an epiphysis.

Reactive new bone is formed along the periphery of the lesion and is demonstrated radiographically as "onion skinning" (Fig. 28-16, *A*). Other neoplasms such as osteosarcoma may mimic this x-ray finding.[78] In later stages of the disease, gross destruction of the bone is evident. The lesion is extremely vascular, and metastases travel primarily through the vascular system.

The predominant complaint is pain, which increases in frequency and severity with time. Associated signs and symptoms include localized edema or diffuse extremity swelling. Pathologic fractures are not uncommon. Depending on the location, paresthesia or extremity weakness may occur. The child will have a palpable, tender mass. Elevation of body temperature is usual, and an elevated sedimentation rate and anemia are not uncommon.

Initial radiographs may demonstrate only superficial cortical erosion that is often accompanied by a honeycombed appearance in a diaphyseal or metaphyseal area. At this point the differential diagnosis should include osteogenic sarcoma and possibly Hodgkin's lymphoma. The onion skin appearance of layered periosteal reactive bone formation may be confused with osteomyelitis or osteogenic sarcoma. In the more advanced lesions, gross bony destruction is evident and is associated with a large soft tissue mass (Fig. 28-16, *B*). A major portion of the metaphysis and diaphysis will be stippled with areas of focal bone lysis.[54]

Treatment should be instituted quickly and in a tertiary care center. The treatment of Ewing's sarcoma traditionally relied on a combination of radiation therapy and chemotherapy,[40] but recent studies have suggested that surgical excision may favorably alter the outcome. A lesion of the axial

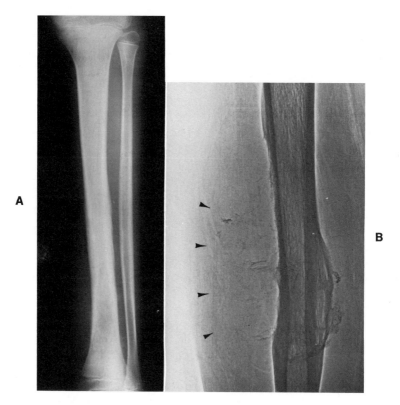

Fig. 28-16. Ewing's sarcoma. **A,** Midshaft tibial lesion demonstrating repeated episodes of periosteal new bone formation: "onion skinning." **B,** Xeroradiogram of a more advanced lesion of the midfemur. There is bony destruction and a large soft tissue mass.

skeleton and onset below age 10 years are poor prognostic signs. Presently, combination treatment yields 5-year disease-free rates of approximately 30% to 60%.[63]

BACK PAIN

As in the adult, back pain in children is merely a symptom, and many disease processes will express themselves in this way. Several of the conditions that may present as back pain in the adolescent are dealt with in other chapters of this text. These include spinal dysraphism (p. 272), juvenile discs (p. 564), kyphosis (Scheuermann's disease) (p. 466), bone tumors (p. 554), and spinal cord tumors (p. 399). The rule of thumb that painful scoliosis is a spinal cord tumor until proved otherwise is a useful reminder that careful neurologic assessment is required when any child has back pain. Finally, children do suffer from stress, and back pain may be its presenting symptom, as it is with many adults. However, the diagnosis of a functional complaint must be based on positive criteria and should not be assumed to exist simply because an organic cause is not apparent.

Spondylolysis and spondylolisthesis

In this discussion we will deal only with the most common form of spondylolisthesis, which is the lytic, isthmic spondylolisthesis. The term itself is descriptive: *spondylo* means vertebra, and *olisthesis* refers to slipping or sliding down a pathway. In this condition, there is a defect in the pars interarticularis, a portion of the lateral column of the vertebra connecting the inferior and superior articulating processes, that allows the body, pedicles, and transverse processes of the superior vertebra to slip forward in relationship to the next caudal vertebra (Fig. 28-17). The posterior elements (lamina, spinous process, and inferior articular process) are "loose" and left behind. The actual slipping is probably a mechanical event. However, there is a strong developmental and genetic predisposition involved in the occurrence of the underlying pars defect,[81] and there is a strong genetic

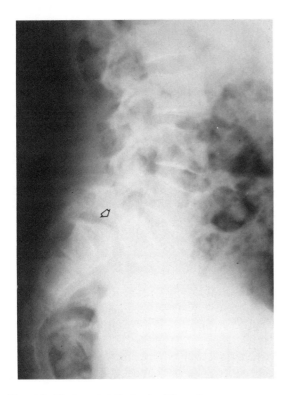

Fig. 28-17. Spondylolisthesis. There is severe antero-listhesis of L-5 on S-1.

association with other developmental abnormalities at the lumbosacral junction, including facet tropism, abnormalities of segmentation, and spina bifida occulta.[3,86]

The typical, lytic pars defect never appears before the age of 5 years. Radiographic surveys of older children in the North American white population demonstrate the defect in as many as 1 in 20 of all children examined. There is an increased incidence in female gymnasts and football interior linemen, and in some instances the lytic defect is believed to represent an acute or stress fracture of the pars interarticularis.[84] However, even when trauma precedes the radiographic identification of the lesion and when the lesion heals after immobilization, it is still presumed that there is an antecedent predisposition.

Symptoms are rare before the child is 10 years old; more commonly, they appear in the teenage years. Pain, the most common symptom, is activity related, is relieved by rest, and recurs with resumption of activity. The pain is usually diffuse

or midlumbar in location but may radiate down the leg, suggesting nerve root irritation. The patient with spondylolisthesis may be more comfortable in the flexed position and therefore prefers a soft bed, a large cushioned chair, or even a hammock to hard beds or the floor. This contrasts markedly with the typical patient with a ruptured intervertebral disc, and such a history will be confusing unless the possibility of spondylolisthesis is kept in mind.

In the milder cases of spondylolisthesis, in which the forward displacement is less than one half of the width of the vertebral body, physical examination may yield only local tenderness to palpation and percussion, and in a thin patient a palpable step between the L-4 and L-5 spinous processes. A careful neurologic examination may reveal mild weakness of the muscles innervated by the L-5 nerve root. Hamstring spasticity is common and may severely limit straight leg raising and should not be confused with sciatic irritation.

When the slip becomes more severe, the child develops remarkable shortening of the torso, as if the trunk had telescoped within the pelvis. There is an acute gibbus at the lumbosacral junction, marked lumbar lordosis just cephalad to the level of the slip, and a transverse crease across the back at the level of the iliac crest. The pelvis is tilted, the hamstrings are severely tightened, and the sacrum is prominent. The gait is marked by an extremely short stride and crouching.

Diagnosis requires AP, lateral, spot lateral, and right and left oblique views of the lumbosacral spine and L-S junction to demonstrate the defect in the pars interarticularis and minor degrees of displacement. A standing lateral view of the lumbosacral junction will make the full extent of the slip apparent.

Treatment. Treatment considerations depend on the extent of the slip at initial diagnosis and some estimate of its rate of progression. It is thought that girls develop severe degrees of slippage more frequently than boys.

Wiltse and Jackson[82] have studied a large number of children longitudinally, and we have generally followed their recommendations for observation and timing of intervention. In the child below the age of 10 years, particularly when symptoms are mild and the degree of slippage small, observation is all that is required and the child is allowed full activity. Radiographic follow-up is mandatory every 4 to 6 months until spinal growth is completed. The child should be guided toward a vocation that does not require heavy physical activity.

If the slip approaches 50% of the width of the vertebral body, some limitation of vigorous athletics such as diving, gymnastics, football, and other contact sports is indicated, particularly in any child who has become symptomatic.

When the slip extends to more than 50% of the width of the vertebral body, the child will almost invariably have the spondylolisthesis posture as well as pain. Conservative management includes limitation of activity, analgesics, anti-inflammatory agents, and such local measures as heat and massage. If this program fails, further immobilization with bed rest, a corset, or even a cast is indicated. If conservative measures fail, if pain recurs, or if there is definite progression, a surgical procedure is indicated.

The surgery most commonly performed is fusion of the fifth lumbar vertebra to the sacrum, but if the slip is severe, the fusion may need to be extended to the fourth lumbar vertebra for mechanical stability. If there are radicular symptoms, nerve root exploration and decompression can be performed at the time of fusion.

Following any spinal fusion, there is a period of ileus that resolves in 1 to 3 days, after which ambulation may begin. After decompression and fusion there is often a dramatic reduction in pain, hamstring spasticity, and gait deviation. However, the child's activity should be severely restricted until the fusion solidifies over a period of 3 to 6 months and vigorous athletic activity should be restricted until maturation of the fusion mass occurs, which takes at least a year.

Other, less common causes of back pain
Ankylosing spondylitis

The discovery of the high degree of association between the HLA antigen B27 and ankylosing spondylitis has focused a great deal of medical attention on the so-called latex-negative spondyloarthropathies.[8] Most forms of inflammatory spondylitis present in young adulthood, but the symptoms often extend as far back as the early teenage years. Some adolescent patients who are thought to have pauciarticular juvenile rheumatoid arthritis subsequently develop the classic picture of ankylosing spondylitis,[5] and an even smaller group develops the full-blown picture of ankylosing spondylitis as early as 13 years of age[9] (Fig. 28-18). Peripheral arthritis is common, and heel pain is a

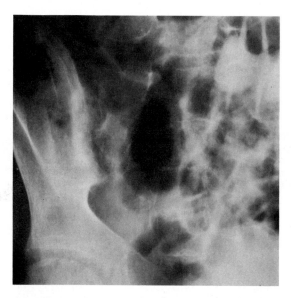

Fig. 28-18. Sacroiliac joint changes in a 14-year-old with a juvenile form of ankylosing spondylitis. There is irregularity, sclerosis, and subchondral cyst formation.

frequent presenting symptom in the teenager. Pain that radiates into the buttocks and thighs may occur, mimicking a herniated intervetebral disc.

The initial treatment of ankylosing spondylitis is primarily medical and includes postural exercises, alterations in sleeping habits, straight-backed chairs, and breathing exercises, all aimed at preventing fusion of the spine in a flexed posture. Surgical intervention, either for reconstruction of involved large joints or for treatment of spinal deformity, is reserved for the late stages of the disease and is rarely necessary in the adolescent.

Clacified intervertebral disc

Spontaneous calcification of an intervertebral disc is actually more common before the teenage years. Its cause is unknown. Asymptomatic calcification may be noted in the thoracic or lumbar spine, but the condition is most often seen in the lower segments of the cervical spine.[27] Pain and torticollis may precede noticeable calcification on x-ray films by 2 to 3 weeks. This seems to be a self-limiting disorder, but the calcification may persist for months after the symptoms resolve. Treatment is symptomatic and usually consists of traction for severe discomfort, flexible neck supports, and analgesics. Rarely, the calcific mass extrudes, causing dysphagia with anterior extrusion and neurologic symptoms with posterior ex-

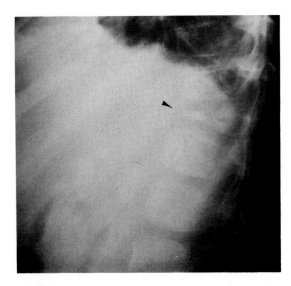

Fig. 28-19. Vertebra plana is most commonly caused by eosinophilic granuloma. In this instance, the vertebral collapse was the result of actinomycosis infection in a child with chronic granulomatous disease.

trusion.[79] Surgical excision should then be considered.

Infection

Vertebral osteomyelitis develops, as it does in most bones, by hematogenous spread. *Staphylococcus aureus* is the most frequent organism, but gram-negative infections develop as a result of the rich epidural venous plexus that drains the pelvic area. Tuberculous and fungal infections still occur, even in the United States, and are most common in children with chronic granulomatous disease (Fig. 28-19) or some other abnormality of the immune system. Destructive vertebral lesions have been seen in sarcoidosis.[35] Involvement of the sacroiliac joint should be considered in any child with vague low back or pelvic pain where the systemic findings suggest infection.[22]

Involvement of the intervertebral disc with infection can occur by direct extension from a vertebral osteomyelitis. Unlike in the adult, the child's intervertebral disc has an intrinsic blood supply that persists until the age of 20 years. Hematogenous disc space infection can and does occur, but often an organism cannot be isolated.[59]

Affected children are usually in the younger age groups but may be teenagers. The pain is localized to the involved vertebral area with no specific pattern of radiation. Rarely is the child acutely ill, but such systemic findings as low-grade fever, elevated sedimentation rate, and increased white blood cell count are typical. As the infection progresses, pain and paravertebral muscle spasm may become severe and the child will be exquisitely sensitive to any motion or jarring; he may refuse to walk, stand, or sit. Radiographically, there is narrowing of the involved disc space, perhaps with some irregularity of the adjacent vertebral endplates.

Treatment. Isolation of an organism is desirable, and throat cultures and blood cultures should be obtained along with needle aspiration or biopsy of the involved interspace. Specific antibiotics are indicated for a period of 3 to 6 weeks and probably should be instituted even in cases where no organism is identified. However, the first principle of treatment is immobilization, and many children will respond to bed rest in a plaster body cast, even without antibiotic therapy. Recumbency is continued until pain, fever, and the sedimentation rate begin to decline; immobilization is then continued for 2 to 3 months. In older patients spontaneous fusion of the interspace may take place, but often the radiographic residual is a narrowed interspace with sclerotic adjacent vertebrae. If narrowing of the interspace or vertebral involvement has led to a localized gibbus, prolonged bracing may be indicated.

REFERENCES

1. Aergerter, E., and Kirkpatrick, J. A., Jr.: Orthopaedic diseases, ed. 4, Philadelphia, 1975, W. B. Saunders Co.
2. Albright, F., and others: Syndrome characterized by osteitis fibrosa disseminata, areas of pigmentation and endocrine dysfunction with precocious puberty in females, N. Engl. J. Med. **216:**727, 1937.
3. Amos, D. B., and others: Linkage between HLA and spinal development, Transplant. Proc. **7**(1):93, 1975.
4. Anderson, R. L., Ropowitz, L., and Li, J. K. H.: An unusual sarcoma arising in a solitary osteochondroma, J. Bone Joint Surg. **51A:**1199, 1969.
5. Ansell, B. M., and Wood, P. H. N.: Prognosis in juvenile chronic polyarthritis, Clin. Rheum. Dis. **2**(2):397, 1976.
6. Bailey, G. L., and others: Avascular necrosis of the femoral head in patients on chronic hemodialysis, Trans. Am. Soc. Artif. Intern. Organs **18:**401, 1972.
7. Bick, E. M.: Surgical pathology of synovial tissue, J. Bone Joint Surg. **12:**33, 1930.
8. Bluestone, R.: Ankylosing spondylitis. In Hollander, J. L., and McCarty, D. J., editors: Arthritis and allied conditions, Philadelphia, 1979, Lea & Febiger.
9. Bywaters, E. G. L.: Ankylosing spondylitis in childhood, Clin. Rheum. Dis. **2**(2):387, 1976.
10. Cassells, S. W.: The arthroscope in the diagnosis of disorders of the patellofemoral joint, Clin. Orthop. **144:**45, 1979.

11. Cattell, H. S., and others: Reconstructive surgery in children with azotemic osteodystrophy, J. Bone Joint Surg. **57A:**516, 1971.

12. Chiroff, R. T., Sears, K. A., and Slaughter, W. H., III: Slipped capital femoral epiphysis and parathyroid adenoma, J. Bone Joint Surg. **56A:**1063, 1974.

13. Chrisman, O. D., Snook, G. A., and Wilson, T. C.: A long-term prospective study of the Hauser and Roux-Goldthwait procedures for recurrent patellar dislocation, Clin. Orthop. **144:**27, 1979.

14. Codman, E. A.: Epiphyseal chondromatous giant cell tumors of the upper end of the humerus, Surg. Gynecol. Obstet. **52:**543, 1931.

15. Cohen, J.: Unicameral bone cysts: a current synthesis of reported cases, Orthop. Clin. North Am. **3**(4):715, 1977.

16. Companacci, M., Desessa, L., and Bellando-Randone, P.: Bone cysts: review of 275 cases—results of surgical treatment and early results of treatment by methylprednisolone acetate injections, Chir. Organi. Mov. **62:**471, 1976.

17. Crosby, E. B., and Insall, J.: Recurrent dislocation of the patella, J. Bone Joint Surg. **58A:**9, 1976.

18. Cruess, R. L.: Cortisone-induced avascular necrosis of the femoral head, J. Bone Joint Surg. **59B:**308, 1977.

19. Dablin, D. C.: Bone tumors, ed. 3, Springfield, Ill., 1978, Charles C Thomas, Publisher.

20. Dablin, D. C., and Coventry, M. B.: Osteogenic sarcoma: a study of six hundred cases, J. Bone Joint Surg. **49A:**101, 1967.

21. Dabska, M., and Buraczewski, J.: Aneurysmal bone cyst: pathology, clinical course and radiologic appearances, Cancer **23:**371, 1969.

22. Delbarre, F., and others: Pyogenic infection of the sacro-iliac joint, J. Bone Joint Surg. **57A:**819, 1975.

23. Donaldson, W. F.: Aneurysmal bone cyst, J. Bone Joint Surg. **49A:**25, 1962.

24. Drennan, D. B., Fahey, J. S., and Maylahn, D. J.: Fractures through large non-ossifying fibromas, J. Bone Joint Surg. **54A:**1794, 1972.

25. Enneking, W. F.: Principles of musculoskeletal pathology, (lithoprinted), Gainesville, Fla. 1970, Starter Printing Co.

26. Enneking, W. F., and Springfield, D. S.: Osteosarcoma, Orthop. Clin. North Am. **3**(4):785, 1977.

27. Eyering, E. J., Peterson, C. A., and Bjornson, D. R.: Intervertebral disc calcification in childhood, J. Bone Joint Surg. **46A:**1432, 1964.

28. Ficat, R. P., Philippe, J., and Hungerford, D. S.: Chondromalacia patellae: a system of classification, Clin. Orthop. **144:**55, 1979.

29. Gaines, R. W., and Goldner, J. L.: Adult and juvenile hallux valgus: analysis and treatment, Orthop. Clin. North Am. **7**(4):863, 1976.

30. Galway, H. R., and MacIntosh, D. L.: The lateral pivot shift: a symptom and sign for anterior cruciate ligament insufficiency, Clin. Orthop. **147:**45, 1980.

31. Gray, D. J., and Gardner, E.: Prenatal development of the human knee and superior tibio-fibular joints, Am. J. Anat. **86:**235, 1950.

32. Green, W. T., and Banks, H. H.: Osteochondritis dissecans in children, J. Bone Joint Surg. **35A:**26, 1953.

33. Haas, S. L.: The localization of the growing point in the epiphyseal cartilage plate of bones, Am. J. Orthop. Surg. **15:**563, 1917.

34. Hardaker, W. T., Whipple, T. L., and Bassett, F. H.: Diagnosis and treatment of the plica syndrome of the knee, J. Bone Joint Surg. **62A:**221, 1980.

35. Harrelson, J. M.: Personal communication, 1980.

36. Harris, W. H., Dudley, H. R., Jr., and Barry, R. J.: The natural history of fibrous dysplasia, J. Bone Joint Surg. **44A:**207, 1962.

37. Harris, W. R.: The endocrine basis for slipping at the upper femoral epiphysis, J. Bone Joint Surg. **32B:**5, 1950.

38. Hoppenfeld, S.: Physical examination of the spine and extremities, New York, 1976, Appleton-Century-Crofts.

39. Hughes, E. S. R.: Osgood-Schlatter's disease, Surg. Gynecol. Obstet. **86:**323, 1948.

40. Hustu, O. H., Pinkel, D., and Pratt, C. B.: Treatment of clinically localized Ewing's sarcoma with radiotherapy and combination chemotherapy, Cancer **30:**1522, 1972.

41. Jaffe, H. L.: Tumors and tumorous conditions of the bones and joints, Philadelphia, 1958, Lea & Febiger.

42. Johnson, L. C.: Personal communication.

43. Johnson, L. C., Vetter, H., and Putschar, W. G. J.: Sarcomas arising in bone cysts, Virchows Arch. (Pathol. Anat.) **335:**428, 1962.

44. Johnston, J.: Giant cell tumor of bone: the role of the giant cell in orthopaedic surgery, Orthop. Clin. North Am. **3**(4):751, 1977.

45. Kaplan, E. B.: Discoid lateral meniscus of the knee joint: nature, mechanism and operative treatment, J. Bone Joint Surg. **39A:**77, 1957.

46. Kelikian, H.: Hallux valgus, allied deformities of the forefoot and metatarsalgia, Philadelphia, 1965, W. B. Saunders Co.

47. Kelsey, J. L., Reggi, R. J., and Southwick, W. O.: The incidence and distribution of slipped capital femoral epiphysis in Connecticut and Southwestern United States, J. Bone Joint Surg. **52A:**1203, 1970.

48. Kennedy, J. C.: The injured adolescent knee, Baltimore, 1972, The Williams & Wilkins Co.

49. Key, J. A.: Epiphyseal coxa vara or displacement of the capital epiphysis of femur in adolescence, J. Bone Joint Surg. **8:**52, 1926.

50. Larson, R. L.: Combined instabilities of the knee, Clin. Orthop. **147:**68, 1980.

51. Laurent, L. E., and Osterman, K.: Operative treatment of spondylolisthesis in young patients, Clin. Orthop. **117:**85, 1976.

52. Lindbom, A., and others: Angiography in osteoid osteoma, Acta Radiol. **54:**327, 1960.

53. Linden, B.: Osteochondritis dissecans of the femoral condyles, J. Bone Joint Surg. **59A:**769, 1977.

54. MacIntosh, D. J., Price, C. H. G., and Jeffree, G. M.: Ewing's tumour, J. Bone Joint Surg. **57B:**331, 1979.

55. Marcove, R. C., Martini, N., and Rosen, G.: The treatment of pulmonary metastasis in primary osteosarcoma, J. Bone Joint Surg. **57A:**145, 1975.

56. Marcove, R. C., and others: Giant cell tumors treated by cryosurgery: a report of twenty-five cases, J. Bone Joint Surg. **55A:**1633, 1973.

57. McFarland, G. B., and Morden, M. L.: Benign cartilaginous lesions, Orthop. Clin. North Am. **3**(4):737, 1977.

58. McKenna, R. J., and others: Sarcomata of the osteogenic series (osteosarcoma, fibrosarcoma, chondrosarcoma,

parosteal osteogenic sarcoma, and sarcomata arising in abnormal bone), J. Bone Joint Surg. **48A:**1, 1966.

59. Menelaus, M. B.: Discitis: an inflammation affecting intervertebral discs in children, J. Bone Joint Surg. **46B:**16, 1964.

60. Moorefield, W. G., and others: Acquired hypothyroidism and slipped capital femoral epiphysis, J. Bone Joint Surg. **58A:**705, 1976.

61. Morrissy, R. T.: What's new in slipped capital femoral epiphysis. In The Hip Society: The hip; proceedings of the sixth open scientific meeting of The Hip Society, 1978, St. Louis, 1978, The C. V. Mosby Co., p. 253.

62. Niemann, K. M.: Diseases related to the hematopoietic system. In Lovell, W. W., and Winter, R. B., editors: Pediatric orthopaedics, Philadelphia, 1978, J. B. Lippincott Co.

63. Pomeroy, T. C., and Johnson, R. E.: Combined modality therapy of Ewing's sarcoma, Cancer **35:**36, 1975.

64. Pritchard, D., and others: Ewing's sarcoma, J. Bone Joint Surg. **57A:**10, 1975.

65. Pyper, J. B.: The flexor-extensor transplant operation for clawtoes, J. Bone Joint Surg. **40B:**528, 1958.

66. Rosen, G., and others: The rationale for multiple drug therapy in the treatment of osteogenic sarcoma, Cancer **35:**936, 1975.

67. Ruderman, R. J., and others: Orthopedic complications of renal transplantation in children, Transplant. Proc. **11**(1):104, 1979.

68. Schajowicz, F., and Slullitel, J.: Eosinophilic granuloma of bone and its relationship to Hand-Schüller-Christian and Letterer-Siwe syndrome, J. Bone Joint Surg. **55B:**545, 1973.

69. Schwartz, D. T., and Alpert, M.: The malignant transformation of fibrous dysplasia, Am. J. Med. Sci. **247:**350, 1964.

70. Selby, S.: Metaphyseal cortical defects in the tubular bones of growing children, J. Bone Joint Surg. **43A:**393, 1961.

71. Sim, F. H., Dahlin, D. C., and Beaboub, J. W.: Osteoid osteoma; diagnostic problems, J. Bone Joint Surg. **47A:**154, 1975.

72. Smillie, I. S.: Injuries of the knee joint, Baltimore, 1951, The Williams & Wilkins Co.

73. Smillie, I. S.: Osteochondritis dissecans, Edinburgh, 1960, E. & S. Livingstone, Ltd.

74. Solomon, L.: Hereditary multiple exostosis, Am. J. Hum. Genet. **16:**351, 1964.

75. Southwick, W. O.: Osteotomy through the lesser trochanter for slipped capital femoral epiphysis, J. Bone Joint Surg. **49A:**807, 1967.

76. Tachdjian, M. O.: Pediatric orthopaedics, Philadelphia, 1972, W. B. Saunders Co.

77. Trott, A.: Hallux valgus in the adolescent. In American Academy of Orthopaedic Surgeons: Instructional Course Lectures, vol. 21, St. Louis, 1972, The C. V. Mosby Co., p. 262.

78. Vohra, V. G.: Roentgen manifestations in Ewing's sarcoma: a study of 156 cases, Cancer **20:**727, 1967.

79. Walker, C. S.: Calcification of intervertebral discs in children, J. Bone Joint Surg. **36B:**601, 1954.

80. Wiberg, G.: Roentgenographic and anatomic studies on the femoropatellar joint, Acta Orthop. Scand. **12:**319, 1941.

81. Wiltse, L. L.: Etiology of spondylolisthesis, J. Bone Joint Surg. **39A:**447, 1957.

82. Wiltse, L. L., and Jackson, D. W.: Treatment of spondylolisthesis and spondylolysis in children, Clin. Orthop. **117:**92, 1976.

83. Wiltse, L., Newman, P. H., and McNab, I.: Classification of spondylolysis and spondylolisthesis, Clin. Orthop. **117:**24, 1976.

84. Wiltse, L. L., Widell, E. H., and Jackson, D. W.: Fatigue fracture: the basic lesion in isthmic spondylolisthesis, J. Bone Joint Surg. **57A:**17, 1975.

85. Woolfrey, B. F., and Chandler, E. F.: Manifestations of Osgood-Schlatter's disease in late teenage and early adulthood, J. Bone Joint Surg. **42A:**327, 1960.

86. Wynne-Davies, R., and Scott, J. H. S.: Inheritance and spondylolisthesis, J. Bone Joint Surg. **61B**(3):301, 1979.

Index

A

Abdomen
  blunt trauma to, 353-356
  distention of, in newborn, significance of, 41-42
  emergencies involving
    acute, in infant and toddler, 206-215
    in child from 2 to 12, 316-324
  examination of, in child from 2 to 12, 316-319
  exploration of, neonatal lesions requiring, 239-240
  lesions of, in newborn, surgery for, follow-up of, 239-240
  masses in
    in child from 2 to 12, 329-330, 332-336
      benign, 335-336
      complications of, 334
      evaluation of, 332-333
      follow-up of, 334-335
      postoperative course of, 334
      referral for, 333
      surgical options for, 333-334
      treatment of, 333
      uncommon, 335
    in infant and toddler, 221-222
  surgically oriented examination of, in infant and toddler, 201
  wall of
    deformities of
      long-term complications of, 369
      in newborn, 38,104-111
    musculature of, absent, 111, 131-132
    perforation of, complicating shunting for hydrocephalus, 271
Abdominal cryptorchid testicle, surgery for, 378-379
Abscess(es)
  intracranial, 392-399; see also Intracranial infections, localized
  subhepatic, complicating appendicitis, 322
  subphrenic, complicating appendicitis, 322
  suture, complicating surgical wounds, 34
Absent abdominal wall musculature syndrome, 111, 131-132
Abuse, child, fractures in, 426-427
Achondroplasia, diagnosis of, in newborn, 171
Acoustic neuroma, 392
Adenoma(s)
  cystic, 248
  islet cell, 350

Adhesions, intestinal obstruction due to, complicating abdominal surgery, 361-362
Adhesive in ostomy management, 31-32
Adolescent bunion, 551
Adolescent; see Teenager
Adrenal genital syndrome, intersex problems and, 134
Aganglionic megacolon, 81-86; see also Hirschsprung's disease
Agenesis, renal, 135
Air block syndrome in newborn, 52-54
"Airdrome sign" in neonatal necrotizing enterocolitis, 89
Airway
  clearing of, in resuscitation following trauma, 351
  involvement of, in burns, 357-358
  maintenance of, for pediatric anesthesia, 8
  obstruction of
    and deformities of, long-term complications of, 369
    in newborn, 54-55
Alimentation
  central, for neonatal necrotizing enterocolitis, 90
  peripheral, for neonatal necrotizing enterocolitis, 90
Alphafetoprotein, maternal serum, in prenatal diagnosis of myelomeningocele, 164
Ambulation, difficulties with, in spinal cord tumors, 399
Ampicillin for appendicitis, 321
Amputation(s)
  acquired, 305-306
  congenital, 306
  Syme's, for fibular hemimelia, 308
Amylase, serum level of, in pancreatic injury, 355
Anastomosis in newborn
  bowel, for jejunoileal atresia, 74-75
  for intestinal duplications, 93
  for mesenteric cysts, 93
Anencephaly, 152
Anesthesia, pediatric, 7-10
  intravenous line for, establishment of, 7-8
  local, 10
  procedures for, 7-10
    special considerations for, 10
Anesthesiologist, preoperative visit from, 7
Aneurysmal bone cyst, 559-560
Aneurysms
  intracranial, 491-492; see also Intracranial aneurysms
  of vein of Galen in newborn, heart failure in, 488-490
Angiography
  cerebral, in evaluation of vascular lesion of brain, 493
  in Meckel's diverticulum evaluation, 341

Page numbers in *italics* indicate illustrations; page numbers followed by *t* indicate tables.

571

DATE DUE

JULY 1983		
JULY 1984		
JULY 1985		
JULY 1986		
LORD		PRINTED IN U.S.A